Endocrine Oncology (Clinical Cases in Endocrinology)

Endocrine Oncology (Clinical Cases in Endocrinology)

Editor: Elaina Lloyd

AMERICAN
MEDICAL PUBLISHERS
www.americanmedicalpublishers.com

AMERICAN
MEDICAL PUBLISHERS
www.americanmedicalpublishers.com

American Medical Publishers,
41 Flatbush Avenue,
1st Floor, New York,
NY 11217, USA

Endocrine Oncology (Clinical Cases in Endocrinology)
Edited by Elaina Lloyd

ISBN 979-8-88740-635-0 (Hardback)

Contents

Preface

The endocrine system consists of various glands in the body that produce hormones, including the thyroid, adrenal glands, pancreas, and pituitary gland. The field of oncology that focuses on the diagnosis, treatment, and management of cancers related to the endocrine system is known as endocrine oncology. Cancers that develop in these glands or involve the production of hormones are referred to as endocrine tumors or endocrine neoplasms. Some of the major types of endocrine tumors are thyroid cancer, adrenal cancer and pituitary tumors. Thyroid cancer originates in the cells of the thyroid gland and can include types such as papillary, follicular, medullary, and anaplastic thyroid cancer. Adrenal cancer develops in the adrenal glands, which produce hormones such as cortisol and adrenaline. This book brings forth some of the most innovative concepts and elucidates the unexplored aspects of endocrine oncology. It will serve as a reference to a broad spectrum of readers.

This book is a result of research of several months to collate the most relevant data in the field.

When I was approached with the idea of this book and the proposal to edit it, I was overwhelmed. It gave me an opportunity to reach out to all those who share a common interest with me in this field. I had 3 main parameters for editing this text:

1. Accuracy - The data and information provided in this book should be up-to-date and valuable to the readers.

2. Structure - The data must be presented in a structured format for easy understanding and better grasping of the readers.

3. Universal Approach - This book not only targets students but also experts and innovators in the field, thus my aim was to present topics which are of use to all.

Thus, it took me a couple of months to finish the editing of this book.

I would like to make a special mention of my publisher who considered me worthy of this opportunity and also supported me throughout the editing process. I would also like to thank the editing team at the back-end who extended their help whenever required.

Editor

1

Two Cases of Armour Thyroid Interference in Thyroglobulin Monitoring for Thyroid Cancer

Michelle Ponder,[1] **Elizabeth Lamos**,[2] **and Kashif Munir**[2]

[1]*University of Maryland Medical Center, 22 S Green St., RM N3E09, Baltimore, MD 21201-1554, USA*
[2]*Division of Endocrinology, Diabetes, and Nutrition, University of Maryland School of Medicine, 827 Linden Avenue, 2nd Floor, Baltimore, MD 21201, USA*

Correspondence should be addressed to Kashif Munir; kmunir@medicine.umaryland.edu

Academic Editor: J. Paul Frindik

Thyroglobulin (Tg) monitoring is the biochemical standard for surveillance of recurrent differentiated thyroid cancer (DTC). Several assays are available to quantify Tg levels: immunometric assay (IMA), radioimmunoassay (RIA), and the newer liquid chromatography tandem mass spectrometry (LC-MS). It is well known that a number of entities can interfere with the accuracy of testing, and at this point in time, no one assay perfectly balances high sensitivity with low risk of interference. In this case study, we present two cases in which treatment with desiccated thyroid extract (Armour thyroid) led to a sudden elevation in Tg, which resolved when Armour thyroid was discontinued. This elevation occurred when Tg was measured with both IMA and LC-MS, which suggests direct interference from porcine Tg rather than heterophilic or thyroglobulin antibody (TgAb) interference. We suggest that patients with a history of DTC not be treated with desiccated thyroid extracts consistent with guidelines. Furthermore, more advances need to be made in the area of Tg testing to improve specificity and avoid detection of nonhuman Tg and other similar proteins.

1. Introduction

After successful treatment for differentiated thyroid cancer (DTC), patients are traditionally monitored for biochemical disease recurrence with serial thyroglobulin (Tg) levels [1, 2]. Tg is a protein synthesized by both healthy thyroid follicles and DTC cells. A rising serum Tg is usually the first detectable sign of DTC recurrence [3]. This noninvasive test has remained the preferred surveillance strategy for many years; however, the test is not without drawbacks. Notably, the presence of both antithyroglobulin antibodies (TgAb) and heterophilic antibodies can interfere with accuracy of the test [4]. Additionally, different assays can result in discordant results for the same sample, even in the absence of antibody interference [5, 6]. Over the years, strides have been made to mitigate these issues, including tandem monitoring of TgAb along with Tg, and attempts at standardization of assays to CRM45 [7]. Additionally, several new assays have emerged over the years in hopes of finding a new reference standard.

Tg testing is primarily performed via either the immunometric assay (IMA) or radioimmunoassay (RIA). Tg monitored via IMA is often underestimated in the presence of TgAb, as these antibodies competitively bind to Tg and prevent detection by reagent antibodies [8]. In contrast, heterophilic antibodies can result in Tg overestimation by binding directly to reagent antibodies and stimulating a response [9]. RIA in contrast is less prone to interference from TgAb and is unaffected by heterophilic antibodies; however, it is also a less sensitive test [3]. Thus, liquid chromatography tandem mass spectrometry (LC-MS) has been introduced in hopes of improving sensitivity and decreasing antibody interference. Proponents claim that this new method is free from TgAb interference, though this has been called into question by several studies [10]. Regardless, discrepancies persist among all three assays, namely, due to

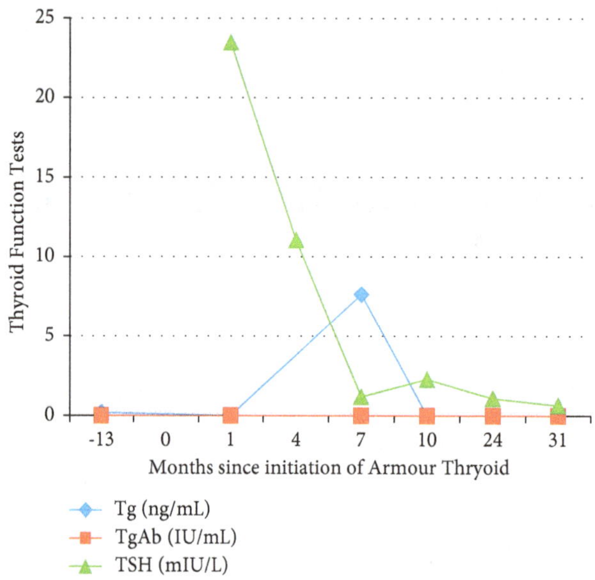

FIGURE 1: Trend of TSH and thyroglobulin results over time in case 1.

pre and posttranslational modification of Tg mRNA, which results in multiple different isoforms of Tg that will be detected with varying accuracy by each test [11].

After initial DTC treatment, patients are supplemented with thyroid hormone to prevent any unnecessary stimulation of thyroid tissue that could result in disease recurrence. The vast majority of patients are treated with synthetic levothyroxine (T4) per guideline recommendations. However, desiccated thyroid hormones have gained recent popularity, with individuals desiring "natural" thyroid hormone replacement, and claims that these formulations provide an advantage over synthetic T4 [12]. Additionally, patients with more longstanding disease may present on preprescribed desiccated thyroid extracts. It has not been explored whether porcine thyroid extracts, such as Armour thyroid, can affect the accuracy of Tg testing.

Here, we present two cases of patients who experienced sudden and unexpected elevations in Tg with both IMA and LC-MS testing while on suppressive therapy with Armour thyroid. In both cases, Tg levels normalized after switching to levothyroxine. This raises concerns that desiccated thyroid extract (including brands such as Armour and nature thyroid) may interfere with Tg testing.

2. Case Presentation

A 53-year-old woman with toxic multinodular goiter in the 1990s was treated with radioactive iodine. A new thyroid nodule developed several months after treatment and subsequently continued to grow. Fine needle aspiration was consistent with thyroid cancer. Total thyroidectomy revealed a 2 cm papillary thyroid cancer. Treatment ensued with levothyroxine 150 mcg PO daily and 100 mCi I-131 postoperatively. Initial postradioiodine whole body imaging showed uptake in the thyroid bed, with multiple subsequent diagnostic whole body scans showing no evidence of abnormal uptake. Periodic sonography and testing of Tg and Tg antibody showed no evidence of biochemical or structural disease recurrence for over 10 years. The patient requested to switch to Armour thyroid. Tg level one month later was <0.1 ng/ml and Tg antibody <1 IU/ml, performed utilizing the Quest Diagnostics Beckman Coulter IMA method (Figure 1). TSH was initially elevated at 23.47 mIU/l. Armour thyroid was adjusted to goal TSH suppression, and 7 months later, repeat testing showed Tg level of 7.62 ng/ml and Tg Ab < 1 IU/ml, performed utilizing the Quest Diagnostics Beckman Coulter IMA method. Concurrent TSH was 1.19 mIU/l on Armour thyroid 180 mg daily. The same sample was sent for LC-MS by Quest Diagnostics, which measured Tg at 9.7 ng/ml. Suspecting Armour thyroid interference with the assay, Armour thyroid was discontinued and levothyroxine therapy was initiated. Three months after restarting levothyroxine, Tg level was <0.1 ng/ml and TgAb < 1 IU/ml, performed utilizing the Quest Diagnostics Beckman Coulter IMA method. TSH was 2.29 mIU/l.

3. Case 2

A 45-year-old woman with a long history of Graves' disease treated initially with methimazole underwent a total thyroidectomy after a fine needle aspiration of a cold nodule revealed multifocal, bilateral micropapillary thyroid cancer (largest focus 5.5 mm, classic variant). Two of 12 lymph nodes were positive for metastatic disease. Postoperative testing revealed an undetectable Tg and TgAb levels and no evidence of structural disease recurrence by thyroid ultrasound and CT of the chest, abdomen, and pelvis. The patient also preferred Armour thyroid after feeling poorly on initial levothyroxine replacement. Her Tg and TgAb remained undetectable for a year after initiation. 19 months later, Tg was <0.1 ng/ml and TgAb was 1 IU/ml performed utilizing the Quest Diagnostics Beckman Coulter IMA method while on Armour thyroid (Figure 2). Her TSH was 0.45 mIU/l at that time. 30 months after initiation, her Tg level rose to

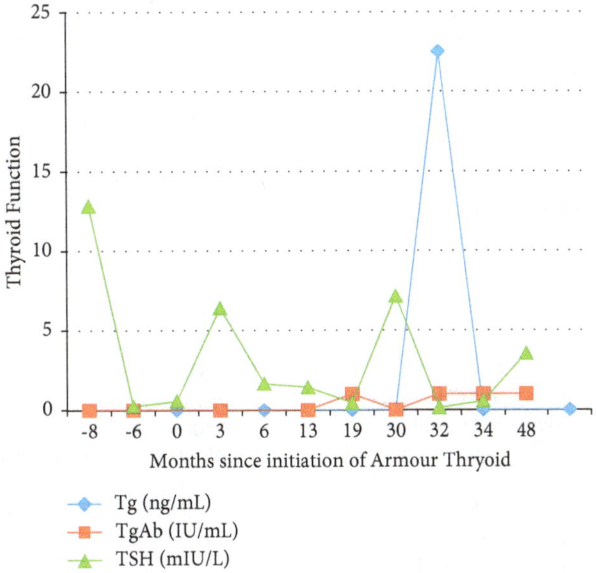

Figure 2: Trend of TSH and thyroglobulin results over time in case 2.

22.5 ng/ml with Tg antibody <1 IU/ml performed utilizing the Quest Diagnostics Beckman Coulter IMA method. TSH at the time was 7.17 mIU/l. Again, the same specimen was sent for testing by LC-MS, and Tg level was 28.6 ng/ml. Armour thyroid was discontinued, and six weeks after restarting levothyroxine, Tg level was <0.1 ng/ml and TgAb was 1 IU/ml performed utilizing the Quest Diagnostics Beckman Coulter IMA method. TSH was 0.15 mIU/l.

4. Discussion

A sudden elevation in Tg level in any patient with a history of DTC can be alarming. However, it is always important to consider the clinical context of any lab abnormality. In the two cases described above, the sudden elevation in Tg after initiating treatment with Armour thyroid raised suspicion for interference with the test. As expected, Tg normalized after switching back to levothyroxine.

One possibility for the unexpected results may be due to antibody interference, as this is the most common reason for Tg testing inaccuracy. However, TgAb positivity generally leads to underestimation of Tg in IMA, and the opposite was observed here. Furthermore, LC-MS avoids antibody interference via use of trypsin [11], which hydrolyzes antibody complexes. Thus, if heterophilic antibodies were the cause, it is unlikely that any interference would be observed with the use of LC-MS.

A second possibility would be interference from Tg itself. Desiccated thyroid extract contains colloid thyroid tissue and thus Tg. Comparison of the structure between human and porcine Tg shows about 76% homology between the two (including 637 amino acid changes or deletions) [13]. It is unsurprising that IMA would have difficulty differentiating between the two similar molecules, as it only uses a single epitope to recognize and detect Tg [12]. However, it should be noted that a protein the size of Tg is less likely to be absorbed by the GI tract [14], and thus, direct observation of Tg in the bloodstream from Armour thyroid is unlikely.

Another possibility may involve indirect interference with the test itself, as is seen with biotin interference with thyroid function monitoring. In this case, the biotin molecule competitively competes with the binding of radiolabeled antibodies with the TSH molecule, thus resulting in a falsely low TSH level when present in high enough amounts [15]. In a similar way, an antigen present in Armour thyroid may bind with and activate the reagent, making Tg levels appear falsely elevated. Some studies suggest the possibility of larger peptide absorption, which could potentially be exacerbated by "leaky gut" that can be seen in individuals with autoimmune disorders (one case had the history of Graves' disease) [16].

At this time, the true mechanism of dissected thyroid interference with thyroglobulin monitoring is unknown. Any patients taking desiccated thyroid extracts who are suspected of having porcine Tg interference should be switched back to levothyroxine and have Tg retested shortly thereafter. To identify if the elevation in Tg is truly due to cancer recurrence (regrowth of thyroid tissue), rhTSH-stimulated Tg may be done. A physiologic rise in Tg in response to TSH stimulation would suggest that the Tg originates from the patient's own thyroid tissue, rather than from an outside source such as thyroid extract.

Guidelines for treatment for hypothyroidism recommend that patients with primary hypothyroidism be treated with levothyroxine rather than desiccated thyroid extract, as long-term outcome data are lacking [17]. However, some patients will seek the use of desiccated thyroid hormone for a number of reasons including lack of symptom improvement on traditional T4 replacement and seeking a more "natural" option. Others may unknowingly be using over-the-counter supplements containing desiccated thyroid extracts. The two cases here demonstrate desiccated thyroid hormone interference with thyroid cancer monitoring, a potential harm if associated with additional testing, imaging, and the emotional toll of an abnormal test. These cases support the current guidelines advocating for synthetic thyroxine as standard of care for thyroid hormone replacement or suppression in differentiated thyroid cancer.

Consent

Written consent has been obtained from both patients described in the case reports.

References

[1] E. L. Mazzaferri, R. J. Robbins, C. A. Spencer et al., "A consensus report of the role of serum thyroglobulin as a monitoring method for low-risk patients with papillary thyroid carcinoma," *Journal of Clinical Endocrinology & Metabolism*, vol. 88, no. 4, pp. 1433–1441, 2003.

[2] B. R. Haugen, E. K. Alexander, K. C. Bible et al., "American thyroid association management guidelines for adult patients with thyroid nodules and differentiated thyroid cancer: The American thyroid association guidelines task force on thyroid nodules and differentiated thyroid cancer," *Thyroid*, vol. 26, no. 1, pp. 1–133, 2016.

[3] E. Baudin, C. Do Cao, A. F. Cailleux, S. Leboulleux, J. P. Travagli, and M. Schlumberger, "Positive predictive value of serum thyroglobulin levels, measured during the first year of follow-up after thyroid hormone withdrawal, in thyroid cancer patients," *Journal of Clinical Endocrinology & Metabolism*, vol. 88, no. 3, pp. 1107–1111, 2003.

[4] J. Krahn and T. Dembinski, "Thyroglobulin and anti-thyroglobulin assays in thyroid cancer monitoring," *Clinical Biochemistry*, vol. 42, no. 4-5, pp. 416–419, 2009.

[5] C. A. Spencer, L. M. Bergoglio, M. Kazarosyan, S. Fatemi, and J. S. LoPresti, "Clinical Impact of thyroglobulin (tg) and Tg autoantibody method differences on the management of patients with differentiated thyroid carcinomas," *Journal of Clinical Endocrinology & Metabolism*, vol. 90, no. 10, pp. 5566–5575, 2005.

[6] C. Spencer, J. Lopresti, and S. Fatemi, "How sensitive (second-generation) thyroglobulin measurement is changing paradigms for monitoring patients with differentiated thyroid cancer, in the absence or presence of thyroglobulin autoantibodies," *Current Opinion in Endocrinology Diabetes and Obesity*, vol. 21, no. 5, pp. 394–404, 2014.

[7] C. A. Spencer, "Challenges of serum thyroglobulin (tg) measurement in the presence of tg autoantibodies," *Journal of Clinical Endocrinology & Metabolism*, vol. 89, no. 8, pp. 3702–3704, 2004.

[8] S. Mariotti, G. Barbesino, P. Caturegli et al., "Assay of thyroglobulin in serum with thyroglobulin autoantibodies: An unobtainable goal?" *Journal of Clinical Endocrinology & Metabolism*, vol. 80, no. 2, pp. 468–472, 1995.

[9] A. N. Hoofnagle and M. Y. Roth, "Improving the measurement of serum thyroglobulin with mass spectrometry," *Journal of Clinical Endocrinology & Metabolism*, vol. 98, no. 4, pp. 1343–1352, 2013.

[10] U. Azmat, K. Porter, L. Senter, M. D. Ringel, and F. Nabhan, "Thyroglobulin liquid chromatography-tandem mass spectrometry has a low sensitivity for detecting structural disease in patients with antithyroglobulin antibodies," *Thyroid*, vol. 27, no. 1, pp. 74–80, 2017.

[11] J. S. Lopresti and A. Hasan, "Monitoring TgAb-positive patients with differentiated thyroid cancer," *Current Opinion in Endocrine and Metabolic Research*, vol. 2, pp. 34–37, 2018.

[12] T. D. Hoang, C. H. Olsen, V. Q. Mai, P. W. Clyde, and M. K. M. Shakir, "Desiccated thyroid extract compared with levothyroxine in the treatment of hypothyroidism: A randomized, double-blind, crossover study," *Journal of Clinical Endocrinology & Metabolism*, vol. 98, no. 5, pp. 1982–1990, 2013.

[13] COBALT: Multiple alignment tool. National center for biotechnology information. 2020. http://www.ncbi.nlm.nih.gov/tools/cobalt/cobalt.cgi.

[14] B. O. Barnes, A. J. Carlson, and A. M. Riskin, "Studies on thyroglobulin," *American Journal of Physiology-Legacy Content*, vol. 98, no. 1, pp. 86–92, 1931.

[15] A. Ardabilygazir, S. Afshariyamchlou, D. Mir, and I. Sachmechi, "Effect of high-dose biotin on thyroid function tests: Case report and literature review," *Cureus*, vol. 10, no. 6, Article ID e2845, 2018.

[16] W. M. Miner-Williams, B. R. Stevens, and P. J. Moughan, "Are intact peptides absorbed from the healthy gut in the adult human?" *Nutrition Research Reviews*, vol. 27, no. 2, pp. 308–329, 2014.

[17] J. Jonklaas, A. C. Bianco, A. J. Bauer et al., "Guidelines for the treatment of hypothyroidism: prepared by the American thyroid association task force on thyroid hormone replacement," *Thyroid*, vol. 24, no. 12, pp. 1670–1751, 2014.

2

A Tale of Two Hypersecreting Adrenal Neoplasms in the Heartland of COVID-19 Pandemic, Lombardy, Italy

Benedetta Zampetti,[1] **Roberto Attanasio**,[2] **Emanuela Carioni**,[1] **Daniela Dallabonzana**,[1] **Iuliana Pauna**,[3] **Marco Boniardi**,[3] **and Renato Cozzi**[2]

[1]*ASST Grande Ospedale Metropolitano Niguarda, Endocrinology Department, Milan, Italy*
[2]*Scientific Committee Associazione Medici Endocrinologi, International Chapter of Clinical Endocrinology, Milan, Italy*
[3]*ASST Grande Ospedale Metropolitano Niguarda, General Oncologic and Mini-invasive Surgery Department, Milan, Italy*

Correspondence should be addressed to Benedetta Zampetti; benedettazampetti@yahoo.it

Academic Editor: J. Paul Frindik

In this study, we report the management, in Lombardy, Italy, of one patient with Cushing's syndrome due to adrenal adenoma and another one with pheochromocytoma, whose surgeries were deferred owing to the COVID-19 pandemic.

1. Introduction

Surgery is the mainstay of treatment for hypersecreting adrenal lesions, whenever clinically and technically feasible [1, 2].

COVID-19 pandemic obliged physicians to find out alternative options to classical pathways, in order to lower viral spread and related dangers as well as to cope with redeployment of personnel and resources.

We describe here two cases in whom surgery for adrenal Cushing's syndrome (CS) and pheochromocytoma (PHEO) could not be performed as usual and was deferred due to the unavailability of surgical facilities.

2. Case 1

A 69-year-old woman was evaluated for CS.

Her history included arterial hypertension for 10 years, hyperlipidemia, and euthyroid multinodular goiter.

In 2017, type 2 diabetes mellitus was diagnosed, and a 35 mm right adrenal mass was incidentally found at US at another hospital. No endocrine work-up was performed. Due to high density (40 HU) of the lesion, a ^{18}F-FDG-PET scan was performed with negative results. The size of the lesion was unchanged at CT follow-up in the following two years.

In December 2019, clinical picture worsened with progressive loss of independence and self-care ability up to walking impairment. Physical examination was suggestive of hypercortisolism (central obesity, muscle atrophy, moon facies, buffalo hump, and leg ulcers). Endocrine work-up showed ACTH-independent hypercortisolism: UFC was 214 nM/24 h (by LC-MS/MS, nv <168), serum cortisol after overnight 1 mg dexamethasone test was 240 μg/L (nv <18), and ACTH 1 ng/L (normal value: 7–63 ng/L). Urinary metanephrines were within the normal range. CT scan confirmed a 35 mm right adrenal mass.

In July 2020, during the full-blown pandemic period, glucometabolic derangement required hospitalization in our hospital. Nasal swab was negative for SARS-CoV-2, fasting glucose was 300 mg/dL, HbA1c 12.5%, eGFR 34 mL/min/1.73 m^2, AST 39 U/L, ALT 60 U/L, and gamma-GT 608 U/L. Abdominal CT did not show additional lesions beyond the known 36 × 33 mm right adrenal nodule; in particular, the liver and biliary tree were normal. Screening for complications of CS ruled out vertebral fractures and disclosed hypertrophic cardiomyopathy with outflow obstruction.

The whole picture was so severe that she was not considered suitable for surgery that was anyway inaccessible due to pandemic. The impairment in the liver function test (LFT) was attributed to steroid hepatitis.

Initial daily treatment included bisoprolol 5 mg, perindopril 10 mg, amlodipine 10 mg, doxazosin 4 mg, furosemide 50 mg, spironolactone 37 mg, atorvastatin 20 mg, and acetylsalicylic acid 100 mg. Antidiabetic treatment was uptitrated with insulin (total daily dose: 84 U; degludec, 38 U, fast-acting aspart, 14 + 18 + 14 U), dapagliflozin 10 mg/day, and long-acting exenatide 2 mg/week.

Medical treatment with ketoconazole (KCZ) was then cautiously administered, starting with 200 mg/day and then uptitrated to 400 mg/day. The choice of KCZ was due to transient unavailability of metyrapone (osilodrostat was not yet marketed). The patient complained nausea, and KCZ dose was downtitrated to 200 and 400 mg every other day. UFC values progressively decreased to 38 μg/24 h (nv 35–137) as well as transaminase and gamma-GT values, and cortisone acetate 12.5 mg/day was added. This block-and-replace schedule was well tolerated, clinical picture improved, and insulin dose was progressively reduced to 70 U/day due to the continuous occurrence of hypoglycemic episodes.

She was discharged home clinically improved, with the indication to weekly control of LFT, insulin dose tapering according to glucose automonitoring and medical advice, and quick glucocorticoid dose increase in case of fever or stress. Adrenal resection should have been planned as soon as possible in relation to clinical improvement and pandemic evolution.

After one month, she was hospitalized in another ward owing to syncope for acute adrenal failure due to symptomatic febrile urinary infection without a timely quick increase of glucocorticoid dosage. The daily block-and-replace schedule was adjusted to KCZ 400 mg plus cortisone acetate 25 mg. This treatment induced a progressive amelioration of clinical picture, including healing of leg ulcers, mood improvement, and restoring of the ability to walk. LFT normalized, antihypertensive drug dosage was reduced, HbA1c dropped to 6.2%, and insulin dose was reduced to 26 U/day owing to frequent hypoglycemic episodes. UFC was now normal (ranging 31–52 μg/24 h).

Due to the persistence of the COVID-19 pandemic in our region and the unavailability of any surgical facilities for not urgent surgeries, despite our pressing on surgeon and hospital management, the patient is still scheduled for adrenal resection. She is carrying on KCZ plus cortisone acetate therapy at fixed dose, with the advice to quickly increasing the steroid dose as soon as any suspect of impending infection occurs. A progressive improvement in clinical and biochemical picture has been observed on this medical treatment that is aimed to keep a good control of arterial pressure and a fair control of the glucose metabolism while avoiding any hypoglycemia.

In July 2021, abdomen CT scan did not show any change in tumor size; the values of UFC and ACTH were 35 μg/24 h and 1.5 ng/L, respectively, on a block-and-replace treatment (KCZ 400 mg plus cortisone acetate 25 mg/day).

3. Case 2

An 83-year-old woman was evaluated for cardiogenic shock.

Her history was remarkable for hyperlipidemia, gastroesophageal reflux, right breast cancer (in 2000 with negative annual follow-up), and surgically treated autonomous thyroid adenoma (in 1980). In addition, she had undergone cholecystectomy in 2018 that was complicated by severe hypertensive crisis with acute heart failure.

In September 2019, abdominal plastic surgery was complicated by severe hypertensive crisis with acute pulmonary edema, cardiogenic shock, and acute renal failure. She was thus transferred to ICU for suspected acute coronary syndrome. Multiple noncritical stenoses were disclosed at coronary angiography and reverse Takotsubo at ventriculography. Chest CT disclosed a left adrenal lesion consistent with PHEO. Conservative therapies (ramipril, lercanidipine, atenolol, and furosemide) induced recovery of systolic function (ejection fraction increased from 5% to 62%).

Endocrine work-up confirmed PHEO: urinary adrenaline was 34 μg/24 h (nv <22), noradrenaline 81 μg/24 h (nv <85), metanephrines 1932 μg/24 h (nv <297), and normetanephrines 2009 μg/24 h (nv <354). At retrospective inquiring, the patient reported palpitations, tremors, diaphoresis, headaches, anxiety, and panic attacks. Fasting plasma glucose was 79 mg/dL and HbA1c 5.2%.

Abdominal CT and MRI confirmed a 45 × 31 mm left adrenal lesion, with irregular margins and inhomogeneous contrast enhancement, whose density was 30 HU, without other remarkable lesions.

The planning of adrenal resection was postponed due to an adrenal hematoma developed while on LMWE treatment. Pressure control was maintained with doxazosin (in addition to ongoing treatment) titrated up to 8 mg bid. In January 2020, CT showed hematoma reabsorption, but while waiting for scheduled surgery, there was the outbreak of pandemic. The patient was monitored throughout Spring and Summer with frequent telemedicine controls that confirmed optimal pressure control, without any side effect of antihypertensive treatment.

In October 2020, nasal swab was negative for SARS-CoV-2, and she underwent laparoscopic left adrenalectomy, taking advantage of a transient decrease of pandemic burden.

Postoperative recovery was uneventful, no hypotension occurred, and the patient was discharged home on atenolol and doxazosin that were quickly tapered and finally discontinued within one month. Histologic examination confirmed the diagnosis of PHEO: the lesion infiltrated the perivisceral adipose tissue due to the previous hematoma, but there was no angioinvasion, Ki-67 was <1%, and PASS score was 7.

One month later, urinary metanephrines were normalized, namely, 93 and 282 μg/24 h for metanephrine and normetanephrine, respectively, and remained normal at the following control.

A recent CT did not disclose any tumor remnant or relapse.

4. Discussion

CS is a life-threatening disease, with vascular disease and infections representing the most common cause of death, mainly in elderly patients. Both diagnosis and management of CS might be cumbersome even in ordinary times, mostly in patients with a cyclic disease. The diagnosis in patient 1 was straightforward but the management was not, due to the COVID-19 pandemic. Surgery is the first-line treatment for CS, regardless of its etiology [1], but in some extremely frail patients, it should be postponed even in ordinary times, in order to ameliorate clinical picture with steroidogenesis inhibitors according to clinical status. Furthermore, surgery should be considered with caution during the pandemic because cortisol hypersecretion may lead to a lessening of immune reaction. In addition, following an issue of hospital management, only urgent cases should be admitted to surgery unit due to the shortage of intensive care units and healthcare personnel.

We followed thus successfully the recommendations of the European Society of Endocrinology [3] that points to surgery only in patients who cannot be controlled with medical therapy or in those requiring biopsy or resection because of possible cancer.

The infective risk is indeed increased by defective innate and adaptive immune response due to chronic glucocorticoid exposure [4]. The increased susceptibility to infection is further increased by visceral obesity, hypertension, and diabetes that are characteristics of the disease and hugely heighten the risk of death. Furthermore, CS patients have high risk of thromboembolic events due to many alterations of coagulation and fibrinolysis that in turn worsen the prognosis in the case of COVID-19 infection. We opted thus for drug treatment to get control of the disease while waiting for more propitious times for a surgical approach.

Among the different steroidogenesis inhibitors, we had to choose KCZ because osilodrostat was not marketed yet, and there was a temporary shortage of metyrapone supply. Keeping in mind the liver toxicity of KCZ, reportedly occurring in 3–19% of treated patients [5], this choice might have been regarded as hazardous in a patient with severe derangement of LFT. Anyway, the severity of clinical picture prompted us to start treatment with a tight monitoring. Treatment obtained actually a quick and progressive improvement in clinical and biochemical picture. No escape was observed, on the contrary adrenal failure developed prompting the use of a block-and-replace schedule. This option has proved effective beyond all our expectations.

In patient 2, the diagnosis of PHEO was neglected for a long time, until catastrophic acute worsening of cardiac function occurred that required intensive treatment.

According to Endocrine Society guidelines, the treatment for PHEO is surgical adrenalectomy after a brief period of medical preparation (7–14 days) with alpha-adrenergic receptor blockade to minimize perioperative complications [2].

The unusual circumstances created by the pandemic necessitated a more prolonged preoperative period of medical management, as already described in other 4 cases recently reported [6, 7]. At last, the adrenal tumor was successfully resected after a prolonged pharmacologic control of blood pressure, and the patient is doing well off antihypertensive treatment.

This effort of progressive continuous adjustment should always take into account both the epidemiological environment with its constraints and the individual clinical picture.

Abbreviations

ACTH: Adrenocorticotropic hormone
ALT: Alanine transaminase
AST: Aspartate transaminase
COVID-19: Corona-virus disease 2019
CS: Cushing's syndrome
CT: Computerized tomography
eGFR: Estimated glomerular filtration rate
gamma-GT: Gamma-glutamyl-transferase
HbA1c: Glycated hemoglobin
HU: Hounsfield units
KCZ: Ketoconazole
LC-MS/MS: Liquid chromatography-tandem mass spectrometry
LFT: Liver function test
LMWE: Low molecular weight heparin
MRI: Magnetic resonance imaging
Nv: Normal values
PASS: Pheochromocytoma of the Adrenal Gland Scaled Score
PET: Positron emission tomography
PHEO: Pheochromocytoma
UFC: Urinary free cortisol
US: Ultrasonography.

Consent

The patients have given informed consent for the publication of their medical history.

References

[1] L. K. Nieman, B. M. K. Biller, J. W. Findling et al., "Treatment of Cushing's syndrome: an endocrine society clinical practice guideline practice guideline," *Journal of Clinical Endocrinology & Metabolism*, vol. 100, no. 8, pp. 2807–2831, 2015.

[2] J. W. M. Lenders, Q.-Y. Duh, G. Eisenhofer et al., "Endocrine Society. Pheochromocytoma and paraganglioma: an Endocrine Society clinical practice guideline," *Journal of Clinical Endocrinology & Metabolism*, vol. 99, no. 6, pp. 1915–1942, 2014.

[3] J. Newell-Price, L. K. Nieman, M. Reincke, and A. Tabarin, "Endocrinology in the time of COVID-19: management of Cushing's syndrome," *European Journal of Endocrinology*, vol. 183, no. 1, pp. G1–G7, 2020.

[4] V. Guarnotta, R. Ferrigno, M. Martino et al., "Glucocorticoid excess and COVID-19 disease," *Reviews in Endocrine & Metabolic Disorders*, vol. 22, no. 4, pp. 703–714, 2020.

[5] R. Pivonello, M. De Leo, A. Cozzolino, and A. Colao, "The treatment of Cushing's disease," *Endocrine Reviews*, vol. 36, no. 4, pp. 385–486, 2015.

[6] E. A. Japp, A. Leiter, E. A. Tsomos, S. A. Reda, and A. C. Levine, "Management of 3 cases of pheochromocytoma during the COVID-19 pandemic in New York City: lessons learned," *Journal of the Endocrine Society*, vol. 5, no. 2, pp. 1–6, 2021.

[7] R. Yu, "Successful management of pheochromocytoma and thyroiditis with fever by telemedicine during the COVID-19 pandemic," *Endocrine Practice*, vol. 26, no. 9, pp. 1042-1043, 2020.

3

Case Report of Rare Parathyroid Tumor with Atypical Presentation and Early Diagnosis

Érika Mayumi Ikeda Cavamura,[1] **Fabiane Karen Miyake**,[2] **Jéssica Yachio Wiezel**,[2] **Laura Schwartz Maranho**,[3] **Luis Felipe Inglês Takada**,[2] **Renata Cassitas Mendonça**,[3] **and Tamila Sohn Fagundes**[3]

[1]*Academic of the Faculdade Pequeno Príncipe, Curitiba, Brazil*
[2]*Academics of the Faculdade Evangélica Mackenzie Paraná, Curitiba, Brazil*
[3]*Medical Residents of the Endocrinology Service at Hospital Universitário Mackenzie Paraná, Curitiba, Brazil*

Correspondence should be addressed to Érika Mayumi Ikeda Cavamura; ki.mayumi@hotmail.com

Academic Editor: J. Paul Frindik

Parathyroid carcinoma is a rare condition, accounting for 1% of cases of hyperparathyroidism. Other causes of hyperparathyroidism main group are single adenoma and parathyroid hyperplasia. The clinics presented by the patients are typical of hyperparathyroidism (fatigue, weakness, weight loss, and anorexia), bone impairment, pain, and fractures, in addition to affecting the renal system The diagnosis of parathyroid carcinoma is most often done postoperatively by means of a histological study. The case report is a 49-year-old male patient who came to the emergency room of Mackenzie Evangelical University Hospital complaining of progressive "muscle weakness" and "joint" that started about 2 months ago. To raise the suspicion of parathyroid carcinoma, it is essential to perform the correlation of the clinical picture, biochemical values, and imaging exams, but to obtain the definitive diagnosis, intraoperative recognition of the tumor and the result of the histopathological examination of the resected tumor are necessary.

1. Introduction

Parathyroid carcinoma is a rare condition, accounting for 1% of cases of hyperparathyroidism [1], being described in the literature, less than 600 cases registered up to the year 2001 [2]. Other causes of hyperparathyroidism main group are single adenoma and parathyroid hyperplasia [3].

The patients presented to the clinic are typical of hyperparathyroidism (fatigue, weakness, weight loss, and anorexia), bone impairment, pain, and fractures, in addition to affecting the renal system (nephrolithiasis, nephrocalcinosis, renal colic, and hypercalcemia) [4].

The diagnosis of parathyroid carcinoma is most often done postoperatively by means of a histological study. It can be suspected in the preoperative period through laboratory and clinical findings such as palpable cervical mass (30–76% of cases), vocal fold paralysis, or presence of regional or distance metastasis (lung and liver) [5]. Laboratory tests show hypercalcemia (above 14 mg/dl or 3- 4 mg/dl above normal), parathyroid hormone (PTH) 3–10 times above the normal value, and alkaline phosphatase often increased [4, 6]. The hypothesis of parathyroid carcinoma should be considered in the presence of severe hyperparathyroidism, parathyroidosis, and serum calcium greater than or equal to 14 mg/dl, especially if associated with cervical mass [7]. Fine needle puncture should be avoided in the suspicion of parathyroid carcinoma due to the risk of metastatic local [8].

The importance of suspecting preoperative carcinoma is mainly due to its management being different from adenoma [9]. Major differences between carcinoma and other benign parathyroid diseases include mean age (48 and 55 years, respectively), tumor size >3 cm frequent in carcinoma and rare in benign diseases, very high PTH in carcinoma and slightly elevated in disease benign, palpable cervical mass present in carcinoma, and rare in benign diseases [10].

The treatment is surgical, with extensive resection with tumor block whenever malignant neoplasia is suspected. It should include the parathyroid, the ipsilateral thyroid lobe, the isthmus, and the lymph nodes of the central compartment. Cervical emptying should be performed in the presence of metastasis. In the postoperative period, it is important to control hipocalcemia [5]. Metabolic complications such as hypercalcemic crisis, bone, or renal abnormalities are the most common [11].

2. Case Report

A 49-year-old male came to the emergency room of Mackenzie Evangelical University Hospital complaining of progressive "muscle weakness" and "joint" that started about 2 months ago. The pain occurs in the lumbar spine region associated with nausea, diarrhea (6 episodes), hyporexia, fluctuating fecal acholia, and unintentional weight loss of about 20 kilograms (kg) within 3 months. He denies allergies, smoking, drinking, and other comorbidities. Physical examination showed arthralgia in the lumbar spine without pain on palpation, but painful with flexion and extension of the spine. He also had pain on palpation of the right lower thoracic region and right hypochondrium and a slightly enlarged and slow base gait with a palpable thyroid nodule in the left lobe region. He refers to an uncle with a history of bone carcinoma. Patient was admitted to the intensive care unit (ICU) with optimized analgesia, hydration, and furosemide.

Chest (1), contrast abdomen (2), and skull (3) computed tomography (CT) and CPK scans were ordered, which showed the following, respectively. (Figures 1–3)

(1) Lytic lesion in costa arch and right trochanter, sprouting tree-like lung tissue with calcified granulomas, and absence of pulmonary lymph nodes or nodules

(2) Diffuse lytic lesions in the bilateral pelvis and right fender head, associated with no obstructive bilateral nephrolithiasis

(3) Reduction of diffuse bone density of skull cap without lytic lesions

Serious calcium was also measured with results greater than 17.1 mg/dl, PTH of 2627 pg/ml, and 558 alkaline phosphatase and hypophosphatemia, as well as protein electrophoresis, creatine phosphokinase test (CPK), prostate-specific antigen (PSA), and partial urine.

Due to hypercalcemia, pamidronate was prescribed with relative improvement of calcium level investigation followed with USG of the cervical region demonstrating a mass in the cervical region on the left, quite delimited, heterogeneous, predominantly hypoechoic, with macrocalcifications and beam fibrotics in between, presenting exuberant flow to the study doppler with apparent plan of cleavage and thyroid measuring 3.0 × 3.5 × 3.0 cm, without being possible to remove the possibility of injury of nature parathyroid among the hypotheses.

Endocrinology follow-up indicates daily dosages of calcium (Ca), phosphorus (P), magnesium (Mg), albumin, and correction as needed, vitamin D dosage, and electrocardiogram (EKG), indication for postoperative ICU parathyroidectomy due to the risk of severe hypocalcemia ("bone hunger"), preoperative examinations, and dosage intraoperating of PTH, besides immediate beginning of calcitriol (dose attacks 2 mcg/day) and cholecalciferol 50.000 UI for 3 consecutive days before the surgery and to maintain maintenance dose with 10.000 UI in a week and magnesium and furosemide replacement.

A parathyroidectomy of the lower left lobe associated with level VI lymphadenectomy was performed. The lesion was highly adhered posteriorly to the sternal part of the sternocleidomastoid muscle and was extremely solid. The level of PTH and vitamin D in the preoperative one was of 2657 pg/ml and 24 ng/ml and in the immediate postoperative thing of 325 pg/ml and 36 ng/mL. Calcium gluconate, EV, and bicarbonate were maintained, as well as vitamin D2 and calcium carbonate replacement with neurological surveillance (epilepsy/tetany/paresthesias), cardioscopy, and prevention of hyperventilation/alkalosis with guidance not to perform loop diuretics and prophylactic cefazolin. The material sent to anatomopathological showed epithelial neoplasia, sometimes trabecular, and sometimes nodular with rounded nucleus cells and macronucleolus, presenting capsule infiltration, without invasion of adjacent tissue or necrosis, with 3 mitoses in 50 GCA.

In immunohistochemistry, it is neoplasia with focal perivascular neoplastic extension that corresponds to vascular invasion and observes capsular transposition and fibrous bands in a trabecular pattern amidst neoplasia. These parameters may correlate with more aggressive clinical behavior, including the occurrence of metastases. The possibility of parathyroid carcinoma should be clinically positive and researched with appropriate evolutionary, clinical, and laboratory monitoring, despite presenting histological aspects that can be correlated with atypical parathyroid adenoma and presenting the following immunohistochemical panel. (Table 1)

Calcitriol 0.25 mcg 3 cp/day associated with cholecalciferol 10,000 IU/week was maintained, and calcium IV replacements were performed; serum calcium, phosphate, and magnesium measurements were performed for follow-up, which showed progressive improvement. The patient was referred to the room after 3 days of ICU with a suspension of calcium IV replacement and started calcium citrate associated with oral vitamin D3. At the seventh postoperative day, PTH was 26 pg/ml and continued improvement in other laboratory tests. New skull tomography demonstrated calcification in the right frontal lobe with signs of bone thinning in skull cap. (Table 2)

Hospital discharged the patient after 42 days of hospitalization. The patient was referred for follow-up at the endocrinology outpatient clinic, where he presented weight gain and muscle strength, but maintaining the need for a walking stick and with asymptomatic hypocalcemia. (Figures 4–6)

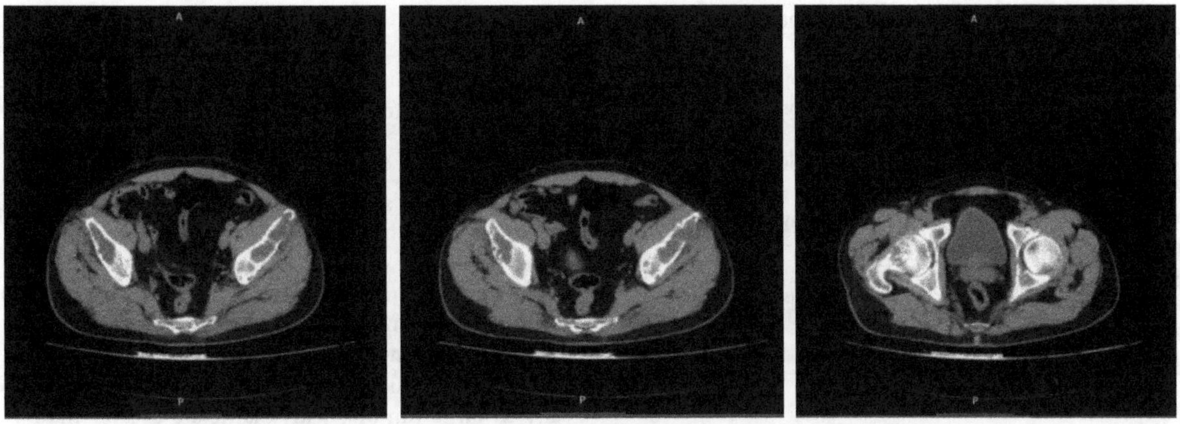

FIGURE 1: Chest CT scans.

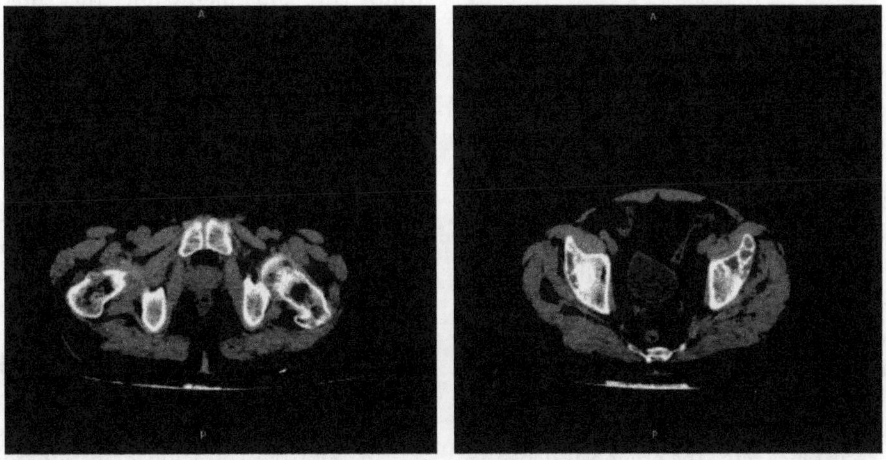

FIGURE 2: Contrast abdomen CT scans.

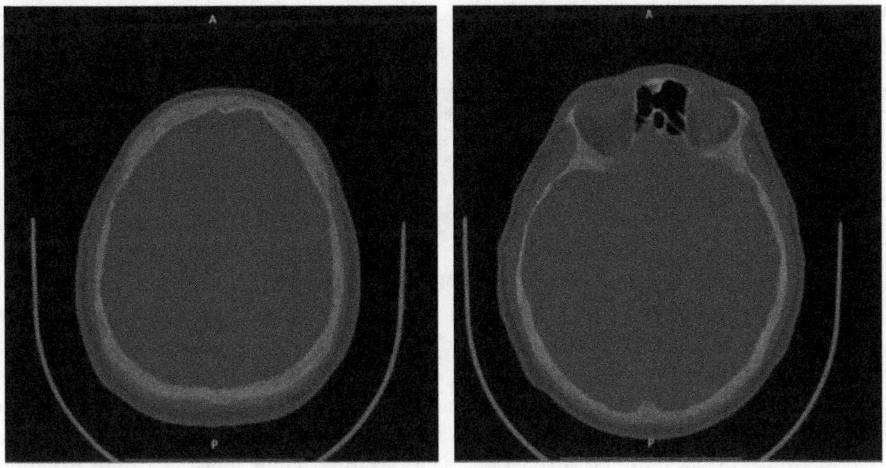

FIGURE 3: Cranial CT scans.

3. Discussion

The parathyroid gland consists of a set of glands that are located mainly in the apex and in the inferior poles of the right and left lobes of the thyroid, usually in a total of four [12]. They originate from the third and fourth branchial arches in the embryonic period. The involvement of this gland by neoplasia is defined as parathyroid carcinoma, an endocrine tumor that has unknown etiology and is associated with mutations in the HRPT2/CDC73 gene [13]. The present case proved to be a parathyroid carcinoma located in the inferior left lobe of the thyroid, requiring parathyroidectomy associated with lymphadenectomy level VI.

Table 1: Immunohistochemical panel.

AE1/AE3	Positive
Calcitonin	Negative
CD31	Positive in vessel
Chromogranin A	Negative
ERG	Positive in vessel
GATA3	Positive
Ki-67	Positive in 10% of cells
Paratormon	Positive
PAX-8	Positive focal
Synaptophysin	Positive focal
Thyroglobulin	Negative
TTF-1	Negative

Table 2: Evolution of the patient's level of albumin, PTH, creatinine, and vitamin D in the preoperative and postoperative periods.

12/02-17H		ALB: 3.7
12/02-20H		ALB: 3.3, CR: 1.48
14/02		PTH: 325
17/02		CR: 1.16
18/02		CR: 1.20
PTH	Pre-op: 2657	Immediate postoperative period: 325 7oPO: 26
Vitamin D	Pre-op: 24	Post-op: 36

The involvement of this carcinoma is not predisposed by sex [14]. The age range of patients at diagnosis varies between 28 and 72 years, with a higher frequency at 40–50 years [8]. The patient in the reported case was male and 49 years old, that is, within the most frequent range of the tumor. The evolution of the neoplasm is slow and progressive with a high recurrence rate. The prognosis depends on the success of the surgical procedure and early detection. The case demonstrates carcinoma discovered at earlier stages in which the moment of follow-up at the endocrinology outpatient clinic showed no recurrence. According to data from the National Cancer Database, the estimated 5 year survival is 49% [15].

In the physical examination of most cases, as well as in the reported case, the tumor is a palpable—a rare differential in cases of benign adenoma hyperparathyroidism. Laboratory tests show elevated calcium levels greater than 14.0 mg/dL or an increase of 3-4 mg/dL in normal index, parathyroid hormone levels of 500 ng/dL or an increase of 3–10 times higher than normal values, and hypophosphatemia [10]. The reported tumor presented levels around 17 mg/dL at the time of diagnosis and a significant increase in parathyroid hormone levels with a preoperative 2657 pg/ml, in addition to hypophosphatemia.

When a diagnosis of parathyroid carcinoma is suspected, at least two imaging tests are recommended to obtain the precise location of the tumor. The most common techniques are cervical ultrasound and Sestamibi, 99m Tc scintigraphy [9, 16]. Ultrasound examination is used to locate the disease, analyze local recurrence, and as a guide for fine needle aspiration (FNA) when regional lymph node metastasis is suspected. However, the FNAB technique should be performed with caution or avoided, since there is a risk of tumor spread in the biopsy path [9].

Already, the scintigraphy with Sestamibi, 99m Tc can indicate the place that the disease affects, however, though it is not possible to distinguish carcinoma from a benign disease. Computed tomography (CT) and magnetic resonance imaging (MRI) may indicate metastases and recurrence cases [17].

Radiography shows bone changes in the hands in 83% of the patients, in the skull in 71%, and in the spine and long bones in 90% of them [18]. Radiological changes are consistent with fibrous osteitis and subperiosteal resorption. The imaging exams in this case were chest, abdomen, and skull scans, all showing radiological alterations. From the anatomopathological point of view, they present macroscopically as large tumors, with diameters greater than 1.5 cm, adherent to adjacent tissues and frequently presenting invasion of the ipsilateral thyroid lobe and cervical musculature [14]. On microscopy, they present thick acellular fibrous bands, mitotic activity, vascular invasion, and capsular invasion [19]. The anatomopathological observation involves the difficulty of differentiating carcinoma from parathyroid adenoma, as in both situations, nuclear pleomorphism, hyperchromatism, free tumor cells in blood vessels, mitosis, and giant cells can be found [20]. Thus, achieving an accurate diagnosis is difficult due to the diversity of clinical presentations and examination findings [21]. The material sent to the anatomopathological presented fields of trabecular and nodular epithelial neoplasia with round nucleus cells and macronucleolus, presenting capsule infiltration, without adjacent tissue invasion or necrosis. This shows that despite the capsule infiltration, the diagnosis was early, since it did not present adjacent tissue invasion.

To raise the suspicion of parathyroid carcinoma, it is essential to perform the correlation of the clinical picture, biochemical values, and imaging exams, but to obtain the definitive diagnosis, intraoperative recognition of the tumor and the result of the histopathological examination of the resected tumor are necessary [22].

The intraoperative macroscopic characteristics of the tumor can be evaluated. Thus, in benign tumors such as parathyroid, adenomas have characteristics such as oval shape, elastic consistency, and reddish color. Already, carcinoma tends to present as a firm mass with gray-white fibrous capsule adhering to the thyroid lobe and other cervical tissues—laryngeal nerve, infrahyoid muscles, esophagus, and trachea [17, 22].

However, the absence of local invasion or regional metastasis makes differentiation difficult [17]. In addition, in freezing analysis, the histopathological aspects of carcinoma may overlap with those of parathyroid adenoma. Therefore, when there is a high preoperative suspicion for carcinoma and absence of suspicious intraoperative findings, en bloc resection of the tumor is recommended [17, 22].

It is not uncommon for a patient with parathyroid carcinoma to be diagnosed only when local recurrence or distant metastasis occurs [22]. Thus, in cases of severe hyperparathyroidism, carcinoma should always be investigated to make an early diagnosis when there is still a possibility of cure.

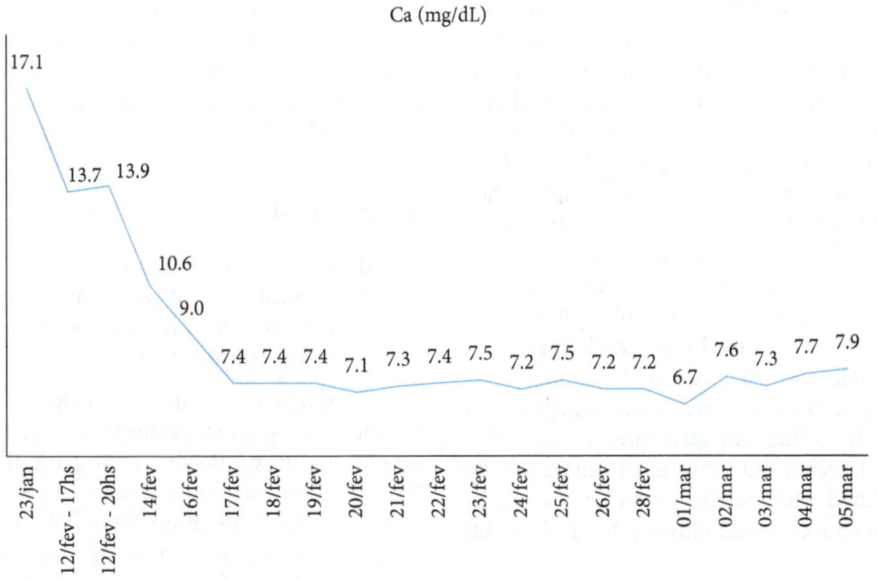

FIGURE 4: Evolution of the patient's calcium level.

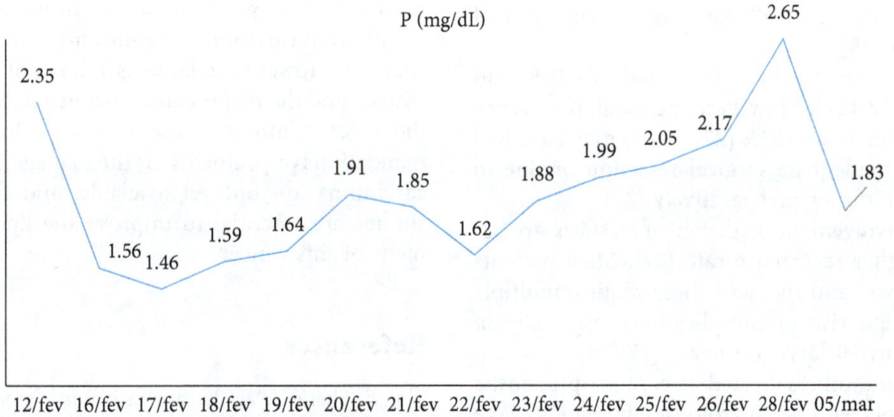

FIGURE 5: Evolution of patient's phosphate level.

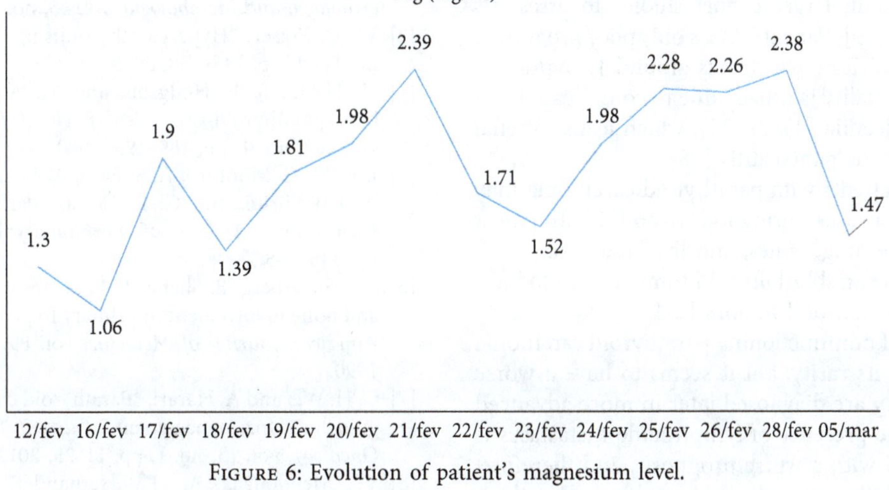

FIGURE 6: Evolution of patient's magnesium level.

Adjuvant irradiation of the neck and mediastinum has recently been reported to be useful in reducing the risk of locoregional disease progression and improving survival [23, 24] as well as for palliative symptoms of hypercalcemia in inoperable patients [2]. In this case, the patient was considered healed and is on watch for possible relapse.

When there is no possibility of surgical correction, clinical treatment can be performed to reduce hypercalcemia and minimize bone resorption. The therapy is aimed at inhibiting bone release of calcium and increasing urinary excretion, and the three targets for treatment are the tumor, osteoclast, and kidney. Initial treatment includes vigorous saline hydration. Loop diuretics, calcitonin, bisphosphonates, plicamycin or mitramycin, and calciomimetic agents [2] may be used. In this case, hydration, loop, diuretic, calcitriol, cholecalciferol, magnesium, calcium, parathyroidectomy, and serial serum calcium, phosphate, and magnesium dosages were performed until discharge.

Metastases occur late, with lymphatic and hematogenous spread, and may occur in the lung, liver, bones, and pancreas [11]. Local invasion to contiguous structures is more frequently observed [18]. Death usually results from metabolic complications associated with hypercalcemia [14], which in this case was of great concern and follow-up by the hospital service.

Follow-up aimed at early detection of locoregional recurrence and/or distant metastases [25, 26]. It should be done by monitoring calcium and PTH every 2 years for the first 5 years and then annually associated with annual cervical ultrasound [25].

The 5 and 10-year survival rate is around 77–100% and 66–80%, respectively [27]. However, the local recurrence rate is common, from 40% to 63% [27]. Many may have had recurrence due to inadequate surgical resection or due to nondiagnosis of the tumor preoperatively [27].

Lymph node involvement or distant metastasis are associated with a higher recurrence rate [27]. Most patients have local recurrence, and many of these require multiple surgeries with a high risk of complications, especially in relation to the recurrent laryngeal nerve [27, 28].

Silva-Figueroa and others created a score for prognostic assessment in patients with parathyroid carcinoma [29]. Age greater than 65 years, serum calcium >15 mg/dl, and vascular invasion were negatively correlated with relapse-free survival after initial parathyroidectomy [29]. Further validation of this score is still needed in larger cohort studies to assess its clinical applicability [29]. Patient W.G.'s only poor prognostic factor was serious calcium, which was around 17 mg/dl.

The cause of mortality is usually due to complications of intractable hypercalcemia [25, 27–29], which leads to renal failure, arrhythmias, or pancreatitis [28].

Up to 25% of patients with parathyroid carcinoma may develop distant metastases during follow-up [27]. The most affected sites are the lung, bones, and liver [26, 27].

The prognosis is variable, but solid tumors seem to have better survival than nonsolid tumors [27].

The prognosis of nonfunctioning parathyroid carcinoma is uncertain due to its rarity, but it seems to have a worse prognosis, since they are diagnosed later in more advanced staging [25, 27]. The presence of lymph node metastases is generally associated with a worse prognosis, and therefore, appropriate cervical dissection should be performed in these patients [27]. The patient in the reported case had an early diagnosis in which he was associated with lymphadenectomy.

Other prognostic factors include age, gender, time to first relapse, elevated serum calcium on recurrence, number of relapses, number of medications used to decrease calcium, inability to completely resect the tumor, and tumor aneuploidy [27, 29].

4. Conclusion

Parathyroid carcinoma is a rare malignant tumor that tends to have clinical signs of severe hypercalcemia. Because it is an uncommon cancer, it is difficult to access consistent data on morbidity and mortality.

The diagnosis is difficult, being necessary the suspicion of the disease preoperatively or even during surgery to enable the most effective treatment, and the definitive diagnosis is not rare only when there is metastasis or recurrence, which highlights the follow-up of these patients. Surgical treatment at an early stage of the disease is an important factor for disease control. Complete block resection with eventual hemithyroidectomy and ipsilateral centrocervical lymphadenectomy should represent the minimal oncologic approach in all patients with suspected parathyroid carcinoma, significantly improving disease-free survival. However, relapse is often not the cause of poor course, and the major cause uncontrollable hypercalcemia is the most common cause of death. In addition, recommendations or protocols for the management of parathyroid carcinoma are not yet available, and further multicenter studies are essential to improve the knowledge and treatment of this cancer.

References

[1] E. Shane, "Parathyroid carcinoma," *Journal of Clinical Endocrinology and Metabolism*, vol. 86, no. 2, pp. 485–493, 2001.

[2] L. K. Morimitsu, M. N. O. Uyeno, M. L. Goulart et al., "Carcinoma de paratiróide: características clínicas e anátomo-patológicas de cinco casos," *Arquivos Brasileiros de Endocrinologia and Metabologia*, vol. 45, no. 2, pp. 148–156, 2001.

[3] W. D. Fraser, "Hyperparathyroidism," *The Lancet*, vol. 374, no. 9684, pp. 145–158, 2009.

[4] H. Heath, S. F. Hodgson, and M. A. Kennedy, "Primary hyperparathyroidism," *New England Journal of Medicine*, vol. 302, no. 4, pp. 189–193, 1980.

[5] J. R. M. C. Montoro, A. S. Fava, A. L. Sartini, L. R. Mattiola, A. J. P. Brito, and G. P. Costa, "Parathyroid carcinoma," *International Archives of Otorhinolaryngology*, vol. 12, no. 1, pp. 145–148, 2008.

[6] S. J. Silverberg, E. Shane, T. P. Jacobs et al., "Nephrolithiasis and bone involvement in primary hyperparathyroidism," *The American Journal of Medicine*, vol. 89, no. 3, pp. 327–334, 1990.

[7] C. H. Wei and A. Harari, "Parathyroid carcinoma: update and guidelines for management," *Current Treatment Options in Oncology*, vol. 13, no. 1, pp. 11–23, 2012.

[8] V. Mendonza, A. F. Hernandez, M. L. Marquez, M. A. Delgadillo, J. Penã, and M. Mercado, "Primary hyperparathyroidism due to parathyroid carcinoma," *Archives of Medical Research*, vol. 28, pp. 303–306, 1997.

[9] M. Abrahao, O. Cervantes, M. Lazaretti-Castro, M. C. Neves, I. S. Kunii, and D. Orlandi, "Parathyroid carcinoma and hungry bone syndrome," *Arquivos Brasileiros de Endocrinologia e Metabologia*, vol. 57, no. 1, pp. 79–86, 2013.
[10] K. E. Levin, M. Galante, and O. H. Clark, "Parathyroid carcinoma versus parathyroid adenoma in patients with profound hypercalcemia," *Surgery*, vol. 101, no. 6, pp. 649–660, 1987.
[11] M. H. d. F. Silva, P. O. D. R. Morais, T. A. d. Souza et al., "Parathyroid carcinoma: case report," *Medicina*, vol. 50, no. 6, pp. 390–397, 2018.
[12] B. Castleman and S. I. Roth, *Tumors of the Parathyroid Glands. Atlas of Tumor Pathology*, Armed Force Institute of Pathology, Washington, DC, 1978.
[13] A. Barbosa and J. C. Costa, "Carcinoma da Paratiróide," *Revista portuguesa de cirurgia cardio-torácica e vascular*, vol. 44, pp. 25–36, 2018.
[14] C.-A. Wang and R. D. Gaz, "Natural history of parathyroid carcinoma," *The American Journal of Surgery*, vol. 149, no. 4, pp. 522–527, 1985.
[15] S. A. Hundahl, I. D. Fleming, A. M. Fremgen, and H. R. Menck, "Two hundred eighty-six cases of parathyroid carcinoma treated in the U.S. between 1985–1995. The American College of Surgeons Commission on Cancer and the American Cancer Society," *Cancer*, vol. 86, no. 3, pp. 538–544, 1999.
[16] F. R. Bringhurst, M. B. Demay, and H. M. Kronenberg, "Hormones and disorders of mineral metabolism," in *Williams Textbook of Endocrinology*, S. Melmed, K. S. Polonsky, P. R. Larsen, and H. M. Kronenberg, Eds., pp. 1255–1277, Elsevier, Philadelphia, 12th ed. edition, 2011.
[17] A. Mohebati, A. Shaha, and J. Shah, "Parathyroid carcinoma," *Hematology-Oncology Clinics of North America*, vol. 26, no. 6, pp. 1221–1238, 2012.
[18] A. G. Wynne, J. V. Heerden, J. A. Carney, and L. A. Fitzpatrick, "Parathyroid carcinoma," *Medicine*, vol. 71, no. 4, pp. 197–205, 1992.
[19] A. Schantz and B. Castleman, "Parathyroid carcinoma.A study of 70 cases," *Cancer*, vol. 31, no. 3, pp. 600–605, 1973.
[20] F. L. D. M. Montenegro, M. R. Tavares, M. D. Durazzo, C. R. Cernea, A. C. Cordeiro, and A. R. Ferraz, "Clinical suspicion and parathyroid carcinoma management," *Sao Paulo Medical Journal*, vol. 124, no. 1, pp. 42–44, 2006.
[21] E. Kebebew, "Parathyroid carcinoma," *Current Treatment Options in Oncology*, vol. 2, no. 4, pp. 347–354, 2001~.
[22] G. Ricci, M. Assenza, M. Barreca et al., "Parathyroid carcinoma: the importance of high clinical suspicion for a correct management," *International journal of surgical oncology*, vol. 2012, Article ID 649148, 2012.
[23] G. L. Clayman, H. E. Gonzalez, A. El-Naggar, and R. Vassilopoulou-Sellin, "Parathyroid carcinoma: evaluation and interdisciplinary management," *Cancer*, vol. 100, no. 5, pp. 900–905, 2004.
[24] N. D. Munson, R. L. Foote, R. C. Northcutt et al., "Parathyroid carcinoma: is there a role for adjuvant radiation therapy?" *Cancer*, vol. 98, no. 11, pp. 2378–2384, 2003.
[25] A. S. Salcuni, F. Cetani, V. Guarnieri et al., "Parathyroid carcinoma," *Best Practice & Research Clinical Endocrinology and Metabolism*, vol. 32, no. 6, pp. 877–889, 2018.
[26] J. M. P. Fernandes, C. Paiva, R. Correia, J. Polónia, and A. Moreira da Costa, "Parathyroid carcinoma: from a case report to a review of the literature," *International Journal of Surgery Case Reports*, vol. 42, pp. 214–217, 2017.
[27] J. Goswamy, M. Lei, and R. Simo, "Parathyroid carcinoma," *Current Opinion in Otolaryngology and Head and Neck Surgery*, vol. 24, no. 2, pp. 155–162, 2016.
[28] P. Libánský, S. Adámek, P. Broulík et al., "Parathyroid carcinoma in patients that have undergone surgery for primary hyperparathyroidism," *In Vivo*, vol. 31, no. 5, pp. 925–930, 2017.
[29] F. Cetani, E. Pardi, and C. Marcocci, "Parathyroid carcinoma," *Parathyroid Disorders*, vol. 51, pp. 63–76, 2019.

4

Cushing Syndrome Secondary to Primary Neuroendocrine Lung Carcinoma

A. Zainal, O. Akinsola, and K. Rajamani

Rochester Regional Health/Unity Hospital, USA

Correspondence should be addressed to A. Zainal; abir.zainal@rochesterregional.org

Academic Editor: Eli Hershkovitz

Cushing syndrome (CS) is a disorder characterized by a result of chronic exposure to excessive glucocorticoids. This article describes a case of a 30-year-old female presenting with fatigue, abdominal striae, unintentional weight gain, and lipodystrophy. A rare diagnosis of ectopic adrenocorticotropic-dependent CS was determined and a neuroendocrine lung tumor (NET) was discovered on chest x-ray. After surgical resection, pathology confirmed lung NET that stained positive for adrenocorticotropic hormone (ACTH). The patient's symptoms fully resolved. The authors aim to urge clinicians to maintain a high index of suspicion for ectopic ACTH secretion (EAS) through a multimodal approach when caring for patients with CS.

1. Background

Adrenocorticotropic hormone (ACTH) overproduction leads to elevated levels of cortisol and subsequently causes Cushing syndrome (CS). CS is a constellation of symptoms and signs including central obesity, abdominal striae, round face, lipodystrophy, fatigue, hypertension, myopathy, osteoporosis, acne, hirsutism, and oligomenorrhea or amenorrhea [1]. Cognitive dysfunction including depression and memory loss can also occur. The most common cause is iatrogenic from glucocorticoid therapy [1]. Another cause is ACTH-independent from an adrenal gland tumor producing cortisol. The second most common cause is ACTH-dependent CS secondary to ACTH-secreting pituitary adenoma, which stimulates cortisol release from the adrenal glands [1]. This is referred to as Cushing disease. ACTH-dependent CS from ectopic ACTH secretion (EAS) accounts for only 10% of those cases [1, 2]. Locating the ACTH source and treating patients can be incredibly challenging.

Investigations including elevated morning glucose, serum cortisol, 24-hour urine cortisol, and midnight plasma cortisol can aid in the diagnosis of CS. Low dose dexamethasone suppression testing failing to suppress endogenous cortisol secretion is confirmatory. A high dose dexamethasone suppression test is more likely to exert negative feedback on ACTH-producing pituitary cells but less likely with ectopic ACTH-producing cells or adrenal cells. Discriminating between EAS and CD can be convoluted. Misdiagnosis can occur due to discordant imaging and biochemical investigations. Current guidelines recommend that inferior petrosal sinus sampling (IPSS) is the gold standard in distinguishing CD from EAS if pituitary MRI is negative [1, 2]. IPSS is limited by the expertise required, its invasive nature, high cost, and risk for thromboembolic complications. As such, utilizing clues from lab investigations can help physicians to consider EAS and promptly search for ectopic sources. Pulmonary neuroendocrine tumors tend to be occult, less likely to metastasize, and carry a good prognosis when diagnosed in a timely manner [2]. We herein report a rare case of ectopic ACTH producing neuroendocrine lung tumor causing CS.

2. Case Presentation

A 30-year-old Vietnamese female presented to the clinic with fatigue, muscle weakness, memory loss, unintentional weight gain, hair loss, and amenorrhea. She has a past medical history of microprolactinoma discovered on recent pituitary magnetic resonance imaging (MRI) treated with cabergoline. A follow-up pituitary MRI was normal and her cabergoline

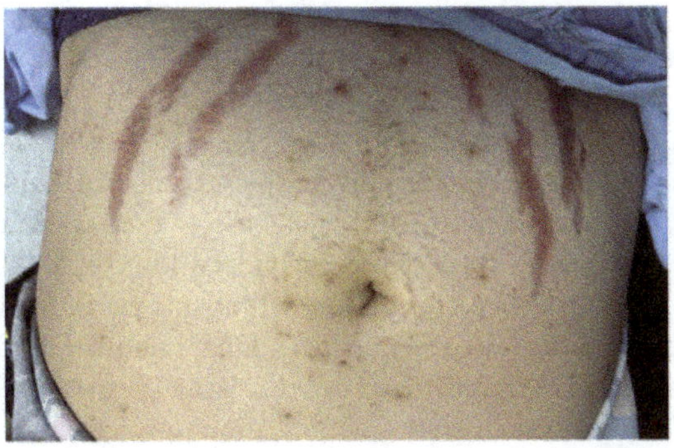

FIGURE 1: Abdominal striae.

was discontinued. She is not taking any medications and has no known allergies. She has a family history of diabetes and coronary artery disease. She has not had any previous surgeries.

On physical examination, her blood pressure was 132/80 and other vital signs were normal. She had facial acne, hirsutism, round face, lipodystrophy, central obesity, and muscle wasting in her lower extremities. She had no evidence of thyromegaly. Auscultation revealed normal heart sounds and no murmurs. Lung auscultation revealed normal breath sounds. Her abdomen was distended, nontender, with thick purple striae (Figure 1). She had ecchymosis and upper extremity striae.

Her morning cortisol was 53.6 (4.3-22.4mcg/dl) and ACTH was 147 (0-46pg/ml). Her midnight salivary cortisol level was 2.54 (<0.09mcg/dL) and urine 24-hour cortisol was 4405 (4-55mcg/24h). Corticotropin releasing factor was 1.9 (<10pg/ml). She had a white cell count of 13 (4.0-10.0 $x10^9$) and TSH 0.05 (0.55-4.78 mIU/L) with normal free T4 1.1 (0.9-1.8ng/dl), likely secondary to excessive glucocorticoid levels or sick euthyroid syndrome. Her serum potassium was 3.3 (3.5-4.5mmol/L). Her glycosylated hemoglobin was 6.4% and her insulin-like growth factor was normal. Prolactin, luteinizing hormone, and follicular stimulating hormone levels were all normal. Other labs including electrolytes, renal function, and blood counts were normal. A low-dose 1mg and a high-dose 8mg dexamethasone suppression test failed to suppress cortisol, raising our suspicion for EAS. Surprisingly, upon review of her brain magnetic resonance imaging (MRI) from Vietnam at the time of diagnosis and posttreatment with cabergoline by our neuroradiologist, this did not reveal a microprolactinoma indicating misdiagnosis. The patient's screening for multiple endocrine neoplasia (MEN) syndrome was negative.

Given our high clinical suspicion for EAS, we performed a chest x-ray, which identified two left upper lobe lung masses (Figure 2). A computed tomography (CT) guided lung biopsy confirmed well-differentiated NET (Figure 3). The lung biopsy stained positive for synaptophysin, chromogranin, and pancytokeratin (Figure 4). The Ki-67 proliferation index was low <2% (Figure 5). Positron emission tomography showed hypermetabolic activity within the lung masses, left hilum, and mediastinal lymph nodes (Figure 6). Hypermetabolic activity in the right anterior second rib was evident raising concern for a fracture. Mild metabolic activity in the medial limb of the left adrenal gland was present, possibly showing evidence of a small adenoma. DEXA scan was normal, but her spontaneous rib fracture confirmed a diagnosis of osteoporosis as a result of excess endogenous glucocorticoid production. Octreotide scan showed increased radiotracer uptake within the lung masses and corresponding lymph nodes. She underwent wedge resection of her left upper lobe and was treated with a steroid taper perioperatively (Figure 7). The patient's surgical margins were clear. She required intermittent insulin therapy for hyperglycemia.

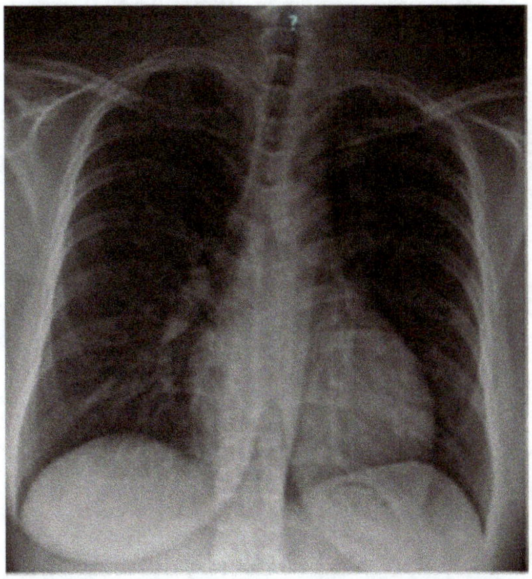

FIGURE 2: Chest X-Ray showing 2 left upper lobe lung masses.

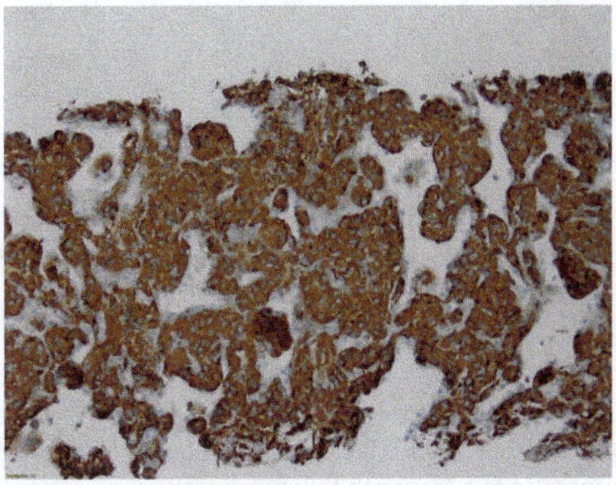

FIGURE 3: Neuroendocrine lung tumor biopsy staining positive for synaptophysin.

3. Outcome and Follow-Up

After surgical resection of the neuroendocrine lung tumor, her labs normalized. Her ACTH levels were 40.9 (0-46pg/ml) and morning cortisol was 10.2 (4.3-22.4mcg/dl). Her glucose levels normalized and her insulin was discontinued. She lost

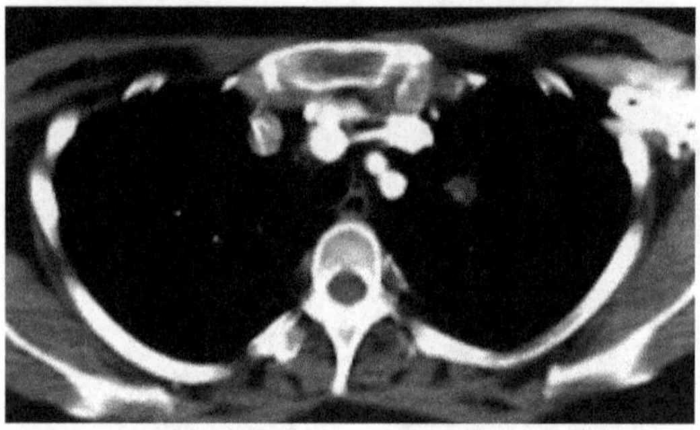

FIGURE 4: Commuted tomography showing 2 left upper lobe lung masses.

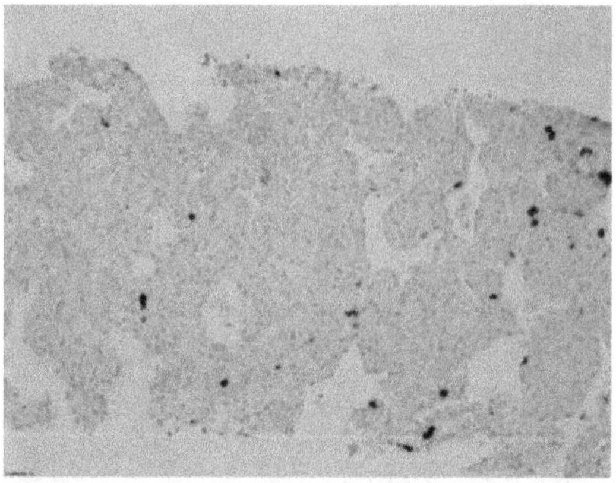

FIGURE 5: Neuroendocrine lung tumor biopsy with <2% Ki-67 proliferation index.

8 pounds and gained more energy. Her cognitive dysfunction resolved and her menstrual cycles regulated. She remained asymptomatic at a 6-month follow-up visit.

4. Discussion

Endogenous CS is uncommon with an incidence of 0.7-2.4 cases per million per year [1]. Differentiating between ACTH-dependent CS secondary to pituitary and ectopic ACTH production can be exceptionally complex.

10% of ACTH-dependent CS can be overly sensitive to dexamethasone suppression testing exhibiting false negative results [3]. 31% of patients with EAS that respond appropriately to dexamethasone suppression have pulmonary carcinoids [2]. Hypokalemia is found in 10% of patients with CD and 90% of patients with EAS due to mineralocorticoid receptor activation as seen in our patient [2, 3]. EAS must be suspected if a pituitary adenoma is not visible on MRI; however, up to 40% may not have a visualizable adenoma [2, 4]. On the other hand, 10% can have incidental pituitary tumors unrelated to CS [3]. Although IPSS carries a sensitivity and specificity of 96% and 100%, respectively, and per guidelines should be the next step, it is invasive and operator dependent [3]. When IPSS is negative, EAS is suspected and initial screening for bronchopulmonary malignancies with CT scan of the chest/mediastinum is recommended. Studies have shown that pulmonary NETs are up to 4 cm in size, which prompted us to commence with a chest x-ray instead [2].

Lung neuroendocrine tumors (NETs) represent a rare 1.2% of all lung malignancies [2]. The surveillance, epidemiology, and end result (SEER) database is the largest case-series looking at cases of CS secondary to ectopic ACTH secretion over a 20-year duration. 90 patients were identified, of which 35 had neuroendocrine lung tumors [2]. Their annual incidence has climbed over the last 50 years to 1.49 per 100,000 persons [2]. They are more common in the fifth and sixth decades of life unlike our younger patient. The incidence of lung NETs is not affected by environmental factors such as tobacco and radiation exposure [2]. Biochemical findings in those patients showed potassium levels as low as 2.0 (ranging from 3.3 to 5.1meq/L) and average urine cortisol levels at 3189 (24-108 mcg/24hr) and serum ACTH 205 (9-52pg/ml) [2]. 17 cases were localized, 17 had lymphadenopathy, and only 1 case was metastatic. Approximately 50% of localized cases were curative. Lung NETs are mostly considered to have low-grade malignancy with good prognosis and rarely metastasize [2, 5].

Somatostatin receptor-based imaging is the functional imaging of choice in the workup of NETs and it is based upon the binding of a radiolabeled ligand to the somatostatin receptor (SSR).

Haug et al. made the first study that evaluated the role of ^{68}Ga-DOTATATE PET/CT in suspected neuroendocrine tumors and correlated it with gold standard pathology [6]. ^{68}Ga-DOTATATE PET/CT was found to have a sensitivity of 81% and specificity of 90%. In another study, Haug et al. investigated the role of ^{68}Ga-DOTATATE PET/CT in detection of metastatic lesions in patients with neuroendocrine cancer and compared it to gold standard pathology [7]. ^{68}Ga-DOTATATE PET/CT was found to have 90% sensitivity and 82% specificity.

Neuroendocrine cancers are slow growing and ^{18}F-FDG PET/CT is not commonly used for initial evaluation of the neuroendocrine cancers. Due to slow metabolic activity of the NETs in initial stages, they are not well visualized on ^{18}F-FDG PET/CT but rather they demonstrate high uptake with ^{68}Ga-DOTATATE because neuroendocrine tumors express significant SSR-2. In high grade NETs, when the tumor becomes poorly differentiated the uptake pattern changes to low ^{68}Ga-DOTATATE uptake due to less expression of SSR-2 and high ^{18}F-FDG PET/CT uptake. Kayani et al. reported a sensitivity of 82% for ^{68}Ga-DOTATATE PET/CT and 66% for ^{18}F-FDG PET/CT.

Interestingly, the etiology of pulmonary NETs remains largely unknown. In the majority of cases, they are sporadic in nature. MEN-1 mutations have been implicated in 5% of lung NETs [1, 2]. The majority of MEN-1 tumors have a loss of heterozygosity (LOH) of chromosome 11q13 [2]. LOH involving chromosomes 3p, 5q21, 9p, 13q13, and 7p13 have also been reported. The accurate diagnosis and characterization of CS requires a multifaceted diagnostic approach to facilitate timely and appropriate treatment.

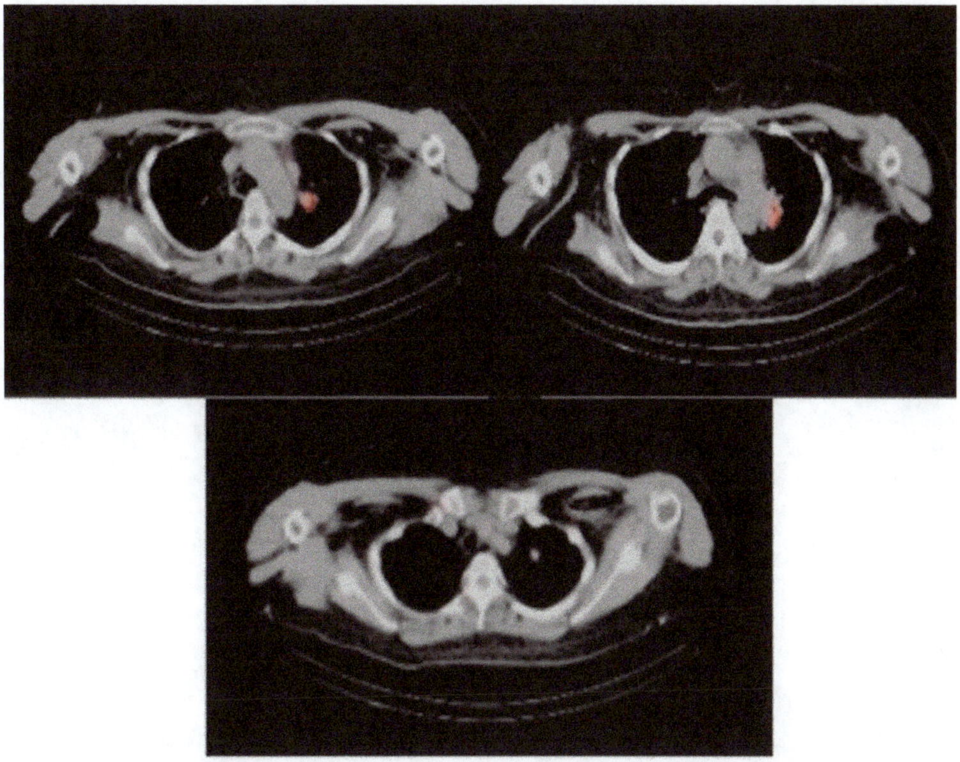

FIGURE 6: Positron emission tomography/commuted tomography showing 2 left upper lobe lung masses.

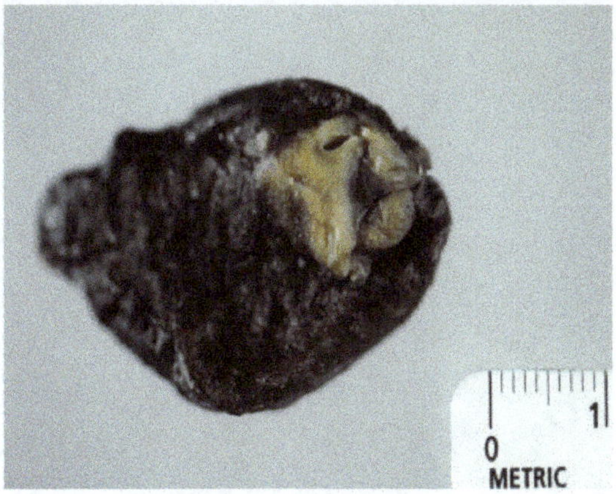

FIGURE 7: Surgical specimen of one of the resected lung masses.

5. Learning Points/Take Home Messages

(i) EAS accounts for 10% of ACTH-dependent CS.

(ii) Diagnosing EAS can be challenging and a high index of clinical suspicion is required if high dose dexamethasone 8mg fails to suppress ACTH/cortisol secretion.

(iii) 90% of EAS will have hypokalemia.

(iv) Pulmonary NETs are up to 4cm in size.

(v) MEN-1 mutations have been implicated in 5% of lung NETs.

References

[1] S. T. Sharma, L. K. Nieman, and R. A. Feelders, "Cushing's syndrome: epidemiology and developments in disease management," *Journal of Clinical Epidemiology*, vol. 7, pp. 281–293, 2015.

[2] I. Ilias, D. J. Torpy, K. Pacak, N. Mullen, R. A. Wesley, and L. K. Nieman, "Cushing's syndrome due to ectopic corticotropin secretion: twenty years' experience at the National Institutes of Health," *The Journal of Clinical Endocrinology & Metabolism*, vol. 90, no. 8, pp. 4955–4962, 2005.

[3] P. Makras, G. Toloumis, D. Papadogias, G. A. Kaltsas, and M. Besser, "The diagnosis and differential diagnosis of endogenous Cushing's syndrome.," *Hormones*, vol. 5, no. 4, pp. 231–250, 2006.

[4] D. Yogi-Morren, M. A. M. Habra, C. Faiman et al., "Pituitary mri findings in patients with pituitary and ectopic acth-dependent cushing syndrome: does a 6-mm pituitary tumor size cut-off value exclude ectopic acth syndrome?" *Endocrine Practice*, vol. 21, no. 10, pp. 1098–1103, 2015.

[5] S. Hashemzadeh, A. Asvadi Kermani, A. Ali-Asgharzadeh, M. Halimi, M. Soleimani, and A. Ladan, "Ectopic cushing's syndrome secondary to pulmonary carcinoid tumor," *The Annals of Thoracic Surgery*, vol. 95, no. 5, pp. 1797–1799, 2013.

[6] A. R. Haug, A. Rominger, M. Mustafa et al., "Treatment with octreotide does not reduce tumor uptake of 68Ga-DOTATATE as measured by PET/CT in patients with neuroendocrine tumors," *Journal of Nuclear Medicine*, vol. 52, no. 11, pp. 1679–1683, 2011.

[7] P. Sharma, H. Singh, C. Bal, and R. Kumar, "PET/CT imaging of neuroendocrine tumors with (68)Gallium-labeled somatostatin analogues: an overview and single institutional experience from India," *Indian Journal of Nuclear Medicine*, vol. 29, no. 1, p. 2, 2014.

5

An Adrenocortical Carcinoma Associated with Non-Islet Cell Tumor Hypoglycemia and Aberrant ACTH Production

M. D. S. A. Dilrukshi,[1] A. W. Wickramarachchi,[2] D. D. K. Abeyaratne,[1] Brian Shine,[3] Bahram Jafar-Mohammadi,[4] and N. P. Somasundaram[1]

[1]*Diabetes and Endocrinology Unit of National Hospital of Sri Lanka, Colombo 10, Sri Lanka*
[2]*National Hospital of Sri Lanka, Colombo, Sri Lanka*
[3]*Clinical Biochemistry, John Radcliffe Hospital, Oxford OX3 9DU, UK*
[4]*Oxford Centre for Diabetes, Endocrinology and Metabolism, Churchill Hospital, Oxford University Hospitals NHS Foundation Trust, Oxford, UK*

Correspondence should be addressed to M. D. S. A. Dilrukshi; dilrukmatharage@gmail.com

Academic Editor: Toshihiro Kita

Introduction. Adrenocortical carcinomas (ACCs) are infrequently reported to present with severe hypoglycemia syndrome resulting from the secretion of insulin-like growth factor II (IGF-II) by tumor cells. Adrenocorticotropic hormone- (ACTH) independent hypercortisolism is the norm of hormonally active ACCs, but aberrant ACTH production by tumor cells can theoretically cause ACTH-dependent hypercortisolism. The purpose of this report was to present a case of an ACC manifested with the co-occurrence of two extremely rare presentations. *Case Description.* We present a rare case of a 43-year-old male patient admitted with recurrent episodes of severe non-ketotic and non-insulin-mediated hypoglycemia due to IGF-II mediated disease and ACTH-dependent Cushing's syndrome. He was diagnosed with a diffusely disseminated adrenocortical carcinoma with immunohistochemistry of tumor cells showing focal ACTH immunostain positivity. *Conclusion.* Non-islet cell tumor hypoglycemia and ACTH-dependent Cushing's syndrome are extremely rare presentations of an ACC, and co-occurrence of these entities in a single patient is never reported in the literature.

1. Introduction

Adrenocortical carcinomas (ACCs) are rare but aggressive tumors which show an incidence of 1-2 cases per million populations per year [1]. Non-islet cell tumor hypoglycemia (NICTH) is a rare paraneoplastic syndrome of ACCs which was described first by Anderson in 1930 and a handful of cases reported thereafter [2]. Cushing's syndrome due to ectopic adrenocorticotropic hormone (ACTH) secretion was first described by Hurst Brown in 1928 [3] in association with bronchial carcinoma. Though non-ACTH-dependent hypercortisolism is the norm of adrenal malignancies, ectopic ACTH secretion by adrenal tumor cells can theoretically result in ACTH-dependent Cushing's syndrome. To the best of our knowledge, the co-occurrence of NICTH and ACTH-dependent hypercortisolism due to aberrant ACTH producing tumor cells is never reported in the medical literature. We report a unique case of a 43-year-old man with disseminated adrenocortical carcinoma presenting with these two rare disease manifestations coincidentally.

2. Case Report

A 43-year-old Sri Lankan male presented to a tertiary care hospital of Sri Lanka (SL) in January 2019 with recurrent episodes of early morning dizzy spells of six-month duration and a history of resistant hypertension and intra-abdominal malignancy for which he received several types of treatment abroad and locally until 3 months before.

He started to experience recurrent episodes of early morning dizzy spells which were associated with excessive hunger, sweating, and palpitations that were resolving with a sugary drink or food in July 2018. These episodes were confirmed to be hypoglycemia at a local hospital with positive Whipple's triad while awaiting surgery for the aforementioned malignancy. There was some improvement of these symptoms after resection of the tumor; hence, no further evaluation was performed. However, hypoglycemia symptoms recurred in September 2019 and gradually progressed thereafter with increasing frequency and severity, up until 2 weeks, when he started to develop episodes of disorientation and confusion, which prompted him to seek medical attention. There were no episodes of coma or seizures to report, and he denied symptoms of overt liver or renal failure apart from the loss of appetite. He neither had features of clinical depression nor history to suggest abuse of oral hypoglycemic agents, insulin, recreational drugs, or alcohol. He was off from any medication over 3 months before the admission.

His past medical history revealed poorly controlled hypertension since mid-2017 which was not properly controlled as he went for employment abroad. According to his medical records, he admitted to a hospital abroad in January 2018, with subacute onset moderate to severe retrosternal chest pain with difficulty in breathing. Additionally, he complained of progressive abdominal distension, nonspecific abdominal pain, significant loss of appetite, loss of weight of 2 months, and chronic watery stools without blood or mucus discharge of similar duration. He also had recurrent nonspecific headaches and palpitations but no episodes of flushing. Examination findings on admission recorded pulse rate (PR) of 96 beats per min with a blood pressure (BP) of 170/100 mmHg. Laboratory workup showed hypokalemia (K^+ 2.8 mmol/l), normal blood counts, renal, and liver functions. He was noted to have heart failure with an ejection fraction of 38% with a concentric left ventricular hypertrophy. His abdominal ultrasonography and subsequent whole-body PET/CT had shown a left suprarenal mass of 22 cm × 13 cm × 23 cm in size with coeliac and para-aortic lymphadenopathy (maximum diameter of 3 cm), and hepatic, lung parenchymal, and subpleural metastasis. Biopsy of abdominal mass had shown tumor cells with a high degree of anaplasia, and immunohistochemistry was compatible with probable adrenocortical malignancy. He had received 3 cycles of chemotherapy according to the records, but no details were mentioned regarding the types or names of medications.

He had received 5 months of Ayurveda treatment after returning to SL before admitting to a local hospital in July 2018, with an uncontrolled blood pressure of 180/90 mmHg. Apart from the recurrent episodes of early morning hypoglycemia, he was otherwise well with normal systemic review and had stable weight. Basic Lab workup was normal except for mild anemia, hypokalemia, and mildly elevated transaminase levels (Table 1).

Contrast-enhanced CT (CECT) scan of the chest, abdomen, and pelvis showed previously detected heterogeneously enhancing left suprarenal mass with central necrosis and foci of calcifications without significant interval change in size. There were multiple liver, lymph node, and pulmonary metastasis to note (Figure 1).

Table 1: Basic laboratory data performed at the local hospital.

Test	Result	Reference range
Hemoglobin	10.9 g/L	13–17 g/L
FBS	78.8 mg/dl	70–99 mg/dl
Na^+	137 mmol/L	136–146 mmol/L
K^+	3.2 mmol/L	3.5–5.1 mmol/L
Serum creatinine	0.48 mg/dl	0.7–1.2 mg/dl
AST	110	5–34 U/L
ALT	40	0–35 U/L

He underwent resection of abdominal mass in July 2018 and made an uneventful and complete recovery after the surgery with improvement in symptoms of hypoglycemia. However, histology of the tumor cells showed a high degree of anaplasia and basic immunohistochemistry pattern was more in favor of a malignant pheochromocytoma. Nevertheless, the patient defaulted from follow-up diverting back to Ayurveda treatment without waiting for further evaluation and management.

He had no significant family history of malignancy or chronic diseases to note. He was a social drinker and a nonsmoker.

On examination at our center, he was seemingly well with a BMI of 25.2 kg/m^2. His PR was 96 beats per minute, and BP was 180/90 mmHg. He had large tender hepatomegaly and a well-healed midline abdominal scar. The rest of the clinical examination was unremarkable with no edema, generalized pigmentation, or other discriminatory features of Cushing's syndrome except for significant proximal myopathy.

During the hospital stay, his vital parameters were stable, and the lowest recorded blood sugar level was 15 mg/dL with symptoms. His laboratory workup revealed neutrophil leukocytosis, anemia, mildly elevated transaminases, and normal renal functions (Table 2).

Further biochemical evaluation of persistently low blood sugar was favoring non-ketotic and non-insulin-dependent hypoglycemia (Table 3). Considering the high probability of IGF-II-mediated hypoglycemia, we sent a serum sample to a reference laboratory in the United Kingdom since the facility to perform IGF-II is not available in SL. Lab results showed serum IGF-II level of 108.8 nmol/L and markedly elevated IGF-II : IGF-I ratio favoring non-islet cell tumor hypoglycemia (NICTH).

Moreover, CECT chest, abdomen, and pelvis showed recurrence of the previously detected tumor (42 mm × 37 mm, 85 × 68 mm and 73 × 86 mm size tumor masses intra-abdominally) with multiple liver (largest of the metastases being 12 × 11 cm in size in segment VII and VIII), renal (40 × 62 mm), and lung metastases (Figure 2). But there were no metastases in the right adrenal gland to note.

Adrenal hormone analysis was performed as the clinical picture was suggestive of a biologically active tumor, in addition to the dilemma created by the initial histology report (Table 4). The hormone profile revealed Cushing's syndrome with nonsuppressed ACTH levels favoring ACTH-dependent Cushing's syndrome. Additionally, adrenal androgens were also elevated with normal urine metanephrines favoring a tumor of adrenocortical origin.

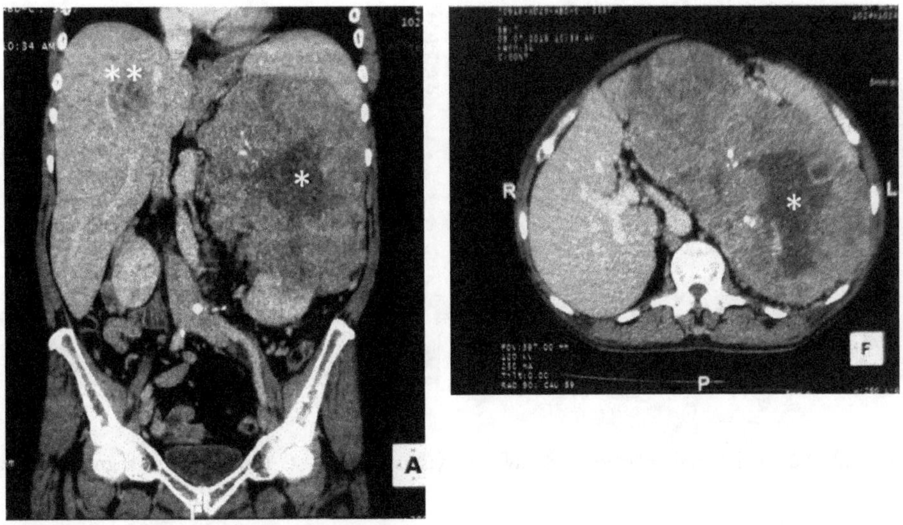

(a) (b)

FIGURE 1: Contrast-enhanced CT abdomen, chest, and pelvis: (a) coronal image and (b) axial image showing heterogeneously enhancing left suprarenal mass ($21 \times 18 \times 24$ cm)* with central necrosis and foci of calcifications. Focal liver metastasis** is also seen.

TABLE 2: Basic laboratory data performed at the tertiary care hospital.

Test	Result	Reference range
WBC	14.72×10^3	$4–10 \times 10^3/\mu L$
Neutrophils	11.28×10^3	$2–7 \times 10^3/\mu L$
Hemoglobin	9.3	11–16 g/dL
AST	127	5–34 U/L
ALT	43	0–35 U/L
Serum creatinine	56	80–115 μmol/L
Na^+	140	136–145 mmol/L
K^+	3.4	3.5–5.1 mmol/L
PT	13.6 seconds	11–15 seconds

TABLE 3: Evaluation of hypoglycemia performed at the tertiary care hospital.

Test	Result	Reference range
Random blood sugar	35 mg/dl	80–140 mg/dl
Urine/serum ketone bodies	Negative	—
Serum insulin (when random blood sugar of 35 mg/dl)	<0.5 mU/L	2.9–25 mU/L
C-peptide	0.09 ng/ml	0.61–3.85 ng/ml
IGF-I	2.8 nmol/L	8.5–27.3 nmol/L
IGF-II	108.8 nmol/L	—
IGF II : IGF-I ratio	38.9	<10

We reassessed tumor tissues in parallel to the above evaluation with extended immunohistochemistry (IHC) profiles. Histology (Figure 3) showed an encapsulated multinodular tumor composed of solid sheets and nests of tumor cells with thick fibrous bands separating them, containing pleomorphic vesicular nuclei with coarse chromatin and eosinophilic cytoplasm. Mitoses were present >30/50 per high power field including atypical forms. There were areas of high nuclear pleomorphism with prominent nucleoli and bizarre multinucleated cells (Fuhrman grade 4). Tumor necrosis and vascular invasion were present. However, clear cell areas were not seen in the examined section.

The IHC staining profile (Figure 4) showed patchy positivity for synaptophysin and focal cytoplasmic positivity for inhibin. Tumor cells were immunonegative for chromogranin, melan A, and pan CK. Overall, the negativity of cytokeratin and chromogranin with the focal positivity of inhibin was in favor of a tumor of adrenal cortical origin. The absence of clear cell areas also favors against pheochromocytoma. The sheet-like diffuse growth pattern, areas with

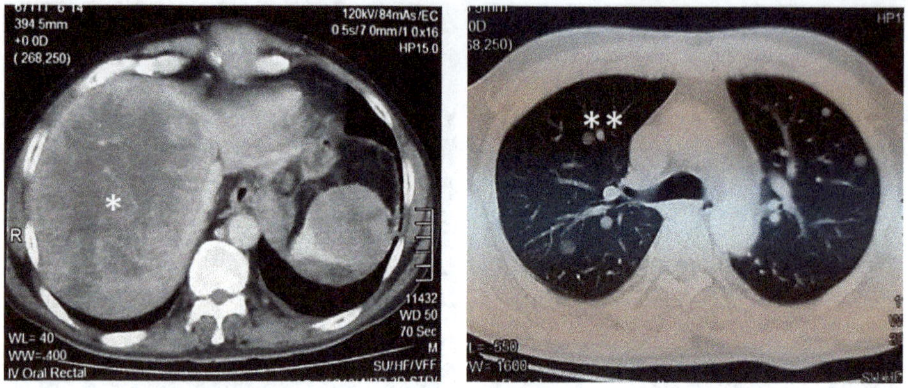

(a) (b)

FIGURE 2: CECT chest and abdomen (axial image): large liver metastasis* (largest: 12 × 11 cm in segment VII and VIII) and lung metastases**.

TABLE 4: Hormone profile performed at the tertiary care hospital.

Test	Result	Reference range
Random cortisol (9am)	>1000 nmol/L	138–635 nmol/L
Serum ACTH (9am)	40.3 pg/ml	7–50 pg/ml
ODST	748.5 nmol/l	<50 nmol/L
LDDST	668 nmol/L	<50 nmol/L
Total testosterone	595 ng/dl	300–1000 ng/dL
Androstenedione	>10 ng/ml	0.7–3.6 ng/ml
DHEAS	>40.71 μmol/l	3.8–13.1 μmol/l
24 hr urinary VMA	8.5 mg/24h	1–11 mg/24 h
24 hr urinary fractionated metanephrine	0.17 mg/24 hours	<1 mg/24 hours

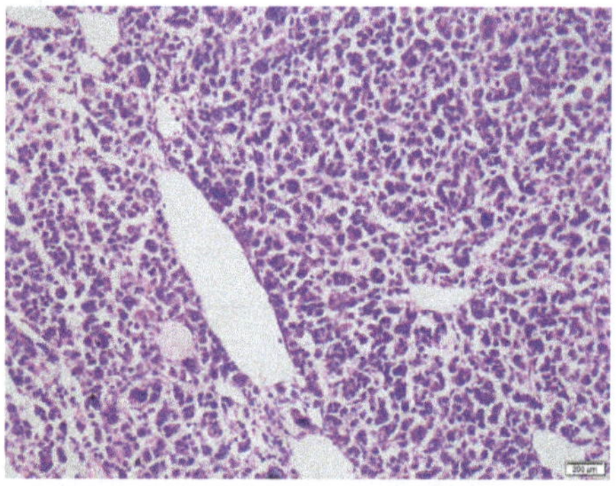

FIGURE 3: H&E stain (high power): solid sheets and nests of tumor cells, containing pleomorphic vesicular nuclei with coarse chromatin and eosinophilic cytoplasm.

a high nuclear grade, high mitotic rate with atypical forms, absence of clear cells, presence of tumor necrosis, venous invasion, and capsular invasion are correlating with the malignant behavior of the adrenocortical tumor with Weiss criteria of 8/9 [4].

As the patient had ACTH-dependent Cushing's syndrome with a theoretical possibility of tumor cells secreting ACTH, we included ACTH immunostain to the IHC profile. Tumor cells showed granular cytoplasmic positivity for ACTH favoring aberrant ACTH production by ACC cells (Figure 5).

Alleviation of the troublesome hypoglycemia to improve quality of life was a priority of this patient's management. He was offered frequent meals and intermittent oral dextrose but failing that commenced on continuous intravenous dextrose infusions with frequent monitoring of blood sugar. Oral diazoxide seemed not effective. Subsequently, the patient was commenced on subcutaneous recombinant growth hormone (rhGH) 3 mg/daily and rapidly increased up to 4 mg/daily for which he showed a significant reduction of severity and frequency of hypoglycemia, hence could limit dextrose infusions. After extensive discussions with the oncologist, patient, and the family, he was opted for palliative chemotherapy believing that reduction of tumor burden to some degree would further help to alleviate symptoms of hypoglycemia. Unfortunately, the patient succumbed to the illness while receiving palliative chemotherapy.

3. Discussion

This patient was diagnosed to have an aggressive, functional adrenocortical carcinoma with diffuse metastasis, which was complicated with paraneoplastic severe NICTH and ACTH-dependent Cushing's syndrome resulting from aberrant ACTH secretion.

This patient had hypercortisolism, hyperandrogenemia and negative urine metanephrines in the presence of disseminated adrenal malignancy favoring a tumor of adrenocortical origin.

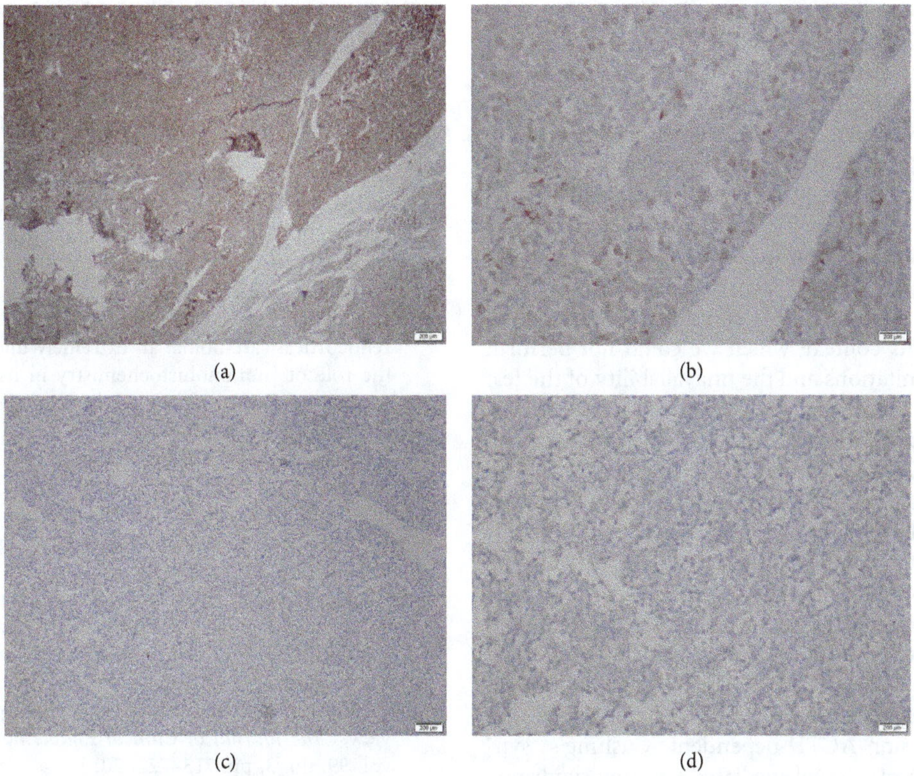

Figure 4: Immunohistochemical staining: (a) synaptophysin stain (patchy positivity), (b) inhibin stain (focal cytoplasmic positivity), (c) Chromogranin stain (negative), and (d) Pan CK stain (negative).

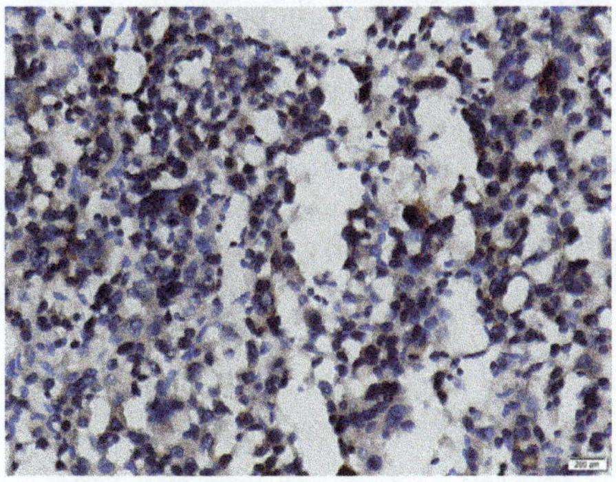

Figure 5: ACTH Immunostaining: few scattered tumor cells showing granular cytoplasmic positivity.

But there was a misclassification of the tumor in the initial histology report. The considerable difficulty associated with differentiation between adrenocortical (ACC) and medullary (pheochromocytoma) tumor with a high degree of anaplasia was previously noted in the medical literature [5]. Even though comparatively higher nuclear pleomorphism and the presence of hyaline globules in the cytoplasm are characteristics of pheochromocytoma those are not specific for the tumor [6]. IHC studies are useful ancillary tests to the differentiation of tumors in this context. Immunopositivity for inhibin is suggestive of an adrenocortical tumor, while strong and diffuse positivity of chromogranin A is expected in pheochromocytoma [7]. The IHC profile of our patient was suggestive of the diagnosis of an ACC which was further strengthened by supportive clinical and laboratory data.

NICTH is a rare paraneoplastic syndrome that is only second to insulinoma as a cause for tumor-induced hypoglycemia [8]. This is commonly seen in tumors of mesenchymal and epithelial cell origin, and approximately 290 cases reported related to this topic so far in the medical literature. NICTH associated with adrenocortical carcinoma is even rarer [9]. The major pathophysiological mechanism behind this syndrome is tumor secretion of abnormal high molecular weight or "big" IGF-II (molecular weight of "big" IGF-II is 10-20 kDa as compared to normal IGF-II which is a 7.5 kDa peptide) which has insulin-like activity [9]. Tumors with aberrant IGF-II gene transcription and gene expression produce this big IGF-II due to abnormal processing. Normal IGF-II molecules circulate as a ternary complex after binding with IGF-binding protein-3 (IGFBP-3) and acid-labile subunit (ALS) thus are incapable of traversing epithelial barriers to bind to insulin receptors. In NICTH, elevated total IGF-II leads to a greater concentration of free form as well as abnormal high molecular weight precursor big IGF-II cannot be bound to ALS due to steric hindrance and thus stay in binary complex binding to IGFBP-3 which could easily go through vascular barriers to act on insulin receptors exerting hypoglycemic effects. Additionally, the activity of IGF-II suppresses both insulin and growth hormone (GH) with resultant low insulin and IGF-I. Low GH also leads to low ALS and IGFBP-3, further elevating the free IGF-II forms [9]. In this condition, serum levels of IGF-II may be elevated or normal and levels of IGF-II precursors are often elevated, and hence elevated IGF-II : IGF-I ratio is used for the diagnosis purpose. The normal molar ratio of IGF-II : IGF-I in plasma is about 3 : 1 and in the presence of recurrent hypoglycemia ratios of 10 : 1 are virtually diagnostic for IGF-II-mediated hypoglycemia [10]. Our patient had significantly elevated IGF-II : IGF-I ratio of 38.9 (<10) in the presence of non-ketotic non-insulin-dependent hypoglycemia and disseminated ACC, favoring this diagnosis. IHC staining of tumor cells for IGF-II could further strengthen the diagnosis in this context, which we could not perform due to financial limitations and the unavailability of the test locally.

Definitive management of ACC is the mainstay of therapy for NICTH after the acute management of hypoglycemia, which seemed impossible to achieve with the extensive tumor burden of this patient. Glucocorticoids [9, 11], glucagon [9, 12], and rhGH [1] were reported in the literature [9] as possible therapeutic options for NICTH. Our patient was commenced on a supraphysiological dose of recombinant growth hormone which helped to alleviate hypoglycemia for a considerable degree when combined with frequent small meals and oral/IV dextrose.

Furthermore, non-ACTH-dependent Cushing's syndrome is the norm of adrenal-mediated Cushing syndrome commonly seen in association with hormonally active ACC. However, our patient had biochemically confirmed Cushing's syndrome with non-suppressed serum ACTH levels. ACCs were never reported to be associated with ectopic ACTH production in the medical literature thus far. But, we hypothesized that this could be a possibility since there was no obvious clinical or imaging evidence to suggest pituitary disease or other ectopic focus. This hypothesis was proved by the immunopositivity of tumor cells for ACTH, indicating aberrant ACTH production.

4. Conclusion

Non-islet cell tumor hypoglycemia is an extremely rare presentation of ACCs. Though non-ACTH-dependent hypercortisolism is the norm of ACC, it can be associated with ACTH-dependent Cushing's syndrome with aberrant ACTH production by tumor cells. To the best of our knowledge, the co-occurrence of these presentations associated with ACC is never reported in the literature. Increased level of suspicion and broad-minded approach in the evaluation of this type of rare endocrine malignancies would help in diagnosing its rare presentations.

References

[1] M. Fassnacht, M. Kroiss, and B. Allolio, "Update in adrenocortical carcinoma," *The Journal of Clinical Endocrinology & Metabolism*, vol. 98, no. 12, pp. 4551–4564, 2013.

[2] J. Michael, T. Eymont, G. Gwinup, F. A. Kruger, D. E. Maynard, and G. J. Hamwi, "Cushing' syndrome with hypoglycemia caused by adrenocortical carcinoma," *The Journal of Clinical Endocrinology & Metabolism*, vol. 25, no. 1, pp. 46–52, 1965.

[3] W. H. Brown, "A case of pluriglandular syndrome: "diabetes of bearded women"," *The Lancet*, vol. 212, no. 5490, pp. 1022-1023, 1928.

[4] M. Papotti, R. Libè, E. Duregon, M. Volante, J. Bertherat, and F. Tissier, "The Weiss score and beyond-histopathology for adrenocortical carcinoma," *Hormones and Cancer*, vol. 2, no. 6, pp. 333–340, 2011.

[5] S. A. Jain, L. Agarwal, A. Goyal et al., "Adrenocortical carcinoma posing as a pheochromocytoma: a diagnostic dilemma," *Journal of Surgical Case Reports*, vol. 2014, no. 5, Article ID rju030, 2014.

[6] G. Gogoi, M. P. Baruah, P. Borah, and M. Borgohain, "Adrenocortical carcinoma: an extremely uncommon entity and the role of Immunohistochemistry in its diagnosis," *Indian Journal of Endocrinology and Metabolism*, vol. 16, no. 2, pp. S373–S375, 2012.

[7] M. Jorda, B. De Madeiros, and M. Nadji, "Calretinin and inhibin are useful in separating adrenocortical neoplasms from pheochromocytomas," *Applied Immunohistochemistry & Molecular Morphology*, vol. 10, no. 1, pp. 67–70, 2002.

[8] S. W. Kim, S. E. Lee, Y. L. Oh, S. Kim, S. P. Park, and J. H. Kim, "Non-islet cell tumor hypoglycemia in a patient with adrenal cortical carcinoma," *Case Reports in Endocrinology*, vol. 2016, Article ID 5731417, 4 pages, 2016.

[9] T. W. Bodnar, M. J. Acevedo, and M. Pietropaolo, "Management of non-islet-cell tumor hypoglycemia: a clinical review," *The Journal of Clinical Endocrinology & Metabolism*, vol. 99, no. 3, pp. 713–722, 2014.

[10] Y. Dynkevich, K. I. Rother, I. Whitford et al., "Tumors, IGF-2, and hypoglycemia: insights from the clinic, the laboratory, and the historical archive," *Endocrine Reviews*, vol. 34, no. 6, pp. 798–826, 2013.

[11] J. D. Teale and V. Marks, "Glucocorticoid therapy suppresses abnormal secretion of big IGF-II by non-islet cell tumours inducing hypoglycaemia (NICTH)," *Clinical Endocrinology*, vol. 49, no. 4, pp. 491–498, 1998.

[12] K. K. Pun, R. T. T. Young, C. Wang, C. F. Tam, and P. W. M. Ho, "The use of glucagon challenge tests in the diagnostic evaluation of hypoglycemia due to hepatoma and insulinoma," *The Journal of Clinical Endocrinology & Metabolism*, vol. 67, no. 3, pp. 546–550, 1988.

6

An Unusual Simultaneous Existence of Parathyroid Carcinoma and Papillary Thyroid Carcinoma: Case Report and Review of Literature

César Ernesto Lam-Chung,[1] Diana Lizbeth Rodríguez-Orihuela,[2] Jazmín De Anda González,[2] and Armando Gamboa-Domínguez[2]

[1]*Department of Endocrinology and Metabolism, Instituto Nacional de Ciencias Médicas y Nutrición Salvador Zubirán, Vasco de Quiroga 15, Sección XVI, Tlalpan, México City 14000, Mexico*
[2]*Department of Pathology, Instituto Nacional de Ciencias Médicas y Nutrición Salvador Zubirán, Vasco de Quiroga 15, Sección XVI, Tlalpan, México City 14000, Mexico*

Correspondence should be addressed to Armando Gamboa-Domínguez; agamboad@gmail.com

Academic Editor: J. Paul Frindik

Synchronous parathyroid and papillary thyroid carcinoma are extremely rare. To our knowledge, only 15 cases have been reported in the last four decades. We describe a 50-year-old female without significant past medical or family history and no previous trauma presented with left heel pain that prompted her to seek medical attention. Physical examination was notable for a painless nodule at the left thyroid lobe. Laboratory evaluation showed a serum calcium level of 14.3 mg/dL (8.6–10.3 mg/dL) and intact parathyroid hormone level of 1160 pg/mL (12–88 pg/mL). 99Tc-sestamibi dual-phase with single-photon emission computed tomography fused images showed increased uptake at the left-sided inferior parathyroid gland. Neck ultrasound showed a 1.4 cm heterogeneous nodule in the middle-third of the left thyroid gland and a solitary 1.9 cm vascularized and hypoechoic oval nodule that was considered likely to represent a parathyroid adenoma. Due to its clinical context (severe hypercalcemia and very high levels of PTH), parathyroid carcinoma (PC) was suspected although imaging studies were not characteristic. The patient underwent en bloc resection of the parathyroid mass and left thyroid lobe and central neck compartment dissection. Pathology analysis revealed classical papillary thyroid carcinoma of classical subtype and parathyroid carcinoma. Immunohistochemical staining was positive for cyclidin D1 and negative for parafibromin. High clinical suspicion is required for parathyroid carcinoma diagnosis in the presence of very high level of parathyroid hormone, marked hypercalcemia, and the existence of any thyroid nodule should be approached and the coexistence of other carcinomas should be considered.

1. Introduction

Less than 1% of all cancers and primary hyperparathyroidism (PHPT) can be attributed to parathyroid carcinoma (PC) [1, 2]. The vast majority of cases are sporadic, whereas the rest occur in the context of genetic syndromes such as multiple endocrine neoplasia type 1 (MEN1) or hyperparathyroidism-jaw tumor syndrome (HPT-JT) [3, 4]. It has equal frequency in both genders and usually occurs during the fifth decade of life [1, 2]. Very high serum levels of intact parathyroid hormone (iPTH) and severe hypercalcemia are the main biochemical findings and clinical manifestations are due to its excessive secretion [5, 6]. It is usually diagnosed postoperatively with histology assessment given its absence of specific clinical and biochemical features [2].

Papillary thyroid cancers (PTCs) account the majority (80–85%) of thyroid cancer cases, specifically papillary thyroid microcarcinomas (PTMs) [7–9]. Radiation exposure and genetics are the known risk factors for PTCs. However, only 5% of PTC cases account for familial PTC [10]. It occurs predominantly in female, and the median age at presentation is 50 years [11]. An asymptomatic thyroid mass is usually the main clinical finding, and it can be accompanied with or without cervical lymph node enlargement. However, vocal cord paralysis and tracheal compression can be present in about 20% of PTC cases, and it is manifested as hoarseness and dysphagia [12]. Biochemical tests are of limited usefulness because most patients have normal thyroid function [13].

The coexistence of thyroid and parathyroid carcinoma is extremely infrequent. Here, we describe a patient with this unusual presentation.

2. Case Presentation

A 50-year-old female without significant past medical or family history and no previous trauma presented with pain on her left heel that prompted her to seek medical attention. Initial evaluation was notable for serum concentration of calcium 14.3 mg/dL (normal range 8.6–10.3 mg/dL), alkaline phosphatase of 339.4 U/L (normal range 34–104 U/L), creatinine of 1.8 mg/dL (normal range 0.3–0.7 mg/dL), and iPTH level of 1160 pg/mL (normal range 12–88 pg/mL). Biochemical data of the patient are summarized in Table 1. Because of the concern for chronic kidney disease, a renal ultrasound was performed and showed both kidney medullary nephrocalcinosis and thinning of the renal parenchyma. Bone densitometry revealed osteoporosis at the anteroposterior spine (T score −2.7) and femoral neck (T score −2.9) and osteopenia at the total hip (T score −2.3). A presumptive diagnosis of parathyroid carcinoma (PC) was made and referred to endocrinology department for further evaluation. Physical examination revealed a hardened and painless nodule at the left thyroid lobe without vocal cord paralysis. Thyroid function test values were within the reference ranges.

A 99mTc-sestamibi dual-phase fusion imaging with single-photon emission computed tomography/computed tomography (SPECT/CT) was performed, and a possible left-sided inferior parathyroid was identified (Figure 1(a)). Neck ultrasonography showed a 1.4 cm heterogeneous nodule and central vascularity in the middle-third of the left thyroid gland (Figures 2(a) and 2(b)). At the same area depicted by SPECT/CT, a 1.9 cm vascularized and hypoechoic oval nodule was present and considered likely to represent a parathyroid adenoma (Figure 1(b)). Due to its clinical context (severe hypercalcemia and very high levels of PTH), PC was suspected although imaging studies were not characteristic. At surgical intervention, a normal-appearing inferior parathyroid gland was identified and preserved in situ. An en bloc resection of the parathyroid mass and left thyroid lobe and central lymph node compartment dissection was performed. On the fourth postoperative day, the iPTH value was 84.6 pg/mL.

Gross examination of the surgical specimen revealed a 4.8 × 2.6 × 2.3 cm left thyroid lobe and a 2.4 × 1.8 × 1.4 cm left superior parathyroid gland. Histological examination revealed a 1.3 × 1.2 cm mass at the left thyroid lobe consistent of PTC of classical subtype (Figure 3) and PC, 2.5 cm in widest tumor dimension, with capsular and vascular space invasion (Figure 4). Immunohistochemical staining was positive for cyclidin D1 and negative for parafibromin. Ki-67

TABLE 1: Laboratory at admission and at two months postoperative.

Laboratory values (normal range)	At admission	At two months postoperatively
Calcemia (8.6–10.3 mg/dL)	14.3	9.5
Ionized calcemia (4.36–5.2 mg/dL)	7.06	4.83
Magnesium (1.9–2.7 mg/dL)	2.1	1.94
Creatinine (0.3–0.7 mg/dL)	2	1.77
Albumin (3.5–5.7 g/dL)	3.68	3.24
Alkaline phosphatase (34–104 U/L)	381	399
PTH (12–88 pg/mL)	1160	7.4
Phosphatemia (2.5–5 mg/dL)	2.73	3.28
25(OH) vitamin D (30–100 ng/mL)	10.1	43
FT4 (0.63–1.34 ng/dL)	0.72	0.97
T3T (0.64–1.81 ng/mL)	1.07	0.79
TSH (0.3–5 mIU/L)	1.8	4.14

index was 2%. Six examined lymph nodes from central compartment were negative for metastasis. Her thyroid carcinoma was staged pT1bN0M0 (TNM AJCC 2018).

On the sixth postoperative day, the patient presented hypocalcemic symptoms (calcium 6.9 mg/dL) consistent with hungry bone syndrome. She received intravenous and oral calcium and vitamin D supplementation. Subsequently, she was discharged with oral calcium treatment and remained well, with the latest serum calcium level being 8.6 mg/dL (6 weeks postoperatively).

3. Discussion

The simultaneous presence of thyroid and parathyroid carcinoma is extremely rare with only 15 documented cases [14–30] in the last 41 years, and no correlation, up to date, has been discovered between these entities [31]. Comparison of the previous cases and ours are described in Table 1. The average age was 52 years (range 21–79), and the vast majority were female (80%). According to Surveillance, Epidemiology, and End Results (SEER) database, PTCs usually occur during the fourth and fifth decades of life and have a 2.5 : 1 female-to-male ratio [32], while the reported mean age for PC presentation was 44 to 45 years with an even distribution between genders [33–35]. As a result, the coexistence of thyroid and parathyroid carcinoma may have an impact on the gender distribution and age presentation. Notably, the youngest patient reported had Hürthle cell thyroid carcinoma and PC [21]. Hürthle cell carcinoma is associated with poorer prognosis and higher recurrence rate in local lymph nodes [36, 37].

Almost all patients had functional PC (including our patient) as outlined in Table 2. Nonfunctional PC is much more infrequent than functional PC, and it has a decreased survival due to its absence of symptoms and perhaps to its aggressive biology [16, 39]. To our knowledge, only one case of nonfunctional PC occurring with PTM was reported [40]. Interestingly, all cases with reported PC localization including the one here reported had a preponderance for the left lower side.

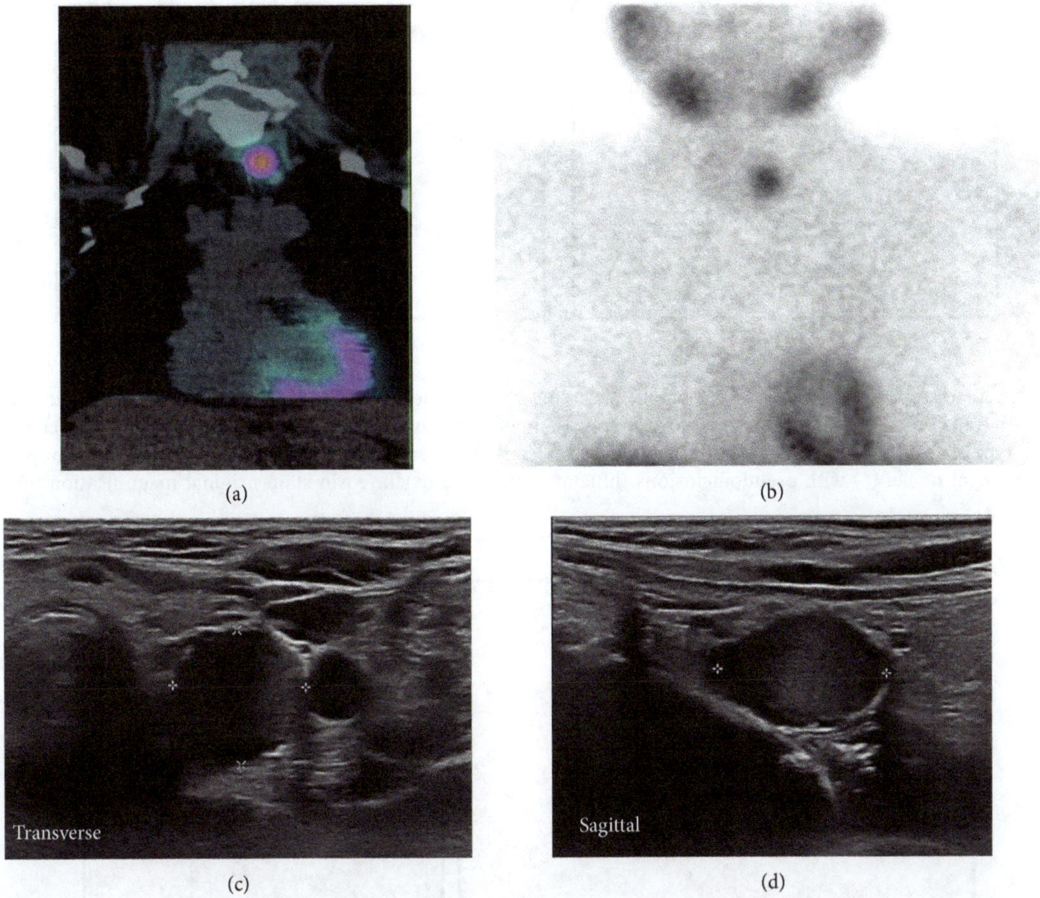

FIGURE 1: (a, b) 99mTc-sestamibi dual-phase with single-photon emission computed tomography/computed tomography fused images, showing uptake within middle to inferior left lobe of the thyroid. (b, c) Ultrasonograms revealing an oval-shaped hypoechoic solid nodule ($1.40 \times 1.39 \times 1.92$ cm) at the same area.

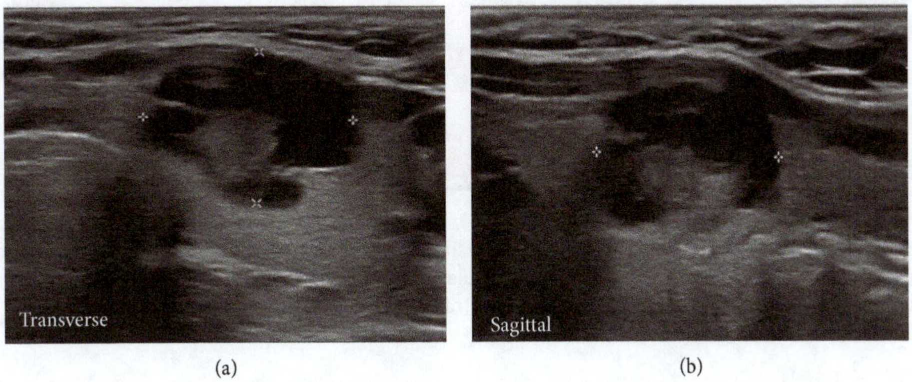

FIGURE 2: (a, b) Ultrasonograms (transverse and sagittal views), demonstrating a fairly oval-shaped solid isoechoic nodule with mixed solid and cystic components ($1.38 \times 1.14 \times 1.36$ cm) in the middle portion of the left thyroid lobe.

A common but not diagnostic features of PC include trabecular architecture of the parenchymal cells, a thick capsule, fibrous trabeculae traversing the gland, nuclear atypia, and high mitotic rates [41–43]. Criteria for definitive diagnosis of PC consist of capsular and vascular invasion, adjacent tissues invasion, involvement of regional lymph nodes, and distant metastatic lesions. Because cell seeding can occur due to the rupture of capsule in the operative field, locally recurrent disease is not diagnostic. Our patient had a clear capsular and vascular invasion (Figures 2(b) and 2(c)),

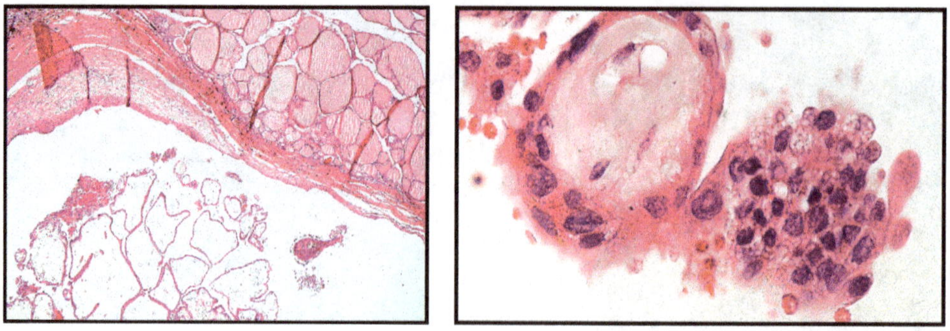

(a) (b)

Figure 3: (a) Histologic appearance of the 1.3 cm papillary carcinoma in the left thyroid lobe, demonstrating a cystic neoplasia with a papillary pattern in transition with residual thyroid normal tissue (hematoxylin-eosin stain original magnification ×4). (b) Histopathological section showing typical features of papillary carcinoma: fibrovascular stalk covered with follicular cells depicting eosinophilic cytoplasm follicular cells and oval nuclei (*) with pseudoinclusions (blue arrow) (hematoxylin-eosin stain original magnification ×40).

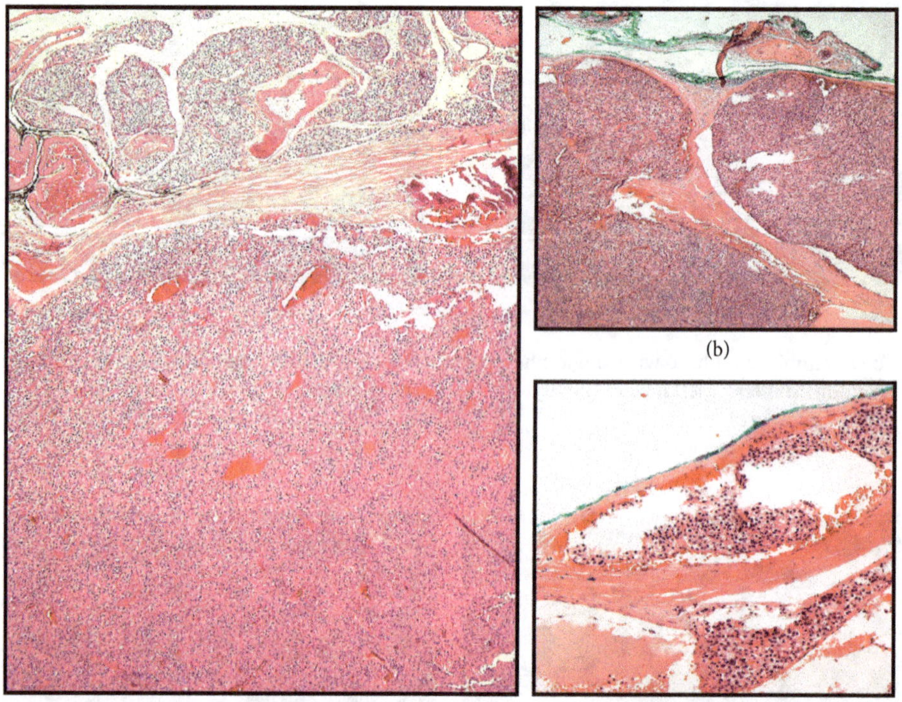

(a) (b) (c)

Figure 4: (a) Histology appearance of parathyroid carcinoma in transition with papillary thyroid carcinoma removed from the left thyroid lobe. The neoplastic cells are represented by the monomorphic cellular proliferation with discrete atypia and mitosis (hematoxylin-eosin stain original magnification ×4). (b) Histopathologic section demonstrating capsular invasion and (c) vascular invasion (hematoxylin-eosin stain original magnification ×10).

making the diagnosis of PC unequivocal. It has been reported that extracapsular vascular invasion correlates best with the diagnosis [33].

Risk factors for PC include history of neck irradiation, long-standing secondary hyperparathyroidism (HPT), end-stage renal disease, and hereditary HPT-jaw tumor syndrome. Additionally, mutation of parafibromin (HRPT2, also known as CDC73) and cyclin D1 (CCND1) plays an important role in the molecular pathogenesis of PC [1, 44, 45]. Our patient has no history of neck irradiation and has not underwent genetic testing.

Here, we describe a case of a PTH-secreting PC that had an appearance of parathyroid adenoma in imaging studies. It was suspected due to marked hypercalcemia and a very high iPTH and renal and bone disease. PTC was only diagnosed postoperatively with histological examination.

Radical surgery provides the best possibility of cure. However, more than 50% of the patients have persistent or recurrent disease. The main cause of morbidity and mortality is due to hypercalcemia complications [34] and less frequently to metastasis [46].

Table 2: Clinical and biochemical features of 15 patients with coexistence of parathyroid and thyroid carcinoma.

Reference	Age	Gender	Calcium (mg/dL)	PTH (pg/mL)	Parathyroid gland size (cm)	Carcinoma location	Thyroid carcinoma	Associated parathyroid disease	Surgical treatment	Outcome
Kurita et al. [38]	68	F	12.2	6300	$4.2 \times 3.2 \times 2.4$	Left lower	Papillary	None	En bloc resection	Postoperative normocalcemia
Christmas et al. [26]	62	F	Hypercalcemia	Unknown	Unknown	Unknown	Follicular	None	Unknown	Died from metastatic parathyroid carcinoma
Savli et al. [22]	47	F	Normal	Normal	Normal	Unknown	Papillary	Hyperplasia	Total thyroidectomy parathyroidectomy (excision of 2 hyperplastic glands)	Normocalcemia (1 year)
Bednarek-Tupikowska et al. [27]	42	F	15.4	1655	5 cm in diameter	Left lower	Follicular	None	En bloc resection	Persistent hypercalcemia
Schoretsanitis, 2002 [24]	55	F	14.2	>1000	3×3	Left lower	Papillary	None	En bloc resection	Normocalcemia (6 years)
Kern et al. [28]	54	F	Unknown	465	$2.5 \times 1.8 \times 1.6$	Right lower	Papillary and follicular	None	Right parathyroidectomy; total thyroidectomy with local lymph node resection; corticectomy in the right superior frontal gyrus	Died from intracranial metastatic parathyroid carcinoma
Lin et al. [25]	38	M	16.5	351	$4 \times 3 \times 3$	Left lower	Papillary	Two enlarged parathyroid glands on contralateral side	Total thyroidectomy and left parathyroidectomy	Normocalcemia (6 years)
Goldfarb et al. [16]	58	M	14.4	2023	$3.4 \times 3.3 \times 2.2$	Left lower	Papillary	Contralateral parathyroid adenoma	En bloc resection	Persistent hypercalcemia after resection of parathyroid carcinoma; normocalcemia after excision of contralateral parathyroid adenoma (1 year)

Table 2: Continued.

Reference	Age	Gender	Calcium (mg/dL)	PTH (pg/mL)	Parathyroid gland size (cm)	Carcinoma location	Thyroid carcinoma	Associated parathyroid disease	Surgical treatment	Outcome
Marcy et al. [17]	42	F	14.1	383	1.3	Right lower	Papillary	None	Total thyroidectomy, right parathyroidectomy, and central and lateral neck dissection	Normocalcemia (14 months)
Chaychi et al. [18]	79	F	10.4	89	$1.1 \times 1.2 \times 4.8$	Left superior	Papillary	None	Total thyroidectomy and left parathyroidectomy	Normocalcemia (6 months)
Amoodi et al. [19]	48	F	Unknown	186	>5	Left lower	Papillary	None	En bloc resection	Persistent hypercalcemia after resection of parathyroid carcinoma; hypoparathyroidism after completion of parathyroidectomy
Zakerkish et al. [21]	21	M	13	1311	Unknown	Unknown	Hürthle	None	Total thyroidectomy and parathyroidectomy	Persistent hypercalcemia and died due to its complications
Song et al. [30]	45	F	17	1455	$4.28 \times 3.09 \times 2.54$	Left lower	Papillary	None	Left parathyroidectomy and left thyroid lobectomy plus left neck dissection	Persistent hypercalcemia after left parathyroidectomy; normocalcemia after left thyroid lobectomy plus left neck dissection (6 months)
Baek et al. [23]	68	F	12.8	1247	$4.2 \times 3.3 \times 3.1$	Left lower	Papillary	None	Left inferior parathyroidectomy and left thyroid lobectomy	Postoperative normocalcemia
Kuzu et al. [29]	52	F	11.4	208	Unknown	Unknown	Papillary	None	Right parathyroidectomy and right thyroid lobectomy	Postoperative normocalcemia
Our case	50	F	13.9	1160	$2.4 \times 1.8 \times 1.4$	Left superior	Papillary	None	Left inferior parathyroidectomy and left thyroid lobectomy	Postoperative normocalcemia

4. Conclusion

The presented case emphasizes the requirement of high clinical suspicion of parathyroid carcinoma in the presence of very high level of iPTH, marked hypercalcemia, and overt skeletal and renal involvement. The existence of any thyroid nodules should be approached and coexistence of other carcinomas should be considered. Although imaging studies assist in the localization, reliable distinction of parathyroid carcinoma from adenoma cannot be made. Radical surgery is the only effective and curative treatment and should consist of initial en bloc resection of the tumor with ipsilateral thyroidectomy and central neck dissection.

Acknowledgments

The authors thank the Department of Endocrinology and Metabolism and Pathology of the Instituto Nacional de Ciencias Médicas y Nutrición Salvador Zubirán.

References

[1] E. Shane, "Parathyroid carcinoma," *The Journal of Clinical Endocrinology & Metabolism*, vol. 86, no. 2, pp. 485–493, 2001.
[2] F. Cetani, E. Pardi, and C. Marcocci, "Update on parathyroid carcinoma," *Journal of Endocrinological Investigation*, vol. 39, no. 6, pp. 595–606, 2016.
[3] E. Kebebew, "Parathyroid carcinoma," *Current Treatment Options in Oncology*, vol. 2, no. 4, pp. 347–354, 2001.
[4] J. M. Sharretts and W. F. Simonds, "Clinical and molecular genetics of parathyroid neoplasms," *Best Practice & Research Clinical Endocrinology & Metabolism*, vol. 24, no. 3, pp. 491–502, 2010.
[5] L. Wang, D. Han, W. Chen et al., "Non-functional parathyroid carcinoma: a case report and review of the literature," *Cancer Biology & Therapy*, vol. 16, no. 11, pp. 1569–1576, 2015.
[6] B. J. Wilkins and J. S. Lewis Jr., "Non-functional parathyroid carcinoma: a review of the literature and report of a case requiring extensive surgery," *Head and Neck Pathology*, vol. 3, no. 2, pp. 140–149, 2009.
[7] S. Guth, U. Theune, J. Aberle, A. Galach, and C. M. Bamberger, "Very high prevalence of thyroid nodules detected by high frequency (13 MHz) ultrasound examination," *European Journal of Clinical Investigation*, vol. 39, no. 8, pp. 699–706, 2009.
[8] L. Dal Maso, C. Panato, S. Franceschi et al., "The impact of overdiagnosis on thyroid cancer epidemic in Italy, 1998–2012," *European journal of cancer*, vol. 94, pp. 6–15, 2018.
[9] L. Davies, L. G. T. Morris, M. Haymart et al., "American Association of Clinical Edocrinologists and American College of Endocrinology Disease State Clinical Review: the increasing incidence of thyroid cancer," *Endocrine Practice*, vol. 21, no. 6, pp. 686–696, 2015.
[10] M. Mileva, B. Stoilovska, A. Jovanovska et al., "Thyroid cancer detection rate and associated risk factors in patients with thyroid nodules classified as bethesda category III," *Radiology and Oncology*, vol. 52, no. 4, pp. 370–376, 2018.
[11] H. Lim, S. S. Devesa, J. A. Sosa, D. Check, and C. M. Kitahara, "Trends in thyroid cancer incidence and mortality in the United States, 1974–2013," *JAMA*, vol. 317, no. 13, pp. 1338–1348, 2017.
[12] F. Rahmat, A. Kumar Marutha Muthu, N. S. R. Gopal, S. Jo Han, and A. S. Yahaya, "Papillary thyroid carcinoma as a lateral neck cyst: a cystic metastatic node versus an ectopic thyroid tissue," *Case Reports in Endocrinology*, vol. 2018, Article ID 5198297, 3 pages, 2018.
[13] S. Suzuki, T. I. Bogdanova, V. A. Saenko et al., "Histopathological analysis of papillary thyroid carcinoma detected during ultrasound screening examinations in Fukushima," *Cancer Science*, vol. 110, no. 2, pp. 817–827, 2019.
[14] S. Tseleni-Balafouta, H. Gakiopoulou, N. Kavantzas, G. Agrogiannis, N. Givalos, and E. Patsouris, "Parathyroid proliferations," *Cancer*, vol. 111, no. 2, pp. 130–136, 2007.
[15] H. Mazeh, D. Prus, and H. R. Freund, "Incidental non-functional parathyroid carcinoma identified during thyroidectomy," *Israel Medical Association Journal*, vol. 10, no. 8-9, p. 659, 2008.
[16] M. Goldfarb, P. O'Neal, J. Shih, P. Hartzband, J. Connolly, and P.-O. Hasselgren, "Synchronous parathyroid carcinoma, parathyroid adenoma, and papillary thyroid carcinoma in a patient with severe and long-standing hyperparathyroidism," *Endocrine Practice*, vol. 15, no. 5, pp. 463–468, 2009.
[17] P.-Y. Marcy, J. Thariat, A. Sudaka, and G. Poissonnet, "Synchronous parathyroid and papillary thyroid carcinomas," *Thyroid*, vol. 19, no. 10, pp. 1131–1133, 2009.
[18] L. Chaychi, K. Belbruno, A. Golding, and V. Memoli, "Unusual manifestation of parathyroid carcinoma in the setting of papillary thyroid cancer," *Endocrine Practice*, vol. 16, no. 4, pp. 664–668, 2010.
[19] H. A. Amoodi, F. M. Makki, S. Mark Taylor, M. J. Bullock, R. D. Hart, and J. R. Trites, "Synchronous thyroid/parathyroid carcinomas," *Journal of Otolaryngology—Head & Neck Surgery*, vol. 39, no. 5, pp. E42–E47, 201.
[20] S. Basceken, V. Genc, S. Ersoz, Y. Sevim, S. Celik, and I. Bayram, "Is local resection sufficient for parathyroid carcinoma?" *Clinics*, vol. 70, no. 4, pp. 247–249, 2015.
[21] M. Zakerkish, E. Rajaei, M. Dargahi, and M. Bahadoram, "A rare constellation of Hürthle cell thyroid carcinoma and parathyroid carcinoma," *Journal of Clinical and Diagnostic Research*, vol. 9, no. 12, 2015.
[22] H. Savli, A. Sevinc, R. Sari, S. Ozen, S. Buyukberber, and E. Ertas, "Occult parathyroid carcinoma in a patient with papillary thyroid carcinoma and Hashimoto's thyroiditis," *Journal of Endocrinological Investigation*, vol. 24, no. 1, pp. 42–44, 2001.
[23] C.-O. Baek, K. H. Kim, and S. K. Song, "Synchronous parathyroid carcinoma and papillary thyroid carcinoma in a patient with long-standing schizophrenia," *The Korean Journal of Internal Medicine*, vol. 32, no. 6, pp. 1104–1107, 2017.
[24] G. Schoretsanitis, J. Melissas, M. Kafousi, N. Karkavitsas, and D. D. Tsiftsis, "Synchronous parathyroid and papillary thyroid carcinoma: a case report," *American Journal of Otolaryngology*, vol. 23, no. 6, pp. 382–385, 2002.
[25] S.-D. Lin, S.-T. Tu, S.-R. Hsu, J. H.-M. Chang, K.-T. Yang, and L.-H. Yang, "Synchronous parathyroid and papillary thyroid carcinoma," *Journal of the Chinese Medical Association*, vol. 68, no. 2, pp. 87–91, 2005.
[26] T. J. Christmas, C. R. Chapple, J. G. Noble, E. J. G. Milroy, and A. G. A. Cowie, "Hyperparathyroidism after neck irradiation," *British Journal of Surgery*, vol. 75, no. 9, pp. 873-874, 1988.
[27] G. Bednarek-Tupikowska, T. Tolloczko, W. Tupikowski et al., "Coexistence of parathyroid carcinoma and non-medullary carcinoma of the thyroid," *Medical Science Monitor*, vol. 7, no. 3, pp. 448–456, 2001.

[28] M. Kern, G. Lee, P. Robbins, M. Bynevelt, and P. Watson, "Intracranial metastatic parathyroid carcinoma," *Journal of Neurosurgery*, vol. 101, no. 6, pp. 1065–1069, 2004.

[29] F. Kuzu, A. Cinkaya, M. Ekici, H. Kodaz, and A. Deger, "Synchronous parathyroid carcinoma and multifocal papillary thyroid carcinoma: a case report," *Eurasian Journal of Medicine and Oncology*, vol. 1, no. 1, pp. 49–52, 2017.

[30] C. Song, J. Wang, X. Cai, and L. Gao, "Synchronous parathyroid carcinoma and papillary thyroid carcinoma : a case study and review of literature," *International Journal of Clinical and Experimental Pathology*, vol. 9, no. 1, pp. 302–309, 2016.

[31] A. Campennì, S. Giovinazzo, S. A. Pignata et al., "Association of parathyroid carcinoma and thyroid disorders: a clinical review," *Endocrine*, vol. 56, no. 1, pp. 19–26, 2017.

[32] http://seer.cancer.gov/statfacts/html/thyro.html.

[33] C. E. Quinn, J. Healy, A. H. Lebastchi et al., "Modern experience with aggressive parathyroid tumors in a high-volume New England referral center," *Journal of the American College of Surgeons*, vol. 220, no. 6, pp. 1054–1062, 2015.

[34] T. Obara and Y. Fujimoto, "Diagnosis and treatment of patients with parathyroid carcinoma: an update and review," *World Journal of Surgery*, vol. 15, no. 6, pp. 738–744, 1991.

[35] E. Shane and J. P. Bilezikian, "Parathyroid carcinoma: a review of 62 patients*," *Endocrine Reviews*, vol. 3, no. 2, pp. 218–226, 1982.

[36] Y. Kushchayeva, Q.-Y. Duh, E. Kebebew, A. D'Avanzo, and O. H. Clark, "Comparison of clinical characteristics at diagnosis and during follow-up in 118 patients with hurthle cell or follicular thyroid cancer," *The American Journal of Surgery*, vol. 195, no. 4, pp. 457–462, 2008.

[37] S. K. G. Grebe and I. D. Hay, "Follicular thyroid cancer," *Endocrinology and Metabolism Clinics of North America*, vol. 24, no. 4, pp. 761–801, 1995.

[38] S. Kurita, S. Mihashi, M. Hirano, T. Nakashima, and A. Tanimura, "Hyperfunctioning parathyroid carcinoma combined with papillary carcinoma of the thyroid gland—report of a case (author's transl)," *Nihon Gan Chiryo Gakkai Shi*, vol. 14, no. 7, pp. 1127–1135, 1979.

[39] J. B. Koea and J. H. F. Shaw, "Parathyroid cancer: biology and management," *Surgical Oncology*, vol. 8, no. 3, pp. 155–165, 1999.

[40] K. Dikmen, H. Bostanci, H. Gobut et al., "Nonfunctional double parathyroid carcinoma with incidental thyroid micropapillary carcinoma: a rare case," *The Pan African Medical Journal*, vol. 27, p. 241, 2017.

[41] G. G. Fernandez-Ranvier, E. Khanafshar, K. Jensen et al., "Parathyroid carcinoma, atypical parathyroid adenoma, or parathyromatosis?" *Cancer*, vol. 110, no. 2, pp. 255–264, 2007.

[42] A. Schantz and B. Castleman, "Parathyroid carcinom: a study of 70 cases," *Cancer*, vol. 31, no. 3, pp. 600–605, 1973.

[43] B. Givi and J. P. Shah, "Parathyroid carcinoma," *Clinical Oncology*, vol. 22, no. 6, pp. 498–507, 2010.

[44] A. Arnold, "Genetic basis of endocrine disease 5: molecular genetics of parathyroid gland neoplasia," *Journal of Clinical Endocrinology & Metabolism*, vol. 77, no. 5, pp. 1108–1112, 1993.

[45] T. M. Shattuck, S. Välimäki, T. Obara et al., "Somatic and germ-line mutations of theHRPT2Gene in sporadic parathyroid carcinoma," *New England Journal of Medicine*, vol. 349, no. 18, pp. 1722–1729, 2003.

[46] A. Campennì, R. M. Ruggeri, A. Sindoni et al., "Parathyroid carcinoma presenting as normocalcemic hyperparathyroidism," *Journal of Bone and Mineral Metabolism*, vol. 30, no. 3, pp. 367–372, 2012.

Microangiopathic Hemolytic Anemia and Fulminant Renal Failure: A Rare Manifestation of Pheochromocytoma

Nishant Sharma, Divya Ravi, Mehvish Khan, Metlapalli Venkata Sravanthi, and Mark M. Aloysius

The Wright Center for Graduate Medical Education, 111 N Washington Ave, Scranton, PA 18503, USA

Correspondence should be addressed to Nishant Sharma; sharman@thewrightcenter.org

Academic Editor: Toshihiro Kita

Pheochromocytoma is a rare adrenal tumor that is classically associated with the triad of paroxysmal tachycardia, diaphoresis, and headaches. However, it can have myriad manifestations. We present a case of a 31-year-old male who presented with abdominal pain, hypertensive emergency, and renal failure. Abdominal imaging demonstrated a left adrenal mass. Plasma metanephrines (153 pg/ml, $n < 57$) and normetanephrines (1197 pg/ml, $n < 148$) were noted to be elevated, leading to the diagnosis of pheochromocytoma. Intravenous antihypertensives were utilized to control his blood pressure. Hemodialysis was initiated given the degree of renal dysfunction. The patient subsequently developed hemolytic anemia, requiring the transfusion of multiple units of packed red cells. He developed acute respiratory failure leading to intubation, but was thereafter liberated from the ventilator following clinical stabilization. Uncontrolled hypertension precipitated by pheochromocytoma can cause microangiopathic hemolytic anemia and renal insufficiency. This case is notable not only for the occurrence of this rare presentation, but also for the severity of manifestations in a young male with no known significant comorbidities.

1. Introduction

Pheochromocytoma is a rare form of catecholamine-secreting adrenal tumor with an estimated annual incidence of about three to eight per million [1]. About 30 percent of pheochromocytoma occur in association with familial neuroendocrine syndromes, while a majority are sporadic. Pheochromocytoma typically presents in the fourth or fifth decade of life, with no specific gender predilection [2]. Historically, pheochromocytoma has been outlined by the classic triad of paroxysmal tachycardia, diaphoresis, and headaches in the setting of uncontrolled hypertension. However, most patients do not manifest with these typical symptoms; pheochromocytoma has been labelled "the great mimic" [3] that can rarely present with dramatic multiorgan crisis or a "pheochromocytoma crisis", as described in our case below.

2. Case Presentation

The patient is a 31-year-old African American male who presented to the ED with a chief complaint of upper abdominal pain. This abdominal pain had begun two weeks prior and was progressively worsening. He described it as a mid-epigastric dull ache, aggravated by eating, and lacking in radiation or alleviating factors. He reported associated nausea, vomiting, and nonbloody diarrhea, as well as a weight loss of 8 pounds over the same period of time, which is something he attributed to poor oral intake. A complete review of systems was limited as the patient was lethargic and slow to answer questions. His medical history was limited to an episode of pancreatitis about 5 years prior to presentation. He had not seen a doctor for years prior to presentation, but was told that he had high blood pressure at a plasma donation center a few years before. He took no medications apart from over the counter ibuprofen as needed for pain. His family history was significant only for hypertension in his mother. He had a 10-pack year smoking history, and biweekly use of marijuana. He denied consumption of alcohol and other illicit drugs.

At presentation, he was found to have a blood pressure of 223/142 mm Hg. Physical exam was notable for moderate epigastric tenderness. His lab work was most notable for leukocytosis ($12.2 \times 109/\mu L$, $n < 10$), normocytic anemia (Hb 7.8 g/dL, $n = 14-17$), thrombocytopenia ($100 \times 109/L$,

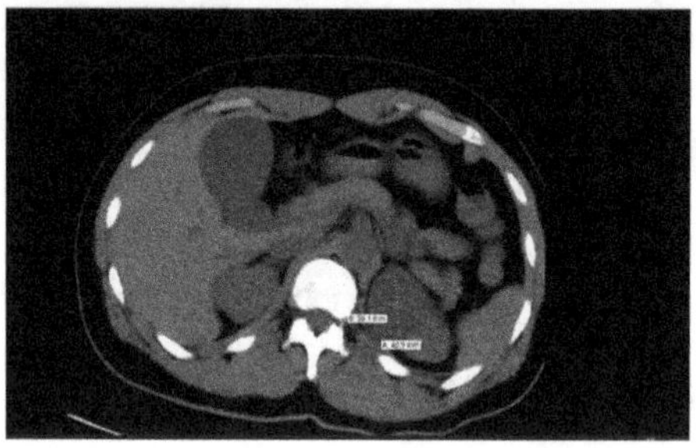

Figure 1: CT abdomen demonstrating adrenal tumor.

$n = 150-450$), deranged renal function (BUN 124 mg/dL, $n < 20$, creatinine 21.6 mg/dL, $n < 1.3$), proteinuria (≥ 500 mg/dL, $n < 20$), mild hematuria with metabolic acidosis (pH of 7.25), and anion (gap of 20). A CT scan of the abdomen demonstrated acute colitis, and a low density left adrenal mass measuring $4.4 \times 4.4 \times 4.5$ cm (Figure 1).

The patient was admitted to the intensive care unit; nicardipine drip was initiated to lower the patient's blood pressure and broad-spectrum antibiotic coverage was started for ongoing colitis. A comprehensive workup for secondary causes of hypertension was ordered, including plasma metanephrines, plasma normetanephrines, plasma renin, plasma angiotensin, a 24-hour urine cortisol, thyroid function tests, and a renal ultrasound. A tunnelled catheter was placed for urgent initiation of dialysis given his severe degree of uremia and possible encephalopathy. The next day, he developed worsening anemia necessitating the transfusion of two units of packed red cells. Additionally, he had an elevated LDH, undetectable haptoglobin, elevated reticulocyte count, negative Coomb's test, and thrombocytopenia. A peripheral smear was notable for the presence of schistocytes. He was transitioned off the nicardipine infusion to oral amlodipine and labetalol. An MRI of the abdomen assisted in confirming and further characterizing the adrenal lesion (Figure 2).

The following day, during a session of hemodialysis, the patient developed acute respiratory distress requiring intubation for airway support and resumption of nicardipine infusion for hypertensive emergency. A chest X-ray demonstrated bilateral alveolar infiltrates and pleural effusion. High sensitivity troponin was found to be elevated and a transthoracic echocardiogram showed mildly impaired left ventricular function with an ejection fraction of 50% and no significant valvular abnormalities. Over the next 48 hours, his oxygen needs improved and he was subsequently extubated. The workup for secondary hypertension revealed elevated plasma metanephrines (153 pg/ml, $n < 57$) and normetanephrines (1197 pg/ml, $n < 148$), thus confirming the diagnosis of pheochromocytoma presenting as hypertensive emergency. Hemodialysis was resumed and he was started on the appropriate antihypertensive medications. Once deemed clinically stable, the patient was transferred to a tertiary care center for evaluation of surgical resection of the tumor.

3. Discussion

Pheochromocytoma is a rare catecholamine secreting tumor, occurring in less than 0.5% of patients with hypertension [4], which classically presents with hypertension, headache, palpitations, sweating, and diaphoresis. It can, however, rarely have more dramatic presentations, including cardiogenic shock [5, 6], myocardial infarction [7], cardiomyopathy [8], rhabdomyolysis [9–12], acute renal failure [5, 13–16], pulmonary haemorrhage [7], arrhythmia, and microangiopathic hemolysis [13, 14, 17]. An acute and severe presentation of pheochromocytoma involving end organ damage or dysfunction brought on by catecholamine-induced hemodynamic instability is referred to as a pheochromocytoma crisis (PCC). While there is a wide variation in mortality estimates, a recent review estimates it to be 15% [18]. One proposed classification system describes two types of crises-Type A, characterized by hemodynamic instability and end organ damage of one or more organ systems, and Type B, characterized by sustained hypotension, or shock, and multiorgan system damage [18]. This case of PCC was notable not only for the presence of two rare manifestations of pheochromocytoma—microangiopathic hemolytic anemia and renal failure—but also for their severity. The patient had severe renal insufficiency with a serum creatinine of 21.6 and estimated GFR of 3 mL/min per 1.73 m^2, and a degree of hemolysis that produced a precipitous drop in hemoglobin.

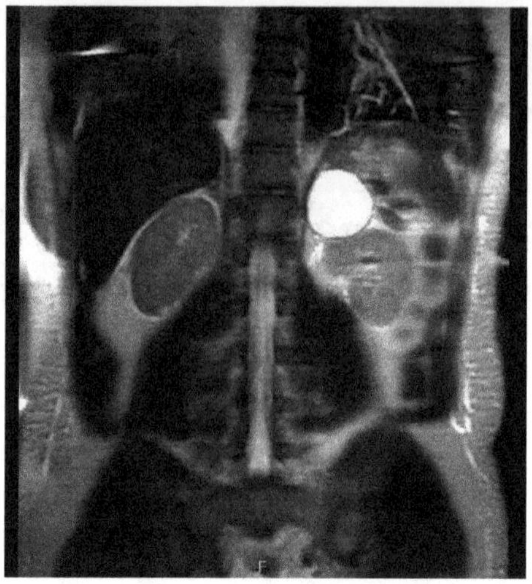

Figure 2: MRI abdomen demonstrating left adrenal mass.

There are multiple possible mechanisms of renal insufficiency in a patient with pheochromocytoma. There have been several case reports detailing the occurrence of acute renal failure as a consequence catecholamine induced vasoconstriction [9, 10]. Another mechanism for renal dysfunction in the setting of pheochromocytoma is hypertension induced intimal thickening of glomerular vasculature, and glomerulosclerosis. It is also important to note the concentric left ventricular hypertrophy on ECHO and the EKG, which is a manifestation of sustained uncontrolled hypertension. Given these findings and lack of medical visits since his remote presentation of elevated BP in a blood donation center few years prior, we propose that this patient's severe renal insufficiency was the result of hypertensive nephropathy possibly complicated by rhabdomyolysis. A renal biopsy, which could have confirmed this hypothesis, was deemed high risk in this patient given the atrophic nature of his kidneys. The co-occurence of rhabdomyolysis as a consequence of catecholamine induced vasoconstriction and resultant muscle ischemia might have made a minor contribution to this patient's renal insufficiency; urinalysis did demonstrate a positive result for blood and only a few RBC on microscopy. A creatine kinase level was not obtained as a part of initial work up; this is one limitation of this case report. Due to the degree of uremia, a tunnelled catheter was placed on an emergent basis for the initiation of dialysis.

Another distinguishing feature of this case is the severe degree of hemolytic anemia, which can be attributed to one or more of the following mechanisms. Uncontrolled hypertension, in itself has been shown to cause microangiopathic hemolytic anemia (MAHA) and thrombocytopenia due to endothelial injury and subsequent destruction of RBCs and platelets [19]. The subnormal haptoglobin coupled with elevated LDH and reticulocyte count, and schistocytes on peripheral smear favor MAHA. There is also some evidence to suggest the role of elevated plasma renin activity (PRA), as noted in this case, in causing accelerated vascular damage and renal dysfunction resulting in microangiopathic hemolysis [20]. Lastly, a high normal vitamin B12 level, negative complement panel and negative Coombs test make other mechanisms of hemolysis less likely.

A review of literature shows us several cases of reported renal failure in the setting of pheochromocytoma secondary to rhabdomyolysis [9, 10] or cardiogenic shock [5]. The concurrence of pheochromocytoma, malignant hypertension, renal failure and microangiopathic hemolytic anemia appears to a rare presentation, with only two reported cases found in our literature review [13, 14]. Our case adds to the body of literature by demonstrating the extent of severity to which pheochromocytoma can cause hematological and renal insults through a combination of mechanisms in a young patient with no significant comorbidities. Schweizer et al. suggest that plasmapheresis can lead to favorable outcomes in pheochromocytoma with thrombotic microangiopathy [14]. However, since the ADAMTS13 activity in our patient was found to be normal, we suggest that the optimum management of both renal failure and microangiopathic hemolytic anemia in a case like ours involves prompt control of hemodynamics, renal replacement therapy, and treatment directed towards the adrenal tumor itself.

A final note must be made on the diagnostic utility of plasma metanephrine and normetanephrine in pheochromocytoma. The Endocrine Society (ES), in their clinical practice guidelines for pheochromocytoma and paraganglioma (PPGL) [21] recommend the measurement of plasma free metanephrines or urinary fractionated metanephrines in the initial biochemical testing for PPGL. However, being metabolites of catecholamines, their levels in the plasma can be elevated in conditions of physiological stress, such as an acute illness [22]. They can be elevated in up to 75% of patients with acute cardiomyopathy [23]. Additionally, renal dysfunction itself may contribute to the elevation of these metabolites [24]. The aforementioned ES guidelines reports a low probability of false positivity in case with elevations of both normetanephrine and metanephrine, or an isolated elevation 3-fold or more above upper cutoffs in either metabolite. In this case, both metanephrine and normetanephrine were found to be elevated, with the latter being 8 fold the upper limit of normal. The coincident identification of an adrenal mass, and characteristic symptoms imparts a high probability for the diagnosis of pheochromocytoma in this patient. A clonidine suppression test may be employed for the differentiation of true-positive from false-positive borderline elevation of normetanephrine [21].

Pheochromocytoma is a disease with a myriad of possible presentations. In a previously healthy young patient, presenting with a triad of malignant hypertension, hemolytic anemia and renal failure, pheochromocytoma must be considered as part of the differential.

References

[1] C. M. Beard, S. G. Sheps, L. T. Kurland, J. A. Carney, and J. T. Lie, "Occurrence of pheochromocytoma in Rochester, Minnesota, 1950 through 1979," *Mayo Clinic Proceedings*, vol. 58, no. 12, pp. 802–804, 1983.

[2] M. A. Guerrero, J. M. J. Schreinemakers, M. R. Vriens et al., "Clinical spectrum of pheochromocytoma," *Journal of the American College of Surgeons*, vol. 209, no. 6, pp. 727–732, 2009.

[3] C. Yucha and N. Blakeman, "Pheochromocytoma. the great mimic," *Cancer Nursing*, vol. 14, no. 3, pp. 136–140, 1991.

[4] V. L. Martucci and K. Pacak, "Pheochromocytoma and paraganglioma: diagnosis, genetics, management, and treatment," *Current Problems in Cancer*, vol. 38, no. 1, pp. 7–41, 2014.

[5] G. V. Raman, "Phaeochromocytoma, presenting with cardiogenic shock and acute renal failure," *Journal of Human Hypertension*, vol. 1, no. 3, pp. 237–238, 1987.

[6] H. A. Mohamed, M. O. Aldakar, and N. Habib, "Cardiogenic shock due to acute hemorrhagic necrosis of a pheochromocytoma: a case report and review of the literature," *The Canadian Journal of Cardiology*, vol. 19, no. 5, pp. 573–576, 2003.

[7] M. Park, K. Hryniewicz, and J. F. Setaro, "Pheochromocytoma presenting with myocardial infarction, cardiomyopathy, renal failure, pulmonary hemorrhage, and cyclic hypotension: case report and review of unusual presentations of pheochromocytoma," *The Journal of Clinical Hypertension*, vol. 11, no. 2, pp. 74–80, 2009.

[8] M. N. Attar, P. K. Moulik, G. D. Salem, E. L. Rose, and A. A. Khaleeli, "Phaeochromocytoma presenting as dilated cardiomyopathy," *International Journal of Clinical Practice*, vol. 57, no. 6, pp. 547–548, 2003.

[9] H. Celik, O. Celik, S. Guldiken, V. Inal, F. O. Puyan, and A. Tugrul, "Pheochromocytoma presenting with rhabdomyolysis and acute renal failure: a case report," *Renal Failure*, vol. 36, no. 1, pp. 104–107, 2014.

[10] D. Shemin, P. S. Cohn, and S. B. Zipin, "Pheochromocytoma presenting as rhabdomyolysis and acute myoglobinuric renal failure," *Archives of Internal Medicine*, vol. 150, no. 11, pp. 2384–2385, 1990.

[11] I. Anaforoglu, M. E. Ertorer, F. E. Haydardedeoglu, T. Colakoglu, N. Tokmak, and N. G. Demirag, "Rhabdomyolysis and acute myoglobinuric renal failure in a patient with bilateral pheochromocytoma following open pyelolithotomy," *Southern Medical Journal*, vol. 101, no. 4, pp. 425–427, 2008.

[12] X. Zhou, C. Zhao, X. Feng et al., "Continuous renal replacement therapy for haemodynamic collapse and rhabdomyolysis induced by pheochromocytoma crisis," *ESC Heart Failure*, vol. 3, no. 4, pp. 282–287, 2016.

[13] M. J. Gillett, R. V. Arenson, M. K. Yew, I. J. Thompson, and A. B. Irish, "Diagnostic challenges associated with a complex case of cystic phaeochromocytoma presenting with malignant hypertension, microangiopathic haemolysis and acute renal failure," *Nephrology Dialysis Transplantation*, vol. 20, no. 5, pp. 1014–1014, 2005.

[14] H. Schweizer, J. Boehm, J. T. Winterer et al., "Phaeochromocytoma and thrombotic microangiopathy: favourable outcome despite advanced renal failure," *Journal of Clinical Pathology*, vol. 63, no. 8, pp. 754–756, 2010.

[15] F. M. Brouwers, G. Eisenhofer, J. W. M. Lenders, and K. Pacak, "Emergencies caused by pheochromocytoma, neuroblastoma, or ganglioneuroma," *Endocrinology and Metabolism Clinics of North America*, vol. 35, no. 4, pp. 699–724, 2006.

[16] L. Q. Gu, L. Zhao, J. M. Liu, T. W. Su, W. Q. Wang, and G. Ning, "Phaeochromocytoma presenting with coexisting acute renal failure, acidosis and in hyperglycaemic emergency," *British Journal of Biomedical Science*, vol. 65, no. 3, pp. 153–155, 2008.

[17] C. Sakai, T. Takagi, M. Oguro, S. Wakatsuki, and T. Kuwahara, "Malignant pheochromocytoma accompanied by microangiopathic hemolytic anemia: a case report," *Japanese Journal of Clinical Oncology*, vol. 24, no. 3, pp. 171–174, 1994.

[18] B. C. Whitelaw, J. K. Prague, O. G. Mustafa et al., "Phaeochromocytoma [corrected] crisis," *Clinical Endocrinology (Oxford)*, vol. 80, no. 1, pp. 13–22, 2014.

[19] A. Khanna and P. A. McCullough, "Malignant hypertension presenting as hemolysis, thrombocytopenia, and renal failure," *Reviews in Cardiovascular Medicine*, vol. 4, no. 4, pp. 255–259, 2003.

[20] B.-J. H. van den Born, R. P. Koopmans, and G. A. van Montfrans, "The renin-angiotensin system in malignant hypertension revisited: plasma renin activity, microangiopathic hemolysis, and renal failure in malignant hypertension," *American Journal of Hypertension*, vol. 20, no. 8, pp. 900–906, 2007.

[21] J. W. Lenders, Q. Y. Duh, G. Eisenhofer et al., "Endocrine society. pheochromocytoma and paraganglioma: an endocrine society clinical practice guideline," *The Journal of Clinical Endocrinology & Metabolism*, vol. 99, no. 6, pp. 1915–1942, 2014.

[22] L. Amar and G. Eisenhofer, "Diagnosing phaeochromocytoma/ paraganglioma in a patient presenting with critical illness: biochemistry versus imaging," *Clinical Endocrinology (Oxford)*, vol. 83, no. 3, pp. 298–302, 2015.

[23] V. Agarwal, G. Kant, N. Hans, and F. H. Messerli, "Takotsubo-like cardiomyopathy in pheochromocytoma," *International Journal of Cardiology*, vol. 153, no. 3, pp. 241–248, 2011.

[24] G. Eisenhofer, F. Huysmans, K. Pacak, M. M. Walther, F. C. Sweep, and J. W. Lenders, "Plasma metanephrines in renal failure," *Kidney International*, vol. 67, no. 2, pp. 668–677, 2005.

8

Novel *TMEM127* Variant Associated to Bilateral Phaeochromocytoma with an Uncommon Clinical Presentation

Antía Fernández-Pombo ,[1,2] José M. Cameselle-Teijeiro ,[3] Jose A. Puñal-Rodríguez,[4] Lourdes Loidi,[5] Roberto Peinó-García,[1] Paloma Cabanas-Rodríguez,[6] Miguel Garrido-Pumar,[7] Sandra Baleato-González,[8] Enrique Flores-Ríos,[8] and David Araújo-Vilar [1,2]

[1]*Division of Endocrinology, University Clinical Hospital of Santiago de Compostela, Spain*
[2]*UETeM-Molecular Pathology Group, Department of Medicine, IDIS-CIMUS, University of Santiago de Compostela, Spain*
[3]*Division of Pathology, University Clinical Hospital of Santiago de Compostela, Spain*
[4]*Division of Surgery, University Clinical Hospital of Santiago de Compostela, Spain*
[5]*Fundación Galega de Medicina Xenómica, Santiago de Compostela, Spain*
[6]*Division of Pediatrics, University Clinical Hospital of Santiago de Compostela, Spain*
[7]*Division of Nuclear Medicine, University Clinical Hospital of Santiago de Compostela, Spain*
[8]*Division of Radiology, University Clinical Hospital of Santiago de Compostela, Spain*

Correspondence should be addressed to David Araújo-Vilar; david.araujo@usc.es

Academic Editor: Carlo Capella

Phaeochromocytomas and paragangliomas are rare catecholamine-secreting tumours arising from the adrenal medulla or sympathetic paraganglia. It is known that 20–30% of all cases occur as a result of germline variants in several well known genes. The *TMEM127* gene was recently identified as a new phaeochromocytoma susceptibility gene. However, until a larger sample of cases is available, the prevalence, genotype-phenotype correlation, and a clear predominant biochemical pattern of *TMEM127*-related PCC, remain to be defined. We present a woman with the pathogenic variant c.86delG (p.Arg29Leu*fs**52) in the *TMEM127* gene, which has not been previously reported, associated to a bilateral phaeochromocytoma, with an uncommon initial clinical presentation and a biochemical profile that is distinctly adrenergic. Her two young children carry the same variant and are, at present, disease-free. Physicians should be aware that phaeochromocytoma can manifest in an atypical manner, as with episodic hypotension, mainly if the symptoms have no obvious aetiology and they worsen over time. This case also supports the presence of a predominant adrenaline secreting pattern in *TMEM127*-positive tumours, as well as the need to consider multigene panel testing in patients with bilateral phaeochromocytomas.

1. Introduction

Phaeochromocytomas (PCC) and paragangliomas are rare neural crest-derived tumours found respectively in the adrenal medulla or sympathetic paraganglia [1]. These tumours are usually benign and sporadic. However, 20–30% of all cases are part of well characterized hereditary tumour syndromes [2], such as von Hippel-Lindau disease, Multiple Endocrine Neoplasia type 2 and Neurofibromatosis type 1, which occur as a result of germline variants in *VHL, RET, NF1*, and *SDH* (subunits A, B, C, D and AF2) genes [3]. In addition, in 2010–2011, the *TMEM127* and *MAX* genes were also identified as new PCC susceptibility genes [4, 5]. The *TMEM127* gene encodes a transmembrane protein that is linked to the regulation of the mTOR signaling complex. The majority of the variants described so far are associated with truncation of the protein, suggesting that they result in loss of *TMEM127* function [4]. Here, we present a family with a novel pathogenic variant in the *TMEM127* gene, associated to a bilateral PCC.

2. Case Presentation

A 33-year-old woman first consulted at the Division of Cardiology because of presyncopal symptoms, which started just after the delivery of her first child, with acral pallor, associated with pain, tremor and weakness in the lower limbs. In addition, she presented gastrointestinal symptoms with epigastric pain and nausea, accompanied by slow palpitations and significant orthostatic hypotension. During one of the episodes an electrocardiogram showed a nodal rhythm with a ventricular rate of 50. The Holter revealed a clear relation between the symptomatology and these episodes of nodal rhythm. Seven years later, after a routine blood test she showed an impaired fasting glucose of 110 mg/dl and was referred to the Division of Endocrinology. During a thorough anamnesis, the patient reported worsening of the symptoms and an increase in their frequency, with the appearance of pulsating headaches, dizziness, tinnitus and high blood pressure (up to 225/117 mmHg) followed by hypotension (63/36 mmHg on average). As far as her medical history is concerned, she had undergone a thyroid lobectomy with isthmusectomy, with a histological finding of a nodular hyperplasia. There was no family history of endocrine disease. However, her mother had hypertension and her father passed away due to a brainstem stroke. She has two healthy children.

With the clinical suspicion of PCC, an analytical study was requested, which showed: urine adrenalin 367 mcg/24 h (<20 mcg/24 h), urine noradrenalin 81 mcg/24 h (15–80 mcg/24 h), urine metanephrine 2490 mcg/24 h (25–312 mcg/24 h) and urine normetanephrine 816 mcg/24 h (60–757 mcg/24 h). Magnetic resonance imaging (MRI) (Figure 1) revealed bilateral adrenal masses, 37 mm right and 49 mm left. It showed a hyperintense signal of both adrenal glands on fat-suppressed T2-weighted, without the presence of fat. After gadolinium administration these masses enhanced avidly and heterogeneously with regions of no enhancement due to cystic changes. Restricted diffusion ($b = 800$) of hypercellular areas was well demonstrated by ADC map as areas of low intensity signal. In oppossite, cystic components demonstrated high signal. ^{123}I-MIBG SPECT/CT (Figure 2) showed increased uptake foci in both adrenal glands, with right predominance, compatible with the diagnosis of bilateral PCC. No extraadrenal tumour localization was detected.

The patient underwent a laparoscopic bilateral adrenalectomy. The bilateral tumours were circumscribed but unencapsulated, and partially surrounded by a bright-yellow ring of normal adrenal cortical cells. Both tumours also showed a fleshy, tan cut surface, with haemorrhage areas, measuring 4.5 cm and 5.4 cm maximum diameter in the right and left glands respectively (Figure 3).

Genetic testing was carried out. The patient presented the pathogenic variant NM_017849.3: c.86delG (p.Arg29Leufs* 52) in heterozygosis in the *TMEM127* gene. This variant has not been reported in available databases (i.e., dbSNP146, 1000 Genomes, ExAC and GnomAD). This consists of the deletion of one nucleotide in exon 2 of *TMEM127* which alters the reading pattern and leads to the appearance of a premature stop codon. Given that this premature stop codon is 7 nucleotides upstream the next exon-junction complex, it is unlikely that this new transcript is down regulated by nonsense-mediated decay [6]. This result suggests a susceptibility to PCC with an autosomal dominant inheritance pattern (OMIM #171300). Given these findings, a genetic study was performed on her children, aged 9 and 6, who were proved to be carriers of the same variant in the *TMEM127* gene. Plasma and urine catecholamines and metanephrines and total body MRI showed normal results in both children. However, given the risk of developing PCC or other tumours (renal carcinoma) [7], they will require surveillance. In addition, her mother tested negative for the variant.

One year after the adrenalectomy the patient is asymptomatic, with normal metanephrine excretion. As expected, she has primary adrenal insufficiency and is being treated with hydrocortisone.

3. Discussion

To the best of our knowledge, this is the first report of a Spanish patient showing that a *TMEM127* variant plays a pathological role in bilateral PCC. Furthermore, this c.86delG variant has not been previously reported.

Patients carrying *TMEM127* pathogenic variants have a similar age of tumour diagnosis as those who have sporadic lesions (41.5 years vs. 45 years); one-third have bilateral disease; the tumours are usually benign; the occurrence of catecholamine excess with symptoms precede PCC diagnosis by several years, and only 25% have a family history of PCC [4, 8, 9]. In this case, in spite of its paroxysmal occurrence, indicative of PCC, the atypical clinical scenario caused a delay in the diagnosis. It is necessary to consider that the presence of sinus node dysfunction may be an initial manifestation of PCC [10]. Physicians must also be aware that it may likewise present with hypotension (excessive stimulation of beta adrenoceptors by elevated levels of epinephrine), postural hypotension or alternating episodes of high and low blood pressure [11]. However, a clear genotype-phenotype correlation is unlikely to become evident until a larger sample of these families is published. It has also been suggested that these patients can likewise develop cathecholamine-mediated arterial vasospasm, leading to cerebral ischemia [12]. Thus, in this case, it is not unreasonable to think that either the patient has a de novo variant or the variant comes from the deceased father, who passed away due to a brainstem stroke.

Regarding the biochemical profile, while in an international cohort of 990 patients with PCC, of whom 2% presented pathogenic *TMEM127* germline variants, no preference of adrenaline or noradrenaline secretion was reported [8], three other studies have reported a predominant adrenaline secreting pattern [7, 13, 14], which we have also described in this case, further raising the suspicion of an etiology distinct from *VHL* or *SDHB* germline variants [15].

At present, the exact prevalence of *TMEM127*-related PCC is still unknown and will need to be defined by the *TMEM127* genotyping of further large series. Moreover, due to the large number of genes responsible for the development of PCC, genetic testing remains a diagnostic challenge. In addition, it has been reported that 3% of apparently sporadic PCC were

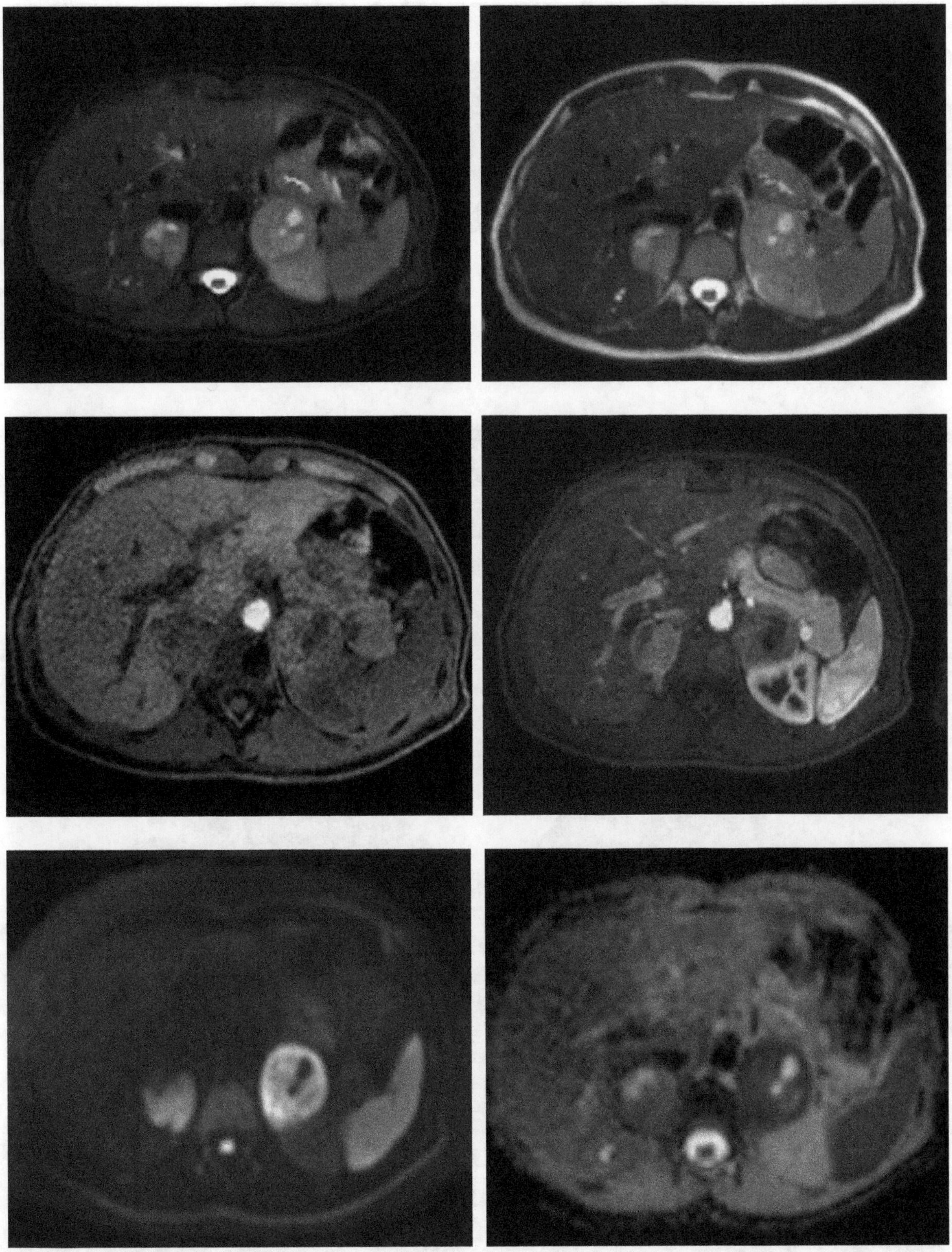

(c)

FIGURE 1: Abdominal MRI scan showing bilateral phaeochromocytoma. (a) axial TSE-T2W images with and without fat suppression; (b) axial GRE-T1W images prior to and 35 s after contrast injection; (c) DWI and ADC map showing restricted diffusion (ADC = 0.6×10^{-3} mm^2/s).

caused by *TMEM127* gene variants [4]. Taking into account the significant implications for patients and their family members, the identification of a possible underlying genetic variant is important. Thus, advances in DNA sequencing technologies that make possible simultaneous testing for multiple genes should be used.

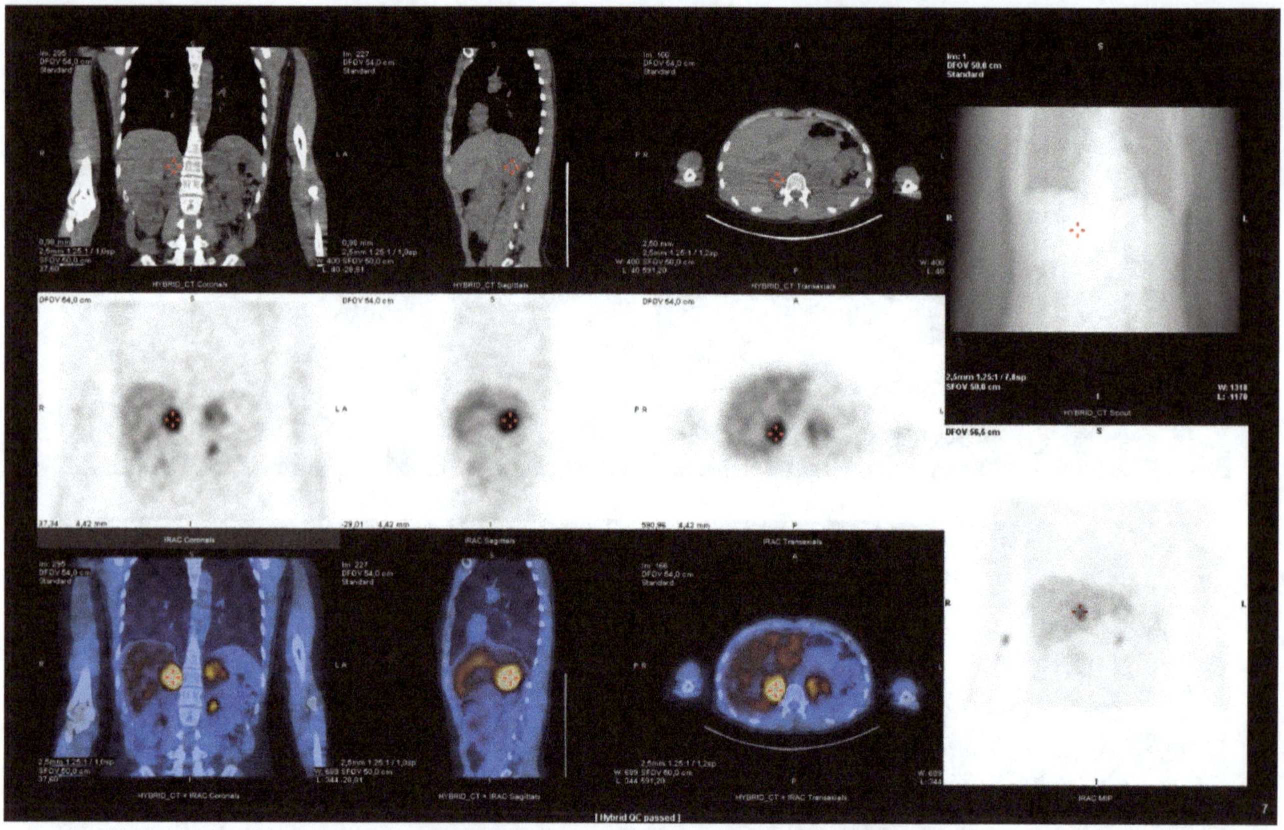

FIGURE 2: ^{123}I-MIBG SPECT/CT showing increased uptake of the tracer in both adrenal glands, with right predominance.

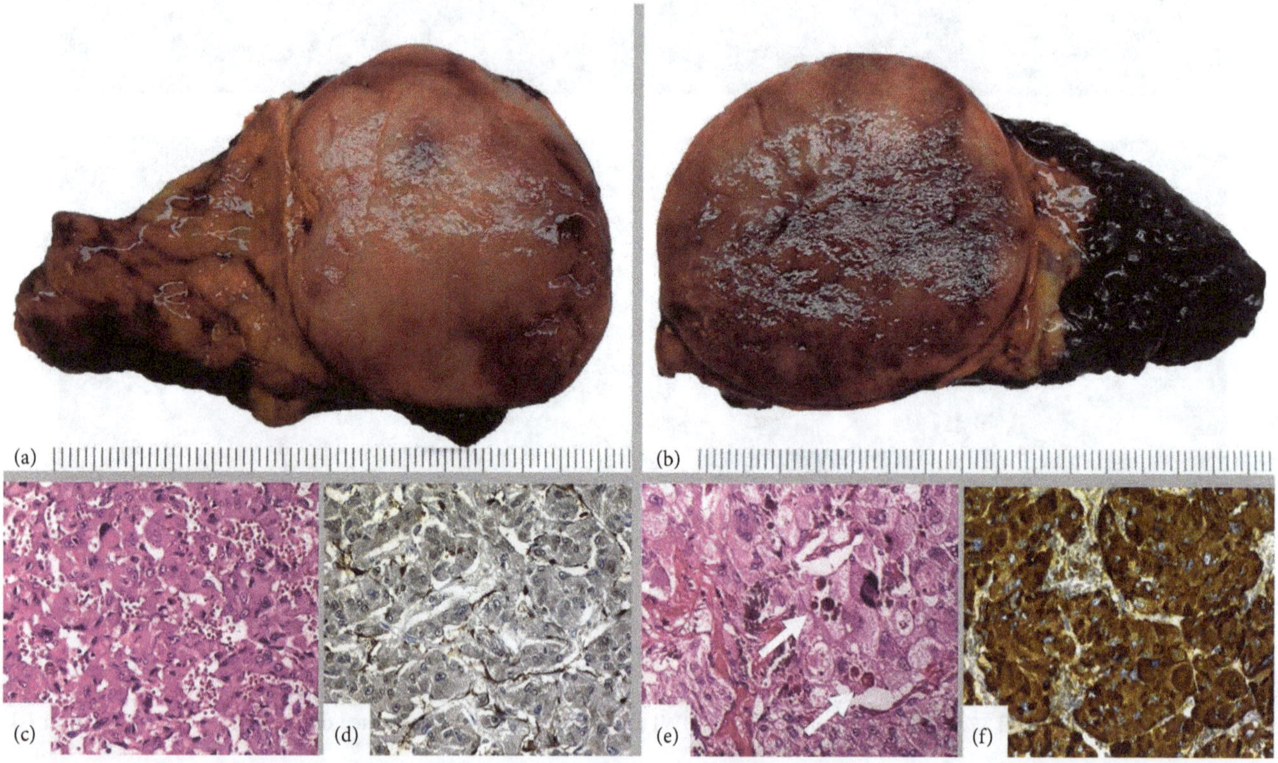

FIGURE 3: Bilateral phaeochromocytoma. Both right (a, c, d) and left (b, e, f) adrenal tumours were similar in the macroscopic and microscopic appearance. Microscopically they showed the typical nested pattern (c, e), moderate pleomorphism and occasional intracytoplasmic hyaline globules (arrows), but no mitotic activity. S100 sustentacular cells (d) and positivity for chromogranin A (f) were demonstrated. The Ki-67 was less than 2%.

This case supports the need to add *TMEM127* to the multigene panel testing in patients with bilateral PCC with a predominant adrenaline secreting pattern, even if there is low suspicion of a hereditary condition.

Consent

Informed consent was obtained from the patient who participated in this study.

Acknowledgments

This work was funded by the Consellería de Industria, Xunta de Galicia (grant number ED341b 2017/19) (D.A-V), and by Grant PI15/0150-FEDER from the Instituto de Salud Carlos III, Ministry of Science, Innovation and Universities, Spain (JMC-T).

References

[1] A. S. Tischler, R. R. de Krijger, and A. Gill, "Phaeochromocytoma world health organization classification of tumours," in *Pathology and Genetics of Tumours of Endocrine Organs*, R. V. Lloyd, R. Y. Osamura, G. Klöppel, and J. Rosai, Eds., pp. 183–189, IARC Press, Lyon, 4th edition, 2017.

[2] H. P. Neumann, B. Bausch, S. R. McWhinney et al., "Germ-line mutations in nonsyndromic pheochromocytoma," *New England Journal of Medicine*, vol. 346, no. 19, pp. 1459–1466, 2002.

[3] D. Astuti, F. Latif, A. Dallol et al., "Gene mutations in the succinate dehydrogenase subunit SDHB cause susceptibility to familial pheochromocytoma and to familial paraganglioma," *The American Journal of Human Genetics*, vol. 69, no. 1, pp. 49–54, 2001.

[4] Y. Qin, L. Yao, E. E. King et al., "Germline mutations in *TMEM127* confer susceptibility to pheochromocytoma," *Nature Genetics*, vol. 42, no. 3, pp. 229–233, 2010.

[5] I. Comino-Mendez, F. Gracia-Aznarez, J. Schiavi et al., "Exome sequencing identifies MAX mutations as a cause of hereditary pheochromocytoma," *Nature Genetics*, vol. 43, no. 7, pp. 663–667, 2011.

[6] B. P. Lewis, R. E. Green, and S. E. Brenner, "Evidence for the widespread coupling of alternative splicing and nonsense-mediated mRNA decay in humans," *Proceedings of the National Academy of Sciences*, vol. 100, no. 1, pp. 189–192, 2003.

[7] K. G. Hernandez, S. Ezzat, C. F. Morel et al., "Familial pheochromocytoma and renal cell carcinoma syndrome: *TMEM127* as a novel candidate gene for the association," *Virchows Archiv*, vol. 466, no. 6, pp. 727–732, 2015.

[8] L. Yao, F. Schiavi, A. Cascon et al., "Spectrum and prevalence of FP/*TMEM127* gene mutations in pheochromocytomas and paragangliomas," *JAMA*, vol. 304, no. 23, p. 2611, 2010.

[9] S. P. Toledo, D. M. Lourenço, T. Sekiya et al., "Penetrance and clinical features of pheochromocytoma in a six-generation family carrying a germline *TMEM127* mutation," *The Journal of Clinical Endocrinology & Metabolism*, vol. 100, no. 2, pp. E308–E318, 2015.

[10] C. Bruch, N. Dagres, H. Wieneke, C. Herborn, K. Brandt-Mainz, and R. Erbel, "Sinus node dysfunction with intermittent sinus arrest and AV-nodal escape rhythm as the first manifestation of pheochromocytoma," *Zeitschrift für Kardiologie*, vol. 91, no. 1, pp. 81–87, 2002.

[11] D. H. Streeten and G. H. Anderson, "Mechanisms of orthostatic hypotension and tachycardia in patients with pheochromocytoma," *American Journal of Hypertension*, vol. 9, no. 8, pp. 760–769, 1996.

[12] T. Majic and V. Aiyagari, "Cerebrovascular manifestations of pheochromocytoma and the implications of a missed diagnosis," *Neurocritical Care*, vol. 9, no. 3, pp. 378–381, 2008.

[13] H. P. Neumann, M. Sullivan, A. Winter et al., "Germline mutations of the *TMEM127* gene in patients with paraganglioma of head and neck and extraadrenal abdominal sites," *The Journal of Clinical Endocrinology & Metabolism*, vol. 96, no. 8, pp. E1279–E1282, 2011.

[14] N. Abermil, M. Guillaud-Bataille, N. Burnichon et al., "*TMEM127* screening in a large cohort of patients with pheochromocytoma and/or paraganglioma," *The Journal of Clinical Endocrinology & Metabolism*, vol. 97, no. 5, pp. E805–E809, 2012.

[15] G. Eisenhofer, J. Lenders, W. Timmers et al., "Measurements of plasma methoxytyramine, normetanephrine, and metanephrine as discriminators of different hereditary forms of pheochromocytoma," *Clinical Chemistry*, vol. 57, no. 3, pp. 411–420, 2011.

9

Solitary Intrathyroid Metastasis Occurring 23 Years after Resection of Renal Cell Carcinoma

X. Vandemergel

Department of Endocrinology, EpiCURA, Boussu, Belgium

Correspondence should be addressed to X. Vandemergel; vandemergel@hotmail.fr

Academic Editor: Osamu Isozaki

A case of solitary intrathyroid metastasis is described in a 60-year-old male patient. He had a history of renal cell carcinoma classified as T1b resected 23 years earlier. A mass was palpable in the right thyroid lobe. Ultrasound showed a hypoechoic polylobular nodule with intense vascularisation in the right lobe. Fine needle aspiration cytology was normal, but thyroidectomy was performed due to mass enlargement, the ultrasound pattern, and the oncological history. Histological examination revealed the presence of an intrathyroid metastasis of renal cell carcinoma. The bone scan and thoracoabdominal CT scan were normal. Postoperative care was uneventful.

1. Introduction

The four main types of primary thyroid cancer are papillary, follicular, medullary, and anaplastic carcinomas, and they represent the majority of newly diagnosed thyroid cancers [1]. The thyroid gland is a rare site of tumour metastasis. Metastatic thyroid tumours account for 1.4–3% of all thyroid neoplasms, are most often related to renal cell carcinoma (RCC) [2], and are frequently asymptomatic. Fine needle aspiration (FNA) is used for the cytological diagnosis of neoplastic lesions in most cases, but they may mimic a poorly differentiated thyroid cancer. We report here the case of a patient with a history of RCC 23 years before presentation, complaining of a palpable nodule in the right lobe. The nodule was classified as EU-TIRADS 5 based on ultrasound. FNA cytology revealed a benign nodule, but due to the ultrasound findings and the oncological history, a surgical procedure was performed. Histology revealed a metastasis of RCC. The patient gave written informed consent. A literature review was also conducted.

2. Case Report

A 60-year-old man was referred to our department of endocrinology for the evaluation of a neck mass. His past medical history included ischemic cardiomyopathy, hypertension, and hyperlipidaemia, and he underwent right nephrectomy 23 years earlier for RCC classified as stage 1 (T1b).

He smoked 20 cigarettes/day, and his treatment included statin, salicylic acid, angiotensin-converting enzyme inhibitor, and diltiazem.

In July 2019, he complained of a right cervical mass. Ultrasound (Figure 1) revealed a large hypoechoic polylobular nodule in the right lobe with a dense central vascularisation, classified as EU-TIRADS 5. FNA cytology was performed and showed normal cells and was classified as Bethesda 2.

The patient was lost to follow-up and came back in July 2020 with the same symptoms. There was no hoarseness. On clinical examination, the thyroid was enlarged and a hard nodule was palpable in the right lobe, without cervical adenopathy. Ultrasound found the same nodule measuring $42 \times 22 \times 28$ mm. There were no microcalcifications.

Biologically, the thyrotropin level was at 0.42 mU/L, the free T4 level was normal, and there were no thyroperoxidase antibodies. The thyroglobulin level was normal at 27 pg/L.

He underwent total thyroidectomy. The histopathological examination showed large clear cells positive for CD10, vimentin, CK19, and PAX 8 with lymphatic and venous metastasis (Figure 2). Thyroid Transcription Factor 1 (TTF1)

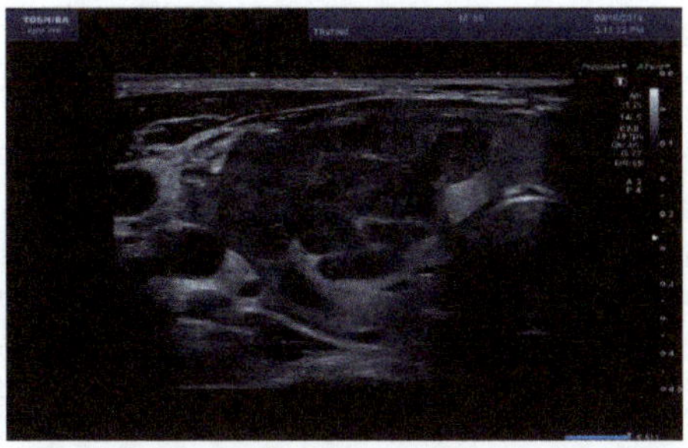

FIGURE 1: Thyroid ultrasound: linear probe and high frequency. Right lobe: hypoechoic polylobular nodule with intense intranodular vascularisation classified as EU-TIRADS 5.

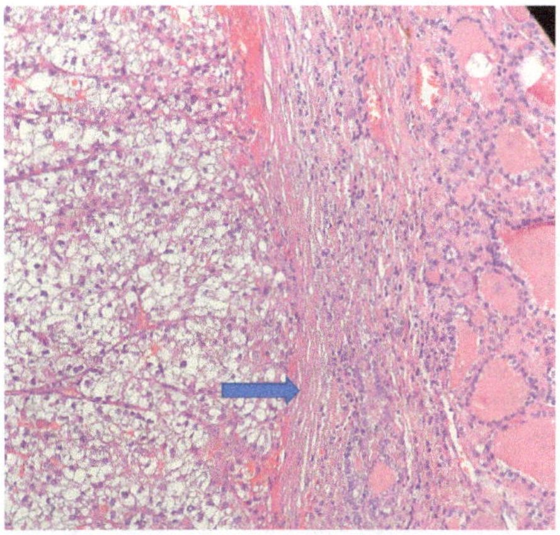

FIGURE 2: Hematoxylin-eosin staining showing large clear cells. A thin fibrovascular network is shown (arrow). Cells have an eosinophilic foamy vacuolated cytoplasm.

was completely negative, ruling out a primary tumour of the thyroid.

The postoperative course was uneventful, and bone scintigraphy and computed tomography also revealed the absence of any other metastases. External radiation completed the treatment. Radiation was delivered to a total dose of 50 Gy in 25 fractions at 2 Gy per day 5 days per week.

Six months later, the patient remained free of recurrence.

3. Discussion

Intrathyroid metastases (ITM) of RCC are very rare despite the fact that RCC are hypervascularised tumours associated with multiple arteriovenous shunts leading to the subsequent growth of metastases through the vascular route and that the thyroid is the second most vascularised organ after the adrenal gland [3]. While clinical ITM are rare, their prevalence in autopsied series varies between 1.25 and 24.4% in patients who died from primary or metastatic malignancies [4]. After the diagnosis of RCC, the risk of recurrence is higher in the first three years, and the local recurrence-free survival rate 15 years after surgery and the distant metastasis-free survival rate at 15 years have been estimated at 95% and 86%, respectively [5]. The risk factors associated with a late recurrence are the tumour stage, the tumour size, and RCC with clear cell histology. The most common sites of metastases are the lung, bone, and liver [6].

When present, thyroid metastases are often secondary to RCC. In a retrospective surgical series including 11 patients with thyroid metastases, Dequanter et al. found that they originated from an RCC in 2 cases, from a pulmonary squamous cell carcinoma in 5 cases, and from an oesophageal, oropharynx, or breast carcinoma and a leiomyosarcoma in 1 case each [7]. In 25 cases of ITM, Calzolari et al. [2] found that they originated from an RCC in 15 cases (60%) followed by lung and colonic cancers.

The symptoms include a palpable thyroid nodule, but ITM is often an incidental finding [2]. ITM may appear many years, or even decades, after the primary lesion, and times to onset ranging between a few months and more than 27 years have been reported [8].

Kobayashi et al. [9] studied the ultrasonographic features of metastatic RCC to the thyroid. Ten patients were included (4 men and 6 women) with a mean age at the time of thyroid surgery of 67 years. The primary site was the right kidney in 9 cases. The metastatic tumour was located in the right thyroid lobe in 9 cases and in the left lobe in 3 cases (two metastases in 2 cases). The tumour shape was irregular and well demarcated with a hypoechoic solid pattern without a capsule-like structure and direct contact with the normal thyroid tissue in all cases, classically classified as EU-TIRADS 5. There were no calcifications. The intratumour vascularity was intense in 8 cases. In our case, we found the same features. Also, while microcalcifications are rarely described, they may be present [10].

In most series, FNA cytology allowed diagnosing a neoplastic lesion in most cases. In the study by Calzolari et al. [2], FNA cytology revealed the presence of neoplastic cells in 8 out of 17 patients. Case reports have focused on the positivity of FNA cytology for the diagnosis of cancer [10–13]. In a series published by Dequanter, ten patients underwent preoperative FNA and the cytological results suggested a metastatic disease in nine of these patients. Bula et al. [14] assessed the usefulness of FNA cytology for the diagnosis of tumour metastases to the thyroid gland in 733 patients with thyroid cancer (metastatic tumours in 10 cases, 7 of them of RCC origin). In all cases, FNA cytology was abnormal and showed a follicular tumour in 3 cases, tumour cells in 2 cases, and atypical cells in the remaining patients. In the study by Kobayashi et al. [9], FNA cytology showed a metastatic carcinoma of RCC in 4 cases, an indeterminate nodule in 2 cases, a benign nodule in 3 cases, and a follicular neoplasm in 1 case for a total of 10 FNA performed. FNA cytology was strictly normal in our case, showing that despite normal FNA cytology, patient history and the ultrasound appearance of the lesion should be taken into account in the surgical decision making.

The 5-year overall survival of patients with ITM varies greatly depending on whether a single metastasis is present and only located in the thyroid or whether multiple metastases are present. In the study by Calzolari et al. [2], 50% of patients had a single ITM while 50% had multiple ITM. The actuarial 5-year overall survival was 31% (median: 48 months). The median survival of patients with multiple lesions was 30 months, and that of patients with a single metastasis in the thyroid gland was 60 months. Also, while the 5-year survival of patients with a single lesion was 48%, none of the patients with multifocal cancer was alive at 5 years.

Treatment is based on surgery. It is not known whether total thyroidectomy is always needed or if partial thyroidectomy may be useful in the management. Radiotherapy may be used for the treatment of RCC metastases [15] despite the fact that RCC have been shown to be radioresistant. It may be indicated in case of painful bone metastases, brain metastases, and painful recurrence in the renal bed [16, 17]. The usefulness of radiation is not established, but some case report concluded that irradiation may be effective at higher level of radiation [18–20].

In conclusion, we reported the case of a 60-year-old patient experiencing an isolated intrathyroid metastasis 23 years after resection of a right-sided renal cell carcinoma. Despite the usefulness of FNA cytology, the ultrasound pattern and the clinical history should be taken into account in the surgical decision making.

Acknowledgments

We thank Dr. S. Drisis and S. Saadi for pictures.

References

[1] F. Pacini, M. Schlumberger, H. Dralle et al., "European consensus for the management of patients with differentiated thyroid carcinoma of the follicular epithelium," *European Journal of Endocrinology*, vol. 154, no. 6, pp. 787–803, 2006.

[2] F. Calzolari, P. V. Sartori, C. Talarico et al., "Surgical treatment of intrathyroid metastasis: preliminary results of a multicentric study," *Anticancer Research*, vol. 28, pp. 2885–2888, 2008.

[3] R. C. R De Stefano, E. Zanni, D. Marchiori et al., "Anticancer research," *International Journal of Cancer Research and Treatment*, vol. 29, pp. 473–476, 2009.

[4] K. Wood, L. Vini, and C. Harmer, "Metastases to the thyroid gland: the royal marsden experience," *European Journal of Surgical Oncology*, vol. 30, no. 6, pp. 583–588, 2004.

[5] S. P. Kim, C. J. Weight, B. C. Leibovich et al., "Outcomes and clinicopathologic variables associated with late recurrence after nephrectomy for localized renal cell carcinoma," *Urology*, vol. 78, no. 5, pp. 1101–1106, 2011.

[6] B. Ljungberg, F. Alamdari, T. Rasmuson, and G. Ross, "Follow-up guidelines for nonmetastatic renall cell carcinoma based on the occurrence of metastases after radical nephrectomy," *BJU International*, vol. 84, pp. 405–411, 1999.

[7] D. Dequanter, P. Lothaire, D. Larsimont, N. d. S.-A. d. Somerhausen, and G. Andry, "Métastases intrathyroïdiennes: série de 11 cas," *Annales d'Endocrinologie*, vol. 65, no. 3, pp. 205–208, 2004.

[8] J. C. Janser, C. Rodier, J. Pusel, and D. Rodier, "Intrathyroidal metastases of a nephroepithelioma: reflections on 5 operated cases," *Journal de Chirurgie (Paris)*, vol. 123, pp. 574–577, 1986.

[9] K. Kobayashi, M. Hirokawa, T. Yabuta et al., "Metastatic carcinoma to the thyroid gland from renal cell carcinoma: role of ultrasonography in preoperative diagnosis," *Thyroid Research*, vol. 8, no. 1, p. 4, 2015.

[10] H. Seki, T. Ueda, Y. Shibata, Y. Sato, and N. Yagihashi, "Solitary thyroid metastasis of renal clear cell carcinoma: report of a case," *Surgery Today*, vol. 31, no. 3, pp. 225–229, 2001.

[11] A. Roux, A. M. Alzharani, C. Rousselot, P. Beutter, and D. Bakhos, "Late metastasis from renal cell carcinoma to the thyroid and nasal cavity: report of a case," *Revue de Laryngologie Otologie Rhinologie*, vol. 134, pp. 101–103, 2013.

[12] H. Chen, T. L. Nicol, and R. Udelsman, "Clinically significant, isolated metastatic disease to the thyroid gland," *World Journal of Surgery*, vol. 23, no. 2, pp. 177–181, 1999.

[13] J. Bertin, D. Rhamani, H. Maurice, and H. Pujol, "Intrathyroid metastasis of kidney cancer: a rare case and diagnostic trap," *Annales d'Endocrinologie*, vol. 60, pp. 45–47, 1999.

[14] G. Bula, J. Waler, A. Niemiec, H. Koziolek, and W. Bichaslki, "Diagnosis of metastatic tumours to the thyroid gland by fine needle aspiration biopsy," *Endokrynologia Polska*, vol. 61, pp. 427–429, 2016.

[15] S. Hosaka, H. Katagiri, M. Niwakawa et al., "Radiotherapy combined with zoledronate can reduce skeletal-related events in renal cell carcinoma patients with bone metastasis," *International Journal of Clinical Oncology*, vol. 23, no. 6, pp. 1127–1133, 2018.

[16] R. Finney, "The value of radiotherapy in the treatment of hypernephroma-a clinical trial," *British Journal of Urology*, vol. 45, no. 3, pp. 258–269, 1973.

[17] M. Kjaer, P. L. Frederiksen, and S. Engelholm, "Postoperative radiotherapy in stage II and III renal adenocarcinoma: a randomized trial by the copenhagen renal cancer study group," *International Journal of Radiation Oncology, Biology, Physics*, vol. 13, no. 5, pp. 665–672, 1987.

[18] V. Onuffrey and M. Mohiuddin, "Radiation therapy in the treatment of metastatic renal cell carcinoma," *International Journal of Radiation Oncology, Biology, Physics*, vol. 11, pp. 2007–2009, 1985.

[19] K. Riaz, M. A. Tunio, M. Alasiri, A. A. E. Mohammad, and M. M. Fareed, "Renal cell carcinoma metastatic to the thyroid gland, presenting like anaplastic carcinoma of the thyroid," *Case Reports in Urology*, vol. 2013, Article ID 651081, 4 pages, 2013.

[20] J. Cho, G. E. Kim, K. H. Rha et al., "Hypofractionated high-dose intensity-modulated radiotherapy (60 Gy at 2.5 Gy per fraction) for recurrent renal cell carcinoma: a case report," *Journal of Korean Medical Science*, vol. 23, no. 4, pp. 740–743, 2008.

10

Central Diabetes Insipidus Induced by Acute Myeloid Leukemia with DNMT3A Mutation

Priyanka Lakshmanan[1], **Heena Asnani**[2] **and David Knorr**[3]

[1]*Department of Medicine Mount Sinai Morningside, Mount Sinai West Icahn School of Medicine, New York, NY, USA*
[2]*Pravara Institute of Medical Sciences, Ahmednagar, India*
[3]*Memorial Sloan Kettering Cancer Center, New York, NY, USA*

Correspondence should be addressed to Priyanka Lakshmanan; priyanka.lakshmanan@mountsinai.org

Academic Editor: Osamu Isozaki

Central diabetes insipidus (CDI) is an uncommon complication of acute myeloid leukemia (AML). Patients present with polyuria either preceding or at the time of diagnosis of AML. We describe the case of a 36-year-old male who presented with a subacute onset of polyuria, polydipsia, nocturia, and fatigue. After an extensive workup, he was diagnosed with AML/CMML (chronic myelomonocytic leukemia) with a normal karyotype with DNMT3A, CBFB, and PTPN11 mutations. Further workup of the polyuria with a water deprivation test helped confirm the diagnosis of CDI along with MRI findings suggestive of hypophysitis. In this report, we analyze the clinical workup for AML and CDI and report the possibility of extramedullary leukemic infiltration associated with DNMT3A mutation, which has been reported as one of the mechanisms in the existing literature. We also discuss other theories hypothesized to cause CDI in AML patients with abnormal karyotypes. Our patient progressed to AML from CMML-2 after a cycle of decitabine, with confirmed gingival and presumed central nervous system (CNS) involvement. He is in minimal residual disease (MRD)-negative complete remission after induction with a CNS-active acute lymphoblastic leukemia-2 regimen. He also received double umbilical cord blood transplantation, conditioned with cyclophosphamide, fludarabine, thiotepa, and total body irradiation (TBI) of 4 Gy. This was complicated by engraftment syndrome for which he is currently being managed. CDI of the patient was corrected by desmopressin administration.

1. Introduction

Pituitary involvement has been reported in 0.6% of leukemia cases; however, because pituitary involvement and the presence of diabetes insipidus are not necessarily correlated, the true prevalence of leukemia-associated central diabetes insipidus is unknown [1]. Diabetes insipidus is a condition in which polyuria occurs as the body is unable to maintain the water balance due to either deficiency of ADH (antidiuretic hormone) which is secreted by the pituitary gland or resistance to ADH in the collecting duct of the kidneys. When it occurs in patients with acute leukemia; it is often a poor prognostic indicator [2]. The gene for ADH is located at the cytogenetic location 20p13; however, most reports of patients with acute myeloid leukemia (AML) and diabetes insipidus (DI) describe cytogenetic aberrations of chromosomes 3 and 7 such as inv (3) (q21.3q26.2) and monosomy 7 [2, 3]. Several mechanisms have been proposed to result in pituitary damage [4]. Certain antineoplastic agents have also been implicated in the causation of diabetes insipidus. Here, we report a unique case in which the patient developed central diabetes insipidus with acute myeloid leukemia.

2. Case Presentation

This is the case of a 36-year-old healthy male who presented with subacute onset of excessive fatigue, polydipsia, polyuria associated with nocturia, and cold intolerance. On initial workup, his urinalysis was normal with no signs of infection.

His complete blood count was significant for leukocytosis (white blood cell: 40,600/μL with 32% neutrophils and 17% blasts in peripheral blood), anemia (hemoglobin: 8.9 g/dl), and a normal platelet count. He was admitted and started on hydroxyurea 500 mg daily, and allopurinol 100 mg daily. A bone marrow aspirate (BMA) and biopsy were performed, and he was discharged on the same day. However, because of increased bleeding from the bone marrow site, he returned to the hospital the day after. The BMA/biopsy results were consistent with chronic myelomonocytic leukemia (CMML-2)/acute myeloid leukemia (AML) with normal karyotype with DNMT3A, CBFB, and PTPN11 mutations. After the course of hydroxyurea, the patient was started on decitabine. He also received continuous intravenous hydration with isotonic fluids and was noted to have a urine output amounting to 12–16 litres per day. The polyuria and polydipsia in conjunction with hypernatremia raised concerns for DI. At baseline, he had a serum osmolality of 297 mOsm/kg, a urine osmolality of 99 mOsm/kg, and the urine sodium was less than 20 mEq/L. The patient underwent a water deprivation test along with administration of one dose of desmopressin acetate (0.05 mg) following which his urine osmolality was found to be 260 mOsm/kg establishing a diagnosis of CDI. Further workup with an MRI (magnetic resonance imaging) of the brain showed focal nodular enhancement at the proximal pituitary infundibulum with a measured value of 0.4 cm with slight effacement of the infundibular recess. The pituitary gland also demonstrated heterogeneous enhancement, and these findings were collectively suggestive of hypophysitis. Additionally, there was a loss of the normal posterior pituitary high-intensity signal on a pre-enhanced T1WI which reflects decreased storage of vasopressin that has a T1-shortening effect in patients with CDI. He was treated with desmopressin and symptomatically improved in the coming months. His urine output during his initial inpatient admission amounted to almost 13-14 liters/day (while receiving maintenance intravenous fluids). With desmopressin, fluid restriction, and diligent follow-up by endocrinologists, his urine output decreased to 5-6 liters/day. He reported improvement in nocturia and polydipsia with the treatments. He also received pituitary radiation for secondary prophylaxis.

3. Discussion

AML is a hematologic malignancy contributing to a considerable number of cancer-related deaths. It accounts for approximately 25% of all leukemias in adults in the Western world. The malignancy typically shows 2 peaks in occurrence in early childhood and later adulthood. The etiology for most cases of AML is unclear. A few conditions associated with this neoplasm include genetic disorders (e.g., Down's syndrome, Li-Fraumeni syndrome, and Fanconi Syndrome), exposure to ionizing radiation, chemotherapeutic agents (alkylating agents), certain RNA retroviruses, and secondary AML in the context of a prior history of myelodysplastic syndromes [5].

The combination of AML and DI is unique, and the diagnosis of DI is mostly made either before the diagnosis of AML or at the time of diagnosis of AML [2, 6]. DI with AML is typical of pituitary origin which is supported by the fact that many patients respond to desmopressin [1, 2]. Antidiuretic hormone (ADH) such as vasopressin is produced in the supraoptic nucleus, and it is transported to the posterior pituitary via hypothalamic-neurohypophyseal fibers. DI may result because of infiltration, infarction, infection, hemorrhage, or thrombosis of the pituitary gland [7].

Typically, a bright spot is seen on T1-weighted MRI, due to vasopressin that is stored in the posterior pituitary. It is not necessary for all the patients with central diabetes insipidus (CDI) and AML to have MRI findings; however, patients can have a loss of the neurohypophysis (posterior pituitary) bright spot, which is suggestive of hypothalamic-pituitary dysfunction [2]. Although patients with AML in combination with CDI may have normal MRI findings, it is not necessary that AML patients who have infiltrates in the pituitary always develop CDI [1]. In the case described by Muller et al, the patient with an MRI previously showing absence of the bright spot of the neurohypophysis had reappearance of the bright spot after 2nd dose of induction therapy with FLAG-Ida protocol before allogeneic stem cell transplantation. This encouraged the idea that the infiltrating cells were destroyed due to chemotherapy implicating that infiltration of leukemic cells may be the cause of CDI in AML [8]. A similar finding was seen in our patient's MRI which was suggestive of hypophysitis, pointing towards leukemic infiltration of the posterior pituitary as the cause of CDI.

According to the report of Müller et al, out of 18 cases that were evaluated cytogenetically, 89% had abnormal chromosome 7, 44% had abnormal chromosome 3, and 39% had abnormalities of both chromosome 3 and 7 [8]. In another study conducted by Ladigan et al., cytogenetic analysis of 41/51 patients revealed that monosomy 7 was the most common abnormality, followed by inversion of chromosome 3. Many patients had abnormalities of both chromosomes simultaneously [2].

It is hypothesized that monosomy 7 may lead to abnormal expression of the neutrophil migration gene which causes neutrophil chemotaxis, in turn causing infiltration of the posterior pituitary leading to DI [1, 9]. Further data are needed to determine the role of other molecular phenotypic markers which contribute to leukemic infiltration.

Based on a study, 90% of ADH is bound to platelets, and only 10% is free in the plasma. This is consequential to ADH uptake by platelets from plasma [10]. It is hypothesized that inversion of chromosome 3 causes thrombocytosis due to overexpression of the EVI1 gene eventually leading to interference with ADH levels. When the platelet levels reach the baseline following treatment of the malignancy, the symptoms of DI subside. This stipulates another possible mechanism of DI induced by AML [2, 11, 12]. One case report of CDI with AML had a deletion of chromosome 20q. The latter has a role in the synthesis of ADH, oxytocin, and their carrier protein [7]. Although there has not been enough documentation of this aberration, it is a potential area for upcoming research.

A study by Xu et al. explored the possibility of extramedullary leukemic infiltration mediated by TWIST1 in patients with DNMT3A mutation (which was seen in our patient); however, a definite causal relationship is still unclear [13].

Cytogenetic abnormalities can be detected in approximately 50% to 60% of newly diagnosed AML [14]. Clinical, cytogenetic, and molecular factors have prognostic value. They also help predict treatment resistance which in turn guides therapeutic decisions [15]. A few examples of cytogenetics associated with unfavorable outcomes include monosomies or deletions of part or all of chromosomes 5 or 7 (−5/−7 AML), trisomy 8, and deletion of the long arm of chromosome 20 [14].

Analogously, CDI with AML is an unfavorable association and some reports have documented poor clinical outcomes [2, 6, 16]. Intensive induction chemotherapy and allogeneic stem cell transplantation have been proven to be beneficial in prolonging survival in a few cases [6]. Owing to the polyuria, inaccessibility to water, or inability to drink, patients may develop dehydration and hypotension and patients should be closely monitored for these side effects especially if they are scheduled to receive chemotherapy [1].

From a leukemia standpoint, he progressed to AML from CMML-2 after a cycle of decitabine, with confirmed gingival and presumed central nervous system (CNS) involvement. He is in minimal residual disease (MRD)-negative complete remission after induction with a CNS-active acute lymphoblastic leukemia-2 regimen with high dose cytarabine, mitoxantrone, and intrathecal methotrexate. Most recently, he received double umbilical cord blood transplantation, conditioned with cyclophosphamide, fludarabine, thiotepa, and total body irradiation (TBI) of 4 Gy. This was complicated by engraftment syndrome for which he is currently being managed.

4. Conclusion

Endocrine manifestations can be seen in patients with hematologic malignancies. They can be a direct consequence of the malignancy or because of certain chemotherapeutic agents. Their recognition is crucial for prompt management. CDI can be one of the manifestations of AML and carries both therapeutic and prognostic implications. CDI can be managed with desmopressin as seen with our patient. The role of intrathecal chemotherapy and radiation therapy in the pituitary needs to be explored further in adult patients with this presentation.

References

[1] P. Dy, P. Chua, J. Kelly, and S. Liebman, "Central diabetes insipidus in the setting of acute myelogenous leukemia," *American Journal of Kidney Diseases*, vol. 60, no. 6, pp. 998–1001, 2012.

[2] S. Ladigan, T. Mika, A. Figge et al., "Acute myeloid leukemia with central diabetes insipidus," *Blood Cells, Molecules, and Diseases*, vol. 76, pp. 45–52, 2019.

[3] M. Bardin, D. Ritchie, R. McLachlan, and C. J. Yates, "Acute myeloid leukaemia presenting with diabetes insipidus," *Internal Medicine Journal*, vol. 49, no. 6, pp. 785–788, 2019.

[4] Y. Ino, H. Tsurumi, T. Yamada, N. Murakami, H. Moriwaki, and Y. Muto, "Acute myelogenous leukemia with diabetes insipidus without desmopressin administration by anti-leukemic chemotherapy," *[Rinsho Ketsueki] The Japanese Journal of Clinical Hematology*, vol. 36, no. 12, pp. 1359–1364, 1995.

[5] B. Deschler and M. Lübbert, "Acute myeloid leukemia: epidemiology and etiology," *Cancer*, vol. 107, no. 9, pp. 2099–2107, 2006.

[6] S. L. Pritzl, D. R. Matson, M. B. Juckett, and D. J. Ciske, "Concurrent central diabetes insipidus and acute myeloid leukemia," *Case Reports in Hematology*, vol. 2021, Article ID 8898671, 5 pages, 2021.

[7] R. Sun, C. Wang, X. Zhong, and Y. Wu, "Diabetes insipidus as an initial presentation of myelodysplastic syndrome: diagnosis with single-nucleotide polymorphism array-based karyotyping," *Tohoku Journal of Experimental Medicine*, vol. 238, no. 4, pp. 305–310, 2016.

[8] C. I. Müller, M. Engelhardt, J. Laubenberger, R. Kunzmann, R. Engelhardt, and M. Lübbert, "Myelodysplastic syndrome in transformation to acute myeloid leukemia presenting with diabetes insipidus: due to pituitary infiltration association with abnormalities of chromosomes 3 and 7," *European Journal of Haematology*, vol. 69, no. 2, pp. 115–119, 2002.

[9] H. H. Lê, J. P. Lengelé, M. Henin, S. Toffoli, and P. Mineur, "Diabetes insipidus and acute myeloid leukemia harboring monosomy 7: report of two cases and literature review," *Acta Clinica Belgica*, vol. 76, no. 2, pp. 132–135, 2021.

[10] S. S. Nussey, V. T. Y. Ang, D. H. Bevan, and J. S. Jenkins, "Human platelet arginine vasopressin," *Clinical Endocrinology*, vol. 24, no. 4, pp. 427–433, 1986.

[11] M. Sonmez, N. Erkut, T. S. Tat, F. Celep, U. Cobanoglu, and H. O. Ersoz, "Can a high platelet count be responsible for diabetes insipidus in acute myelogenous leukemia with monosomy 7 and inversion 3 (q21q26)?" *International Journal of Hematology*, vol. 90, no. 2, pp. 273-274, 2009.

[12] H. Ma, J. Yang, B. Xiang, and Y. Jia, "Acute myeloid leukemia with monosomy 7, ectopic virus integration site-1 overexpression and central diabetes insipidus: a case report," *Oncology Letters*, vol. 9, no. 6, pp. 2459–2462, 2015.

[13] J. Xu, W. Zhang, X.-J. Yan et al., "DNMT3A mutation leads to leukemic extramedullary infiltration mediated by TWIST1," *Journal of Hematology and Oncology*, vol. 9, no. 1, p. 106, 2016.

[14] C. C. Kumar, "Genetic abnormalities and challenges in the treatment of acute myeloid leukemia," *Genes and Cancer*, vol. 2, no. 2, pp. 95–107, 2011.

[15] U. Y. Malkan, G. Gunes, A. Isik et al., "Rebound thrombocytosis following induction chemotherapy is an independent predictor of a good prognosis in acute myeloid leukemia patients attaining first complete remission," *Acta Haematologica*, vol. 134, no. 1, pp. 32–37, 2015.

[16] C. Castagnola, M. Morra, B. Bemasconi, C. Astori, S. Santagostino, and C. Bemasconi, "Acute myeloid leukemia and diabetes insipidus: results in 5 patients," *Acta Haematologica*, vol. 93, no. 1, 1995.

11

Thyroid-Associated Ophthalmopathy after Radioactive Iodine Therapy for Metastatic Follicular Thyroid Carcinoma

Daisuke Murayama,[1] **Soji Toda**,[1] **Yoichiro Okubo**,[2] **Hiroyuki Hayashi**,[3] **Ai Matsui**,[1] **Mio Yasukawa**,[1] **and Hiroyuki Iwasaki**[1]

[1]*Department of Breast and Endocrine Surgery, Kanagawa Cancer Center, 2-3-2 Nakao Asahi-ku, Yokohama, Kanagawa 241-8515, Japan*
[2]*Department of Pathology, Kanagawa Cancer Center, 2-3-2 Nakao Asahi-ku, Yokohama, Kanagawa 241-8515, Japan*
[3]*Department of Pathology, Yokohama Municipal Citizen's Hospital, 1-1 Mitsuzawanishicho Kanagawa-ku, Yokohama, Kanagawa 221-0855, Japan*

Correspondence should be addressed to Daisuke Murayama; murayama.dr@gmail.com

Academic Editor: Désirée Deandreis

Thyroid-associated ophthalmopathy (TAO) is an inflammation of the extraocular muscles and periorbital connective tissue caused by autoantibodies against common antigens to both the thyroid and orbit. The release of antigens and induction of hypothyroidism caused by radioactive iodine (RAI) therapy may exacerbate TAO. Here, we present the case of a 67-year-old-woman treated with RAI therapy for metastatic follicular thyroid carcinoma who presented with TAO during the course of sorafenib administration. Tg and TgAb levels were gradually decreased with sorafenib and lenvatinib treatment, and TAO was improved without any ophthalmologic treatment.

1. Introduction

Thyroid-associated ophthalmopathy (TAO) is an inflammation of the extraocular muscles and periorbital connective tissue caused by autoantibodies against common antigens to both the thyroid and orbit such as thyroid-stimulating hormone receptor (TSH-R) [1]. Several reports suggest that the release of antigens and induction of hypothyroidism caused by radioactive iodine (RAI) therapy may exacerbate TAO [2]. Sorafenib is an orally administered inhibitor of vascular endothelial growth factor receptor- (VEGFR-) 1, 2, and 3, RET, RAF, and platelet-derived growth factor receptor (PDGFR)-β [3]. Lenvatinib is also an orally administered inhibitor of VEGFR-1, -2, and -3, fibroblast growth factor receptor-1 to -4, PDGFR-α, RET, and KIT [4]. TAO after RAI for thyroid carcinoma after total thyroidectomy has been reported in a few studies [5–7]; however, the improvement in TAO during the course of sorafenib and lenvatinib treatment for metastases of RAI-refractory differentiated thyroid carcinoma after total thyroidectomy has not been reported.

2. Case Presentation

A 67-year-old-woman who presented with back pain was referred to our institution to evaluate the cause. Computed tomography (CT) revealed a thyroid tumor and multiple vertebral bone metastases (C5, L4, S1, and left acetabular cartilage) (Figure 1). Biopsy of L4 was performed, and pathological findings showed metastasis of follicular thyroid carcinoma. Denosumab was initiated to address multiple bone metastases, and the patient underwent total thyroidectomy and central neck dissection. Pathological diagnosis was poorly differentiated carcinoma derived from follicular thyroid carcinoma with minimal invasion (Figure 2). After the surgery, the patient received TSH-suppressive therapy with levothyroxine sodium hydrate 100 μg daily and treated with RAI therapy (3.7 GBq). However, no uptake was

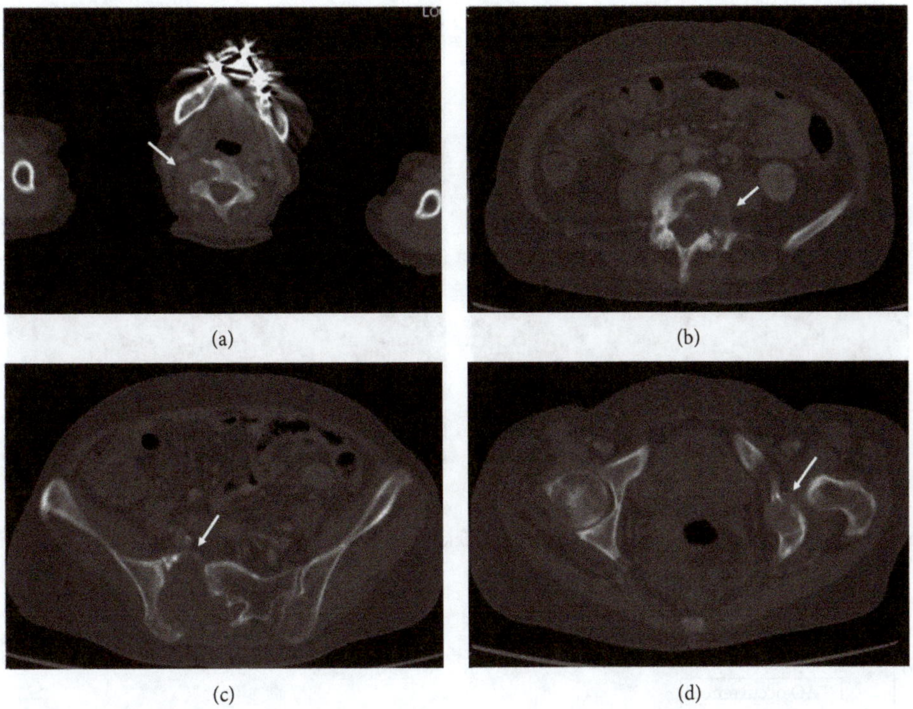

FIGURE 1: Computed tomography revealing bone metastasis (arrow). (a) C5, (b) L4, (c) S1, and (d) left acetabular cartilage.

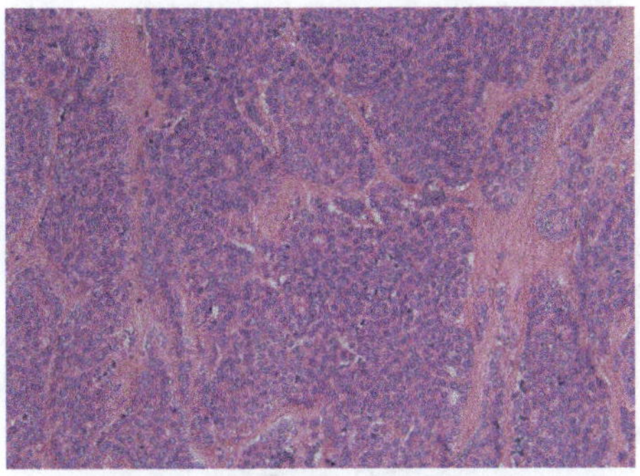

FIGURE 2: Pathological diagnosis of poorly differentiated carcinoma derived from follicular thyroid carcinoma with minimal invasion; Victoria Blue hematoxylin and eosin staining, 200x.

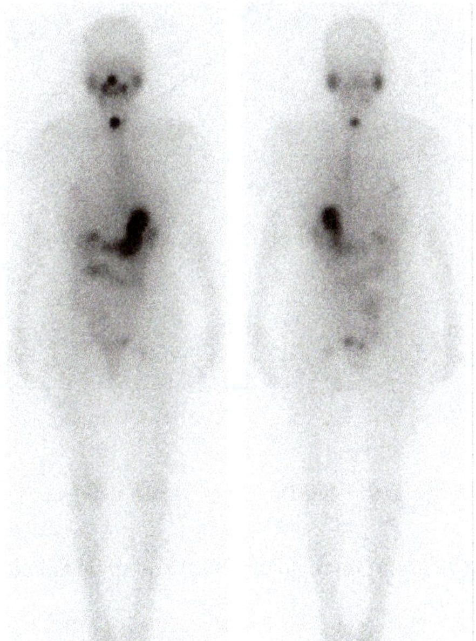

FIGURE 3: Iodine-131 scintigraphy after radioactive iodine therapy. No uptake was observed in the metastatic lesions.

observed in the metastatic lesions (Figure 3). Three months after RAI therapy, external beam radiation therapy (36 Gy/12F) was performed to the lumbar spine and sacrum. Six months after RAI, sorafenib 800 mg was initiated with gradually decreasing dosage because of diarrhea. One year after RAI, the patient presented with diplopia, and magnetic resonance imaging revealed a thickening of the right inferior rectus muscle (Figure 4). Laboratory data obtained the following findings: thyrotropin receptor antibody (TRAb) 11.8 IU/L, euthyroid, thyroglobulin (Tg) 37700 ng/mL, and thyroglobulin antibody (TgAb) 215 IU/L (the normal value of TRAb, Tg, and TgAb are 2.0 IU/L or less, 33.7 ng/mL or less, and 28.0 IU/mL or less, respectively). Lumbar puncture and cytology found no abnormalities, and the patient was diagnosed with TAO. Despite the recommendation of an ophthalmologist, she refused treatment for TAO. However, Tg and TgAb gradually decreased with sorafenib and lenvatinib administration, and TAO was improved two years after occurrence (Figure 5). At the time of TAO improvement, Tg and TgAb levels were 1620 ng/mL and 13 IU/L, respectively. During the course of treatment, no changes in bone metastasis were observed on CT.

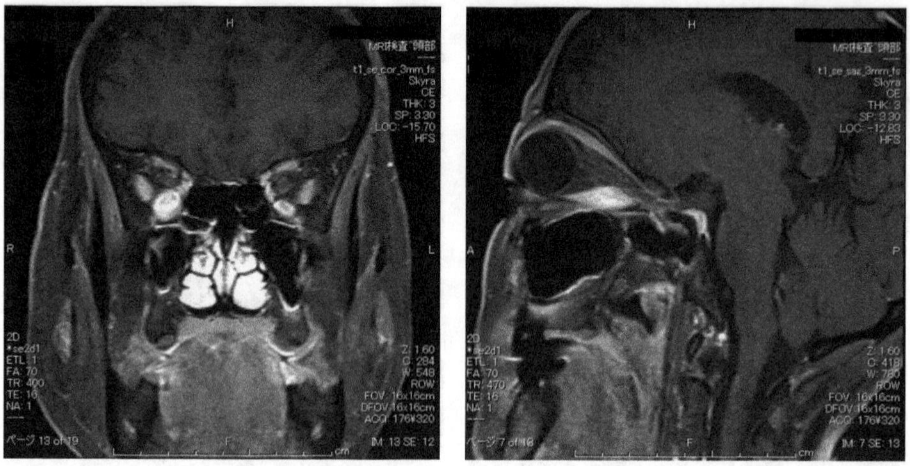

(a) (b)

Figure 4: Magnetic resonance imaging revealing thickening of the right inferior rectus muscle (asterisk).

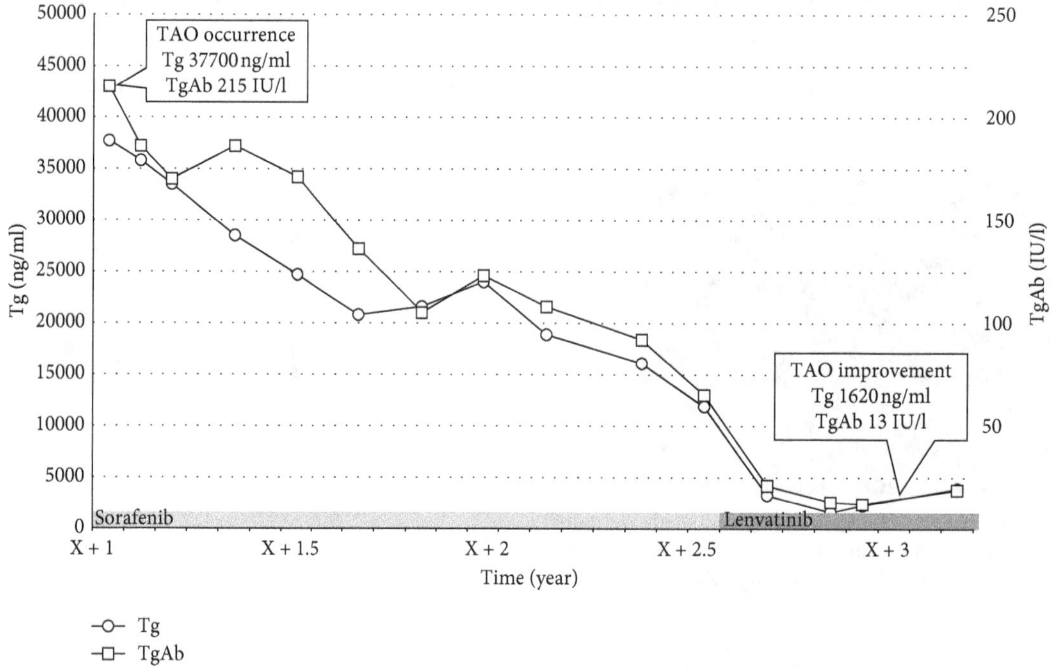

Figure 5: Change of thyroglobulin (Tg) and thyroglobulin antibody (TgAb) levels (from thyroid-associated ophthalmopathy occurrence to improvement).

3. Discussion

In 1967, Kriss et al. [8] initially reported the exacerbation of TAO after RAI therapy. Radiation injury appears to induce thyroid antigen leakage, leading to an increased production of TSH-R antibodies [9], which may cause orbital injury, since TSH-R is expressed in orbital tissue [10]. TAO may develop at any time 1–24 months after RAI for Grave's disease [11]. However, Bartalena and Tanda [12] reported that TAO may occur in patients with no thyroid dysfunction.

Only three case reports of TAO after RAI for thyroid carcinoma have been reported [5–7], and all were treated with an ablative dose (2.2 to 3.7 GBq). Despite the absence of thyroid tissue after total thyroidectomy for nonmetastatic thyroid carcinoma, TAO occurred after RAI [6, 7]. The time period from RAI to TAO onset is 3–34 years [5–7]. All three previous cases demonstrated no thyroid dysfunction, as with our case.

Lahooti et al. [13] reported a significant positive correlation between serum Tg levels and the presence and severity of ophthalmopathy in patients with Graves' disease. As for our case, the decline of thyroid antigen (Tg and TgAb) with sorafenib and lenvatinib administration resulted in TAO improvement (Figure 5). However, TRAb was evaluated only once at TAO onset, and we could not establish whether TRAb was improved with sorafenib and lenvatinib treatment.

In conclusion, our case presented with TAO after RAI. Tg and TgAb levels were gradually decreased with sorafenib and lenvatinib treatment, and TAO was improved without any ophthalmologic treatment.

Consent

Written informed consent was obtained from the patients for their anonymized information to be published in this article.

Acknowledgments

The authors would like to thank Enago (http://www.enago.com) for the English language review.

References

[1] I. M. M. J. Wakelkamp, O. Bakker, L. Baldeschi, W. M. Wiersinga, and M. F. Prummel, "TSH-R expression and cytokine profile in orbital tissue of active vs. inactive Graves' ophthalmopathy patients," *Clinical Endocrinology*, vol. 58, no. 3, pp. 280–287, 2003.

[2] F. Träisk, L. Tallstedt, M. Abraham-Nordling et al., "Thyroid-associated ophthalmopathy after treatment for Graves' hyperthyroidism with antithyroid drugs or iodine-131," *The Journal of Clinical Endocrinology and Metabolism*, vol. 94, no. 10, pp. 3700–3707, 2009.

[3] M. S. Brose, C. M. Nutting, S. I. Sherman et al., "Rationale and design of decision: a double-blind, randomized, placebo-controlled phase III trial evaluating the efficacy and safety of sorafenib in patients with locally advanced or metastatic radioactive iodine (RAI)-refractory, differentiated thyroid cancer," *BMC Cancer*, vol. 11, no. 1, p. 349, 2011.

[4] M. Schlumberger, M. Tahara, L. J. Wirth et al., "Lenvatinib versus placebo in radioiodine-refractory thyroid cancer," *New England Journal of Medicine*, vol. 372, no. 7, pp. 621–630, 2015.

[5] P. B. Rogers, N. Gupta, G. E. Rose, and P. N. Plowman, "Thyroid eye disease associated with athyria," *British Journal of Ophthalmology*, vol. 84, no. 4, p. 439, 2000.

[6] A. Antonelli, P. Fallahi, S. Tolari, S. M. Ferrari, and E. Ferrannini, "Thyroid-associated ophthalmopathy and TSH receptor autoantibodies in nonmetastatic thyroid cancer after total thyroidectomy," *The American Journal of the Medical Sciences*, vol. 336, no. 3, pp. 288–290, 2008.

[7] L. Giovansili, G. Cayrolle, G. Belange, G. Clavel, and M.-L. Herdan, "Graves' ophthalmopathy after total thyroidectomy for papillary carcinoma," *Annales d'Endocrinologie*, vol. 72, no. 1, pp. 42–44, 2011.

[8] J. P. Kriss, V. Pleshakov, A. L. Rosenblum, M. Holderness, G. Sharp, and R. Utiger, "Studies on the pathogenesis of the ophthalmopathy of Graves' Disease1," *The Journal of Clinical Endocrinology & Metabolism*, vol. 27, no. 4, pp. 582–593, 1967.

[9] K. A. Ponto, S. Zang, and G. J. Kahaly, "The tale of radioiodine and Graves' orbitopathy," *Thyroid*, vol. 20, no. 7, pp. 785–793, 2010.

[10] A. Feliciello, I. Ciullo, G. F. Fenzi, G. Bonavolontà, A. Porcellini, and E. V. Avvedimento, "Expression of thyrotropin-receptor mRNA in healthy and Graves' disease retro-orbital tissue," *The Lancet*, vol. 342, no. 8867, pp. 337-338, 1993.

[11] S. H. Acharya, A. Avenell, S. Philip, J. Burr, J. S. Bevan, and P. Abraham, "Radioiodine therapy (RAI) for Graves' disease (GD) and the effect on ophthalmopathy: a systematic review," *Clinical Endocrinology*, vol. 69, no. 6, pp. 943–950, 2008.

[12] L. Bartalena and M. L. Tanda, "Graves' ophthalmopathy," *New England Journal of Medicine*, vol. 360, no. 10, pp. 994–1001, 2009.

[13] H. Lahooti, T. Shanmuganathan, B. Champion, and J. R. Wall, "Serum thyroglobulin levels in patients with thyroid autoimmunity with and without ophthalmopathy or isolated upper eyelid retraction," *Trends in Immunology*, vol. 3, pp. 22–27, 2015.

12

Ectopic Cushing's Syndrome Unveiling a Metastatic Parotid Carcinoma

Sofia Castro Oliveira,[1,2,3] João Sérgio Neves,[1,2,3] Pedro Souteiro,[1,2,3] Sandra Belo,[1] Ana Isabel Oliveira,[1] Helena Moreira,[4] Paulo Mergulhão Gomes,[4] Lígia Coelho,[5] Cristina Sarmento,[6] Elsa Fonseca,[2,7,8] Celestino Neves,[1,2] Paula Freitas,[1,2,3] and Davide Carvalho[1,2,3]

[1]*Department of Endocrinology, Diabetes and Metabolism, Centro Hospitalar Universitário de São João (CHSJ), Porto, Portugal*
[2]*Faculty of Medicine of Universidade do Porto (FMUP), Porto, Portugal*
[3]*Instituto de Investigação e Inovação em Saúde, Universidade do Porto (i3S), Porto, Portugal*
[4]*Unidade Polivalente de Cuidados Intermédios Geral (UPCIG), Centro Hospitalar Universitário de São João (CHSJ), Porto, Portugal*
[5]*Department of Maxillofacial Surgery, Centro Hospitalar Universitário de São João (CHSJ), Porto, Portugal*
[6]*Department of Medical Oncology, Centro Hospitalar Universitário de São João (CHSJ), Porto, Portugal*
[7]*Department of Pathology, Centro Hospitalar Universitário de São João (CHSJ), Porto, Portugal*
[8]*Instituto de Patologia e Imunologia Molecular, Universidade do Porto (IPATIMUP), Porto, Portugal*

Correspondence should be addressed to Sofia Castro Oliveira; sofiacastro.oliveira@gmail.com

Academic Editor: Michael P. Kane

Introduction. Adrenocorticotropic hormone (ACTH) ectopic production is a rare cause of Cushing syndrome (CS). The most commonly associated tumours are small-cell lung carcinoma along with bronchial and thymic carcinoids. To date, only 5 cases have been published in the literature featuring ectopic ACTH secretion from metastatic acinic cell carcinoma (ACC) of the parotid gland. We hereby describe a very uncommon case of ectopic CS (ECS) unveiling a metastatic parotid ACC. *Case Presentation.* A 46-year-old man with hypertension and dyslipidemia diagnosed 4-months before, as well as new-onset diabetes mellitus unveiled 1-month earlier, was referred to emergency department for hypokalemia. Hormonal study and dynamic biochemical tests performed indicated ECS. Imaging and cytological findings pointed toward a likely primary right parotid malignancy with liver metastases. Somatostatin receptor scintigraphy has shown an increased uptake in the parotid gland and mild expression in liver metastasis. The patient underwent right parotidectomy, and histopathologic examination confirmed ACC. Meanwhile, hypercortisolism was managed with metyrapone, ketoconazole, and lanreotide. Despite chemotherapy onset, a rapid disease progression and clinical course deterioration was observed. *Conclusion.* The present report highlights a rare ECS, exposing a metastatic parotid ACC, with an aggressive and challenging clinical course, representing the first case whose diagnosis of ECS came prior to ACC.

1. Introduction

Adrenocorticotropic hormone (ACTH) ectopic production is a rare cause of Cushing syndrome (CS), accounting for only 6% of the cases in a recent multicenter study [1, 2]. The most commonly associated tumours are small-cell lung carcinoma (SCLC) along with bronchial and thymic carcinoids [3, 4]. To date, to the best of our knowledge, only 5 cases have been published in the literature featuring ectopic ACTH secretion from metastatic acinic cell carcinoma (ACC) of the parotid gland. In fact, primary ACC springing up from salivary glands represents a very uncommon, typically low-grade malignant tumour, accounting for 1%–6% of the salivary neoplasms and 15% of all parotid gland malignancies [5–7]. ACC affects mainly mid-age females, metastasize in about 10% of the cases and 35% tends to recur, with a 5-year disease-associated mortality usually less than 10% [5, 7].

We hereby report a rare case of an ectopic CS (ECS) unveiling a metastatic parotid ACC, with an aggressive and defiant clinical course.

Table 1: Hormonal profile.

	Hormonal study	Initial Assessment	After 1-month follow-up	After 1-month tumour ressection	Reference values
Morning	ACTH	206.8	422.3	200.7	<63.3 ng/L
	Cortisol	30.1	54.7	4.4	6.2–19.4 μg/dL
Midnight	Serum cortisol	36.2	36.7	—	<7.5 μg/dL
	Salivary cortisol	4.15	13.4	<0.018	<0.32 μg/dL
	24h-UFC	6210.0	11068.2	14.9	36–137 μg/24h
	1 mg overnight dexamethasone suppression test	42.6	—	—	<1.8 ug/dL

ACTH: adrenocorticotropic hormone; 24h-UFC: 24h-urinary free cortisol.

Table 2: Low- and high-dose dexamethasone suppression tests.

	Low-dose dexamethasone test			High-dose dexamethasone test		End	Reference values
	Baseline	Day 1	Day 2	Day 3	Day 4	Day 5	
Cortisol 8 a.m.	38.3	44.7	44.6	36.9	32.2	32.0	6.2–19.4 μg/dL
Cortisol 16 p.m.	38.1	47.5	38.2	36.5	28.7	—	
ACTH 8 a.m.	209.2	268.3	247.9	228.1	197.3	215.9	<63.3 ng/L
ACTH 16 p.m.	198.8	242.1	181.2	201.7	250.9	—	
24-h UFC	6900.3	3425.4	4148.0	3898.0	3097.7	—	36.0–137.0 μg/24h

ACTH: adrenocorticotropic hormone; 24 h-UFC: 24 h-urinary free cortisol.

2. Case Presentation

We describe a case of a 46-year-old man with hypertension and dyslipidemia diagnosed 4-months before, as well as new-onset diabetes mellitus (DM) unveiled 1 month earlier (on oral anti-diabetic drugs), referred to emergency department for hypokalemia of 2.5 mEq/L [reference value (RV): 3.5–5.1]. He had paresthesias, weakness, anorexia, and asthenia associated with a marked weight loss (about 10 kg) for over a month, along with a suspicion of endogenous hypercortisolism [morning ACTH 146.0 ng/L (RV: 9.0–52.0) and cortisol 44.5 μg/dL (RV: 5.0–25.0)] on ambulatory analysis. The patient also presented mild peripheral oedema, in the absence of striae or typical central obesity. He was then admitted to the Endocrinology department for further investigation.

Hormonal study revealed a midnight serum cortisol level of 36.2 ug/dL (RV: <7.5), midnight salivary cortisol 4.2 ug/dL (RV: <0.3) and 24 h-urinary free cortisol (UFC) 6210.0 ug/24 h (RV: 36.0–137.0). The result of 1 mg overnight dexamethasone suppression test was 42.6 ug/dL (RV: <1.8) (Table 1). The remaining biochemical assessment indicated serum potassium level of 3.0 mEq/L (RV: 3.5–5.1), with no other relevant changes. We subsequently performed a low-dose dexamethasone suppression test, which was compatible with CS, and a further high-dose dexamethasone suppression test showed no suppression of cortisol levels (Table 2).

Initial abdominal ultrasound found multiple nodular lesions in right hepatic lobe, the largest with 65 mm diameter, suggestive of secondary lesions by neoplastic process. Cervico-thoraco-abdominal computed tomography (CT) scan exposed a 16 × 1 × 17 mm nodular image on the right

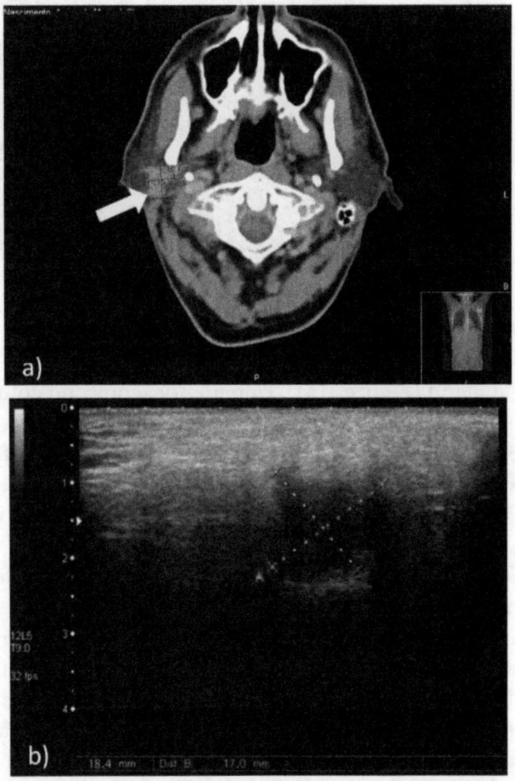

Figure 1: Cervico-thoraco-abdominal CT scan exposed a 16 × 1 × 17 mm nodular image on the right parotid gland (a); Parotid ultrasound documented a non specific 18 mm hypoechogenic nodule in the right parotid gland, with no signs of vascular invasion and no cervical adenomegalies (b).

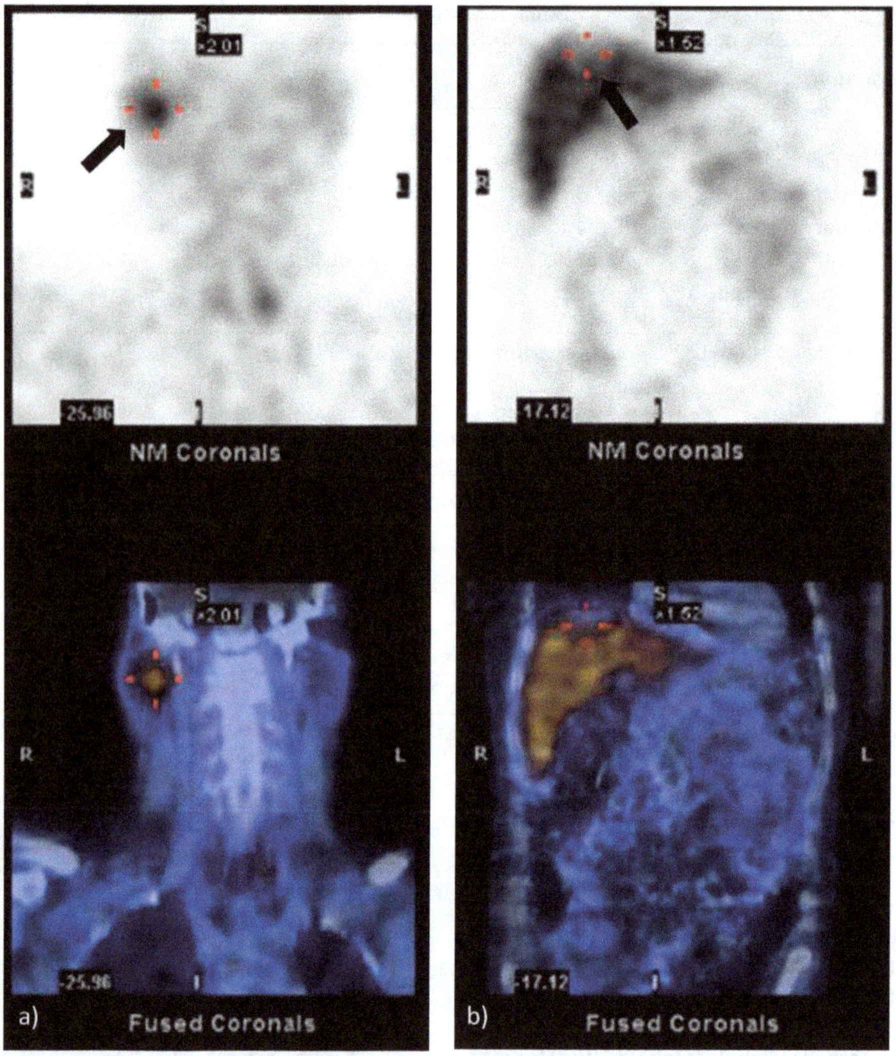

FIGURE 2: Octreoscan revealed increased uptake in the parotid gland (a) and mild expression in liver metastases (b).

parotid gland (Figure 1(a)). Upper endoscopy and colonoscopy showed no significant lesions. Parotid ultrasound, subsequently performed, documented a non specific 18 mm hypoechogenic nodule in the right parotid gland, with no signs of vascular invasion or cervical adenomegalies (Figure 1(b)).

Notably, parotid fine-needle aspiration biopsy revealed carcinoma (primary or metastatic), raising the suspicion of an ACC. A deeper investigation was carried out, with cervical magnetic resonance imaging (MRI) revealing a $17 \times 17 \times 20$ mm spiculated nodule in the superficial lobe of the right parotid, immediately posterior to the mandible angle, with a marked contrast-uptake; in addition, a 9 mm well-circumscribed nodule in the deeper planes of the left submandibular gland was reported, without malignancy features; no other cervical lesions were observed. Liver biopsy confirmed malignancy, with overlapping morphological features of the parotid cytology. Somatostatin receptor scintigraphy (Octreoscan) demonstrated an increased uptake in the parotid gland (Figure 2(a)), whereas liver metastases exhibited mild expression (Figure 2(b)). Meanwhile, ^{68}Gallium (^{68}Ga)-Positron emission tomography (PET) showed no uptake.

The patient underwent right parotidectomy, with concomitant right supraomohyoid neck dissection and left submaxillectomy. The postoperative period was complicated by local hematoma with airway compromise, requiring surgical reintervention which, subsequently, led to an altered state of consciousness. In face of a normal brain CT, a psychosis associated with hypercortisolism was considered. In addition, he also presented infection of the surgical site, solved after antibiotherapy course.

Pathologic examination showed an ACC: solid patterned neoplasia, without glandular features or evidence of mucin secretion, composed by cells with extensive acinic differentiation demonstrated by the presence of diastase-resistant PAS-positive zymogen granules that were immunoreactive for cytokeratins 8/18, DOG1, beta-catenin, and cyclin D1; Ki67 index 70%. There was no evidence of neuroendocrine differentiation (the neoplastic cells were immunonegative for chromogranin A and synaptophysin.). Immunoexpression of ACTH was not detected (Figure 3). Pathologic TNM staging: pT3N0R1.

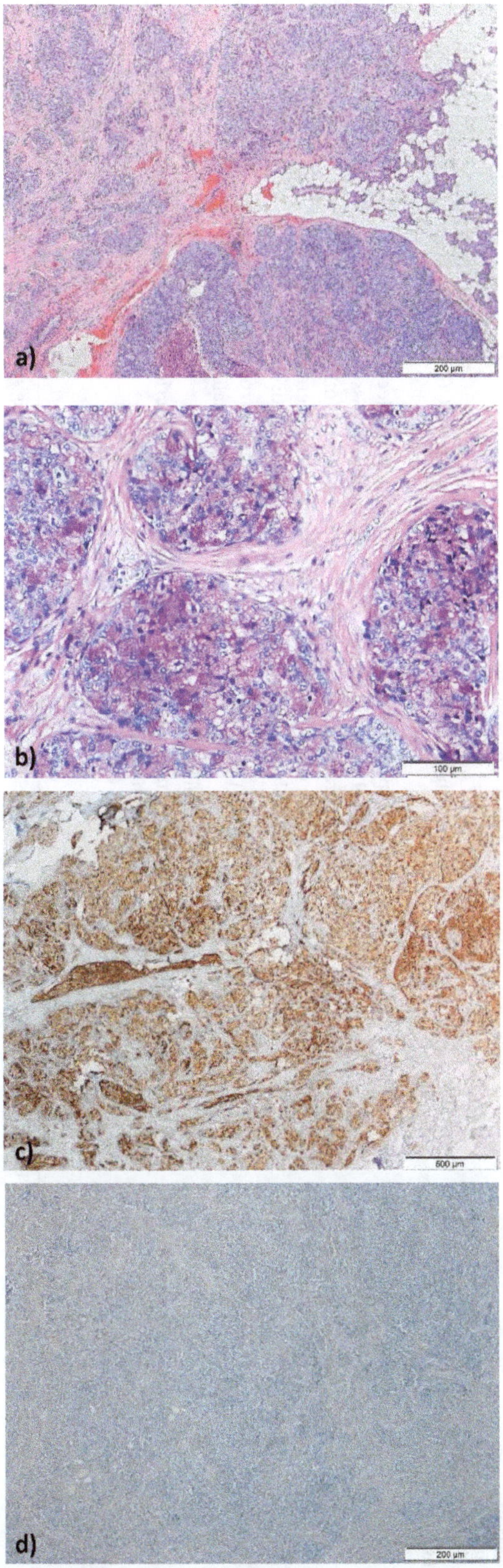

Figure 3: Histology–ACC: solid pattern and necrosis (H&E staining) (a); typical acinar cells with diastase-resistant PAS-positive granules (PAS-D staining) (b). The tumour cells showed strong immunoreactivity for DOG1 (c), being negative for ACTH immunostaining (d). ACC: acinic cell carcinoma; H&E: hematoxylin and eosin; PAS: periodic acid–schiff; PAS-D: PAS–diastase; DOG1: discovered on GIST-1; ACTH: adrenocorticotropic hormone.

Imaging reevaluation indicated disease progression with, additionally, multiple bone metastases in vertebral column. Thereafter, chemotherapy was started with a weekly paclitaxel-carboplatin regimen and hypercortisolism was managed with metyrapone (3 g/day), ketoconazole (400 mg/day) and lanreotide (120 mg/month). Further, high insulin doses were required to maintain an acceptable glycemic control. Posterior to case discussion at multidisciplinary team meeting, the patient was proposed to radiotherapy of symptomatic spinal metastases. Afterwards, a rapid disease progression was depicted by cervico-thoraco-abdominal CT with hepatic, bone, adrenal, and ganglionar metastases. At that time, it was decided to switch chemotherapy regimen to oral vinorelbine in monotherapy. However, in face of the clinical worsening, that treatment was withdrawn and the patient was referred to palliative care. As his condition progressively deteriorated, he eventually passed away, 15-months after initial diagnosis.

3. Discussion

The authors describe an ECS emerging as a paraneoplastic feature, exposing a metastatic parotid ACC, with a challenging and fierce outcome.

Endogenous CS is a rare endocrine entity, with evidence pointing toward an annual incidence of 0.2–5 cases per million people, being about 80% of the cases ACTH-dependent forms [1, 8]. Among these, pituitary corticotroph adenoma (Cushing's disease) is the most common, with extrapituitary (ectopic) tumours standing for up to 20% [9]. Recent data from the large ERCUSYN cohort, points out that only 6% of total CS cases was caused by ectopic ACTH secretion [2]. SCLC along with pancreatic, thymic and bronchial neuroendocrine tumours (NETs) accounts for the majority of ECS cases. Other less frequently associated tumours comprise medullary carcinoma of thyroid, pheochromocytoma, gastroenteropancreatic and genitourinary tumours [3, 4, 10]. Noteworthy, parotid origin is extremely rare, with only 5 cases drawn in the literature so far (summarized on Table 3) [10–14].

Salivary gland carcinomas constitute rare malignant tumours comprising a diverse set of histopathology features [7]. These entities can be classified as either high-grade or low-grade tumours such as salivary duct carcinomas and conventional ACC, respectively [7]. Among the latter, mostly springs up from the major glands, with about 80% arising in the parotid gland [15]. In effect, parotid ACC is typically a slow-growing tumour, albeit owing the potential to recur locally or metastasize, with the lung, bone and liver typifying the commonest locations affected [15]. The 5-year disease-associated mortality ranges from 1.3% to 26% in the available literature [15].

Whilst parotid ACC etiology is yet to be fully disclosed, ionizing radiation and familiar predisposition represent well-established risk factors [6]. Further, long-term studies have suggested that genetic alterations, environmental triggers, several viruses, and endogenous hormones may also play a role in ACC pathogenesis [6]. Pathological diagnosis stands on the identification of acinic cell differentiation (polyedric cells with abundant basophilic cytoplasm containing diastase-resistant

TABLE 3: Brief summary of the five cases previously published in the literature featuring ectopic ACTH secretion from metastatic ACC of the parotid gland.

	Case 1 [11]	Case 2 [12]	Case 3 [13]	Case 4 [14]	Case 5 [10]
Age (years)	44	62	60	52	60
Sex (M/F)	M	F	M	F	F
Clinical features at presentation	Nervousness, insomnia, night sweats, nocturia, oedema, wasting, weakness, flushed and puffy face, cutaneous hyperpigmentation	Oedema, progressing fatigue, central obesity, mild hypertension	Acute confusional state, paranoid behaviour, hallucinations, oedema	Weakness, wasting, moon-like facies, buffalo hump, supraclavicular fat pads, thin skin, livedo reticularis, hypertension	Fatigue, oedema, weakness, central obesity, plethoric face, thin skin, purplish abdominal striae, exacerbated hypertension
Initial laboratory test	Exacerbated hyperglycemia, hypokalemia and metabolic alkalosis	Glucose intolerance, severe hypokalemia and metabolic alkalosis	Hypokalemia and metabolic alkalosis	Hypokalemia and metabolic alkalosis	Hypokalemia
Serum cortisol (μg/dL)	118 (RV: 12–18) (*morning*)	49.2 (RV: NA) (*morning*)	57.1 (RV:6.2–19.4) (*morning*)	171.6 (RV: <1.8) (*midnight*)	—
Morning serum ACTH (ng/L)	547 (RV: <120)	153 (RV: NA)	106 (RV: <40)	810 (RV: 10–50)	106 (RV: 7–63)
24h-UFC (μg/24h)	10700 (RV: 20–90)	—	5572.5 (RV: 7.2–32.6)	7720.4 (RV: <54.4)	1624.2 (RV: <52.9)
1 mg overnight dexamethasone suppression test (μg/dL)	97.0	—	—	—	28.5
Low- and high-dose dexamethasone suppression tests	—	—	Low-dose: positive	—	Low-dose: positive
Moment of ECS diagnosis	12 months after ACC diagnosis	7 months after ACC diagnosis	2 months after ACC diagnosis	6 months after ACC diagnosis	36 months after ACC diagnosis
Treatment	(i) Total parotidectomy combined with left radical neck dissection; radiotherapy 9 months later for local recurrence (ii) No steroidogenesis inhibitors employed	(i) Right total parotidectomy with sacrifice of the facial nerve and right facial sling; postoperative radiotherapy (ii) No steroidogenesis inhibitors employed	(i) Left parotidectomy and radical neck dissection; postoperative radiotherapy; palliative chemotherapy with gemcitabine and docetaxel (ii) Metyrapone	(i) Total parotidectomy with right neck dissection; postoperative radiotherapy; palliative chemotherapy with single-agent doxorubicin (ii) Ketoconazole, somatostatin analogues	(i) Surgical resection (information about neck dissection or adjuvant therapy NA) (ii) Metyrapone
Clinical course	Rapid clinical deterioration	Rapid clinical deterioration	Clinical and biochemical improvement after 2 cycles of chemotherapy	Rapid clinical deterioration	Rapid clinical deterioration
Time from ECS diagnosis to disease-associated death (weeks)	6	4	NA	3	NA

ACTH: adrenocorticotropic hormone; ACC: acinic cell carcinoma; M/F: male/female; RV: reference value; 24h-UFC: 24h-urinary free cortisol; ECS: ectopic Cushing syndrome; NA: not available.

PAS–positive zymogen granules), similar to the serous cellular elements found in the normal parotid gland [5, 7, 16]. These are epithelial pancytokeratin–positive cells characteristically immunoreactive for DOG1 antibody [16]. No molecular features are described as typical for ACC. High-grade transformation is a rare variant of ACC, anchoring an aggressive clinical behaviour and outcome [17]. Strong membrane beta-catenin and nuclear cyclin D1 immunoreactions have been associated with aggressive high-grade ACCs [16]. Empirical evidence has also shown that poor prognosis relies on blood vessel involvement, invasion to adjacent tissue, undifferentiated histological pattern, facial nerve involvement, and lymph node metastasis [18]. Surgical resection is the mainstay treatment; however, adjuvant radiotherapy may be advised for recurrent and undifferentiated tumours, with positive margins and locoregional dissemination [6]. Radiation monotherapy has also demonstrated effective results, mostly for inoperable tumours [6]. In addition, chemotherapy may be a useful therapeutic tool in cases of advanced ACC [7]. Nevertheless, current literature regarding the chemotherapy regimen of choice for parotid ACC is scarce, given the few cases depicted worldwide [7].

Our case remarkably reports a distinct presentation of parotid ACC, revealed by an ECS. The initial clinical hallmarks were classic of CS from ectopic ACTH-producing tumours, since this patient featured wasting, weakness, asthenia, peripheral oedema, hypertension, severe hypokalemia, and glucose intolerance. Moreover, the rapid onset and progression of symptoms along with the severity of endogenous hypercortisolism has increased the suspicion index, required to an early ECS diagnosis. Dynamic biochemical tests subsequently performed were concordant and confirmed the diagnosis. At this regard, one should bear in mind that ECS frequently represents an arduous diagnostic challenge as none of the biochemical parameters achieves 100% accuracy, and bilateral inferior petrosal sinus sampling (BIPSS) is often necessary, being considered the most reliable tool [3, 19].

Since the election treatment for ECS stands in complete resection of the tumour, localizing the source of ACTH production is crucial and remains a defiant endeavor for the majority of patients, even so for about 12% the source may not be identified [10]. As no single imaging modality has an ideal accuracy, it is recommended to add more than one imaging technique such as conventional CT, MRI, somatostatin receptor scintigraphy, or PET scan [19]. In this patient, a cervico-thoraco-abdominal CT scan revealed the parotid tumour, further depicted by MRI, also confirming liver metastasis. Additionally, octreoscan showed increased uptake in the parotid gland and mild expression in hepatic metastasis, albeit no uptake was observed in ^{68}Ga-PET.

The histological and immunohistochemical examination of surgical specimen revealed an ACC with negative immunostaining for ACTH. At this respect, negative ACTH staining in malignant ectopic Cushing's tumours is thought to be related with a more aggressive pattern and worse prognosis [10, 20]. In effect, tumours owning a high ACTH secretory rate, with concomitant secretion of precursor fragments, can become depleted of its intracellular ACTH leading to a negative immunostaining, even though these patients exhibit high ACTH circulating levels, which may have been the case of our patient [20]. Moreover, herein a marked hypercortisolism was observed adding to the progressive clinical deterioration and adverse outcome. Accordingly, several lines of evidence point out that hypercortisolemia level is also strictly correlated with prognosis of ACTH secreting tumour [1]. Given the severity of hypercortisolism, the patient was kept under metyrapone, ketoconazole, and lanreotide. Actually, medical therapy is often warranted in order to control ECS, mainly until surgery. Current evidence indicates that adrenal steroidogenesis inhibitors as ketoconazole or metyrapone are preferred for their efficacy and safety. Somatostatin analogs have also been used to treat ECS, with controverse results [1]. Meanwhile, bilateral adrenalectomy was not performed in our patient since his clinical condition worsened, increasing the surgical risk. A rapid disease progression was documented despite the instituted chemotherapy, with a downhill clinical course.

In conclusion, the present case highlights an ECS unveiling a metastatic parotid ACC, with an aggressive and defiant behaviour. Noteworthy, contrary to the 5 previous cases published in the literature so far, this report represents the first in whose diagnosis of ECS came prior to ACC. Actually, since there are only few related cases depicted worldwide, current available literature is scarce and its pathophysiology has yet to be fully disclosed, standing this condition as a huge diagnostic and therapeutic challenge. Therefore, sharing these very uncommon cases may broad the knowledge to provide, in the future, a more comprehensive patient care.

Consent

The authors state that written informed consent was obtained from the patient's next of kin (since the case relates to a deceased person) for the publication of this case report.

Acknowledgments

Thanks are due to the Nuclear Medicine and Radiology Departments of Centro Hospitalar Universitário de São João (CHSJ), Porto, Portugal.

References

[1] A. Deldycke, C. Haenebalcke, and Y. Taes, "Paraneoplastic Cushing syndrome, case-series and review of the literature," *Acta Clinica Belgica*, vol. 73, no. 4, pp. 298–304, 2018.

[2] E. Valassi, H. Franz, T. Brue et al., "Diagnostic tests for Cushing's syndrome differ from published guidelines: data from ERCUSYN," *European Journal of Endocrinology*, vol. 176, no. 5, pp. 613–624, 2017.

[3] P. Rodrigues, J. L. Castedo, M. Damasceno, and D. Carvalho, "Ectopic Cushing's syndrome caused by a pulmonary ACTH-secreting tumor in a patient treated with octreotide octreotide," *Arquivos Brasileiros de Endocrinologia & Metabologia*, vol. 56, no. 7, pp. 461–464, 2012.

[4] V. Alcantara, E. Urgell, J. Sancho, and A. Chico, "Severe ectopic Cushing syndrome caused by adenoid cystic carcinoma of a salivary gland," *Endocrine Practice*, vol. 19, no. 5, pp. e118–e121, 2013.

[5] W. Cha, M.-S. Kim, J.-C. Ahn et al., "Clinical analysis of acinic cell carcinoma in parotid gland," *Clinical and Experimental Otorhinolaryngology*, vol. 4, no. 4, pp. 188–192, 2011.

[6] N. Al-Zaher, A. Obeid, S. Al-Salam, and B. S. Al-Kayyali, "Acinic cell carcinoma of the salivary glands: a literature review," *Hematology/Oncology and Stem Cell Therapy*, vol. 2, no. 1, pp. 259–264, 2009.

[7] Y. Khelfa, M. Mansour, Y. Abdel-Aziz, A. Raufi, K. Denning, and Y. Lebowicz, "Relapsed acinic cell carcinoma of the parotid gland with diffuse distant metastasis: case report with literature review," *Journal of Investigative Medicine High Impact Case Reports*, vol. 4, no. 4, 2016.

[8] A. Lacroix, R. A. Feelders, C. A. Stratakis, and L. K. Nieman, "Cushing's syndrome," *The Lancet*, vol. 386, no. 9996, pp. 913–927, 2015.

[9] S. T. Sharma, L. K. Nieman, and R. A. Feelders, "Cushing's syndrome: epidemiology and developments in disease management," *Clinical Epidemiology*, vol. 7, pp. 281–293, 2015.

[10] T. Dacruz, A. Kalhan, M. Rashid, and K. Obuobie, "An ectopic ACTH secreting metastatic parotid tumour," *Case Reports in Endocrinology*, vol. 2016, Article ID 4852907, 4 pages, 2016.

[11] M. Lillian Cox, R. D. Gourley, and A. E. Kitbachi, "Acinic cell adenocarcinoma of the parotid with ectopic production of adrenocorticotropic hormone," *The American Journal of Medicine*, vol. 49, no. 4, pp. 529–533, 1970.

[12] L. Jamieson, S. M. Taylor, A. Smith, M. J. Bullock, and M. Davis, "Metastatic acinic cell carcinoma of the parotid gland with ectopic ACTH syndrome," *Otolaryngology-Head and Neck Surgery*, vol. 136, no. 1, pp. 149–150, 2007.

[13] M. I. Butt, D. S. Rose, and A. M. Robinson, "Cushing syndrome secondary to ectopic acth secretion by dedifferentiated acinic cell carcinoma of the parotid gland," *The Endocrinologist*, vol. 18, no. 4, pp. 161–162, 2008.

[14] V. V. Shenoy, Z. Lwin, A. Morton, and J. Hardy, "Ectopic adrenocorticotrophic hormone syndrome associated with poor prognosis in metastatic parotid acinic cell carcinoma," *Otolaryngology-Head and Neck Surgery*, vol. 145, no. 5, pp. 878–879, 2011.

[15] I. Sepúlveda, M. Frelinghuysen, E. Platin, M. L. Spencer, A. Urra, and P. Ortega, "Acinic cell carcinoma of the parotid gland: a case report and review of the literature," *Case Reports*, vol. 8, no. 1, pp. 1–8, 2015.

[16] B. M. Wenig, *Atlas of head and neck pathology*, Elsevier, Philadelphia, PA, USA, 3rd edition, 2015.

[17] S. S. Al-Otaibi, F. Alotaibi, Y. A. Zaher, N. A. Zaher, and M. A. Dababo, "High-grade transformation (dedifferentiation) of acinic cell carcinoma of the parotid gland: report of an unusual variant," *Case Reports in Otolaryngology*, vol. 2017, Article ID 7296467, 4 pages, 2017.

[18] R. Das, G. Nath, S. Bohara, and S. Raghuvanshi, "Two unusual cases of acinic cell carcinoma: role of cytology with histological corelation," *Journal of Clinical and Diagnostic Research*, vol. 10, no. 8, pp. e21–e22, 2016.

[19] M. S. Zemskova, B. Gundabolu, N. Sinaii et al., "Utility of various functional and anatomic imaging modalities for detection of ectopic adrenocorticotropin-secreting tumors," *The Journal of Clinical Endocrinology & Metabolism*, vol. 95, no. 3, pp. 1207–1219, 2010.

[20] P. J. Coates, I. Doniach, T. A. Howlett, L. H. Rees, and G. M. Besser, "Immunocytochemical study of 18 tumours causing ectopic Cushing's syndrome," *Journal of Clinical Pathology*, vol. 39, no. 9, pp. 955–960, 1986.

Papillary Thyroid Cancer Affecting Multiple Family Members: A Case Report and Literature Review of Familial Nonmedullary Thyroid Cancer

Khaled Ahmed Baagar and Buthina Ibrahim Alowainati

Endocrine Department, Hamad Medical Corporation, Doha, P.O. Box 3050, Qatar

Correspondence should be addressed to Khaled Ahmed Baagar; kbaagar@hamad.qa

Academic Editor: Wayne V. Moore

Familial nonmedullary thyroid cancer (FNMTC) represents 5–10% of NMTC cases. Many controversies are associated with the FNMTC, namely, the minimum required number of affected family members to define the condition, aggressiveness, prognosis, and treatment and screening recommendations. Moreover, the genetic basis of the FNMTC has not yet been identified. We report a family diagnosed with FNMTC and present a comprehensive literature review of the condition. The index case was a 26-year-old male who was diagnosed with locally advanced papillary thyroid cancer (PTC). Then, his family members became worried and asked for a neck ultrasound. Four of his six siblings, in addition to his father, were diagnosed with PTC. In addition, two of his cousins were diagnosed. The patient underwent total thyroidectomy with bilateral neck dissection, and he received 2 doses of radioactive iodine (100 mCi each). Furthermore, one of his siblings required a second surgery with repeated radioactive iodine therapy. The index case genetic screening and whole-exome sequencing did not show any abnormalities. Future genetic and clinical research should focus on kindred with 3 or more affected individuals for better identification of the FNMTC susceptibility genes and to better guide management and screening recommendations.

1. Introduction

Papillary thyroid cancer (PTC) is the most common primary thyroid malignancy and accounts for more than 80% of thyroid cancers [1]. Most PTC cases are sporadic; however, 5–10% are familial [2, 3], and like the sporadic form, females are 2–3 times more affected than males [4–6]. Familial PTC (FPTC) is the most common type of familial nonmedullary thyroid cancer (FNMTC) [7], which is identified, in most studies, when two or more first-degree relatives are diagnosed with the condition in the absence of a history of familial syndromes or risk factors that are commonly associated with NMTC [8–11].

We report a family which was diagnosed with FPTC after the index case (i.e., the first case had been diagnosed in the family) had been diagnosed with a locally advanced PTC. In addition, in this report, we reviewed the topic of FNMTC with its associated controversies in definition, aggressiveness in comparison to sporadic NMTC (SNMTC), latest information about the genetic background, prognosis, screening and management recommendations, and future research requirements to improve our knowledge about the condition.

2. Case Presentation

In February 2015, a 26-year-old male presented to the emergency department with generalized muscle weakness for 1 day. On physical examination, he had normal vital signs except for a pulse rate of 105/minute, a muscle power of 3/5 throughout his extremities, and a multinodular goiter with bilateral cervical lymphadenopathy. His laboratory workup was significant for potassium: 1.8 mmol/L (normal: 3.6–5), TSH: <0.01 mIU/L (normal: 0.45–4.5), FT4: 22.2 pmol/L (normal: 9–20), and FT3: 10 pmol/L (normal: 3.4–6). His muscle power improved with potassium replacement. A thyroid uptake scan showed increased uptake with a cold thyroid nodule. Therefore, carbimazole and propranolol were prescribed.

Neck ultrasound and magnetic resonance imaging showed 1.6 cm and 1.2 cm nodules with calcifications in the right thyroid lobe, with evidence of bilateral lymph node metastases and bilateral extranodal soft tissue metastases. CT chest to assess mediastinal lymphadenopathy or lung metastases was unremarkable. Fine-needle aspiration biopsy (FNAB) from a lymph node metastasis in the neck showed metastatic PTC. Then, FNAB from the right thyroid nodules was performed, and it showed PTC.

The patient underwent total thyroidectomy and bilateral neck dissection. Two foci (2 cm and 1 cm) of classical PTC were found in the right thyroid lobe with lymph node involvement and extranodal metastases. Thereafter, I^{131} 100 mci was given, and the postablation scan showed a remnant in the left thyroid bed (TNM staging: T4aN1bM0 tumor).

The patient's family was worried about themselves and asked for a thyroid evaluation. The patient's brother, in addition to 3 of his 5 sisters, was found to have PTC (see details in Table 1). The remaining 2 sisters (aged 22 and 29 years) and the mother (aged 52 years) underwent a normal initial thyroid ultrasound scan, and then the yearly ultrasound surveillance was unremarkable. The father (aged 55 years) was found to have a thyroid nodule; however, he was reluctant to have FNAB until January 2018 at another institution where he was diagnosed with thyroid cancer, but we do not have any data about his follow-up there (see family pedigree in Figure 1).

There were no other cancers or clinical features indicating a familial syndrome in the family. The patient's genetic screening was negative for pathogenic variants of the PARP4, APC, DICER1, RET, SDHB, and SDHD genes. In addition, the patient underwent whole-exome sequencing, which was unremarkable.

After more than 6 years of follow-up of the index case and his family, two of them, including himself, had a recurrence and required further treatment (see Table 1). In addition, he reported to us that 2 of his paternal cousins, who were not siblings, had developed thyroid cancer.

3. Discussion

In 1955, Robinson and Orr presented the first evidence of the familial clustering of NMTC, where they reported PTC in 2 monozygotic twins [12].

Many controversies are related to the FNMTC, starting from its definition to clinical behavior, outcomes, management recommendations, and screening of the patients' family members. This controversy is mainly because of the small number of studies of FNMTC, mostly retrospective, and their relatively small number of subjects because of the low disease prevalence. In addition, the follow-up duration in these studies was short relative to the nature of the disease.

There is no consensus on whether two [2, 9, 13, 14] or three [15–18] first-degree relatives of a family are the minimum required number to define FNMTC, as SNMTC is very common and it can affect more than one individual in a family. Charkes [5] found that in families with 2 affected individuals, 62–69% of the cases are sporadic, while in families with ≥3 affected members, less than 6% of the cases are sporadic. In one study, it was found that 4.6% of at-risk individuals had thyroid cancer in families with 2 affected members, while 22.7% of at-risk individuals were affected in the families with ≥3 affected members [19].

Despite the recommendation to consider mainly families with ≥3 affected members for clinical and genetic analyses [5], most of the reports are mainly based on families with 2 affected cases. The family we described in this report, with 6 affected first-degree relatives, has very strong evidence of FNMTC.

3.1. Histopathological Features. From a histological viewpoint, there is no specific feature that distinguishes FNMTC from SNMTC [20], except in one report which showed that patients in the FNMTC group had more significantly classic variant PTC than those in the sporadic PTC group (84% vs. 63.3%; $P < 0.001$) [7]. We found that all the affected individuals in the reported family had classic variant PTC, except one who had a follicular variant PTC.

3.2. Clinical Aggressiveness at Presentation. It is the most controversial part, as some studies have shown that FNMTC demonstrates a more aggressive presentation than SNMTC, such as earlier onset, bilateral and multifocal tumors, extrathyroidal invasion, and lymph node metastasis [9, 14, 21–28].

Recently, El Lakis et al. reported that FNMTC patients were diagnosed at an earlier age (62% vs. 49.5%; $P = 0.041$), with a higher rate at the T1 stage (75% vs. 57.8%; $P = 0.01$) and a higher rate of lymph node involvement ($P = 0.002$) [7].In addition, Sezer et al. found that both FPTC and sporadic PTC (SPTC) groups had no difference in age at presentation or tumor size; however, the familial group was found to have more aggressive features, such as higher rates of multifocal tumors ($P = 0.011$), bilateral involvement ($P = 0.004$), extrathyroid extension ($P = 0.040$), and lymph node metastasis ($P = 0.013$) [29]. Furthermore, Kim YS et al. reported more multifocality ($P = 0.020$), benign thyroid nodules ($P = 0.015$), and lateral neck lymph node involvement ($P = 0.021$) in the FNMTC group [10].

The reported family had 6 affected members, with 2 of them (the index case and sibling 3) showing the most aggressive features such as multifocality, capsular invasion, extrathyroid extension, vascular/lymphatic invasion, and lymph node involvement and sibling 3 showing bilateral disease.

Even those with familial papillary microcarcinoma, when compared to their sporadic counterparts, had more multifocal tumors (71%), more vascular invasion (43%), and a higher rate of lymph node involvement (57%) [30]. In the reported family, only sibling 4 had a microscopic PTC with no aggressive features.

On the other hand, a good number of studies did not show any difference in clinical aggressiveness at presentation between FNMTC and SNMTC patients [1, 6, 18, 31–33].

Table 1: Characteristics of the diagnosed thyroid cancer in the family members.

	Index case	Sibling 1	Sibling 2	Sibling 3	Sibling 4	Father
Age at diagnosis (years)	26	30	23	29	33	58
Gender	Male	Male	Female	Female	Female	Male
Nodular goiter (±)	+	−	−	+	+	
Tumor diameter (cm)	2.0	1.0	2.2	2.6	0.12	
Histological variant of PTC	Classic	Classic	Classic	Classic	Follicular	
Laterality (unilateral/ bilateral)	Unilateral	Unilateral	Unilateral	Bilateral	Unilateral	
Focality (unifocal/ multifocal)	Multifocal	Unifocal	Unifocal	Multifocal	Unifocal	
Capsule invasion (±)	+	+	−	+	−	
Extrathyroid extension (±)	+	−	−	+	−	
Vascular/ lymphatic invasion	+	−	−	+	−	
Hashimoto's thyroiditis (±)	−	−	+	−	−	
Central LN involvement (±)	+	−	−	+	−	
Lateral LN involvement (±)	+	Not sampled	Not sampled	Not sampled	Not sampled	
Distant metastasis (±)	−	−	−	−	−	
pTNM classification	T4aN1bM0	T1aN0M0	T2N0M0	T3bN1aM0	T1aN0Mx	
Surgical procedures	Total thyroidectomy with bilateral neck dissection	Total thyroidectomy with central LN dissection	Total thyroidectomy with central LN dissection	Total thyroidectomy with central LN dissection	Total thyroidectomy with central LN dissection	
RAI ablation and dose	+, 100 mCi	+, 100 mCi	−	+, 30 mCi	−	
Persistence/ recurrence of the disease (±)	+	−	−	+	−	
Repeated treatment (surgery and/or RAI and dose)	In February 2017, he received a 2nd dose of RAI (100 mCi) for local recurrence in the thyroid bed	−	−	In April 2019, surgery for thyroid recurrence with bilateral neck dissection and RAI (100 mCi)	−	
Death from the disease (±)	−	−	−	−	−	−
Duration of follow-up	Since April 2015 (75 months)	Since July 2015 (72 months)	Since November 2015 (68 months)	Since May 2016 (62 months)	Since August 2015 (71 months)	Since January 2018 (42 months)

PTC: papillary thyroid cancer, LN: lymph node, and RAI: radioactive iodine. *Note.* There were no data about the father's tumor, as he had the management and follow-up data outside our institution.

Most studies, whether they showed or did not show that FNMTC was more aggressive than SNMTC, did not show a difference in the rate of distant metastasis. However, Sezer et al. reported a higher rate in the familial group ($P \leq 0.0001$) [29], and McDonald et al. [34] found that the FNMTC group had more distant metastasis (8.8%) than the SNMTC group (3.1%) ($P = 0.003$), with more aggregation of the cases in some families with ≥3 affected members.

Some studies have tried to investigate whether there is any difference in the clinical behavior of the FNMTCs when

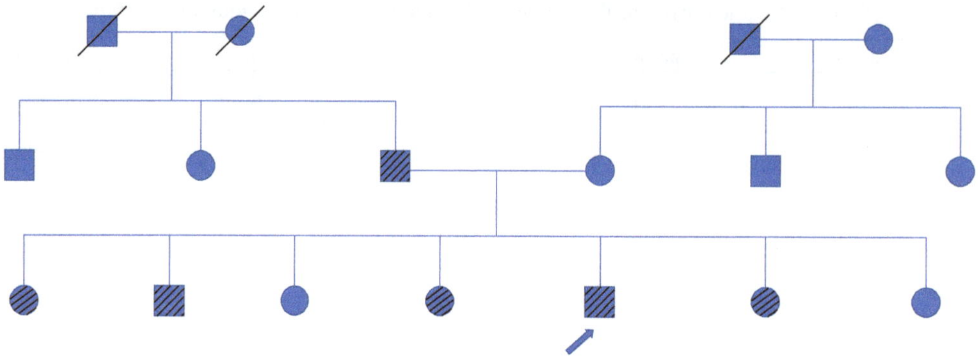

Figure 1: Family pedigree. Squares represent male family members; circles represent female family members; multiple-slashed symbols represent affected members; single-slashed symbols represent deceased members. The arrow points to the proband.

only 2 first-degree relatives are affected and when ≥ 3 first-degree relatives are affected. In the study performed by Zhang et al. [9], the FNMTC subgroup with 2 affected members had more significant multifocal tumors than the SNMTC group. The FNMTC subgroup with ≥3 affected members had more significant thyroid nodular goiter and bilateral and multifocal tumors with extrathyroid extension and lateral lymph node metastasis than both the SNMTC group and the FNMTC subgroup with 2 affected members. On the other hand, Pinto et al. [13] showed that the FNMTC subgroup with ≥3 affected members had no difference from the SNMTC group regarding the clinicopathological features or DNA ploidy, with only a nonsignificant tendency for extrathyroid invasion in that subgroup. In addition, McDonald et al. [34] showed no difference in almost the same surgical pathology features between the SNMTC, 2-member FNMTC, and ≥3-member FNMTC groups.

In more recent studies, El Lakis et al. found no difference between the FNMTC subgroup of 2 affected members and either the SNMTC group or the FNMTC subgroup of ≥3 affected members; however, the latter group presented at a younger age ($P = 0.04$) and had more lymph node metastasis ($P = 0.009$) than the SNMTC group [7]. On the other hand, Sezer et al. showed that the 2-member FPTC group, in comparison to the SPTC group, had more significant bilaterality, multifocality, extrathyroid extension, and distant metastasis [29]. The ≥3-member FPTC group, in comparison to the SPTC group, had more distant metastasis and less extrathyroid extension [29]. The comparison of the 2-member FPTC group and the ≥3-member FPTC group showed that the former had more vascular invasion and extrathyroid extension and lower rates of bilaterality, lymphatic invasion, and distant metastasis [29].

A meta-analysis of 6 retrospective studies, with a relatively small number of subjects, comparing the clinicopathological features between the first and second generations in families with FNMTC found that second-generation patients tend to be younger, male, and have a higher risk of lymph node metastasis. However, there was no difference in tumor size, multifocality, or extrathyroid invasion [8].

One study tried to compare 2 subtypes of FNMTC, namely, parent-offspring type and sibling type versus each other and versus SNMTC [27]. When compared to SNMTC, the sibling FNMTC group had more females, smaller tumor size, and more combined chronic thyroiditis; however, there was no difference in age at the time of diagnosis, lymph node metastasis, extrathyroid invasion, multicentricity, or TNM staging. The parent-offspring FNMTC group had more multicentricity than the SNMTC group. The sibling FNMTC group had only more females than the parent-offspring FNMTC group. Another study found that the sibling FNMTC group was associated with more Hashimoto's thyroiditis and extrathyroid extension than the parent-offspring FNMTC group [14]. Furthermore, in comparison to the SNMTC group, the sibling FNMTC group had more bilateral and multicentric tumors, while the parent-offspring FNMTC group showed more Hashimoto's thyroiditis, central lymph node metastasis, and T3 tumors [14].

Another type of comparison was performed by Rosario et al. [35] between index cases and their affected siblings who were screened by ultrasound. The index cases were found to have an older average age at the time of diagnosis, larger tumors, more lymph node metastases, and more extrathyroid invasion. In addition, McDonald et al. [34] reported that the index cases had a more aggressive disease because the other family members sought screening and they were diagnosed at an earlier stage of the disease. Recent studies reported that the index cases had larger tumor sizes and more lymph node metastases, and because of that, they required more aggressive surgeries and radioactive iodine therapy [7, 19]. The index case in our report had the most aggressive disease (T4aN1bM0) in comparison to his siblings, and he required more extensive initial surgery in addition to 2 radioactive iodine ablation therapy doses of 100 mCi each.

3.3. Prognosis (Recurrence, Disease-Free Survival, and Survival). In general, PTC has good survival rate with only 6% malignancy-related mortality at a median follow-up of 16 years in patients with nonmetastatic disease at presentation [36]. However, the controversy continues with the prognosis of FNMTC, where some studies showed that it has worse outcomes than SNMTC, while others did not show a difference.

The rate of tumor recurrence in FNMTC was higher than that in SNMTC in a number of publications [9, 22, 28, 34], while it did not differ in others [6, 10, 13, 14, 18, 31, 33].

After more than 6 years of follow-up of the reported family, the 2 members who had more aggressive tumors at presentation developed recurrent disease and required more aggressive surgeries and repeated radioactive iodine ablation therapy.

Only a few studies have assessed the disease-free survival (i.e., time to tumor recurrence), and it was shorter in FNMTC [9, 22, 24, 27, 28].

Regarding mortality in association with FNMTC, most of the studies showed no difference from SNMTC [1, 7, 9, 10, 13, 14, 22, 24, 31, 33, 37], except in the study carried out by McDonald et al. [34], where the FNMTC group had more significant mortality (3.3% of 91 cases) than the SNMTC group (0.4% of 521 cases) ($P = 0.01$).

Some studies tried to compare the different subtypes of FNMTC prognostically. For example, in one study [9], the disease-free survival was shorter in families with ≥3 affected members than in families with only 2 victims ($P = 0.045$), while in other studies [18, 27, 33], there was no difference. In addition, there was no difference between these two FNMTC subgroups in persistence or recurrence of the disease or in mortality [9]. Furthermore, there was no difference in the recurrence rate between sibling and parent-offspring subtypes of FNMTC [14, 27] or in a meta-analysis [8] comparing first-generation versus second-generation patients in families with FNMTC.

3.4. Pathogenesis and Genetic Background. Sometimes FNMTC is referred to as syndromic and nonsyndromic [20]. The syndromic group is not consistent with the true definition of the FNMTC, where FNMTC should not be a part of a familial syndrome, e.g., familial adenomatous polyposis, Werner syndrome, Cowden syndrome, Pendred syndrome, and Carney complex. Nonsyndromic FNMTC can be subdivided into different forms, namely, pure familial PTC with or without oxyphilia, familial PTC with papillary renal cell carcinoma, and familial PTC with multinodular goiter [20].

The genetic background of the nonsyndromic FNMTC is still unknown. However, based on the studied kindred, it is thought to be polygenic and autosomal dominant with incomplete penetrance and variable expression [20, 38].

In addition, FNMTC demonstrated the phenomenon of genetic anticipation, where with successive generations, the disease is diagnosed at an earlier age with a more aggressive presentation [14, 16, 39].

The genetic testing of the proband in the reported family did not show any genetic abnormality linked to his phenotype.

Research to identify FNMTC susceptibility genes is still ongoing. There are different potential genetic loci and genes that have been reported, such as multinodular goiter 1 (MNG1; 14q32) [40], thyroid carcinoma with oxyphilia (TCO; 19p13.2) [41], fPTC/papillary renal neoplasia (PRN; 1q21) [42], NMTC1 (2q21) [43], familial thyroid epithelial neoplasia (FTEN; 8p23.1–p22) [44], telomere-telomerase complex [45], TITF-1/NKX2(which encodes thyroid transcription factor-1) [46], SRGAP1 (Slit- Robo Rho GTPase activating protein 1) genes [47], hyaluronan binding protein 2 (HABP2) [48], FOXE1 [49], SRRM2 (serine/arginine repetitive matrix 2 gene) [50], C14orf93 (RTFC) [51], mitogen-activated protein kinase kinase 5 (MAP2K5) [52], CHEK2 and ATM genes [53], ANXA3, NTN4, SERPINA1, FKBP10, PLEKHG5, P2RX5, SAPCD1 [54], and protection of telomeres 1 [POT1] gene [55].

The reason that, until now, no definite FNMTC susceptibility genes have been identified may be related to the inclusion of families with only 2 affected members in the genetic studies, while NMTC is not an uncommon condition in the general population. In addition, other modes of inheritance should be studied, such as the possible role of epigenetics [56].

3.5. Screening and Management Recommendations. There are no randomized controlled trials to guide the screening and management recommendations of FNMTC, and the available evidence only came from observational studies and expert opinion.

We need to take into consideration that recommending a screening program for any cancer condition requires the following[19]:

(1) To be directed to at-risk individuals

(2) To be able to discover the disease early in its course

(3) That early detection of the disease impacts the outcome

(4) To be cost-effective

Currently, the best available screening method is the ultrasound neck [2, 14, 19, 57], as there is no genetic test to definitely diagnose FNMTC and, for example, guide prophylactic thyroidectomy similar to familial medullary thyroid cancer [2].In addition, physical examination alone can miss many cases with nodular thyroid disease [19, 35]. Klubo-Gwiezdzinska et al. reported screening of 109 at-risk individuals, of which 55 (50.5%) had thyroid nodules detected by ultrasound; however, only 7 cases (7/55 = 12.7%) were palpable on physical examination.

Screening can detect FNMTC cases at an earlier stage of the disease; however, there is no consensus on at what age ultrasound screening should start and how frequently it should be performed. The youngest diagnosed patient with FNMTC was aged 8 years [13]. Some authors [14] recommended starting ultrasound screening from the age of 18 years and performing ultrasound screening yearly afterward, while others advised screening from the age of 10 years [2].

Most of the published management recommendations endorse more aggressive treatment, including total thyroidectomy, central lymph node dissection, radioactive iodine ablation therapy, and suppressive thyroid hormone treatment, in almost all patients with FNMTC [9, 10, 14, 58].In addition, the treatment of FNMTC in families with 3 or more affected members should be more aggressive, as they usually have a more hostile disease [7].

Capezzone et al. suggested that management recommendations for FNMTC should depend on controlled studies with comparable groups of FNMTC cases and SNMTC cases in their baseline characteristics [11].Furthermore, as the latest recommendations for less aggressive management of SNMTC were not assessed specifically in those with FNMTC, the authors suggested total thyroidectomy and radioactive iodine ablation therapy, especially for those belonging to families with 3 or more affected members [11].

Mazeh and Sippel [57] suggested an algorithm for screening and management of FNMTC where treatment decisions took into consideration the number of affected family members and the degree of aggressiveness of the disease within the family. They suggested performing a neck ultrasound screening on all family members starting from the age of 20 years or 10 years younger than the youngest affected family member. If there is no nodule, periodic ultrasound should be performed. If the person has benign nodules based on FNAB, prophylactic thyroidectomy could be performed if the family has an aggressive disease or has 3 or more affected members. They justified this recommendation based on families with FNMTC being more likely to have benign and malignant thyroid disease, which lowers the chance to detect cancer. If cancer was identified by FNAB, they recommend total thyroidectomy, routine central neck dissection in almost all patients, radioactive iodine ablation therapy if the family is known to have an aggressive disease or has 3 or more affected members, and thyroid hormone suppressive therapy in all patients.

Recently, Klubo-Gwiezdzinska et al. [19] authored a prospective study using neck ultrasound screening and reported a cancer detection rate of 4.6% in families with 2 members affected, which is similar to the general population (4.5%) [1, 59]. However, in families with ≥3 members affected, the detection rate was 22.7% ($P = 0.01$).In addition, thyroid nodules were documented in 72.2% of the parents of index cases. Furthermore, the FNMTC detected in the screened cases was less aggressive than the index cases and required less aggressive surgery (hemithyroidectomy 23.5% versus 0%; $P = 0.002$) and a lower rate of radioactive iodine ablation therapy ($P \leq 0.001$), with a better response to initial treatment than the index cases ($P = 0.045$). Based on their data, the authors recommended active screening using neck ultrasound only for families with 3 or more affected first-degree relatives. The screening of first-degree relatives should include all generations relative to the index case and involve those at least aged 20 years or 10 years younger than the youngest diagnosed case with NMTC. Neck ultrasound should be performed every 2–3 years.

The latest American Thyroid Association (2015) guidelines did not recommend or discourage using neck ultrasound for FNMTC screening [60]. However, in view of the recent accumulating evidence, families with ≥3 affected first-degree relatives should be considered eligible for ultrasound screening. In addition, to avoid overdiagnosis and overtreatment of clinically insignificant thyroid cancer cases in the population, it is better not to implement a screening program for families with only 2 affected members.

In the reported family, we performed neck ultrasound screening for siblings and parents. In addition, we advised them to start screening their children when they reach the age of 13 years (10 years less than the youngest diagnosed member in the family) and to repeat it yearly for the unaffected family members. All the family members diagnosed after the index case underwent total thyroidectomy with central lymph node dissection, including sibling 4 with microscopic PTC.

3.6. Future Research. Future research should focus on the identification of a solid molecular basis of FNMTC, as this is the best way to diagnose true familial cases. This will help to conduct further studies to develop evidence-based recommendations for patient management and follow-up and for family screening protocols.

Limiting the definition of FNMTC to include only kindred with 3 or more affected members may help in better characterization of the susceptibility genes, and this, in turn, helps to endorse more solid screening and management recommendations.

Because of the low prevalence of FNMTC, research and clinical centers in different countries should collaborate to have enough patients to obtain meaningful results.

4. Conclusions

FNMTC has many controversies in relation to its definition, clinicopathological aggressiveness, prognosis, treatment, and screening of at-risk family members. Different genetic mutations have been investigated; however, none of them was confirmed to be a source of the condition. Based on the available evidence, it is advisable to implement ultrasound neck screening only in families with 3 or more affected members and to be done yearly starting at age 10 years earlier than the youngest affected family member. In addition, the diagnosed cases in those families should have a lower threshold for a more aggressive management decision.

The multidisciplinary team of endocrinologists, surgeons, and genetics specialists at our institution recommended the same for the reported family.

FNMTC is an area that needs to be addressed in future research to resolve its ambiguity and controversial issues and to have screening and management recommendations based on high-quality evidence.

References

[1] W. Moses, J. Weng, and E. Kebebew, "Prevalence, clinicopathologic features, and somatic genetic mutation profile in familial versus sporadic nonmedullary thyroid cancer," *Thyroid*, vol. 21, no. 4, pp. 367–371, 2011.

[2] O. H. Clark, "Controversies in familial thyroid cancer 2014," *Turkish Journal of Surgery*, vol. 30, no. 2, pp. 62–66, 2014.

[3] M. Capezzone, C. Secchi, N. Fralassi et al., "Should familial disease be considered as a negative prognostic factor in micropapillary thyroid carcinoma?" *Journal of Endocrinological Investigation*, vol. 42, no. 10, pp. 1205–1213, 2019.

[4] C. D. Malchoff and D. M. Malchoff, "Familial nonmedullary thyroid carcinoma," *Cancer Control*, vol. 13, no. 2, pp. 106–110, 2006.

[5] N. D. Charkes, "On the prevalence of familial nonmedullary thyroid cancer in multiply affected kindreds," *Thyroid*, vol. 16, no. 2, pp. 181–186, 2006.

[6] K.-C. Loh, "Familial nonmedullary thyroid carcinoma: a meta-review of case series," *Thyroid*, vol. 7, no. 1, pp. 107–113, 1997.

[7] M. El Lakis, A. Giannakou, P. J. Nockel et al., "Do patients with familial nonmedullary thyroid cancer present with more aggressive disease? implications for initial surgical treatment," *Surgery*, vol. 165, no. 1, pp. 50–57, 2019.

[8] Y.-M. Zhou, H. Luo, J.-X. Gou et al., "Second generation of familial nonmedullary thyroid carcinoma: a meta-analysis on the clinicopathologic features and prognosis," *European Journal of Surgical Oncology*, vol. 43, no. 12, pp. 2248–2256, 2017.

[9] Y.-B. Zhang, X.-X. Wang, X.-W. Zhang et al., "Familial nonmedullary thyroid carcinoma," *Chinese Medical Journal*, vol. 131, no. 4, pp. 395–401, 2018.

[10] Y. S. Kim, M. Seo, S. H. Park, S. Y. Ju, and E. S. Kim, "Should total thyroidectomy Be recommended for patients with familial non-medullary thyroid cancer?" *World Journal of Surgery*, vol. 44, no. 9, pp. 3022–3027, 2020.

[11] M. Capezzone, E. Robenshtok, S. Cantara, and M. G. Castagna, "Familial non-medullary thyroid cancer: a critical review," *Journal of Endocrinological Investigation*, vol. 44, no. 5, pp. 943–950, 2020.

[12] D. W. Robinson and T. G. ORR, "Carcinoma of the thyroid and other diseases of the thyroid in identical twins," *Archives of Surgery*, vol. 70, no. 6, pp. 923–928, 1955.

[13] A. E. Pinto, G. L. Silva, R. Henrique et al., "Familial vs. sporadic papillary thyroid carcinoma: a matched-case comparative study showing similar clinical/prognostic behaviour," *European Journal of Endocrinology*, vol. 170, no. 2, pp. 321–327, 2014.

[14] L. Jiwang, L. Zhendong, L. Shuchun, H. Bo, and L. Yanguo, "Clinicopathologic characteristics of familial versus sporadic papillary thyroid carcinoma," *Acta Otorhinolaryngologica Italica: organo ufficiale della Societa italiana di otorinolaringologia e chirurgia cervico-facciale*, vol. 35, no. 4, pp. 234–242, 2015.

[15] L. O'Connell, R. S. Prichard, E. O'Reilly, S. Skehan, D. Gibbons, and E. W. McDermott, "Running in the family: a rare diagnosis of familial papillary thyroid cancer," *International Journal of Surgery Case Reports*, vol. 16, pp. 64–66, 2015.

[16] M. Capezzone, S. Marchisotta, S. Cantara et al., "Familial nonmedullary thyroid carcinoma displays the features of clinical anticipation suggestive of a distinct biological entity," *Endocrine-Related Cancer*, vol. 15, no. 4, pp. 1075–1081, 2008.

[17] S. Lei, D. Wang, J. Ge et al., "Single-center study of familial papillary thyroid cancer in China: surgical considerations," *World Journal of Surgical Oncology*, vol. 13, no. 1, p. 115, 2015.

[18] E. Robenshtok, G. Tzvetov, S. Grozinsky-Glasberg et al., "Clinical characteristics and outcome of familial nonmedullary thyroid cancer: a retrospective controlled study," *Thyroid*, vol. 21, no. 1, pp. 43–48, 2011.

[19] J. Klubo-Gwiezdzinska, L. Yang, R. Merkel et al., "Results of screening in familial non-medullary thyroid cancer," *Thyroid*, vol. 27, no. 8, pp. 1017–1024, 2017.

[20] J. Guilmette and V. Nosé, "Hereditary and familial thyroid tumours," *Histopathology*, vol. 72, no. 1, pp. 70–81, 2018.

[21] V. Nosé, "Familial thyroid cancer: a review," *Modern Pathology*, vol. 24, no. S2, pp. S19–S33, 2011.

[22] S. Uchino, S. Noguchi, H. Kawamoto et al., "Familial nonmedullary thyroid carcinoma characterized by multifocality and a high recurrence rate in a large study population," *World Journal of Surgery*, vol. 26, no. 8, pp. 897–902, 2002.

[23] R. F. Grossman, S. H. Tu, Q. Y. Duh, A. E. Siperstein, F. Novosolov, and O. H. Clark, "Familial nonmedullary thyroid cancer," *Archives of Surgery*, vol. 130, no. 8, pp. 892–897, 1995.

[24] O. Alsanea, N. Wada, K. Ain et al., "Is familial non-medullary thyroid carcinoma more aggressive than sporadic thyroid cancer? A multicenter series," *Surgery*, vol. 128, no. 6, pp. 1043–1051, 2000.

[25] F. Triponez, M. Wong, C. Sturgeon et al., "Does familial nonmedullary thyroid cancer adversely affect survival?" *World Journal of Surgery*, vol. 30, no. 5, pp. 787–793, 2006.

[26] H. Mazeh, J. Benavidez, J. L. Poehls, L. Youngwirth, H. Chen, and R. S. Sippel, "In patients with thyroid cancer of follicular cell origin, a family history of nonmedullary thyroid cancer in one first-degree relative is associated with more aggressive disease," *Thyroid*, vol. 22, no. 1, pp. 3–8, 2012.

[27] Y. J. Park, H. Y. Ahn, H. S. Choi, K. W. Kim, D. J. Park, and B. Y. Cho, "The long-term outcomes of the second generation of familial nonmedullary thyroid carcinoma are more aggressive than sporadic cases," *Thyroid*, vol. 22, no. 4, pp. 356–362, 2012.

[28] X. Wang, W. Cheng, J. Li et al., "Endocrine tumours: familial nonmedullary thyroid carcinoma is a more aggressive disease: a systematic review and meta-analysis," *European Journal of Endocrinology*, vol. 172, no. 6, pp. R253–R262, 2015.

[29] H. Sezer, M. O. Demirkol, D. Yazici, Y. Kapran, and F. Alagöl, "The clinicopathologic characteristics of familial and sporadic papillary thyroid carcinoma in Turkish patients," *Turkish Journal of Medical Sciences*, vol. 44, no. 2, pp. 360–368, 2020.

[30] G. Lupoli, G. Vitale, M. Caraglia et al., "Familial papillary thyroid microcarcinoma: a new clinical entity," *The Lancet*, vol. 353, no. 9153, pp. 637–639, 1999.

[31] E. L. Maxwell, F. T. Hall, and J. L. Freeman, "Familial nonmedullary thyroid cancer: a matched-case control study," *The Laryngoscope*, vol. 114, no. 12, pp. 2182–2186, 2004.

[32] Y. Ito, M. Fukushima, T. Yabuta et al., "Prevalence and prognosis of familial follicular thyroid carcinoma," *Endocrine Journal*, vol. 55, no. 5, pp. 847–852, 2008.

[33] Y. Ito, K. Kakudo, M. Hirokawa et al., "Biological behavior and prognosis of familial papillary thyroid carcinoma," *Surgery*, vol. 145, no. 1, pp. 100–105, 2009.

[34] T. J. McDonald, A. A. Driedger, B. M. Garcia et al., "Familial papillary thyroid carcinoma: a retrospective analysis," *Journal of Oncology*, vol. 2011, Article ID 948786, 8 pages, 2011.

[35] P. W. Rosario, A. F. C. Mineiro Filho, B. S. S. Prates, L. C. O. Silva, R. X. Lacerda, and M. R. Calsolari, "Ultrasonographic screening for thyroid cancer in siblings of patients with apparently sporadic papillary carcinoma," *Thyroid*, vol. 22, no. 8, pp. 805–808, 2012.

[36] E. L. Mazzaferri and S. M. Jhiang, "Long-term impact of initial surgical and medical therapy on papillary and follicular thyroid cancer," *The American Journal of Medicine*, vol. 97, no. 5, pp. 418–428, 1994.

[37] F. Pitoia, G. Cross, M. E. Salvai, E. Abelleira, and H. Niepomniszcze, "Patients with familial non-medullary thyroid cancer have an outcome similar to that of patients with sporadic papillary thyroid tumors," *Arquivos Brasileiros*

de Endocrinologia & Metabologia, vol. 55, no. 3, pp. 219–223, 2011.

[38] A. J. Bauer, "Clinical behavior and genetics of nonsyndromic, familial nonmedullary thyroid cancer," *Endocrine Tumor Syndromes and Their Genetics*, vol. 41, pp. 141–148, 2013.

[39] A. Hillenbrand, J.-E. Varhaug, M. Brauckhoff et al., "Familial nonmedullary thyroid carcinoma-clinical relevance and prognosis. A European multicenter study," *Langenbeck's Archives of Surgery*, vol. 395, no. 7, pp. 851–858, 2010.

[40] G. R. Bignell, F. Canzian, M. Shayeghi et al., "Familial nontoxic multinodular thyroid goiter locus maps to chromosome 14q but does not account for familial nonmedullary thyroid cancer," *The American Journal of Human Genetics*, vol. 61, no. 5, pp. 1123–1130, 1997.

[41] F. Canzian, P. Amati, H. R. Harach et al., "A gene predisposing to familial thyroid tumors with cell oxyphilia maps to chromosome 19p13.2.2," *The American Journal of Human Genetics*, vol. 63, no. 6, pp. 1743–1748, 1998.

[42] C. D. Malchoff, M. Sarfarazi, B. Tendler et al., "Papillary thyroid carcinoma associated with papillary renal neoplasia: genetic linkage analysis of a distinct heritable tumor syndrome," *The Journal of Clinical Endocrinology & Metabolism*, vol. 85, no. 5, pp. 1758–1764, 2000.

[43] J. D. McKay, F. Lesueur, L. Jonard et al., "Localization of a susceptibility gene for familial nonmedullary thyroid carcinoma to chromosome 2q21," *The American Journal of Human Genetics*, vol. 69, no. 2, pp. 440–446, 2001.

[44] B. M. Cavaco, P. F. Batista, L. G. Sobrinho, and V. Leite, "Mapping a new familial thyroid epithelial neoplasia susceptibility locus to chromosome 8p23.1-p22 by high-density single-nucleotide polymorphism genome-wide linkage analysis," *The Journal of Clinical Endocrinology & Metabolism*, vol. 93, no. 11, pp. 4426–4430, 2008.

[45] M. Capezzone, S. Cantara, S. Marchisotta et al., "Telomere length in neoplastic and nonneoplastic tissues of patients with familial and sporadic papillary thyroid cancer," *The Journal of Clinical Endocrinology & Metabolism*, vol. 96, no. 11, pp. E1852–E1856, 2011.

[46] E. S. W. Ngan, B. H. H. Lang, T. Liu et al., "A germline mutation (A339V) in thyroid transcription factor-1 (TITF-1/NKX2.1) in patients with multinodular goiter and papillary thyroid carcinoma," *Journal of the National Cancer Institute: Journal of the National Cancer Institute*, vol. 101, no. 3, pp. 162–175, 2009.

[47] H. He, A. Bronisz, S. Liyanarachchi et al., "SRGAP1Is a candidate gene for papillary thyroid carcinoma susceptibility," *The Journal of Clinical Endocrinology & Metabolism*, vol. 98, no. 5, pp. E973–E980, 2013.

[48] S. K. Gara, L. Jia, M. J. Merino et al., "Germline-HABP2Mutation causing familial nonmedullary thyroid cancer," *New England Journal of Medicine*, vol. 373, no. 5, pp. 448–455, 2015.

[49] J. S. Pereira, J. G. da Silva, R. A. Tomaz et al., "Identification of a novel germline FOXE1 variant in patients with familial nonmedullary thyroid carcinoma (FNMTC)," *Endocrine*, vol. 49, no. 1, pp. 204–214, 2015.

[50] J. Tomsic, H. He, K. Akagi et al., "A germline mutation in SRRM2, a splicing factor gene, is implicated in papillary thyroid carcinoma predisposition," *Scientific Reports*, vol. 5, no. 1, Article ID 10566, 2015.

[51] C. Liu, Y. Yu, G. Yin et al., "C14orf93 (RTFC) is identified as a novel susceptibility gene for familial nonmedullary thyroid cancer," *Biochemical and Biophysical Research Communications*, vol. 482, no. 4, pp. 590–596, 2017.

[52] F. Ye, H. Gao, L. Xiao et al., "Whole exome and target sequencing identifies MAP2K5 as novel susceptibility gene for familial non-medullary thyroid carcinoma," *International Journal of Cancer*, vol. 144, no. 6, pp. 1321–1330, 2019.

[53] Y. Wang, S. Liyanarachchi, K. E. Miller et al., "Identification of rare variants predisposing to thyroid cancer," *Thyroid*, vol. 29, no. 7, pp. 946–955, 2019.

[54] M. Sarquis, D. C. Moraes, L. Bastos-Rodrigues et al., "Germline mutations in familial papillary thyroid cancer," *Endocrine Pathology*, vol. 31, no. 1, pp. 14–20, 2020.

[55] A. Srivastava, B. Miao, D. Skopelitou et al., "A germline mutation in the *POT1* gene is a candidate for familial nonmedullary thyroid cancer," *Cancers*, vol. 12, no. 6, p. 1441, 2020.

[56] S. A. Ammar, W. M. Alobuia, and E. Kebebew, "An update on familial nonmedullary thyroid cancer," *Endocrine*, vol. 68, no. 3, pp. 502–507, 2020.

[57] H. Mazeh and R. S. Sippel, "Familial nonmedullary thyroid carcinoma," *Thyroid*, vol. 23, no. 9, pp. 1049–1056, 2013.

[58] R. S. Sippel, N. R. Caron, and O. H. Clark, "An evidence-based approach to familial nonmedullary thyroid cancer: screening, clinical management, and follow-up," *World Journal of Surgery*, vol. 31, no. 5, pp. 924–933, 2007.

[59] L. Furuya-Kanamori, K. J. L. Bell, J. Clark, P. Glasziou, and S. A. R. Doi, "Prevalence of differentiated thyroid cancer in autopsy studies over six decades: a meta-analysis," *Journal of Clinical Oncology*, vol. 34, no. 30, pp. 3672–3679, 2016.

[60] B. R. Haugen, E. K. Alexander, K. C. Bible et al., "2015 American thyroid association management guidelines for adult patients with thyroid nodules and differentiated thyroid cancer: the American thyroid association guidelines task force on thyroid nodules and differentiated thyroid cancer," *Thyroid*, vol. 26, no. 1, pp. 1–133, 2016.

14

Transient Hypophosphatemia: A Dangerous Event in Multiple Myeloma

Paula Jeffs, Michelle Mangual-García, Alex González-Bóssolo, and Nadyeschka Rivera-Santana

Endocrinology Department, San Juan City Hospital, San Juan, PR 00921, USA

Correspondence should be addressed to Paula Jeffs; paujeffs@gmail.com

Academic Editor: Osamu Isozaki

Patients with malignancies frequently experience multiple electrolyte disturbances. In multiple myeloma, hypercalcemia and hyperphosphatemia are one of the most common metabolic disturbances observed as part of pathogenesis of the disease. However, in rare occasions and during the course of the disease, many patients can develop hypophosphatemia due to multiple factors that affects the phosphate absorption and excretion. We hereby present a 56 y/o woman recently diagnosed with multiple myeloma who developed severe hypophosphatemia during medical treatment. We should note that the following manuscript was presented at the 2019 American Association of Clinical Endocrinologists (AACE) 28th Annual Scientific and Clinical Congress.

1. Introduction

Cancer is the second cause of death in the United States, and multiple myeloma accounts for approximately 1 to 2 percent of all cancers [1]. In such regard, the American Cancer Society estimates that, in 2020, new cases of multiple myeloma will reach 32,270 in the U.S., while deaths could top 12,830 [2]. This disease is characterized by neoplastic proliferation of immunoglobulin-producing plasma cells, and patients may present a variety of signs or symptoms including, without limitation, bone pain, anemia, acute renal failure, high serum proteins, and multiple electrolyte disturbances. Also, in multiple myeloma, hypercalcemia is observed in approximately one-third of patients and could be mediated by parathyroid hormone-related peptide, osteolytic cytokine production, and excess 1,25-dihydroxyvitamin D production [3, 4]. However, in asymptomatic patients, it is important that pseudohypercalcemia associated to paraproteins is excluded; thus, ionized calcium measurement is recommended. On the contrary, hyperphosphatemia is most likely secondary to renal dysfunction. Nonetheless, hypophosphatemia is rare, and there are few reported cases. For instance, Mao and Ong described a case of hypophosphatemia that was due to paraproteins causing assay interference [5]. As you will see in our case, we faced the classic presentation of multiple myeloma with subsequent development of dangerous hypophosphatemia during medical regimen.

2. Case Report

This is the case of a 56-year-old Hispanic woman with a past medical history of arterial hypertension, type 2 diabetes mellitus, and chronic anemia who was transferred from a community medical clinic to our institution for management of symptomatic anemia, severe hypercalcemia, and renal failure. Upon evaluation at our institution, the patient stated that, for the last three months, she had been experiencing fatigue, generalized weakness, back pain, decreased appetite, and unquantified weight loss. Moreover, the day prior to admission, she had an episode of lightheadedness followed by loss of consciousness for which she was taken to the community medical clinic for evaluation. Upon arrival to our institution, her blood pressure was 161/76 mmHg with a heart rate of 78 bpm, respiratory rate of 18 rpm, temperature of 36.5°C, and peripheral oxygen saturation of 99% at room air. The physical examination provided a remarkable perspective for an acutely ill appearance, generalized paleness,

Table 1: Laboratories upon admission.

BUN (mg/dL)	Creatinine (mg/dL)	Calcium (mg/dL)	Albumin (g/dL)	Total protein (g/dL)	Magnesium (mg/dL)	Phosphorous (mg/dL)	Intact PTH (pg/ml)	1,25-Dihydroxyvitamin D (pg/ml)	25-Hydroxyvitamin D (ng/ml)
67.00 (8–21)	7.00 (0.6–1.10)	12.40 (8.8–10.3)	2.30 (3.7–4.9)	11.50 (6.2–7.9)	2.06 (1.8–2.2)	2.50 (2.4–4.2)	25 (11–67)	8.6 (19.9–79.3)	38.1 (30–100)

and dry oral mucosa. Initial laboratories were also remarkable for normocytic normochromic anemia of 6.5 g/dL (12.0–14.0), albumin-corrected calcium of 13.8 mg/dL (8.8–10.3), and elevated creatinine of 6.7 mg/dL (0.60–1.10) with a glomerular filtration rate of 7 min/mL (>60). 25-Hydroxyvitamin D was within normal limits at 38.1 ng/ml (30.0–100.0), whereas 1,25-dihydroxyvitamin D was low at 8.6 pg/mL (19.9–79.3). Notwithstanding, the patient had normal phosphorus level in 2.50 mg/dL (2.40–4.20) and normal intact parathyroid hormone in 25 pg/mL (11–67) (see Table 1). Finally, radiographic images disclosed multiple skeletal lytic lesions. In light of such clinical presentation, the patient was admitted into the internal medicine ward with ongoing diagnosis of symptomatic anemia, acute renal failure, and moderate hypercalcemia.

During the early course of hospitalization, both nephrology and hematology/oncology services were consulted for further recommendations regarding renal function deterioration with multiple electrolyte disturbances and a high suspicion of multiple myeloma. The patient was initially managed with aggressive intravenous hydration with isotonic saline and systemic dexamethasone, with marked improvement in renal function during the course of the first week. The results from bone marrow biopsy were consistent with high-risk IgG/kappa multiple myeloma, reason why she was started on chemotherapy with cyclophosphamide, bortezomib, and dexamethasone (CyBorD).

At this point, it was remarkable that the patient continued with corrected hypercalcemia of 11 mg/dL (8.8–10.3) and developed hypophosphatemia of 1.7 mg/dL (2.40–4.20). During the second week of hospitalization, the patient suffered a pathological fracture of the right humerus for which a single dose of zoledronic acid was administered. Therefore, based on the evidence of the pathological fracture, the patient was evaluated by radiation-oncology specialists and was treated with external beam radiotherapy (IMRT technique) up to about the total dose of 4000 cGy.

Furthermore, at day 20, endocrinology service was consulted for recommendations regarding persistent hypophosphatemia despite oral and intravenous replacement. Consequently, new laboratory workup was ordered and was remarkable for marked elevation of intact PTH in 711 pg/ml (11–67), 1,25-dihydroxyvitamin D of 123.0 pg/mL (19.9–79.3), normal albumin-corrected calcium of 8.9 mg/dl (8.8–10.3), and fractional excretion of phosphorus in 14% with reference range <5%. The ionized calcium level was low at 1.15 mEq/L (1.17–1.58) (see Table 2) and phosphorus in 1.4 mg/dl (2.40–4.20).

In view of the persistent hypophosphatemia and the new laboratory results, we considered secondary hyperparathyroidism and pseudohypercalcemia as the etiology of hypophosphatemia. The patient was initiated on calcitriol, and as a result, electrolytes normalized. She was discharged from our institution after 30 days of hospitalization, with remarkable laboratories at the moment of discharge for normal renal function with creatinine at 0.96 mg/dL (0.6–1.10), albumin-corrected calcium at 9.9 mg/dL (8.8–10.3), and phosphorus at 4.70 mg/dL (2.40–4.20) (see Table 3). Eventually, the patient was successfully treated with an autologous stem cell transplant with excellent response.

3. Discussion

Patients with malignancies are exposed to experience multiple metabolic abnormalities. These disturbances can be part of the original process of the disease, medical treatment, or complications during the progression of the disease.

Multiple myeloma (MM) is characterized by proliferation of monoclonal plasma cells in the bone marrow, resulting thereby in overproduction of monoclonal paraproteins. The excessive plasma cell production results in extensive skeletal destruction with osteolytic lesions and pathologic fractures. Also, the deposition of paraproteins in kidneys affecting the renal function coupled with the lytic lesions can provoke the most common electrolyte disturbances seen in MM, which are hypercalcemia and hyperphosphatemia.

In our case, the patient was diagnosed with multiple myeloma with a typical presentation of the disease. During the first weeks of hospitalization, albumin-corrected calcium showed elevated values until ionized calcium ordered during the workup for persistent hypophosphatemia demonstrated the opposite. This finding coupled with the fact that the patient did not present symptoms of hypercalcemia favored the diagnosis of pseudohypercalcemia.

There is evidence that multiple myeloma can occasionally cause laboratory artifacts due to paraproteinemia, causing thereby confusion among physicians. For instance, Ashrafi et al. and Caras reported laboratory interference in electrolytes due to high levels of paraproteins [6, 7]. The proposed mechanisms of these findings include binding of calcium to abnormal immunoglobulins interfering with immunologic assays [4].

Initially, the patient presented normal intact parathyroid hormone (PTH), which exponentially increased after management of factitious hypercalcemia in multiple myeloma. In the absence of high ionized calcium, elevated PTH is the equivalent to secondary hyperparathyroidism [8]. The main mechanism that explains the secondary hyperparathyroidism in our patient is the expected response to true hypocalcemia. As part of the dynamic of parathyroid secretion in

Table 2: Laboratories at the moment of endocrinology service evaluation.

BUN (mg/dL)	Creatinine (mg/dL)	Calcium (mg/dL)	Albumin (g/dL)	Total protein (g/dL)	Magnesium (mg/dL)	Phosphorous (mg/dL)	Intact PTH (pg/ml)	1,25-Dihroxyvitamin D (pg/ml)	1,25-Dihydroxyvitamin D (ng/ml)	Ionized calcium (mEq/L)
17.0	1.13	7.50	2.20	8.60	1.73	1.40	711	123	31.7	1.15
(8–21)	(0.6–1.10)	(8.8–10.3)	(3.7–4.9)	(6.2–7.9)	(1.8–2.2)	(2.4–4.2)	(11–67)	(19.9–79.3)	(30–100)	(1.17–1.58)

TABLE 3: Laboratories at the moment of discharge.

BUN (mg/dL)	Creatinine (mg/dL)	Calcium (mg/dL)	Albumin (g/dL)	Total protein (g/dL)	Magnesium (mg/dL)	Phosphorous (mg/dL)
8.00 (8–21)	0.96 (0.6–1.10)	8.50 (8.8–10.3)	2.30 (3.7–4.9)	7.80 (6.2–7.9)	1.52 (1.8–2.2)	4.70 (2.4–4.2)

response to the ongoing hypocalcemia and improvement in the renal function, intact PTH and 1,25-dihydroxyvitamin D increased significantly provoking the dramatic changes in the homeostasis of phosphorus, which was observed in our case.

In addition, the patient developed severe hypophosphatemia with persistent inadequate response to medical replacement. The effects of elevated parathyroid hormone (PTH) decreased the activity of sodium phosphate cotransporters at the proximal and distal renal tubules, causing an increase in phosphate excretion [9, 10]. This mechanism was evident in our patient with elevated fractional excretion of phosphate during the course of medical management. The primary cause of transient hypophosphatemia in our patient was the secondary hyperparathyroidism caused by true low ionized calcium.

Moreover, several medical therapies utilized in multiple myeloma including, without limitation, volume expansion, bisphosphonates, and corticosteroids, are mainly associated to the increase in phosphorus excretion. Consequently, the patient was treated with a single dose of zoledronic acid infusion, which is a bisphosphonic acid that inhibits the resorption and remodeling activity of the bones. The manufacturer prescribing information of zoledronic acid describes the incidence of hypophosphatemia in 973 patients treated for multiple myeloma and bone metastasis of solid tumors. Grade 3 hypophosphatemia (serum phosphate less than 2 mg/dL) was 12%, while grade 4 hypophosphatemia (serum phosphate less than 1 mg/dL) was less than 1%. Thus, although the exact mechanism of zoledronic acid-induced hypophosphatemia is not completely understood, the hypothesized explanations are that the adverse effect of hypocalcemia provokes induced hyperparathyroidism aggravating the phosphate excretion. This could be a possibility in our case. However, we need to point out the fact that the 973 patients had a median duration of exposure for a safety period of 12.8 months with zoledronic acid every 3-4 weeks, whereas in our case, the patient was treated with a single dose of zoledronic acid. As mentioned, the combined treatments for factitious hypercalcemia coupled with the original process and complications of the disease can trigger electrolyte disorders that could be very challenging to treat.

4. Conclusion

In summary, this case report highlights different uncommon electrolyte disorders that can be found in patients with multiple myeloma. Pseudohypercalcemia in the setting of elevated total proteins should always be taken under consideration, particularly when the patient does not exhibit signs and symptoms suggestive of elevated calcium level. In such cases, measurement of ionized calcium should be strongly considered to determine the true extracellular calcium levels. Additionally, the combined treatment for factitious hypercalcemia and renal impairment can trigger secondary hyperparathyroidism aggravating thereby other electrolyte disorders.

Finally, the multiple electrolyte disturbances faced in multiple myeloma and medication side effects can precipitate serious metabolic disorders such as hypophosphatemia seen in our patient. There are different mechanisms including an increase in phosphate excretion and intracellular shifting worsening the phosphate level. For that reason, the physician should be able to differentiate between true and spurious electrolyte imbalance in order to prevent unnecessary interventions that could be detrimental to the patient.

References

[1] R. L. Siegel, K. D. Miller, and A. Jemal, "Cancer statistics, 2020," *CA: A Cancer Journal for Clinicians*, vol. 70, no. 1, pp. 7–30, 2020.

[2] American Cancer Society, *Cancer Facts & Figures 2020*, American Cancer Society, Atlanta, GA, USA, 2020.

[3] J. D. Schwab, M. A. Strack, L. D. Hughes, Shaker et al., "Pseudohypercalcemia in an elderly patient with multiple myeloma: report of a case and review of literature," *Endocrine Practice: November*, vol. 1, no. 6, pp. 390–392, 1995.

[4] W. Goldner, "Cancer-related hypercalcemia," *Journal of Oncology Practice*, vol. 12, no. 5, pp. 426–432, 2016.

[5] Z. Mao and A. C. M. Ong, "Spurious hypophosphatemia associated with monoclonal paraproteinemia," *QJM*, vol. 105, no. 7, pp. 693–696, 2012.

[6] F. Ashrafi, B. Iraj, P. Nematollahi, and A Darakhshandeh, "Pseudohypercalcemia in multiple myeloma: a case report," *International Journal of Hematology-Oncology and Stem Cell Research*, vol. 11, no. 3, pp. 246–249, 2017.

[7] J. A. Caras, "Spurious hypophosphatemia associated with multiple myeloma," *Endocrine Practice of Official Journal of the American College of Endocrinology and the American Association of Clinical Endocrinologists*, vol. 3, pp. 135-136, 1997.

[8] R. Freaney, Y. McBrinn, and M. J. McKenna, "Secondary hyperparathyroidism in elderly people: combined effect of renal insufficiency and vitamin D deficiency," *The American Journal of Clinical Nutrition*, vol. 58, no. 2, pp. 187–191, 1993.

[9] M. H. Homer Smith Award, "Cellular mechanisms in proximal tubular Pi reabsorption: some answers and more questions," *J Am Soc Nephrol*, vol. 2, p. 1649, 1992.

[10] H. Murer, M. Lötscher, B. Kaissling, M. Levi, S. A. Kempson, and J. Biber, "Renal brush border membrane Na/Pi-co-transport: molecular aspects in PTH-dependent and dietary regulation," *Kidney International*, vol. 49, no. 6, p. 1769, 1996.

15

Be(a)ware of Leukocytosis in Papillary Thyroid Cancer

Styliani Laskou,[1] Konstantinos Sapalidis,[1] Christos Topalidis,[2] Triantafyllia Koletsa,[2] and Isaak Kesisoglou[1]

[1]3rd Surgical Department, Aristotle University of Thessaloniki, AHEPA Hospital, Thessaloniki, Greece
[2]Department of Pathology, Faculty of Medicine, Aristotle University of Thessaloniki, Thessaloniki, Greece

Correspondence should be addressed to Styliani Laskou; stelaskou@gmail.com

Academic Editor: J. Paul Frindik

Leukocytosis can be present at any time during various malignancies. A 42-year-old male was admitted to our department for surgical management of his metastatic papillary thyroid cancer. Persistent white blood cell (WBC) elevation with left shift led to a thorough investigation. Having excluded other causes, leukocytosis was attributed to thyroid cancer itself. Positive immunostaining for IL-6 and CEA, as well as elevated serum levels, established this connection.

1. Introduction

Tumor-related leukocytosis is associated with advanced tumor-stage and poor patient outcomes. However, it has been largely ignored or misinterpreted. If the underlying malignancy is not clinically evident, leukocytosis could be attributed to myeloproliferative neoplasms, misleading the patient's management. Solid tumors such as lung, genitourinary, gastrointestinal, melanoma, and head and neck may secrete cytokines, mainly granulocyte colony-stimulating factor (G-CSF), granulocyte-macrophage CSF (GM-CSF), and/or interleukins. As far as thyroid cancer is concerned, squamous and anaplastic cancer cases associated with leukocytosis have been reported. We report the rare case of a well-differentiated papillary thyroid carcinoma linked to neoplastic leukocytosis and elevated CEA levels.

2. Case Report/Case Presentation

In February 2021, a 42-year-old male was admitted to our surgical department due to metastatic papillary thyroid carcinoma detected on an outpatient investigation. He had previously visited a maxillofacial surgeon due to palpable right neck lymphadenopathy, who suggested a neck ultrasound (US). The US showed a 21 × 12 mm hypoechoic solid lesion in the thyroid isthmus and a 33 × 32 × 25 mm lesion with abnormal parenchymal composition and calcifications occupying the right lobe. Central and right lateral cervical lymph nodes were highly suspicious. Fine needle aspiration of the two tumors and a region III lymph node suggested the presence of a metastatic multifocal papillary thyroid carcinoma (PTC).

Thyroid function examination and anti-thyroglobulin antibodies were within the normal range while serum thyroglobulin was 176.9 ng/ml (normal range: 0–50 ng/ml). It was noteworthy that his laboratory tests showed leukocytosis with neutrophilia (WBC: 21,390 K/μl, NE: 18,300 K/μl), although further investigation was not considered. The patient underwent thyroidectomy with central and right lateral selective lymph node dissection. Due to the aggressive behavior of the tumor, the right thyroid lobe and specimens from the trachea were sent for intraoperative histologic examination, which confirmed the presence of PTC in the right lobe and neoplastic infiltration of the fibroadipose tissue from the trachea along with a metastatic lymph node. The operation was completed, and the patient had an uneventful recovery.

Gross examination of the thyroid specimen revealed multiple white to tan nodules scattered throughout the gland, both in the lobes, but also in the isthmus, measured from 0.2 cm to 5 cm in diameter. Hematoxylin and eosin-stained sections showed that the described lesions correspond to PTC characterized mainly by papillary structures "(shown in Figure 1(a))". The lining epithelium consisted of medium-sized cells with eosinophilic cytoplasm and distinctive nuclear features, namely, nuclear overlapping, chromatin clearing, irregular nuclear contour, and nuclear grooves and pseudoinclusions "(shown in Figure 1(b))". Psammoma bodies were also present in the adjacent area. Stroma was fibrous with dense collagenous with sparsely inflammatory cells. Despite the multiple sections, areas of low differentiation or anaplastic features were not observed. Cancer cells invaded the thyroid capsule and expanded in the surrounding tissues. In addition, seven cervical lymph nodes displayed metastases from the carcinoma. Histologic findings were consistent with a multifocal PTC of the classic variant pT4aN1b according to the pTNM classification scheme.

The patient was reevaluated on the second postoperative month. The US showed left lateral cervical lymphadenopathy and a recurrence of $24 \times 19 \times 22$ mm in the central region despite the meticulous operation. Cervical computed tomography (CT) depicted the aforementioned pathologic lymph nodes. Chest and abdominal CT did not reveal further metastatic lesions. TSH and TG were elevated (18,1 μIU/ml and 131 ng/ml, respectively) while leukocytosis with neutrophilia (WBC: 23,720 K/μl, NE: 19,800 K/μl) remained. Blasts and immature white blood cells were not found, while erythrocyte sedimentation rate (ESR), C-reactive protein (CRP), and carcinoembryonic antigen (CEA) levels were elevated (22 mm/L, 16 ng/ml, and 18 ng/ml, respectively). After a thorough investigation by the internal medicine department, infectious diseases, leukemia, and myeloproliferative neoplasms were excluded. Searching for the cause of leukocytosis, serum concentrations of granulocyte colony-stimulating factor (G-CSF) and IL-6 were measured. IL-6 levels were found elevated (71 pg/ml, normal range<7), which partially explained the observed leukocytosis.

In June, the patient underwent a second operation with left lateral neck dissection and excision of the recurrence in the central compartment. Histologic examination revealed nine metastatic lymph nodes. After being informed of high serum IL-6 levels, immunohistochemistry with IL-6 antibody was performed, which revealed positivity in a few neoplastic cells "(shown in Figure 2(a))". Few cells were immunoreactive to CEA antibody as well "(shown in Figure 2(b))".

Postoperatively, he received a dose of 120 mCi iodine 131. Whole-body scan showed foci of uptake in the thyroid bed. Appropriate thyroxine suppressive therapy was added and on the second post-iodine month patient new examinations were ordered revealing normalized levels of TSH and TG (0,8 μIU/ML and 0.1 ng/ml respectively). Surprisingly, WBC and neutrophils, ESR, CRP, and CEA were also within the normal range (WBC: 9800 K/μl, NE: 5,000 K/μl, ESR:12, CRP:0,5, CEA: 1,2). IL-6 levels were also measured (2,8 pg/ml). The patient remains under close endocrinologic and surgical surveillance without evidence of recurrence.

3. Discussion

This patient may represent the first established classic papillary thyroid carcinoma case with associated leukocytosis and elevated CEA levels caused by IL-6 and CEA expression by tumor cells. Leukocytosis and malignancy have long been linked and known as paraneoplastic leukemoid reaction [1]. In its formal definition, leukemoid reaction refers to persistent leukocytosis (WBC >40 000/μL) in the absence of a hematologic malignancy. Various infections, intoxications, malignancies, severe hemorrhage, or acute hemolysis may be the etiology [2]. Paraneoplastic leukemoid reaction occurs in the presence of a non-hematolymphoid cytokine-secreting tumor and in the absence of bone marrow infiltration by that tumor [3]. In many malignancies, a less profound leukocytosis may be observed, although.

It seems that irregular cytokine production by tumor cells, such as granulocyte colony-stimulating factor (G-CSF), granulocyte-macrophage colony-stimulating factor (GM-CSF), and interleukins (IL-3, IL-6, and TNF-α) initiate the pathogenesis [4] leading to granulocytosis. This ability may be present along with tumor development or secondarily after dedifferentiation and can also be seen in metastatic sites even if it is absent in the primary tumor [5]. Cytokine-producing tumor foci grow faster than the nonproducing ones due to an autocrine growth induction phenomenon [6]. In addition to stimulating bone marrow granulocytosis, an inhibition of myeloid cell differentiation in the tumor microenvironment may be observed, causing the accumulation of immature myeloid cells. These myeloid-derived suppressor cells "protect" the tumor, contributing also to neoangiogenesis and cancer progression. Such patients seem to have a poor prognosis [3].

A variety of tumors may be associated with elevated WBC. Tumor-related leukocytosis may be present at any time during the disease, simultaneously, late, or even prior to the diagnosis. Although lung and kidney malignancies are commonly associated with leukocytosis, gastrointestinal, hepatobiliary, genitourinary, melanoma, and head and neck cancers [2] have also been reported.

Thyroid malignancies have also been associated with paraneoplastic leukocytosis. Two cases of squamous cell carcinoma [7, 8] and seventeen cases of anaplastic tumor have been reported [9–23]. Both cases of squamous cell carcinoma were related to marked leukocytosis and hypercalcemia. The authors proposed that tumor cells produced G-CSF, IL- 1a, and PTH-rP, suggesting the existence of a new paraneoplastic syndrome. Elevated G-CSF levels were detected in anaplastic thyroid cancer cases. Only a few case reports evaluated IL-6 levels as either elevated or within the normal range [10–12, 23].

A unique case of aggressive papillary thyroid cancer associated with neutrophilia has been published.

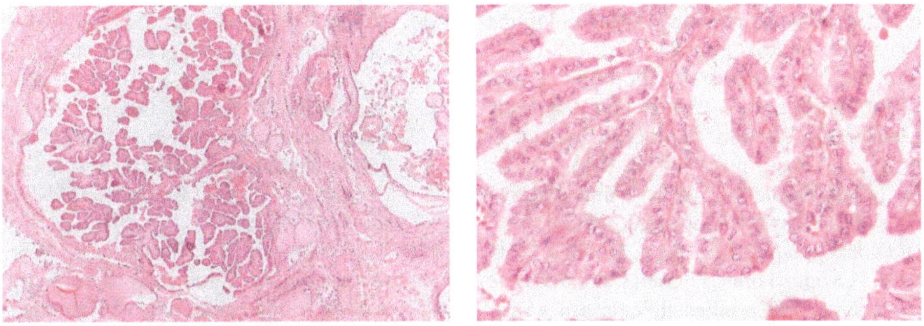

(a) (b)

FIGURE 1: (a) (×40) Papillary structures typical of papillary thyroid carcinoma filling cystic spaces. (b) (×400) Papillary structures are lined by medium-sized cells with eosinophilic cytoplasm and nuclear features typical of papillary thyroid carcinoma.

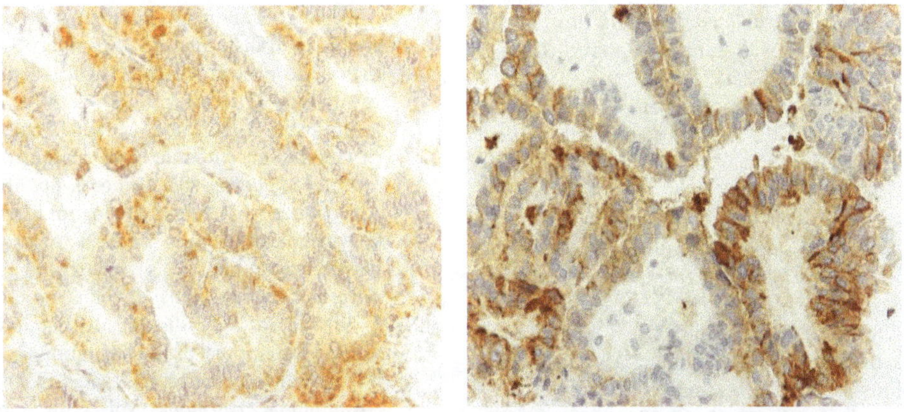

(a) (b)

FIGURE 2: (a) (×400) Immunohistochemical stain for IL-6 proved to be positive in cancer cells. (b) (×400) A small proportion of cancer cells displayed immunoreactivity for CEA.

Vassilatou et al. hypothesized that the presence of CSF-producing tumor was indicated by elevated GM-CSF serum levels. Bone marrow biopsy revealed infiltration by the papillary thyroid carcinoma [24]. Our patient differed from the above since the tumor cells synthesized and secreted IL-6, which seemed to be the cause of leukocytosis. Perhaps, both cases indicate papillary thyroid cancer as a precursor of anaplastic.

Moreover, tumor cells were positive for CEA with elevated CEA serum levels. CEA is produced as an expression of CEA-related cell adhesion molecule 5 gene and is found in 90% of gastrointestinal cancers, 70% of lung cancers, and 50% of breast cancers [25]. Elevated levels may also be seen in ovarian cancer, appendix, mucinous cystadenoma, and medullary thyroid carcinoma. Since only single cases of CEA-positive papillary thyroid cancer have been observed, its significance remains uncertain.

4. Conclusion

Tumor-related leukocytosis is associated with tumor aggressiveness and probably poor prognosis. When dealing with patients with unexplained leukocytosis, a high level of suspicion is required for this entity.

Additional Points

Tumor-related leukocytosis could represent a form of paraneoplastic syndrome caused by cytokine secretion from tumor cells.

Consent

The patient has given written informed consent to publish this case including the publication of images.

Authors' Contributions

S.L. perceived the idea, collected the samples, processed the data, drafted the manuscript, and designed the figures. K.S. was involved in planning and supervised the work. T.K. and C.T. performed the histopathological analysis and designed the histopathologic figures. I.K. was the supervising physician. All authors discussed the results and commented on the manuscript.

References

[1] S. Asano, A. Urabe, T. Okabe, N. Sato, and Y. Kondo, "Demonstration of granulopoietic factor(s) in the plasma of

nude mice transplanted with a human lung cancer and in the tumor tissue," *Blood*, vol. 49, no. 5, pp. 845–852, 1977.

[2] V. Sakka, S. Tsiodras, E. J. Giamarellos-Bourboulis, and H. Giamarellou, "An update on the etiology and diagnostic evaluation of a leukemoid reaction," *European Journal of Internal Medicine*, vol. 17, no. 6, pp. 394–398, 2006.

[3] I. A. Abukhiran, J. Jasser, and S. Syrbu, "Paraneoplastic leukemoid reactions induced by cytokine-secreting tumours," *Journal of Clinical Pathology*, vol. 73, no. 6, pp. 310–313, 2020.

[4] J. M. Granger and D. P. Kontoyiannis, "Etiology and outcome of extreme leukocytosis in 758 nonhematologic cancer patients: a retrospective, single-institution study," *Cancer*, vol. 115, no. 17, pp. 3919–3923, 2009.

[5] R. A. Wilcox, "Cancer-associated myeloproliferation: old association, new therapeutic target," *Mayo Clinic Proceedings*, vol. 85, no. 7, pp. 656–663, 2010.

[6] I. Kasuga, S. Makino, H. Kiyokawa, H. Katoh, Y. Ebihara, and K. Ohyashiki, "Tumor-Related leukocytosis is linked with poor prognosis in patients with lung carcinoma," *Cancer*, vol. 92, no. 9, pp. 2399–2405, 2001.

[7] K. Saito, Y. Kuratomi, K. Yamamoto et al., "Primary squamous cell carcinoma of the thyroid associated with marked leukocytosis and hypercalcemia," *Cancer*, vol. 48, no. 9, pp. 2080–2083, 1981.

[8] P. E. Riddle and H. P. Dincsoy, "Primary squamous cell carcinoma of the thyroid associated with leukocytosis and hypercalcemia," *Archives of Pathology & Laboratory Medicine*, vol. 111, no. 4, pp. 373-374, 1987.

[9] T. Fujita, Y. Ogasawara, M. Naito, H. Doihara, and N. Shimizu, "Anaplastic thyroid carcinoma associated with granulocyte colony-stimulating factor: report of a case," *Surgery Today*, vol. 36, no. 1, pp. 63–67, 2005.

[10] J. S. Saitoh, A. Musha, T. Mizukami, T. Abe, and T. Nakano, "A case of thyroid anaplastic carcinoma presenting marked neutrophilia and eosinophilia due to co-production of GM-CSF, M-CSF and IL-6," *International Journal of Radiology & Radiation Therapy*, vol. 3, no. 2, pp. 203–206, 2017.

[11] T. Sato, M. Omura, J. Saito et al., "Neutrophilia associated with anaplastic carcinoma of the thyroid: production of macrophage colony-stimulating factor (M-CSF) and lnterleukin-6," *Thyroid*, vol. 10, no. 12, pp. 1113–1118, 2000.

[12] S. Yazawa, H. Toshimori, K. Nakatsuru, H. Katakami, J. Takemura, and S. Matsukura, "Thyroid anaplastic carcinoma producing granulocyte-colony-stimulating factor and parathyroid hormone-related protein," *Internal Medicine*, vol. 34, no. 6, pp. 584–588, 1995.

[13] H. Murabe, T. Akamizu, A. Kubota, and S. Kusaka, "Anaplastic thyroid carcinoma with prominent cardiac metastasis, accompanied by a marked leukocytosis with a neutrophilia and high GM-CSF level in serum," *Internal Medicine*, vol. 31, no. 9, pp. 1107–1111, 1992.

[14] K. Iwasa, M. Noguchi, K. Mori et al., "Anaplastic thyroid carcinoma producing the granulocyte colony stimulating factor (G-CSF): report of a case," *Surgery Today*, vol. 25, no. 2, pp. 158–160, 1995.

[15] T. Nakada, H. Sato, F. Inoue, F. Mizorogi, K. Nagayama, and T. Tanaka, "The production of colony-stimulating factors by thyroid carcinoma is associated with marked neutrophilia and eosinophilia," *Internal Medicine*, vol. 35, no. 10, pp. 815–820, 1996.

[16] S. Hoshi, A. Yoshizawa, H. Arioka, N. Kobayashi, K. Kudo, and H. Niino, "Anaplastic thyroid carcinoma with lung metastasis producing CA 19-9 and GM-CSF," *Nihon Kokyuki Gakkai Zasshi*, vol. 38, no. 5, pp. 391-397, 2000.

[17] T. Kitanishi, M. Suzuki, J. Fukui et al., "Two cases of thyroid carcinoma producing granulocyte colony-stimulating factor," *Journal of Otolaryngology*, vol. 29, no. 3, pp. 174–178, 2000.

[18] M. Zweifel, F. Stenner-Liewen, A. Weber et al., "Increased bone marrow activity on F-18-FDG PET/CT in granulocyte colony stimulating factor producing anaplastic thyroid carcinoma," *Clinical Nuclear Medicine*, vol. 35, no. 2, pp. 103-104, 2010.

[19] R. Nakayama, K. Horiuchi, M. Susa et al., "Anaplastic transformation of follicular thyroid carcinoma in a metastatic skeletal lesion presenting with paraneoplastic leukocytosis," *Thyroid*, vol. 22, no. 2, pp. 200–204, 2012.

[20] K. Kang, J. H. Park, J. Y. Ryu, S. Y. Lee, G. J. Ko, and Y. J. Kwon, "Acute pyelonephritis with anaplastic thyroid carcinoma producing granulocyte colony-stimulating factor," *Blood Research*, vol. 48, no. 1, pp. 63–66, Mar. 2013.

[21] H. R. Lee, J. S. Baek, S. H. Lee, A. R. Cho, J. Y. Lee, and J. M. Jang, "Paraneoplastic neutrophilia originating from an anaplastic transformation of papillary thyroid carcinoma in a metastatic pleural lesion," *Medical Journal of Chosun University*, vol. 39, no. 1, pp. 39–42, 2014.

[22] J. Shiraishi, H. Koyama, M. Seki et al., "Anaplastic thyroid carcinoma accompanied by uncontrollable eosinophilia," *Internal Medicine*, vol. 54, no. 6, pp. 611–616, 2015.

[23] A. Polymeris, C. Kogia, D. Ioannidis et al., "Excessive leukocytosis leading to a diagnosis of aggressive thyroid anaplastic carcinoma: a case report and relevant review," *The European Thyroid Journal*, vol. 9, no. 3, pp. 162–168, 2020.

[24] E. Vassilatou, M. Fisfis, G. Morphopoulos et al., "Papillary thyroid carcinoma producing granulocyte-macrophage colony-stimulating factor is associated with neutrophilia and eosinophilia," *Hormones*, vol. 5, no. 4, pp. 303–309, 2006.

[25] K. Wakabayashi-Nakao, K. Hatakeyama, K. Ohshima, K. Ken Yamaguchi, and T. Mochizuki, "Carcinoembryonic antigen-related cell adhesion molecule 4 (CEACAM4) is specifically expressed in medullary thyroid carcinoma cells," *Biomedical Research*, vol. 35, no. 4, pp. 237–242, 2014.

16

Hypokalemic Periodic Paralysis as the First Manifestation of Thyrotropin-Secreting Pituitary Adenoma

Chatchon Kaewkrasaesin,[1,2] Patinut Buranasupkajorn,[2,3] Paisith Piriyawat,[4] Sarat Sunthornyothin ,[2,3] and Thiti Snabboon [2,3]

[1]*Division of Medicine, Taksin Hospital, Medical Service Department, Bangkok Metropolitan Administration, Bangkok, Thailand*
[2]*Department of Medicine, Faculty of Medicine, Chulalongkorn University, Bangkok, Thailand*
[3]*Excellence Center in Diabetes, Hormone and Metabolism, King Chulalongkorn Memorial Hospital, Thai Red Cross Society, Bangkok, Thailand*
[4]*Department of Neurology, Texas Tech University Health Sciences Center El Paso, El Paso, USA*

Correspondence should be addressed to Thiti Snabboon; thiti.s@chula.ac.th

Academic Editor: Hidetoshi Ikeda

Thyrotoxic periodic paralysis is an unusual neurological manifestation of thyrotoxicosis, and even rarer when it occurs in thyrotropin-secreting pituitary adenoma, only 6 cases having been previously reported. We describe a case of pituitary microadenoma with clinical syndromes of thyrotoxicosis complicated with hypokalemic periodic paralysis. Clinical manifestations and proposed management are discussed.

1. Introduction

Thyrotropin-secreting pituitary adenoma (TSHoma) is the rarest subtype among the functioning pituitary adenomas, with its prevalence less than 3% of all pituitary tumors [1]. About 80–85% of TSHomas, at diagnosis, are macroadenoma with local mass effect and mild thyrotoxicosis [2]. Herein, we report an unusual presentation of TSHoma with thyrotoxic periodic paralysis (TPP).

2. Case Presentation

A 42-year-old Thai man presented with quadriparesis upon awakening after having a high-carbohydrate dinner. His two previous episodes were mild and self-limited. He denied history of medication, alcohol use, or family history of weakness. He however noticed palpitations and 3-kg weight loss over the past 6 months. The patient was alert with tachycardia of 108/min. Neurological examination showed proximal muscle weakness grade 2/5 and the distal grade 4/5 of both extremities, while sensation and reflexes were preserved. No dysarthria, nystagmus, or cranial nerve palsy was involved. Thyroid gland was about twice the normal size without bruit or exophthalmos. Laboratory investigation revealed K^+2.7 mEq/L and inappropriate secretion of TSH: TSH 12.96 μIU/mL (0.4–4.1), FT_4 2.17 ng/dL (0.8–1.8), and FT_3 8.41 pg/dL (1.8–4.0). Other pituitary hormone levels as well as electrolytes were unremarkable (Table 1). ECG revealed sinus tachycardia with *U* wave. MRI of the pituitary gland revealed a microadenoma, 6 mm in diameter, without pressure effect on adjacent structures (Figure 1). A diagnosis of TPP from TSHoma was proposed by his dramatic recovery of muscle strength within 6 hours with rebound hyperkalemia after only 100 mEq of potassium replacement. Methimazole (15 mg/d), subcutaneous short-acting octreotide (Sandostatin 100 μg three times a day) and propranolol (40 mg/d) were commenced and trans-sphenoidal surgery (TSS) was performed 4 weeks later. Pathology and immunohistochemistry confirmed the diagnosis of TSHoma, as well as a negative mutation study of the thyroid hormone receptor beta (THRB) gene. During the one-year follow-up, he was in euthyroid state and complete remission of periodic attack (Table 2).

TABLE 1: Laboratory data on admission.

Hematology	
White blood cells (cell/mm^3)	7500
Hemoglobin	13.5
Platelets (×10^3/mm^3)	210
Blood chemistry	
Glucose (mg/dL)	95
Creatinine (0.5–1.0 mg/dL)	0.9
Sodium (135–145 mEq/L)	140
Potassium (3.4–4.5 mEq/L)	2.7
Carbon dioxide (22–29 mEq/L)	24
Calcium (8.5–10.5 mg/dL)	9.0
Phosphate (2.5–4.5 mg/dL)	2.5
Albumin (3.5–4.5 g/dL)	3.9
Magnesium (1.7–2.4 mg/dL)	1.7
CPK (0–190 U/L)	110
Hormonal analysis	
FT_3 (1.6–4.0 pg/mL)	8.41
FT_4 (0.8–1.8 ng/dL)	2.17
TSH (0.3–4.1 μU/mL)	12.96
IGF-I (101–267 ng/mL)	201
Prolactin (3–25 ng/mL)	15
FSH (1.0–8.4 IU/L)	8.8
LH (1.0–10.5 IU/L)	5.6
Testosterone (290–1,300 ng/dL)	452
8 AM. Cortisol (μg/dL)	10.9
Thyroid autoantibody	
Anti-TPO (<50 IU/mL)	34
Anti-Tg (<100 IU/mL)	56

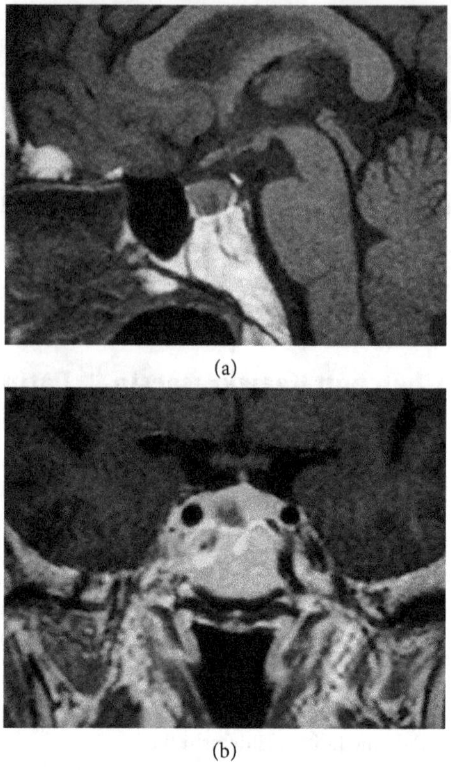

FIGURE 1: MRI pituitary gland (T1-weighted, sagittal view) showed a 6 mm hypointensity sellar lesion with irregular margin (a). On coronal postcontrast T1-weighted image, the lesion remained hypointensity while the gland showed marked homogenous enhancement (b).

TABLE 2: Serum potassium levels and thyroid function tests at admission, during treatment, and follow-up period.

	Admission	6 hour later*	Before operation**	12 month follow up
Serum potassium (3.5–4.5 mEq/L)	2.7	5.9	3.9	4.2
FT_3 (1.6–4.0 pg/mL)	8.41	NA	4.6	2.3
FT_4 (0.8–1.8 ng/dL)	2.17	NA	1.9	1.1
TSH (0.3–4.1 μU/mL)	12.96	NA	8.45	3.77

*After potassium chloride elixir 100 m Eq. **4 weeks later with sandostatin, methimazole, and propranolol. NA: not available.

3. Discussion

At diagnosis, less than 70% of TSHoma patients have thyroid manifestations, most of which are goiter or thyroid nodules, with only 20–30% of them having thyrotoxicosis symptoms [2]. We report here case of a rare neurologic-thyrotoxic concurrence, in a TSHoma patient with microadenoma.

Triad findings of TPP are transient episodes of flaccid muscle weakness, hypokalemia, and thyrotoxicosis [3]. While commonly associated with Graves' disease, it has been also described in any etiology of thyrotoxicosis. Most of TPP patients are male Asian patients despite female preponderance of Graves' disease. The characteristics of weakness are indistinguishable from other types of hypokalemic periodic paralysis which mainly involve in proximal parts of upper and lower extremities and rarely ocular, bulbar, bowel/bladder, or respiratory muscles. The frequency of attacks is variable and duration of episodes ranges from hours to several days. Severity of weakness correlates with the degree of hypokalemia. Muscle strength improves after restoration of serum potassium level and correction of thyrotoxic state. Onset is typically at night or early morning, particularly during the resting time. Myalgia has been described in some cases, while respiratory failure or fatal arrhythmia is very unusual. Predisposing factors are high-carbohydrate diet, heavy exercise, alcohol ingestion, and stress. The exact mechanism of TPP is still elusive. Intracellular shift from upregulation of Na^+-K^+ATPase pump is the main mechanism, whereby its activity is provoked by thyrotoxicosis state and/or various precipitating factors.

Key to prevent periodic attacks is the reestablishment of euthyroid state [3]. In case of TSHoma, administration of medications including somatostatin analog, antithyroid drug and nonselective beta-blocker prior to transsphenoidal surgery (TSS) is recommended [2, 4]. Prompt correction of serum potassium reverses muscle weakness and prevents

TABLE 3: Reported cases of TSH-secreting pituitary tumor with TPP, including our case.

Age (y)/ Ethnicity/Sex	Time to diagnosis (y)	Pituitary tumor (cm)	Symptoms		Serum potassium (mEq/L)	Thyroid function test					Treatment and outcome		
			Thyro-toxicosis	Goiter		FT_3 (pg/dL)	T3 (ng/dL)	FT_4 (ng/dL)	T4 (μg/dL)	TSH (μIU/mL)	TSS	Medication	Remission
27/Asian/M [4]	6	2	+	+	1.3	NA	256 (70–170)	4.1 (0.6–1.8)	23.8 (4.5–12.5)	6.4 (0.2–3.4)	+	+	+
43/Asian/M [5]	1	2	–	+	1.2	NA	430 (84–176)	3.0 (0.7–1.6)	23.3 (5.4–11.6)	4.3 (0.4–4.0)	+	+	+
44/Asian/M [6]	**	1.5	–	–	2.0	NA	227 (100–190)	NA	14.4 (4.4–12.5)	2.10 (0.50–5.15)	+	+	+
31/Asian/M [7]	2	0.3	+	+	2.5–2.8	NA	190 (57.9–158.8)	2.1 (0.6–1.6)	NA	5.55 (0.4–4.0)	+	+	+
40/Asian/M [8]	3 month	macro#	+	–	1.2	19.9 (2.0–4.4)	NA	4.87 (0.8–1.8)	NA	56.8 (0.4–5.5)	–	+	+
28/Asian/M [9]	**	3.1	–	+	2.5	8.0 (2.3–4.0)	NA	2.6 (0.9–1.7)	NA	7.0 (0.5–5.0)	+	+	+
42/Asian/M*	**	0.6	+	+	2.7	8.4 (1.8–4.0)	NA	2.2 (0.8–1.8)	NA	13.0 (0.4–4.1)	+	+	+

*: Our case. **: Presenting symptom. #: Macroadenoma. +: Positive, –: Negative. NA: not available.

cardiopulmonary complications such as cardiac arrhythmias. However, careful dosing of potassium replacement must be exercised to prevent rebound hyperkalemia from extracellular shift of potassium. In addition, precipitating factors should be avoided and nonselective beta blockers should be administered until a euthyroid state is achieved.

Our literature search returned only 6 case reports of TPP from TSHoma [4–9] (Table 3). Concordantly, all patients were Asian men [Japanese (2 cases), Chinese (1 case), Indonesian (1 case), Indian (1 case), and Syrian (1 case)] and most of their tumors (5 from 6 cases) were macroadenoma. Interestingly, all of them had TPP as the presenting symptom; however, their manifestations and responses to treatments, TSS with/without preoperative medications—octreotide and thionamides, did not differ from those of TSHoma without TPP.

4. Conclusion

We are presenting a rare case of TSHoma which manifests initially with TPP. Physician should be cognizant about the concomitant thyrotoxicosis, particularly among Asian male patients.

References

[1] L. Onnestam, K. Berinder, P. Burman et al., "National incidence and prevalence of TSH-secreting pituitary adenomas in Sweden," *The Journal of Clinical Endocrinology & Metabolism*, vol. 98, no. 2, pp. 626–635, 2013.

[2] G. Cossu, R. Daniel, T. Pierzchala et al., "Thyrotropin-secreting pituitary adenomas: a systematic review and meta-analysis of postoperative outcomes and management," *Pituitary*, vol. 22, no. 1, pp. 79–88, 2019.

[3] A. W. Kung, "Clinical review: Thyrotoxic periodic paralysis: a diagnostic challenge," *The Journal of Clinical Endocrinology & Metabolism*, vol. 91, no. 7, pp. 2490–2495, 2006.

[4] Y. Kiso, K. Yoshida, K. Kaise et al., "A case of thyrotropin (TSH)-secreting tumor complicated by periodic paralysis," *Japanese Journal of Medicine*, vol. 29, no. 4, pp. 399–404, 1990.

[5] A. M. Alings, E. Fliers, W. W. de Herder et al., "A thyrotropin-secreting pituitary adenoma as a cause of thyrotoxic periodic paralysis," *Journal of Endocrinological Investigation*, vol. 21, no. 10, pp. 703–706, 1998.

[6] F. S. Hsu, W. S. Tsai, T. Chau, H. H. Chen, Y. C. Chen, and S. H. Lin, "Thyrotropin-secreting pituitary adenoma presenting as hypokalemic periodic paralysis," *The American Journal of the Medical Sciences*, vol. 325, no. 1, pp. 48–50, 2003.

[7] T. Pappa, L. Papanastasiou, A. Markou et al., "Thyrotoxic periodic paralysis as the first manifestation of a thyrotropin-secreting pituitary adenoma," *Hormones*, vol. 9, no. 1, pp. 82–86, 2010.

[8] S. Ghosh, R. Sahoo, S. Rao, and D. Rath, "Pituitary macroadenoma: a rare cause of thyrotoxichypokalaemic periodic paralysis," *BMJ Case Reports*, vol. 2013, no. 1, 2013.

[9] K. Monami, F. Takashi, M. Kunitaka et al., "A rare case of thyrotoxic periodic paralysis caused by TSH-secreting pituitary adenoma: case report and review of the Literature," *Journal of Endocrinology and Thyroid Research*, vol. 1, no. 1, p. 555551, 2017.

17

Langerhans Cell Histiocytosis of the Thyroid Leading to the Diagnosis of a Disseminated Form

Ibtissem Ben Nacef,[1] Sabrine Mekni,[1] Chedi Mhedhebi,[1] Ines Riahi,[2] Imen Rojbi,[1] Mchirgui Nadia,[1] and Karima Khiari[1]

[1]*Department of Endocrinology, Charles Nicolle Hospital, Tunis, Tunisia*
[2]*Department of Otorhinolaryngology-Head and Neck Surgery, Charles Nicolle Hospital, Tunis, Tunisia*

Correspondence should be addressed to Ibtissem Ben Nacef; bennacef.ibtissem@yahoo.com

Academic Editor: Osamu Isozaki

Langerhans cell histiocytosis (LCH) is a rare sporadic proliferative disorder of Langerhans cells. LCH rarely involves the thyroid gland. We report herein a case of a disseminated chronic form of LCH with a diagnosis established by histological examination of the thyroid gland. It is about a 37-year-old female who underwent total thyroidectomy for a thyroid nodule of the right lobe. Histological study showed a granulomatous thyroiditis, and the immunohistochemistry study revealed a strong positivity of histiocytes for the CD1 antigen and for the S100 protein. The incidence of LCH involving the thyroid gland, either as an isolated lesion or as a part of multisystemic disease, is extremely rare.

1. Introduction

Langerhans cell histiocytosis (LCH) is a rare sporadic proliferative disorder of Langerhans cells. It can cause either localized or generalized lesions, leading to the destruction of hard and soft tissues [1]. LCH rarely involves the thyroid gland. We report a case of a disseminated chronic form of LCH with a diagnosis established by histological examination of the thyroid gland.

2. Case Report

A 37-year-old female underwent surgery for a thyroid nodule of the right lobe. The nodule presented as suspicious because of its hard consistency, its adhesion to surrounding tissues, and the presence of calcifications on ultrasound. The patient was euthyroid before surgery. She had a total thyroidectomy. Histological study showed a granulomatous thyroiditis. The granulomas were composed of lymphocytes and histiocytes grouped into clusters. After surgery, the patient was referred to our establishment for investigation of a polyuropolydipsic syndrome and a one-year history of amenorrhea-galactorrhea.

Physical examination was normal except for bilateral galactorrhea. Urine specific gravity before test was 1.005. The water deprivation test results were in favor of a central diabetes insipidus (DI) (Table 1). Hormonal tests revealed pan-hypopituitarism, with a very low follicle-stimulating hormone (FSH) level of 0.9 mIU/mL (reference range 3.9–8.9 mIU/mL) and a luteinizing hormone (LH) level below 0.1 mIU/mL (reference range 2.1–10.9 mIU/mL). Baseline serum cortisol was 240 nmol/L and did not respond to insulin hypoglycemia test. An inappropriate adrenocorticotropic hormone (ACTH) level of 12 pg/mL suggested secondary adrenal insufficiency. Likewise, baseline GH was 0.25 ng/mL and did not respond to insulin hypoglycemia test. Prolactin level was mildly elevated (2520 mIU/mL with a reference range of 71–567 mIU/mL), which was consistent with disconnection hyperprolactinemia. As for the thyroid function tests, they were noninterpretable because the patient had already been on therapy. However, it is important to note that thyroid-stimulating hormone (TSH) level

Table 1: Water deprivation test results.

	Baseline	After water deprivation	After desmopressin
Diuresis (mL/h)	600	210	15
Urine specific gravity	1005	1010	1025
Serum osmolarity (mOsm/L)	303,4	319,4	286
Na (mEq/L)	147	154	138

responded to TRH stimulating test. MRI of the hypothalamic-pituitary axis showed an infiltrative process of the hypothalamus with a loss of the posterior pituitary bright spot. The patient was discharged; she received hormone replacement therapy including desmopressin acetate 20 µg intranasal solution per day, oral hydrocortisone 20 mg per day, and levothyroxine 150 μg per day.

Eight months later, she presented with a left retroauricular bone pain and preauricular and submandibular lymphadenopathies, along with dental pain and tooth mobility. The facial and temporal bones CT-scan revealed a lytic lesion of the horizontal branch of the right mandible and a significant lytic lesion of the left petrous bone, extended to the squama (Figure 1(a)). The diagnosis of LCH was then strongly suspected, which led to re-examination of the excised thyroid gland by the pathology department. The immunohistochemistry study was performed, and it revealed a strong positivity of histiocytes for the CD1 antigen and the S100 protein (Figure 2).

The extension assessment of the disease included a thoracic CT-scan that revealed peripheral pulmonary micronodules, some of which were excavated. The treatment consisted of a chemotherapy combining vinblastine at a dose of 5 mg weekly and prednisone at a dose of 0.5 mg/kg daily. After four months of treatment, favorable evolution was noted, with a good tolerance of treatment, a clear relief of the headache, and disappearance of the left retroauricular pain. The control temporal bones CT-scan showed complete regression of the lytic lesion (Figure 1(b)). Nevertheless, the patient still required the same doses of pituitary hormones replacement therapy.

3. Discussion

Langerhans cell histiocytosis is a rare disease that affects predominantly, but not exclusively, children. It has an incidence of up to 9 cases per million children in Western Europe, dropping to 1-2 cases per million in adults [2]. LCH of the adult preferably affects the bones, lungs, skin, and posterior pituitary gland. The most common endocrinological manifestation of LCH is diabetes insipidus, which is a consequence of posterior pituitary involvement. However, other manifestations such as anterior pituitary deficiency are observed, resulting in secondary or tertiary hypothyroidism [3].

Our patient presented with DI and amenorrhea-galactorrhea syndrome as the clinical feature of disconnection hypothalamic hyperprolactinemia, which is caused by the histiocytic infiltration of the pituitary hypothalamus including stalk.

Pan-hypopituitarism, as in our case, is rare. Pituitary insufficiency is explained by the lack of secretion of hormones from the hypothalamus and pituitary [4].

The incidence of LCH involving the thyroid gland, either as an isolated lesion or as a part of a multisystemic disease, is extremely rare. Thyroid LCH is much more common in adults than in children, especially for females [5–8].

Patten et al. [9] reviewed 66 cases of LCH with thyroid involvement and observed an overall median age of 28 years with the majority of the patients presenting clinically with euthyroid goiter. Of the 66 cases, solitary thyroid involvement was noted in only 17 cases (25.7%) with all, except one, presenting in adulthood. Our patient was 37 years old and presented a solitary thyroid involvement initially.

Hypothyroidism during LCH can be either primary or most commonly secondary. In our case, it was due to a TRH (thyrotropin-releasing hormone) secretion deficiency. The normal response to TRH stimulation test supports this assumption.

Clinically, thyrotropic insufficiency is distinguished from primary hypothyroidism by the absence of myxedema and mainly by the clinical features of other pituitary deficiencies, as it is usually part of an anterior pan-hypopituitarism.

Thyroid gland involvement leads in the majority of cases to confusion and diagnostic mistakes. Lahey et al. (out of 10) reported a case of LCH with thyroid involvement; the diagnosis of thyroiditis was initially suspected in light of the results of the fine needle aspiration (FNA). The diagnosis was corrected after thyroidectomy. El Halabi et al. [10] also reported a case of LCH with thyroid localization. The result of the FNA cytology was in favor of either a lymphocytic thyroiditis or papillary carcinoma. The diagnosis was confirmed after histological study of the thyroidectomy specimen. In our case, thyroid involvement appeared eight months before hypothalamic involvement manifestations, which was unknown.

The initial misdiagnosis of granulomatous thyroiditis is due to the inflammatory character of LCH. In fact, the formation of highly active inflammatory granuloma and the recruitment of additional inflammatory cells such as eosinophils, lymphocytes, and neutrophils are explained by the expression of proinflammatory cytokines in the mutated LCs. This led some authors to the definition of LCH as an *inflammatory myeloid neoplasia* [11].

To establish the diagnosis of LCH, it is required to have histopathological analyses identifying tissue infiltration by histiocytes with characteristics of LCs. Pathologic histiocytes in LCH are mononucleated cells with coffee bean- or kidney-shaped nuclei. Detection of LC markers is mandatory to

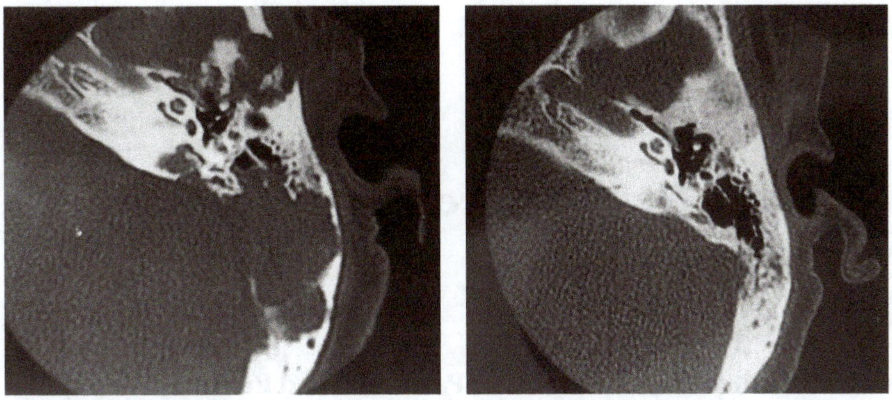

(a) (b)

Figure 1: Scan of the left temporal bone in axial section, bone window. (a) Extensive lytic lesions (arrow). (b) Complete regression of the lytic lesions after treatment.

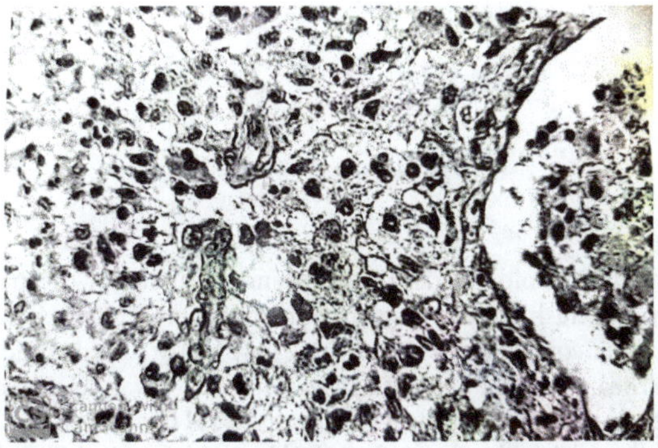

Figure 2: Granulomas of tumor histiocytes with an oval nucleus centered by a small nucleolus; their cytoplasm is weakly eosinophilic.

confirm the diagnosis. In routine practice, detection of Birbeck granules by electron microscopy has been widely replaced by detection of CD1a and CD207 expression, whereas expression of protein S100 is not specific. LCH cells are often associated with abundant eosinophils and multinucleated giant cells [12]. In our case, the diagnosis of histiocytic infiltration of the thyroid was made retrospectively despite the presence of granulomas composed of lymphocytes, plasma cells, and especially histiocytes grouped into clusters. The immunohistochemical study of the thyroidectomy specimen was of a great contribution for the rectification of the diagnosis.

In conclusion, LCH is a rare disease, especially the thyroid gland involvement. The diagnosis is made through histological analysis and immunohistochemical staining. As in our case, the Langerhans cell histiocytosis of the thyroid can easily be missed and only established after typical manifestation of the disseminated form.

References

[1] C. E. Allen and K. L. McCain, "Langerhans cell histiocytosis: a review of past, current and future therapies," *Drugs of Today*, vol. 43, no. 9, pp. 627–643, 2007.

[2] A. Guyot-Goubin, J. Donadieu, M. Barkaoui, S. Bellec, C. Thomas, and J. Clavel, "Descriptive epidemiology of childhood Langerhans cell histiocytosis in France, 2000–2004," *Pediatric Blood & Cancer*, vol. 51, no. 1, p. 71–75, 2008.

[3] V. L Broadbent, R. M. Egeler, and M. E. Nesbit, "Langerhans cell histiocytosis - clinical and epidemiological aspects," *British Journal of Cancer*, vol. 23, pp. 11–16, 1994.

[4] A. Tabarin, J. B. Corcuff, M. Dautheribes et al., "Histiocytosis X of the hypothalamus," *Journal of Endocrinological Investigation*, vol. 14, no. 2, pp. 139–145, 1991.

[5] C.-X. Xia, R. Li, Z.-H. Wang et al., "A rare cause of goiter: Langerhans cell histiocytosis of the thyroid," *Endocrine Journal*, vol. 59, no. 1, pp. 47–54, 2012.

[6] Y.-F. Cai, Q.-X. Wang, C.-J. Ni et al., "A case report: the diagnosis and therapeutic evaluation for a rare disease of Langerhans cell histiocytosis involving thyroid," *Medicine*, vol. 94, no. 44, Article ID e1891, 2015.

[7] O. O. Gul, P. Sisman, S. Cander et al., "An unusual case of adult-onset multi-systemic Langerhans cell histiocytosis with perianal and incident thyroid involvement," *Endocrinology, Diabetes & Metabolism Case Reports*, vol. 2017, pp. 16-0087, 2017.

[8] K. Khiari, N. B. Abdallah, L. Cherif et al., "Histiocytose langerhansienne infiltrant la glande thyroïde : à propos d'une observation," *La Revue de Médecine Interne*, vol. 24, no. 12, pp. 838-839, 2003.

[9] D. K. Patten, Z. Wani, and N. Tolley, "Solitary Langerhans histiocytosis of the thyroid gland: a case report and literature review," *Head and Neck Pathology*, vol. 6, no. 2, pp. 279–289, 2012.

[10] D. A. El-Halabi, M. El-Sayed, W. Eskaf, J. T. Anim, and P. Dey, "Langerhans cell histiocytosis of the thyroid gland a case report," *Acta Cytologica*, vol. 44, no. 5, pp. 805–884, 2000.

[11] M.-L. Berres, M. Merad, and C. E. Allen, "Progress in understanding the pathogenesis of Langerhans cell histiocytosis: back to histiocytosis X?" *British Journal of Haematology*, vol. 169, no. 1, pp. 3–13, 2015.

[12] J.-F. Emile, O. Abla, S. Fraitag et al., "Revised classification of histiocytoses and neoplasms of the macrophage-dendritic cell lineages," *Blood*, vol. 127, no. 22, pp. 2672–2681, 2016.

18

Sporadic Medullary Thyroid Carcinoma with Paraneoplastic Cushing Syndrome

Aleksandra I. Pivovarova ,[1,2] Stephanie Patrick,[1,3] and Punuru J. Reddy[4]

[1]*Alabama College of Osteopathic Medicine, 445 Health Sciences Blvd, Dothan, AL 36303, USA*
[2]*University of Mississippi Medical Center, 2500 N State St., Jackson, MS 39216, USA*
[3]*University of Tennessee Health Science Center, 910 Madison Ave, Memphis, TN 38163, USA*
[4]*Decatur Morgan Hospital, Department of Internal Medicine, 1201 7th St. SE, Decatur, AL 35601, USA*

Correspondence should be addressed to Aleksandra I. Pivovarova; pivovarovaai@acom.edu

Academic Editor: Takeshi Usui

Medullary thyroid cancer (MTC) is a rare form of neoplasm affecting the thyroid gland. This neuroendocrine tumor is capable of releasing active substances causing systemic manifestation in the form of flushing, diarrhea, and uncommonly, Ectopic Cushing's syndrome (ECS). MTC can be hereditary as a part of multiple endocrine neoplasm type 2 syndrome (MEN2) or arise sporadically. We report a case of a 74-year-old female presenting with chronic diarrhea, in whom diagnosis of sporadic MTC was delayed due to previous history of gastrointestinal (GI) disturbances. The patient developed liver metastases yielding ACTH dependent Cushing's Syndrome leading to abnormal clinical presentation and laboratory values driven by elevated cortisol level. Metastatic MTC should be considered in patients presenting with chronic diarrhea and weakness unexplained by other GI related causes.

1. Introduction

Medullary Thyroid Cancer is a neuroendocrine tumor of the C cells and accounts for 1–2% of thyroid cancers in the United States. While nearly all patients with familial MTC have *RET* germline mutation, only half of the sporadic MTC have somatic *RET* mutation present in tumor cells [1]. About 25% of MTCs are a part of familial MEN2 syndrome. Patients with MEN2 syndrome are inclined to develop MTC, pheochromocytoma, and hyperparathyroidism. In some MTC patients the disease can manifest systemically due to overproduction of calcitonin and other substances, such as catecholamines, serotonin, and histamine [2]. Majority of sporadic MTC patients will present with a palpable thyroid nodule, at which point approximately 75% of these patients would already develop cervical and 10% distant metastases [3]. The diagnosis is usually confirmed by a fine needle aspiration. After diagnosis of MTC has been established, measurement of serum calcitonin, carcinoembryonic antigen (CEA), genetic testing for germline *RET* mutations, and biochemical evaluation for coexisting tumors, especially pheochromocytoma should follow [1]. Measurement of calcitonin and CEA levels is used to determine a preoperative baseline and therapeutic response [4]. The first-line treatment for MTC is a surgical resection. Unfortunately, patients with metastatic MTC disease at diagnosis are rarely cured by surgery.

Only 0.7% of patients with MTC develops ECS, while MTC accounts for approximately 2.2–7.5% of patients with ectopic ACTH [5]. Ectopic Cushing's Syndrome from MTC is associated with significant morbidity and mortality, as secondary complications of hypercortisolism account for 50% of the mortality in MTC [6]. In the past, management of hypercortisolism was limited to decreasing metastatic tumor burden and using antiadrenal therapies such as ketoconazole, mitotane, and metyrapone [7]. Surgical intervention with bilateral adrenalectomy is another option available to some patients. However systemic therapy with tyrosine kinase inhibitors offers a further management strategy for disease control of metastatic and is now considered a first line therapy for ECS in the setting of unresectable disease or progressive, metastatic disease [8, 9].

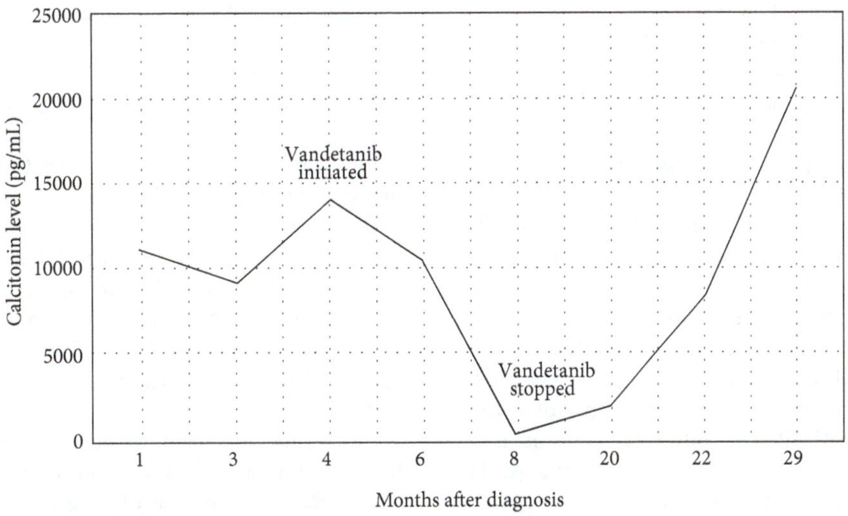

FIGURE 1: Calcitonin levels while on Vandetanib therapy. The graph depicts levels at baseline before the treatment was started, followed by initiation of Vandetanib, and subsequent rise in calcitonin levels after the therapy was stopped.

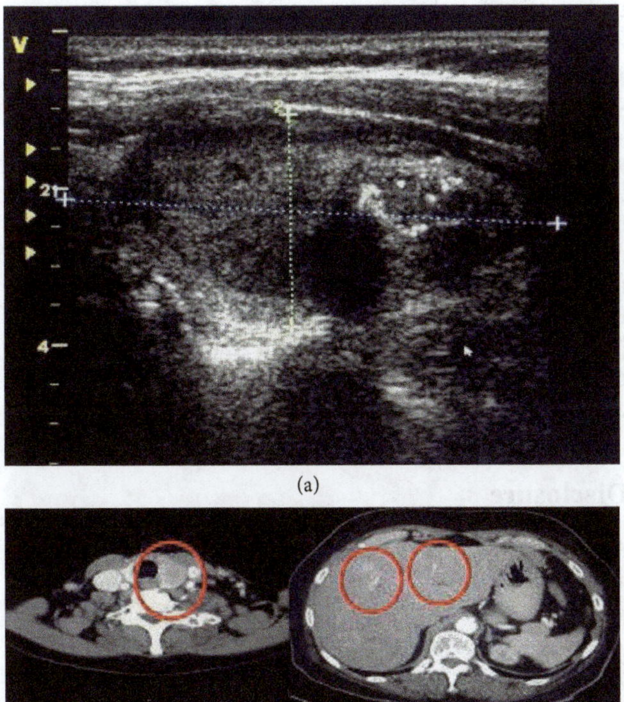

(a)

(b)

FIGURE 2: (a) Thyroid ultrasound demonstrating hypoechoic lesion. (b) Preoperative CT of the neck (left) and the abdomen (right) revealing cervical lymphadenopathy and liver metastasis.

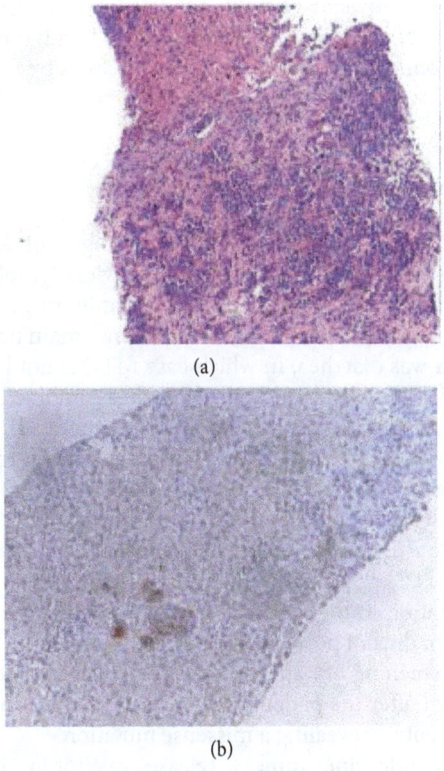

(a)

(b)

FIGURE 3: Liver biopsy showing metastatic medullary thyroid carcinoma cells (×10) (a) H&E stain. (b) Calcitonin stain.

2. Case Presentation

A 74-year-old female presented with chronic diarrhea, weight loss, hematochezia, abdominal cramps, and fever. Her past medical history was significant for hypertension, metabolic syndrome, and perforated diverticulitis. Physical examination identified a nontender mass in her left submandibular area with no thyromegaly. The serological exam was remarkable for elevated chromogranin A level of 299 (normal <93). Suspicion for carcinoid tumor warranted an octreotide scan that identified increased uptake on the right side of the abdomen and left side of her neck. Laboratory tests revealed elevated calcitonin level, 11,290 pg/mL (ref. value <7.6 pg/mL) (Figure 1). Ultrasound of the neck identified a highly suspicious thyroid mass (Figure 2(a)), and a CT scan showed a heterogeneous thyroid nodule, and several enhanced lesions in the liver (Figure 2(b)). A liver biopsy revealed that tumor was of neuroendocrine origin consistent with the medullary carcinoma of the thyroid (Figure 3).

Patient had no family history of MTC or MEN syndrome. She underwent a total thyroidectomy followed by treatment with Vandetanib, which lead to resolution of diarrhea and normalization of bowel function. However, the drug was poorly tolerated, patient developed rash, fatigue, weakness, and nausea, and the dosage had to be tapered down and eventually stopped completely.

Two and a half years after the initial diagnosis of MTC, the patient returned to the clinic with edema, skin acne, elevated blood pressure, hyperglycemia, hypernatremia, and hypokalemia. Her symptoms were consistent with the Cushing syndrome. The Cortisol level was drastically elevated, 120.2 μg/dL (ref. range for A.M. cortisol 6.2–19.4 μg/dL). High dose dexamethasone suppression test was indicative of ectopic ACTH tumor. Brain MRI ruled out pituitary adenoma. It was concluded that liver lesions were the source of ectopic ACTH. To control hypokalemia, Aldactone was started along with a cortisol lowering ketoconazole, potassium, and calcium replacement. The patient was not a good surgical candidate, and bilateral adrenalectomy was not an option. While still in the hospital, the patient developed altered mental status and bleeding of colovaginal fistula. Her calcitonin level increased to 20,503 pg/mL (Figure 1). The patient's family decided in favor of comfort care, and less than two weeks later the patient passed away.

3. Discussion

Among the most common presenting signs of MTC are clinically detectable thyroid nodule, cervical lymph nodes, upper aerodigestive tract compression manifesting as hoarseness and/or dysphagia [1, 10]. Our patient's main presenting symptom was diarrhea, in which case MTC is not high on a differential. Initial presentation of diarrhea combined with the previous history of diverticulosis warranted a GI workup, which eventually lead to an accurate diagnosis of MTC. Unfortunately, diarrhea usually signifies advanced stage of MTC with metastatic disease [11].

While *RET* gene mutation is responsible for majority of familial MTC cases, 50% of sporadic MTC cases have somatic *RET* mutation in the tumor tissue [1]. With that being said, our patient did not possess a germline *RET* mutation, however genetic screening of patient's liver biopsy by NeoGenomics, performed after the patient passed away, demonstrated *RET* involvement by revealing a missense mutation.

Neuroendocrine tumors release calcitonin, calcitonin-gene related peptide, biogenic amines, and sometimes other active substances like ACTH, causing systemic symptoms. Ectopic ACTH secretion by a nonpituitary tumor leads to Cushing's syndrome, which is most commonly caused by corticotropin secreting pituitary tumor. Production of ACTH by MTC metastases is a rare occurrence and represents only about 5–10% of ECS [12]. Likewise, cancers such as small cell lung, thymic, pulmonary, pancreatic carcinoid tumours, and pheochromocytomas have the potential to produce ectopic ACTH [13]. The time between MTC diagnosis and ECS presentation can vary, with some declaring themselves even before MTC diagnosis, and others over 20 years after [14, 15]. In our case, ECS was detected almost three years after the initial diagnosis of MTC.

Once the type of cancer was identified, thyroidectomy and chemotherapy were quickly initiated. During the early stages of disease, the patient was treated with Vandetanib, the first drug approved in the United States for the treatment of progressive symptomatic MTC in patients with unresectable and/or metastatic tumors. Although the treatment with Vandetanib achieved resolution of diarrhea and return of normal bowel function, it had to be stopped due to poor tolerance. Even with the primary lesion being removed, liver metastases produced ectopic ACTH leading to Cushing syndrome, abnormal laboratory results, and overall worsening prognosis.

The Tyrosine kinase inhibitors Vandetanib and Cabozantinib have been approved by the Food and Drug Administration (FDA) for the treatment of progressive metastatic MTC [8]. Sorafenib, another kinase inhibitor, has been used off-label for treatment of metastatic MTC [16]. In a study by Barosso-Sousa, the treatment of metastatic MTC with ectopic ACTH syndrome with Sorafenib, reduced the cortisol and ACTH levels and lead to dramatic clinical improvement [17].

Vandetanib is considered a first-line therapy for ECS and should be used prior to bilateral adrenalectomy. Nonetheless, due to the patient's poor health and prior Vandetanib intolerance, she was not in the position to accept it and was started on comfort care instead. For patients with unresectable tumors and those who are unable to tolerate first line treatment, adrenal enzyme inhibitors such as ketoconazole, metyrapone, and etomidate can be used to control the symptoms along with glucocorticoid receptor blocker mifepristone. However, this is generally considered a suboptimal treatment [7]. Ultimately, late diagnosis due to an unusual presentation of MTC, and other existing comorbidities lead to poor outcome.

Disclosure

An earlier version of this case report was presented as a poster at an annual Society of Hospital Medicine 2019 conference.

Acknowledgments

The authors thank the team of physicians assisting this patient's case: Drs. James Dailey, Virginia Dailey Graham, Heather Shah, Robert Walker, and Khurshid Yousef at Decatur Morgan Hospital.

References

[1] S. A. Wells, S. L. Asa, H. Dralle et al., "Revised American thyroid association guidelines for the management of medullary thyroid carcinoma," *Thyroid*, vol. 25, no. 6, pp. 567–610, 2015.

[2] J. W. de Groot, I. P. Kema, H. van der Breukelman et al., "Biochemical markers in the follow-up of medullary thyroid cancer," *Thyroid*, vol. 16, no. 11, pp. 1163–1170, 2006.

[3] J. F. Moley, "Medullary thyroid carcinoma: management of lymph node metastases," *Journal of the National Comprehensive Cancer Network*, vol. 8, no. 5, pp. 549–556, 2010.

[4] R. Cohen, J. Campos, M. C. Salaün et al., "Preoperative calcitonin levels are predictive of tumor size and postoperative calcitonin normalization in medullary thyroid carcinoma," *The Journal of Clinical Endocrinology & Metabolism*, vol. 85, no. 2, p. 919, 2000.

[5] S. L. Barbosa, P. Rodien, S. Leboulleux et al., "Endocrines ectopic adrenocorticotropic hormone—syndrome in medullary carcinoma of the thyroid: a retrospective analysis and review of the literature," *Thyroid*, vol. 15, no. 6, pp. 618–623, 2005.

[6] A. A. Nella, M. B. Lodish, E. Fox et al., "Vandetanib successfully controls medullary thyroid cancer-related Cushing syndrome in an adolescent patient," *Journal of Clinical Endocrinology and Metabolism*, vol. 99, pp. 3055–3059, 2014.

[7] P. Kamenický, C. Droumaguet, S. Salenave et al., "Mitotane, metyrapone, and ketoconazole combination therapy as an alternative to rescue adrenalectomy for severe ACTH-dependent Cushing's syndrome," *Journal of Clinical Endocrinology and Metabolism*, vol. 96, no. 9, pp. 2796–2804, 2011.

[8] S. A. Wells, B. G. Robinson, R. F. Gagel et al., "Vandetanib in patients with locally advanced or metastatic medullary thyroid cancer: a randomized, double-blind phase III trial," *Journal of Clinical Oncology*, vol. 30, no. 2, pp. 134–141, 2012.

[9] A. C. Paepegaey, B. Cochand-Priollet, E. Louiset et al., "Long-term control of hypercortisolism by vandetanib in a case of medullary thyroid carcinoma with a somatic RET mutation," *Thyroid*, vol. 27, no. 4, pp. 587–590, 2017.

[10] F. Pacini, M. Castagna, G. C. Cipri, and M. Schlumberger, "Medullary thyroid carcinoma," *Clinical Oncology*, vol. 22, no. 6, pp. 475–485, 2010.

[11] J. Fromigué, T. De Baere, E. Baudin, C. Dromain, S. Leboulleux, and M. Schlumberger, "Chemoembolization for liver metastases from medullary thyroid carcinoma," *The Journal of Clinical Endocrinology & Metabolism*, vol. 91, no. 7, pp. 2496–2499, 2006.

[12] M. Boscaro and G. Arnaldi, "Approach to the patient with possible Cushing's syndrome," *The Journal of Clinical Endocrinology & Metabolism*, vol. 94, no. 9, pp. 3121–3131, 2009.

[13] A. Isidori, G. Kaltsas, C. Pozza et al., "Extensive clinical experience: the ectopic adrenocorticotropin syndrome: clinical fea- tures, diagnosis, management, and long-term follow-up," *The Journal of Clinical Endocrinology & Metabolism*, vol. 91, no. 2, pp. 371–377, 2006.

[14] L. Matheny, J. Wilson, and H. Baum, "Ectopic ACTH production leading to diagnosis of underlying medullary thyroid carcinoma," *Journal of Investigative Medicine High Impact Case Reports*, vol. 4, no. 2, Article ID 232470961664398, 2016.

[15] A. Chrisoulidou, K. Pazaitou-Panayiotou, E. Georgiou et al., "Ectopic Cushing's syndrome due to CRH secreting liver metastasis in a patient with medullary thyroid carcinoma," *Hormones*, vol. 7, no. 3, pp. 259–262, 2008.

[16] E. T. Lam, M. D. Ringel, R. T. Kloos et al., "Phase II clinical trial of sorafenib in metastatic medullary thyroid cancer," *Journal of Clinical Oncology*, vol. 28, pp. 2323–2330, 2010.

[17] R. Barroso-Sousa, A. Lerario, M. Evangelista et al., "Complete resolution of hypercortisolism with sorafenib in a patient with advanced medullary thyroid carcinoma and ectopic ACTH (adrenocorticotropic hormone) syndrome," *Thyroid*, vol. 24, no. 6, pp. 1062–1026, 2014.

19

Simultaneous Coexistence of Thyrotropin-Prolactin-Secreting Adenoma and Papillary Thyroid Carcinoma

Somaya Safi,[1,2] **Yousra Benabdelfedil**,[1,2] **Sara Derrou**,[1,2] and **Faycal El Guendouz**[1,2]

[1]*Department of Endocrinology, Moulay Ismail Military Hospital, Meknes, Morocco*
[2]*Department of Fundamental Sciences, Laboratory of Human Pathology Biomedicine and Environment, Faculty of Medicine and Pharmacy of Fez (FMPF), Sidi Mohammed Ben Abdellah University (USMBA), Fez, Morocco*

Correspondence should be addressed to Faycal El Guendouz; el.guendouz@gmail.com

Academic Editor: Mihail A. Boyanov

Background. The thyrotropin-secreting adenomas are very rare and even more rare when they simultaneously coexist with thyroid carcinoma. So far, only sixteen cases have been reported in the literature. Here, we present a unique case of successful management of a concurrent case of thyrotropin-prolactinoma with papillary thyroid carcinoma. *Case Presentation.* A 50-year-old Moroccan woman underwent a total thyroidectomy and complementary totalization by iratherapy for papillary thyroid carcinoma, who presented persistence of an inappropriate secretion of the thyroid-stimulating hormone (TSH > 4 mUI/L) despite of levothyroxine suppressive therapy (300 μg/d). After eliminating noncompliance, interfering medicines, and thyroid malabsorption, a pituitary adenoma (12 mm) was documented at magnetic resonance imaging. The patient has had transsphenoidal pituitary adenomectomy with histology confirming a thyrotropin-prolactin-secreting adenoma. After surgery and lanreotide treatment failures, we noted a complete response (TSH < 0.5) with cabergoline treatment (3 mg/week). *Conclusion.* The unusual association of thyroid adenocarcinoma and TSHoma enriches the hypothesis of a potential link between thyrotropic hypersecretion and thyroid carcinogenesis. Our case also illustrates the difficulty of monitoring thyroid carcinoma in nonremission of a TSHoma.

1. Introduction

The thyrotropin-secreting adenomas (TSHomas) are very rare; their prevalence accounts for 0.5–3% of all pituitary tumors [1]. The sensitive laboratory assays and the accuracy of magnetic resonance imaging currently allow early and precise diagnosis. Simultaneous coexistence of TSHoma and papillary thyroid carcinoma (PTC) is still exceptional, and so far, only sixteen cases have been reported [2–14]. This association suggests the involvement of TSH in thyroid carcinogenesis and raises the difficulty of monitoring levothyroxine suppressive therapy in thyroid carcinoma after a total thyroidectomy.

2. Observation

A 50-year-old Moroccan woman, followed for type 2 diabetes, who underwent a total thyroidectomy with histology confirming papillary thyroid carcinoma (measuring 10 mm) classified T1b Nx M0 (Figure 1). She also received an adjuvant therapy with 100 mCi of radioactive iodine. Posttherapy whole-body scanning revealed fixation in the right thyroid bed compatible with thyroid remnant without metastasis. Cervical ultrasound did not objectify any residue or lymphadenopathy. We noted persistently unrepressed TSH after gradual dose levothyroxine suppressive therapy up to 300 μg per day (4 μg/kg/day); her serum TSH level fluctuating from 4.5 to 50 μIU/mL and thyroglobulin (Tg) level was 6.8 ng/mL. We had quickly eliminated noncompliance, interfering medicines, and thyroid malabsorption, and we suspected a syndrome of inappropriate TSH secretion (SITSH). A pituitary MRI showed a macroadenoma in the sella turcica (10 × 12 mm), without local mass effect on adjacent structures, especially optic chiasm (Figure 2). The specific investigation was in favor of TSHoma, in particular the absence of TSH suppression in the T3

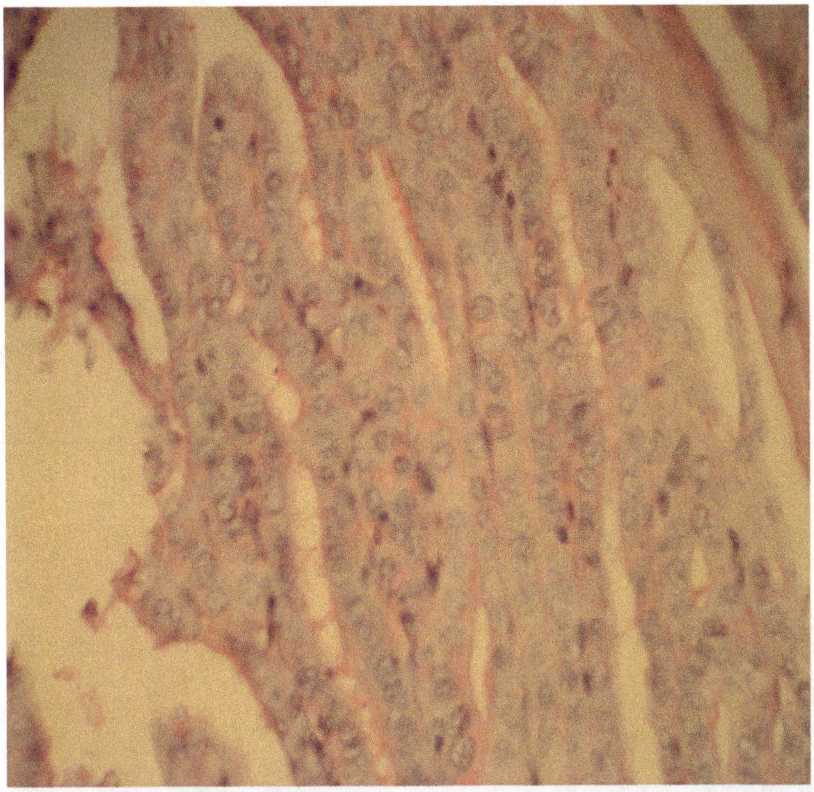

FIGURE 1: Nuclear features of papillary thyroid carcinoma, ground glass appearance, intranuclear grooves, nuclear crowding, and overlapping (x400).

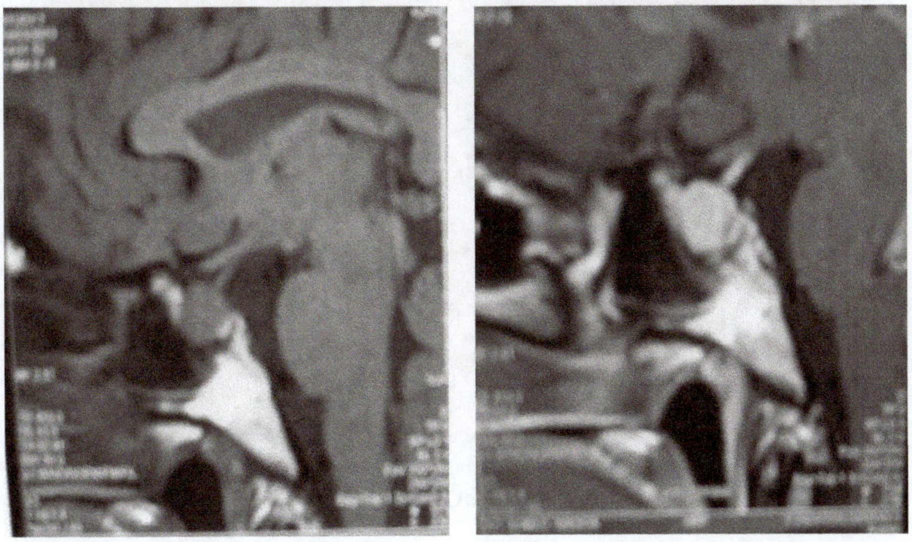

(a) (b)

FIGURE 2: Preoperative pituitary MR images (T1-weighted, contrast, and sagittal view) showing (a) pituitary macroadenoma 12 mm without mass effect on adjacent structures (especially optic chiasm) and (b) strong homogeneous enhancement of the pituitary adenoma after contrast administration.

suppression test (100 μg/day divided in 3 administrations), the serum alpha-subunit levels (α-GSU) was 4.9 ng/mL (normal postmenopausal value 0.6 to 1.5 ng/mL), and α-GSU/TSH molar ratio was 1.4 (normal <1). Other investigations to evaluate pituitary function were normal (Table 1).

Accordingly, the patient has had transsphenoidal pituitary adenomectomy with histology confirming a thyrotropin-prolactin-secreting adenoma (50% of βTSH immunoreactivity and 25% of prolactin immunoreactivity) (Figure 3).

Table 1: Pertinent laboratory findings.

Investigations	Before admission	At admission	After surgery	After lanreotide	After cabergoline	Reference range
TSH (μIU/mL)	4.5–50	35	20	6	0.5	0.35–4.95
FT4 (pmol/L)	—	23	24	22	19	12–22
FT3 (pmol/L)	—	5.3	6.7	6.6	5.9	2.8–7.1
Thyroglobulin (ng/mL)	—	6.8	22.7	8	0.4	<1
α subunit (ng/mL)	—	4.9	—	—	—	0.6–1.5
α-GSU/TSH molar ratio	—	1.4	—	—	—	<1
LH (IU/L)	—	36.8	—	—	—	2.4–12.6
FSH (IU/L)	—	84.1	—	—	—	3.5–12.5
Estradiol (pmol/L)	—	51	—	—	—	46–607
Prolactin (mIU/L)	—	250	230	—	90	72–511
Cortisol (nmol/L)	—	525	—	—	—	171–536
ACTH (pg/mL)	—	40	—	—	—	7–63
IGF1 (μg/L)	—	102	—	—	—	93–245

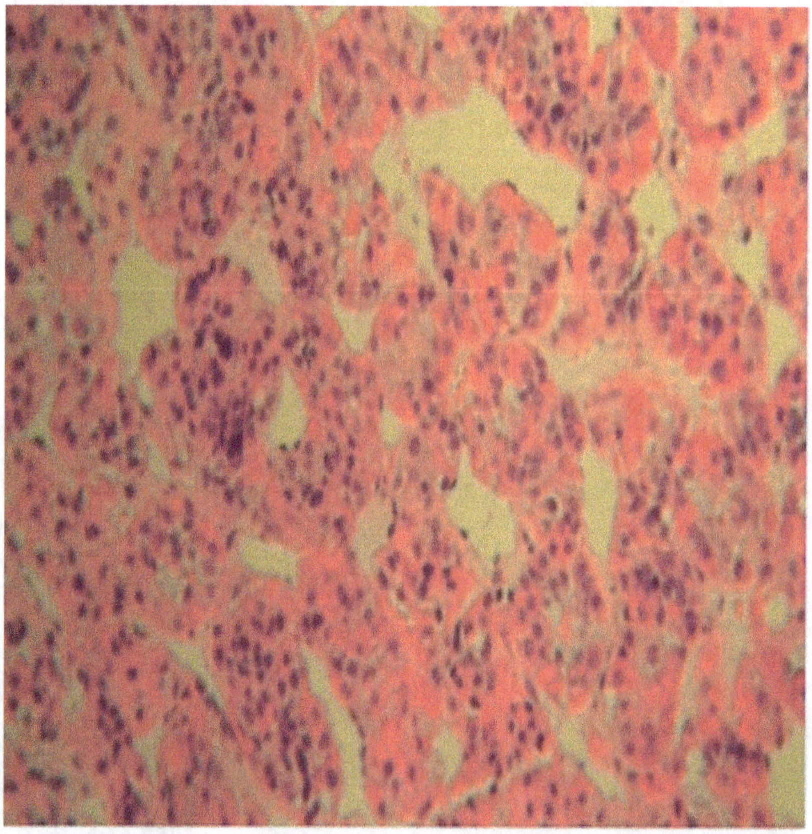

(a)

Figure 3: Continued.

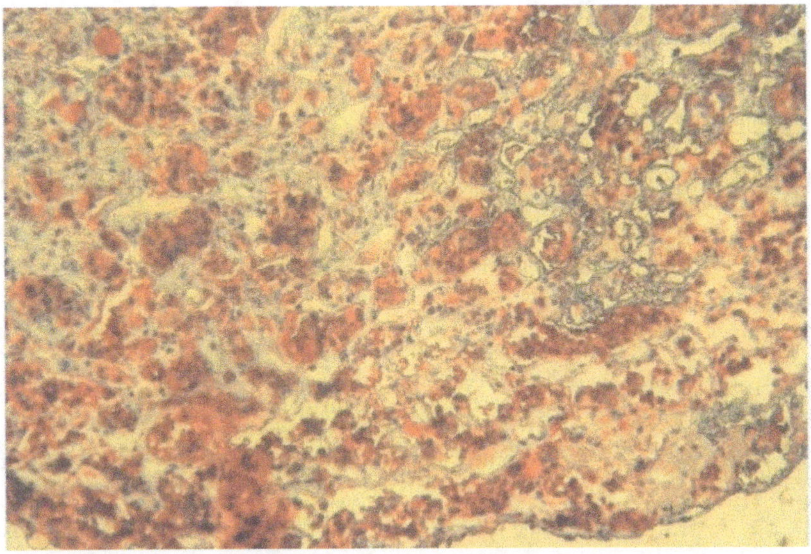

(b)

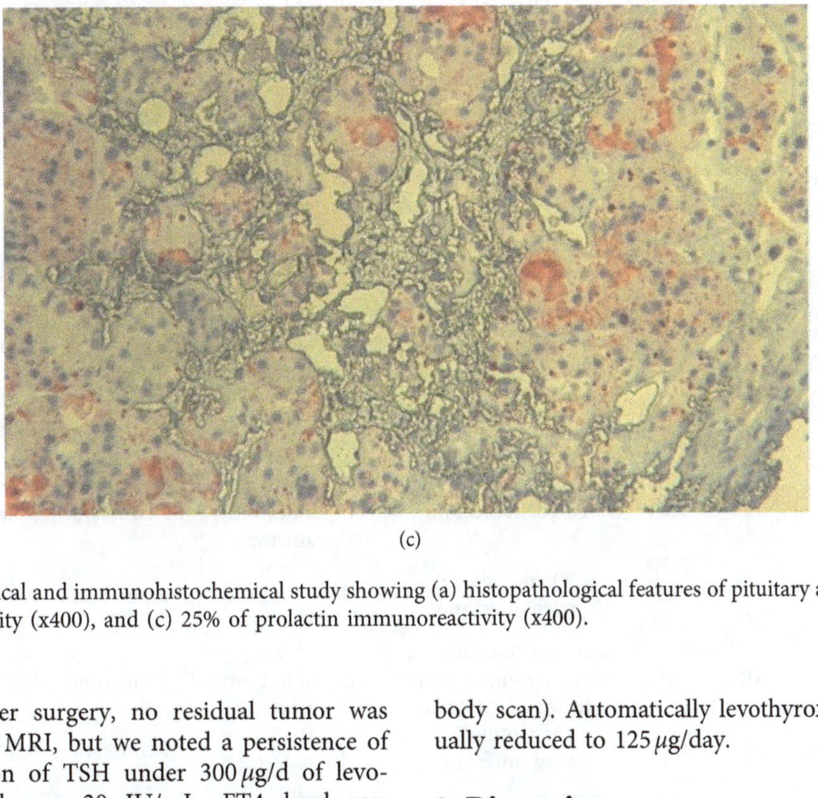

(c)

FIGURE 3: Histopathological and immunohistochemical study showing (a) histopathological features of pituitary adenoma (x200), (b) 50% of ßTSH immunoreactivity (x400), and (c) 25% of prolactin immunoreactivity (x400).

Three months after surgery, no residual tumor was apparent on pituitary MRI, but we noted a persistence of inappropriate secretion of TSH under 300 μg/d of levothyroxine, TSH level was 20 μIU/mL, FT4 level was 22.4 pmol/l, FT3 level was 5.6 pmol/l, and Tg level was 22.7 ng/mL (Table 1). Given the absence of biological remission after surgery, the patient underwent lanreotide therapy at 90 mg per month for three months, but the TSH level was still increased which provokes the stop of lanreotide. The TSH level was lowered for the first time after switching to cabergoline therapy and it allowed a complete response under 3 mg per week (Table 1). The follow-up is eight years after cabergoline therapy with a good cardiac tolerance: the patient has managed to achieve complete remission of thyroid cancer without any biochemical or structural recurrence (low nonstimulated thyroglobulin levels, normal cervical ultrasound, and negative 131I-whole-body scan). Automatically levothyroxine dosage was gradually reduced to 125 μg/day.

3. Discussion

We present here a case of thyroid cancer in coexistence with thyrotropin-prolactin-secreting adenoma. The sixteen published cases are reviewed and compared with our patient at the level of many parameters: age, sex, size of thyroid cancer, size of TSHoma, immunohistochemical study results, therapies used, and observed evolution (Table 2) [2–14].

TSH-suppressive hormonal therapy is a cornerstone of thyroid carcinoma therapy. Unrepressed TSH after levothyroxine suppressive therapy first evokes noncompliance, interfering medicines, thyroid malabsorption, and biological interference, before conducting further investigations for

TABLE 2: Literature review of thyroid cancer with TSHoma.

Case	Age	Sex	Size of TC (mm)	Size of PA (mm)	IHC of PA	Therapies of TSHoma	Therapies of TC	Evolution of TSHoma	Evolution of TC	References (year of publication)
1	55	M	50	30	TSH	TS adenomectomy	Total thyroidectomy/ iratherapy	Remission	Remission	[2] (1991)
2	37	F	20	10	TSH	Refusing treatment	Total thyroidectomy/ iratherapy	NR	Remission	[3] (1998)
3	27	F	30	10	TSH	Octreotide/TS adenomectomy	Partial thyroidectomy	Remission	NR	[4] (2000)
4	45	F	20	15	TSH	Octreotide/TS adenomectomy	Total thyroidectomy	Remission	NR	[5] (2001)
5	47	F	8	4	TSH/ PRL	TS adenomectomy	Total thyroidectomy/ iratherapy	NR	Remission	[6] (2006)
6	50	M	17	3	TSH	Refusing treatment	Total thyroidectomy	Stability	Remission	[7] (2009)
7	57	F	8	26	TSH/ GH	Octreotide	Total thyroidectomy/ iratherapy	Remission	Remission	[8] (2010)
8	38	F	40	14	TSH/ FSH	Octreotide/TS/ radiosurgery	Total thyroidectomy/ iratherapy	Stability	Remission	[9] (2013)
9	27	F	10	28	TSH	TS adenomectomy/ lanreotide	Total thyroidectomy/ iratherapy	Partial response	Remission	[9] (2013)
10	33	F	14	20	TSH/ GH	TS adenomectomy/ cabergoline	Total thyroidectomy/ iratherapy	Remission	Remission	[10] (2014)
11	47	M	15	19	TSH	TS adenomectomy/ lanreotide	Total thyroidectomy/ iratherapy	Remission	Remission	[11] (2015)
12	46	M	12	7	TSH/ GH	TS adenomectomy/ lanreotide	Total thyroidectomy/ iratherapy	Remission	Remission	[11] (2015)
13	42	M	40	12	TSH	TS adenomectomy	Total thyroidectomy/ iratherapy	Remission	Remission	[11] (2015)
14	44	F	30	16	TSH/ GH/ FSH	Octreotide/TS adenomectomy	Total thyroidectomy/ iratherapy	Remission	Remission	[12] (2017)
15	27	F	NR	NR	TSH	Surgical resection for nasopharyngeal tumor (ectopic TSHoma)	Total thyroidectomy/ iratherapy	Remission	Remission	[13] (2017)
16	57	M	NR	30	TSH	Octreotide/TS adenomectomy	Partial thyroidectomy	Remission	Remission	[14] (2018)
Our case	50	F	10	12	TSH/ PRL	TS adenomectomy/ lanreotide/cabergoline	Total thyroidectomy/ iratherapy	Remission	Remission	-(2021)

NR, not reported; TC, thyroid cancer; PA, pituitary adenoma; IHC, immunohistochemistry; TSH, thyrotropin; PRL, prolactin; GH, growth hormone; FSH, follicle-stimulating hormone; TS, transsphenoidal.

SITSH. These diagnoses can be easily excluded by questioning, monitoring of drug intake, testing malabsorption, and repeating serum TSH measurement with several laboratory methods to exclude transitory changes and biological interference [15, 16]. Once these diagnoses are excluded, we are therefore faced with SITSH and the second step is to differentiate between TSHoma and syndromes of thyroid hormone resistance (RTH) [16, 17]. The differential diagnosis is complicated, so clinical presentations, laboratory assessment, and imaging advances may help and guide diagnosis (Table 3). T3 suppression test is the most specific and sensitive test, especially in patients with thyroid ablation. α-GSU may also be used; an elevated α-GSU concentration or a high α-GSU/TSH molar ratio favors the diagnosis of TSHoma in particular, in macroadenoma; these parameters are within the normal range in the case of a

TABLE 3: The differential diagnosis markers between TSH-secreting adenomas (TSHomas) and resistance to thyroid hormones (RTH).

	TSHoma	RTH
Family history of thyroid disease	Absent	85%
Unsuppressed TSH or increased	Present	Present
Elevated thyroid hormone levels	Present	Present
Nycthemeral profile of TSH	Absent	Present
High levels of SHBG (TeBG)	Present	Absent
Increased α subunit	65%	3%
α-GSU/TSH molar ratio	>1%	<1%
Increase in TSH after a TRH	Negative	Positive
T3 suppression test	No TSH suppression	Suppression of TSH
Somatostatin test	FT4 ↓ >30%	FT4 is not affected
Multihormonal production	Possible	Absent
MRI pituitary	98%	10–20%
DNA mutation analysis	–	+

microadenoma [18]. Due to their low sensitivity and high variability in several conditions such as age and menopause, α-GSU and GSU/TSH molar ratio may rarely help in the differential diagnosis [19]. Other tests are useful in the differential diagnosis like the increase of liver parameter such as the sex hormone binding globulin (SHBG) in the case of TSHomas, while it is normal in RTH [20, 21] (Table 3). This test was not performed in our patient because she was under a supraphysiological dose of levothyroxine. In addition, a difficulty of imaging lies in the presence of pituitary incidentalomas in 10–20% of the normal population and they are more frequent than TSHoma, so autonomous TSH production must be established [22, 23]. Finally, an association between TSHoma and RTH has been reported, hence the interest in gathering clinical, hormonal, and morphologic information [24]. In our patient, the radiological findings (pituitary macroadenoma) were associated with clinical data (no family history of thyroid disease) and biological findings (unrepressed TSH in T3 suppression test and elevated α-GSU level and α-GSU/TSH molar ratio), which allowed diagnosis of TSHoma.

Many cases of TSHomas are completely asymptomatic which explains why the majority of TSHomas are macroadenomas as in our patient [20] Therefore, it is important that the clinician be alerted to persistently unrepressed TSH after levothyroxine suppressive therapy in order to be able to carry out investigations and treat TSHoma as early as possible. On the other hand, it is so difficult to control and to monitor the carcinologic side of PTC when it coexists simultaneously with TSHoma as in our case.

The unusual association of PTC with TSHomas enriches the hypothesis of a potential link between thyrotropic hypersecretion and thyroid carcinogenesis. Thus, the role of TSH in carcinogenesis and development of PTC have been suggested in several studies where we noted high incidence of PTC in the patients with TSHomas and a meta-analysis of 28 studies have objectified a significant association between TSH levels and the risk of PTC [20, 25, 26]. Conversely, thyroidectomy when performed first before resection of pituitary adenoma may affect growth rate and secretion of the TSHoma due to diminished negative feedback effect of thyroid hormones [9]. This is the same mechanism described in Nelson's syndrome after adrenalectomy in Cushing's disease.

There are several therapeutic modalities for TSHoma, but the first line therapy is transsphenoidal pituitary surgery in order to remove tumor mass and to normalize TSH, with a success rate of 80% [27, 28]. In our case, surgery allowed removing tumor mass without TSH suppression. Second-line treatments include repeat pituitary surgery, radiation therapy, and medical therapy; they should be considered after failed transsphenoidal surgery and when the patient is not amenable to surgery or he declines it. Radiotherapy (conventional fractional radiotherapy or radiosurgery) may also be indicated in the treatment of TSHoma; however, the benign character of the condition, the potential side effects of radiation in particular hypopituitarism, and the long delay between radiation and efficacy will make its use less frequent, especially when medical therapies provide good control of the disease as we will see below [29]. Somatostatin analogs (SA) are the best choice of medical alternative treatment; they restore normal thyroid function in about 95% and shrink the size of TSHoma in up to 50% of patients [30–32]. Resistance to SA in our case is most likely related to nonexpression of somatostatin receptors. The presence of dopamine receptors on the thyrotroph cells justifies the therapeutic use of dopaminergic agents in TSHomas; however, efficiency in control of TSH secretion and tumor shrinkage was lower compared to SA and the best results were obtained in mixed TSH/prolactin adenomas [30, 31, 33–36]. The immunohistochemical study had objectified an immunofixation for TSH and also for prolactin with the absence of clinical or biological symptoms of prolactinoma on admission (neither amenorrhea nor galactorrhea and normal serum prolactin); this situation defines the true silent prolactinoma. It is a rare entity, especially in macroprolactinoma, most frequently associated with somatotropic adenomas. Discovery of PRL positive staining may provide an option for dopamine agonists in the treatment of recurrent silent prolactinomas as illustrated in our observation [37].

4. Conclusion

The unusual association of PTC with TSHomas enriches the hypothesis of a potential link between thyrotropic hypersecretion and thyroid carcinogenesis. Our observation highlights efficiency of cabergoline in control of TSH secretion, especially in the presence of mixed TSH/

prolactin adenomas, without forgetting the difficulty encountered to control and to monitor the carcinologic side of PTC when it coexists simultaneously with TSHoma.

References

[1] P. Beck-Peccoz, L. Persani, and A. Lania, "Thyrotropin-Secreting Pituitary Adenomas," in *Endotext*, K. R. Feingold, B. Anawalt, A. Boyce et al., Eds., MDText.com, Inc., South Dartmouth, MA, USA, 2019.

[2] A. L. Calle-Pascual, E. Yuste, P. Martin et al., "Association of a thyrotropin-secreting pituitary adenoma and a thyroid follicular carcinoma," *Journal of Endocrinological Investigation*, vol. 14, no. 6, pp. 499–502, 1991.

[3] P. Gasparoni, D. Rubello, L. Persani, and P. Beck-Peccoz, "Unusual association between a thyrotropin-secreting pituitary adenoma and a papillary thyroid carcinoma," *Thyroid*, vol. 8, no. 2, pp. 181–183, 1998.

[4] M. Kishida, F. Otsuka, H. Kataoka et al., "Hyperthyroidism in a patient with TSH-producing pituitary adenoma coexisting with thyroid papillary adenocarcinoma," *Endocrine Journal*, vol. 47, no. 6, pp. 731–738, 2000.

[5] S. Ohta, S. Nishizawa, Y. Oki, and H. Namba, "Coexistence of thyrotropin-producing pituitary adenoma with papillary adenocarcinoma of the thyroid: a case report and surgical strategy," *Pituitary*, vol. 4, no. 4, pp. 271–274, 2001.

[6] A. Gessl, H. Vierhapper, and H. Feichtinger, "Non-suppressible TSH in a patient thyroidectomized due to follicular thyroid carcinoma," *Experimental and Clinical Endocrinology & Diabetes*, vol. 114, no. 07, pp. 389–392, 2006.

[7] M. Poggi, S. Monti, C. Pascucci, and V. Toscano, "A rare case of follicular thyroid carcinoma in a patient with thyrotropin-secreting pituitary adenoma," *The American Journal of the Medical Sciences*, vol. 337, no. 6, pp. 462–465, 2009.

[8] H. D. Nguyen, M. S. Galitz, V. Q. Mai, P. W. Clyde, B. C. Glister, and M. K. M. Shakir, "Management of coexisting thyrotropin/growth-hormone-secreting pituitary adenoma and papillary thyroid carcinoma: a therapeutic challenge," *Thyroid*, vol. 20, no. 1, pp. 99–103, 2010.

[9] U. Ünlütürk, C. Sriphrapradang, M. F. Erdoğan et al., "Management of differentiated thyroid cancer in the presence of resistance to thyroid hormone and TSH-secreting adenomas: a report of four cases and review of the literature," *Journal of Clinical Endocrinology & Metabolism*, vol. 98, pp. 2210–2217, 2013.

[10] B. Feigel-Guiller, "Association entre carcinome papillaire thyroïdien et adénome hypophysaire mixte thyréotrope et somatotrope, observation clinique et revue de la littérature," Université de Nantes, Nantes, France, Thèse de doctorat en médecine, 2014.

[11] F. Perticone, F. Pigliaru, S. Mariotti et al., "Is the incidence of differentiated thyroid cancer increased in patients with thyrotropin-secreting adenomas? Report of three cases from a large consecutive series," *Thyroid*, vol. 25, no. 4, pp. 417–424, 2015.

[12] P. Kiatpanabhikul, S. Shuangshoti, K. Chantra et al., "A case of coexistence of TSH/GH-secreting pituitary tumor and papillary thyroid carcinoma: challenges in pathogenesis and management," *Journal of Clinical Neuroscience*, vol. 41, pp. 78–80, 2017.

[13] J. Yang, S. Liu, Z. Yang, and Y. B. Shi, "Ectopic thyrotropin secreting pituitary adenoma concomitant with papillary thyroid carcinoma," *Medicine*, vol. 96, no. 50, Article ID e8912, 2017.

[14] H. Inoue, N. Shinojima, R. Ueda et al., "A rare case of thyrotropin-secreting pituitary adenoma coexisting with papillary thyroid carcinoma presenting with visual disturbance without hyperthyroidism," *World Neurosurgery*, vol. 119, pp. 394–399, 2018.

[15] O. Koulouri, C. Moran, D. Halsall, K. Chatterjee, and M. Gurnell, "Pitfalls in the measurement and interpretation of thyroid function tests," *Best Practice & Research Clinical Endocrinology & Metabolism*, vol. 27, no. 6, pp. 745–762, 2013.

[16] S. Laboureau-Soraes Barbosa, F. Boux de Casson, and V. Rohmer, "Exploration fonctionnelle de la thyroïde (en dehors de l'imagerie)," *EMC-Endocrinologie-Nutrition*, vol. 4, no. 4, pp. 1–11, 2007.

[17] P. Caron, "Adénomes hypophysaires à TSH ou adénomes thyréotropes," *La Presse Médicale*, vol. 38, no. 1, pp. 107–111, 2009.

[18] H. Socin, P. Chanson, B. Delemer et al., "The changing spectrum of TSH-secreting pituitary adenomas: diagnosis and management in 43 patients," *European Journal of Endocrinology*, vol. 148, no. 4, pp. 433–442, 2003.

[19] A. Tjörnstrand and H. F. Nyström, "Diagnosis OF endocrine disease: diagnostic approach to TSH-producing pituitary adenoma," *European Journal of Endocrinology*, vol. 177, pp. R183–R197, 2017.

[20] P. Beck-Peccoz, C. Giavoli, and A. Lania, "A 2019 update on TSH-secreting pituitary adenomas," *Journal of Endocrinological Investigation*, vol. 42, no. 12, pp. 1401–1406, 2019.

[21] P. Beck-Peccoz, A. Lania, A. Beckers, K. Chatterjee, and J.-L. Wemeau, "2013 European thyroid association guidelines for the diagnosis and treatment of thyrotropin-secreting pituitary tumors," *European Thyroid Journal*, vol. 2, no. 2, pp. 76–82, 2013.

[22] S. Ezzat, S. L. Asa, W. T. Couldwell et al., "The prevalence of pituitary adenomas," *Cancer*, vol. 101, no. 3, pp. 613–619, 2004.

[23] P. Beck-Peccoz, F. Brucker-Davis, L. Persani, R. C. Smallridge, and B. D. Weintraub, "Thyrotropin-secreting pituitary tumors*," *Endocrine Reviews*, vol. 17, no. 6, pp. 610–638, 1996.

[24] J. D. Safer, S. D. Colan, L. M. Fraser, and F. E. Wondisford, "A pituitary tumor in a patient with thyroid hormone resistance: a diagnostic dilemma," *Thyroid*, vol. 11, no. 3, pp. 281–291, 2001.

[25] A. Dorange, S. Triau, S. Mucci-Hennekinne et al., "An elevated level of TSH might be predictive of differentiated thyroid cancer," *Annales d'Endocrinologie*, vol. 72, no. 6, pp. 513–521, 2011.

[26] H. K. Kim, J. H. Yoon, S. J. Kim, J. S. Cho, S.-S. Kweon, and H.-C. Kang, "Higher TSH level is a risk factor for differentiated thyroid cancer," *Clinical Endocrinology*, vol. 78, no. 3, pp. 472–477, 2013.

[27] D. S. A. McLeod, K. F. Watters, A. D. Carpenter, P. W. Ladenson, D. S. Cooper, and E. L. Ding, "Thyrotropin and thyroid cancer diagnosis: a systematic review and dose-response meta-analysis," *Journal of Clinical Endocrinology & Metabolism*, vol. 97, no. 8, pp. 2682–2692, 2012.

[28] P. Beck-Peccoz, L. Persani, D. Mannavola, and I. Campi, "TSH-secreting adenomas," *Best Practice & Research Clinical Endocrinology & Metabolism*, vol. 23, no. 5, pp. 597–606, 2009.

[29] E. Malchiodi, E. Profka, E. Ferrante et al., "Thyrotropin-secreting pituitary adenomas: outcome of pituitary surgery and irradiation," *Journal of Clinical Endocrinology & Metabolism*, vol. 99, no. 6, pp. 2069–2076, 2014.

[30] F. G. Amlashi and N. A. Tritos, "Thyrotropin-secreting pituitary adenomas: epidemiology, diagnosis, and management," *Endocrine*, vol. 52, no. 3, pp. 427–440, 2016.
[31] P. Chanson, J. Orgiazzi, P. J. Derome et al., "Paradoxical response of thyrotropin to L-dopa and presence of dopaminergic receptors in a thyrotropin secreting pituitary adenoma," *Journal of Clinical Endocrinology & Metabolism*, vol. 59, no. 3, pp. 542–546, 1984.
[32] W. Zgliczynski, P. Zdunowski, I. Czajka-Oraniec, W. Jeske, and G. Zielinski, "The role of somatostatin analogues in treatment of TSH secreting pituitary adenomas," *Thyroid Research*, vol. 6, no. Supp 2, p. A64, 2013.
[33] Y.-H. Kao, T.-J. Chang, and T.-S. Huang, "Thyrotropin-secreting pituitary tumor presenting with congestive heart failure and good response to dopaminergic agonist cabergoline," *Journal of the Formosan Medical Association*, vol. 112, no. 11, pp. 721–724, 2013.
[34] T. Kienitz, M. Quinkler, C. J. Strasburger, and M. Ventz, "Long-term management in five cases of TSH-secreting pituitary adenomas: a single center study and review of the literature," *European Journal of Endocrinology*, vol. 157, no. 1, pp. 39–46, 2007.
[35] F. Mouton, F. Faivre-Defrance, C. Cortet-Rudelli et al., "TSH-secreting adenoma improved with cabergoline," *Annales d'Endocrinologie*, vol. 69, no. 3, pp. 244–248, 2008.
[36] J. Mulinda, S. Hasinski, and L. I. Rose, "Successful therapy for a mixed thyrotropin- and prolactin-secreting pituitary macroadenoma with cabergoline," *Endocrine Practice*, vol. 5, no. 2, pp. 76–79, 1999.
[37] J. Drummond, F. Roncaroli, A. B. Grossman, and M. Korbonits, "Clinical and pathological aspects of silent pituitary adenomas," *Journal of Clinical Endocrinology & Metabolism*, vol. 104, no. 7, pp. 2473–2489, 2019.

20

Mediastinal Thyroid Carcinoma and Graves' Disease: A Rare Presentation

Sara Lomelino Pinheiro,[1] Inês Damásio,[1] Ana Figueiredo,[1] Tiago Nunes da Silva,[1,2] and Valeriano Leite[1,2]

[1]*Serviço de Endocrinologia, Instituto Português de Oncologia de Lisboa Francisco Gentil, Rua Professor Lima Basto, 1099-023 Lisboa, Portugal*
[2]*Unidade de Investigação em Patobiologia Molecular, Instituto Português de Oncologia de Lisboa Francisco Gentil, Rua Professor Lima Basto, 1099-023 Lisboa, Portugal*

Correspondence should be addressed to Sara Lomelino Pinheiro; saralomelinopinheiro@gmail.com

Academic Editor: Wayne V. Moore

Background. Mediastinal thyroid carcinoma is extremely rare, with few cases reported in the literature. *Case Report.* A 73-year-old man presented with weight loss for 6 months. Imaging by computed tomography (CT) documented a large mediastinal mass below the thyroid gland and pulmonary metastases. Neck ultrasound found two spongiform nodules in the right thyroid lobe, and fine-needle aspiration citology (FNAC) of these nodules revealed they are benign. Endobronchial ultrasound-guided needle biopsy of the mediastinal mass was compatible with papillary thyroid cancer. A few weeks later, the patient developed overt hyperthyroidism due to Graves' disease, which was treated with antithyroid drugs. ^{99m}Pertechnetate scintigraphy showed increased diffuse uptake in the thyroid parenchyma but the absence of uptake in the paratracheal mass and in the lung nodules. The patient was not considered eligible for surgical intervention or therapy with tyrosine kinase inhibitor due to tracheal and mediastinal vessel invasion and was treated with palliative radiotherapy. Two months later, restaging PET-FDG showed an intense uptake in the right lobe of the thyroid gland, lymph nodes, lungs, bone, muscle, myocardial, kidney, and adrenal gland. *Conclusion.* In this case, thyroid carcinoma presented as a mediastinal mass with concurrent hyperthyroidism due to Graves' disease. Although uncommon, the clinicians should be aware of these situations. Obtaining a prompt histological examination of an intrathoracic mass is crucial to ensure an early diagnosis and treatment.

1. Introduction

Mediastinal thyroid cancer is extremely rare, with few cases reported in the literature [1–3]. Surgical excision of the malignant lesion, whenever possible, is the treatment of choice [4]. In this clinical case, the distinction between ectopic and metastatic thyroid carcinoma is challenging.

We describe a case of papillary thyroid carcinoma (PTC) presenting as an intrathoracic mass with lung metastases. Besides the unique presentation, this case had an atypical course, with subsequent hyperthyroidism due to Graves' disease and widespread cardiac, muscle, and adrenal involvement.

2. Case Presentation

A 73-year-old man presented with a 6-month history of unquantified weight loss. His past medical history included hypertension, type 2 diabetes, and smoking (750 pack-years). There was no record of previous head and neck radiation and no relevant family history. Physical examination showed emaciated appearance. Neck examination revealed a palpable nonadherent nodule in the right lobe of the thyroid gland.

2.1. Diagnosis. Imaging by computed tomography (CT) documented a large mediastinal mass (41 × 29 mm) inferior to the right lobe of the thyroid gland, interposing between the trachea and supra-aortic vessels, with probable tracheal and mediastinal vessel infiltration (Figure 1). The mass was initially considered a mediastinal lymph node due to its clear demarcation from the adjacent thyroid gland (Figure 1). Chest CT demonstrated multiple pulmonary lesions suggestive of metastases. Endobronchial ultrasound-guided needle biopsy of the mediastinal mass was compatible with PTC (papillary structures with nuclear pseudoinclusions) with thyroglobulin (Tg) in the washout of the needle above 30.000 ng/mL. Tumour cells showed positive staining for Tg, transcription factor 1 (TTF1), and PAX8. There were no cytologic features of undifferentiated tumour in this specimen. Serum Tg was 111 ng/mL (NR: <55). Neck ultrasonography (US) showed two spongiform nodules in the right thyroid lobe with 15 mm and bilateral micronodules. Fine-needle aspiration citology (FNAC) of the two spongiform nodules revealed benign lesions. Upper gastrointestinal endoscopy demonstrated oesophageal compression without significant stenosis or mucosal changes. Bronchoscopy was performed and revealed tracheal infiltration by the tumour. Blood tests confirmed a euthyroid state. The patient was diagnosed with metastatic thyroid cancer.

While awaiting the staging exams, the patient referred palpitations, hand tremors, and diarrhoea. Physical examination showed tachycardia without signs of goiter or thyroid ophthalmopathy. Blood tests identified overt hyperthyroidism due to Graves' disease: TSH <0.02 μUI/mL (NR: 0.30–4.20), free thyroxine (FT4) 3.86 ng/dL (NR: 0.90–1.70), free triiodothyronine (FT3) 9.2 pg/mL (NR: 2.0–4.4), and thyroid-stimulating antibodies (TRABS) 21.9 UI/L (NR: <1.8). ^{99m}Pertechnetate scintigraphy showed increased diffuse uptake in the thyroid parenchyma but the absence of uptake in the paratracheal mass and in the lung nodules (Figure 2).

2.2. Treatment. The patient was treated with methimazole (MMI) 30 mg and propranolol 60 mg per day, and there was clinical improvement after correction of the thyroid hyperfunction.

Due to the extension of tracheal invasion and disseminated disease, the patient was not eligible for surgical intervention. Therapy with TKI was also not considered because of the patient's general condition and mediastinal vessels infiltration, given the risk of potentially fatal bleeding in case of significant tumour reduction. The mediastinal mass was treated with 20 gray of palliative radiotherapy.

2.3. Outcome. Two months after completion of radiation treatment, the patient described severe pain in the chest. Restaging fluorodeoxyglucose- (FDG-) positron emission tomography (PET) showed intense uptake in the right lobe of the thyroid gland, lymph nodes, lungs, pleura, bone, muscle, myocardium, liver, kidney, and adrenal gland (Figure 3). These lesions were interpreted as metastases of thyroid cancer. At this moment, serum Tg was 369 ng/mL. Due to headaches and confusional state, head CT was performed and showed a frontal lytic lesion of the skull without endocranial involvement. Pain was managed with opioid treatment, and the patient was considered for palliative care. Eventually, clinical deterioration occurred and the patient died a few weeks later.

3. Discussion

The evaluation of a mediastinal mass is challenging, and obtaining a prompt histological examination is crucial to ensure an early diagnosis and treatment. Thyroid carcinoma can rarely present as an intrathoracic mass, with few cases described in the literature [1–3]. In such situations, it is difficult to differentiate between metastatic occult thyroid carcinoma and malignant transformation of ectopic thyroid tissue [2, 4]. Surgical excision of the malignant lesion is the treatment of choice. Total thyroidectomy is essential to differentiate between ectopic and malignant thyroid carcinoma, but it should be performed based on individualized risk stratification [4].

Our patient presented with an intrathoracic mass with clear demarcation from the adjacent thyroid gland and pulmonary metastases. Histological examination of the mediastinal mass revealed PTC. In this case, distinction between primary intrathoracic goiter based on an ectopic thyroid or a secondary goiter was not possible because the patient did not have access to surgery and autopsy was not performed. The two largest thyroid nodules found through neck US had a spongiform appearance, and the cytologic result was benign. Bilateral micronodules in the thyroid gland were not biopsied. Although it is rare, a few cases of microcarcinomas with metastases have already been reported [5].

Secondly, the histopathological classification of the tumor revealed a differentiated thyroid carcinoma, with positivity of PAX8 and TTF1. The histological images were suggestive of PTC showing papillary structures and nuclear pseudoinclusions. However, this diagnosis has to be interpreted with caution, since the demonstration of PTC requires multiple histological images picked up at different locations, all showing the features of PTC. A biopsy was not obtained due to the location of the tumor and the patient's general condition.

In this case, there was rapid disease progression with PET-FDG showing multiple lesions with intense uptake, regarded as a malignant, less-differentiated disease. This clinical course is rare for highly differentiated PTC, but it seems to be more frequent as an undifferentiated transformation of PTC or as a poorly differentiated thyroid carcinoma. However, PET-FDG was not performed at diagnosis because diagnostic evaluation was initially conducted in another institution. PET-FDG imaging is a useful tool in poorly differentiated thyroid carcinomas in initial staging and in the follow-up to evaluate metastatic disease. In the authors' view, the tumor was probably heterogenous with mixed areas, and the cytological analysis identified the differentiated component only. Tumors based on an undifferentiated transformation of PTC are often observed to have a mixture of undifferentiated and differentiated sites [6]. Nevertheless, the involvement of the myocardium, muscle, and adrenal by thyroid carcinoma is rare, and only few cases have been reported in the literature [7, 8].

Thyroid carcinoma presenting with concurrent hyperthyroidism due to Graves' disease is also uncommon [9, 10].

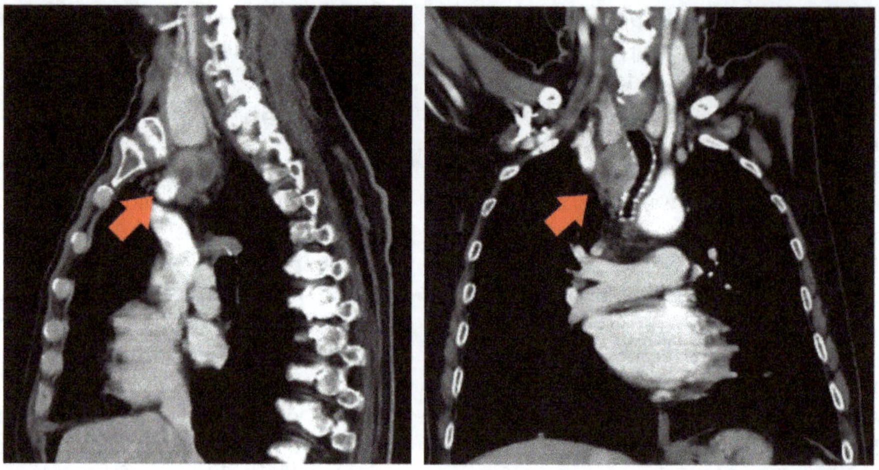

FIGURE 1: Neck and chest CT. The sagittal image revealed a mediastinal mass (41 × 29 mm) with clear demarcation form the right lobe of the thyroid gland. The coronal image shows the mediastinal mass interposing between the trachea and supra-aortic vessels.

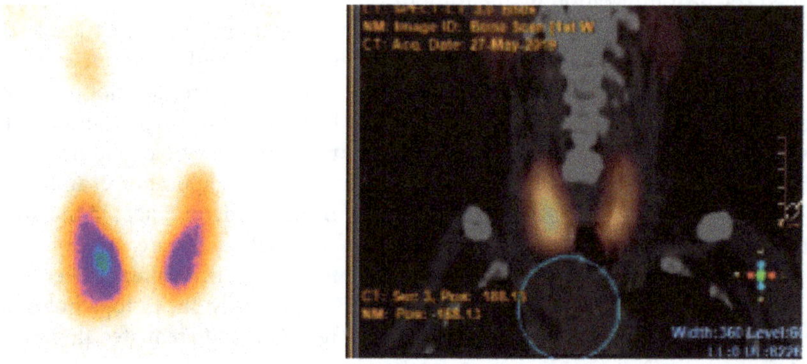

FIGURE 2: ^{99m}Pertechnetate scintigraphy showing increased diffuse uptake in the thyroid parenchyma and the absence of uptake in the mediastinal mass.

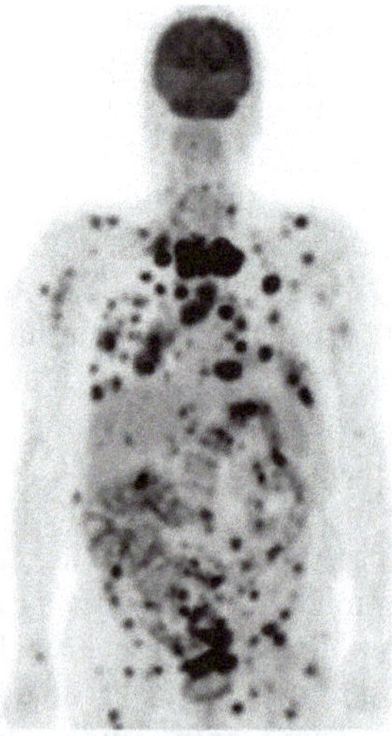

FIGURE 3: FDG-PET revealed multiple lesions with intense FDG uptake due to malignant disease (thyroid, mediastinal lymph nodes, lungs, bone, muscle, heart, liver, and adrenal).

^{99m}Pertechnetate scintigraphy showed diffuse uptake in the thyroid parenchyma but no uptake in the paratracheal mass. One hypothesis is that the increased uptake in the hyperfunctioning thyroid gland probably suppressed the uptake in the mediastinal mass, similar to toxic adenoma or struma ovarii [11]. Another explanation is the dedifferentiation of the mediastinal and lung metastases with subsequent loss of sodium iodide symporter which is needed for pertechnetate to enter the cells.

The authors chose to report this case despite the unfavorable outcome because of its unique and unexpected presentation and symptoms. Thyroid cancer, although rare, is a possible diagnosis to consider in the presence of a mediastinal mass.

Consent

Written informed consent was not obtained because the patient deceased before this work was finished. The patient's wife, the only close family member, was difficult to trace. The authors ensure the anonymity of all the information given about the patient.

Disclosure

This case report was presented as a poster in the 7th EYES (ESE Young Endocrinologists and Scientists) meeting in 2019.

Acknowledgments

The authors acknowledge Dr. Conceição Pereira for the important contribution regarding patient management.

References

[1] T. Imai, Y. Morishita, S. Ito, S. Saijo, and Y. Asada, "A case of ectopic thyroid presenting as a superior mediastinal mass," *Cureus*, vol. 12, no. 8, Article ID e9541, 2020.

[2] S. Shafiee, A. Sadrizade, A. Jafarian, S. Rasoul Zakavi, and N. Ayati, "Ectopic papillary thyroid carcinoma in the mediastinum without any tumoral involvement in the thyroid gland," *A Case report. Asia Oceania Journal of Nuclear Medicine and Biology*, vol. 1, no. 1, pp. 44–46, 2013.

[3] M. Yasuda, T. Osaki, Y. Fukuich, K Kobayashi, T Iwata, and T So, "Anterior mediastinal tumor as a solitary lymph node metastasis of occult thyroid carcinoma," *Journal of Surgical Case Reports*, vol. 2019, no. 2, pp. 1–3, 2019.

[4] J. Klubo-Gwiezdzinska, R. P. Manes, S. H. Chia et al., "Clinical review: ectopic cervical thyroid carcinoma--review of the literature with illustrative case series," *The Journal of Cinical Endocrinology and Metabolism*, vol. 96, no. 9, pp. 2684–2691, 2011.

[5] M. J. Jeon, W. G. Kim, Y. M. Choi et al., "Features predictive of distant metastasis in papillary thyroid microcarcinomas," *Thyroid*, vol. 26, no. 1, pp. 161–168, 2016.

[6] C. Eloy, C. Ferreira, C. Salgado, P. Soares, and M. Sobrinho-Simões, "Poorly differentiated and undifferentiated thyroid carcinomas," *Turk Patoloji Derg*, vol. 31, pp. 48–59, 2015.

[7] D. Giuffrida and H. Gharib, "Cardiac metastasis from primary anaplastic thyroid carcinoma: report of three cases and a review of the literature," *Endocrine-Related Cancer*, vol. 8, no. 1, pp. 71–73, 2001.

[8] C. Valkenborgh, L. Médart, and L. Collignon, "Muscle metastasis from undifferentiated (anaplastic) thyroid carcinoma," *Journal of the Belgian Society of Radiology*, vol. 103, no. 1, Article ID 27, 2019.

[9] B. M. Kadia, C. A. Dimala, N. N. Bechem, and D Aroke, "Concurrent hyperthyroidism and papillary thyroid cancer: a fortuitous and ambiguous case report from a resource-poor setting," *BMC Research Notes*, vol. 9, Article ID 369, 2016.

[10] H. Fu, L. Cheng, Y. Jin, and L. Chen, "Thyrotoxicosis with concomitant thyroid cancer," *Endocrine-Related Cancer*, vol. 26, no. 7, pp. R395–R413, 2019.

[11] C. M. Intenzo, A. E. dePapp, S. Jabbour, J. L. Miller, S. M. Kim, and D. M. Capuzzi, "Scintigraphic manifestations of thyrotoxicosis," *RadioGraphics*, vol. 23, no. 4, pp. 857–869, 2003.

21

Clavicular Metastasis as an Initial Presentation of Papillary Thyroid Cancer

Russell Fung, [1,2] Madeline Fasen, [2] Firas Warda, [1,2] Patrick Natter, [3] Stacey Nedrud, [4] Rui Fernandes, [4] Ahmad Alkhasawneh, [5] and Gunjan Y. Gandhi [1,2]

[1] *Division of Endocrinology, University of Florida College of Medicine-Jacksonville, Jacksonville, FL, USA*
[2] *Department of Medicine, University of Florida College of Medicine-Jacksonville, Jacksonville, FL, USA*
[3] *Department of Radiology, University of Florida College of Medicine-Jacksonville, Jacksonville, FL, USA*
[4] *Department of Oral and Maxillofacial Surgery, University of Florida College of Medicine-Jacksonville, Jacksonville, FL, USA*
[5] *Department of Pathology and Laboratory Medicine, University of Florida College of Medicine-Jacksonville, Jacksonville, FL, USA*

Correspondence should be addressed to Gunjan Y. Gandhi; gunjan.gandhi@jax.ufl.edu

Academic Editor: Lucy Mastrandrea

Objective. We present the case of a 44-year-old man with a large neck mass to highlight the unique presentation of papillary thyroid carcinoma (PTC) metastatic to the clavicle. *Methods.* We reviewed the medical record for a detailed history and physical examination findings. Our radiology colleagues examined the diagnostic imaging studies performed. The pathology team reviewed the neck mass biopsy and the confirmatory surgical pathology after total resection of the mass. *Results.* A 44-year-old man presented with an enlarging neck mass. Initial X-rays revealed a large soft tissue density mass that extended to the midline of the right clavicle. A neck ultrasound established a 5.4 × 3.6 cm mass with increased vascularity and calcification extending from the thyroid. A CT scan noted the extension of the mass into the adjacent sternoclavicular junction with osteolysis of the middle third of the clavicle and the superior aspect of the sternal body. Fine-needle aspiration revealed a thyroid neoplasm with follicular features and positive immunostaining consistent with thyroid carcinoma. The patient underwent a composite resection of the tumor, including a segmental osteotomy of approximately two-thirds of the medial clavicle. The pathology report confirmed PTC with extrathyroidal extension and clavicle involvement (staged pT4a pN0), with further genomic findings showing positive KRAS mutation. *Conclusion.* Clavicular metastasis from differentiated thyroid cancer is rare. While the prognosis is generally favorable, various factors, including age greater than 45 years, poor differentiation, follicular thyroid carcinoma, Hurthle cell variant, and extrapulmonary metastasis, have typically been associated with poorer cancer-specific survival.

1. Introduction

Thyroid cancer is a curable disease that affects approximately 53,000 patients annually in the United States, with more than 2,000 deaths each year [1]. Papillary thyroid carcinoma (PTC) remains the most prevalent form of thyroid malignancy and is usually associated with a good prognosis [2]. While metastatic spread from the thyroid gland to the bone is uncommon [3], it has a better survival rate (10-year survival rates ranging from 13% to 21%) than that of other primary carcinomas metastatic to the bone [4]. However, prognosis generally depends on age, tumor burden, and the number of bony metastases at diagnosis [5].

The hypothesis of "seed and soil" is widely accepted in describing the pathophysiology of thyroid carcinoma metastasizing to the bone [6]. This hypothesis indicates that cancer cells circulating in the blood (seeds) tend to metastasize to organs (soil), advantageous for their growth. Bone is a large organ with high calcium, growth factors, and a robust blood supply. These factors are released during bone resorption and provide a fertile microenvironment for growth [7]. Axial skeleton red marrow has been involved in approximately 80% of differentiated thyroid carcinoma metastases due to its high blood flow.

Up to 10% of patients with papillary and follicular thyroid carcinomas present with distant metastases [8].

While the lung is considered the most common site of metastases from thyroid malignancy, bone metastases, if seen, are usually observed at skeletal sites such as the humerus, pelvis, radius, and scapula. PTC metastases to the clavicular bone as an initial presentation is a rare and unique finding [9]. We present a case of PTC that was first noticed as a growth on the right base of the neck and later found to have metastasized to the right clavicle.

2. Case Report

A 44-year-old man presented to his primary care provider for a right proximal clavicular mass and enlarging neck for six months that he attributed to an injury from Jujitsu. The patient endorsed mild pain in the area but denied dysphagia, dysphonia, choking, or shortness of breath. The patient reported 20 lbs of weight loss. He denied hypoesthesia or motor deficits. On physical examination, a firm 8 cm mass was fixed to his right clavicle. There was palpable thyromegaly, the right lobe more prominent than the left, but there was no cervical lymphadenopathy and no significant motor or sensory deficits. Initial workup with an X-ray of his right clavicle revealed a large soft tissue density mass extended to the midline of the right proximal clavicle. A subsequent soft tissue neck ultrasound confirmed a 5.4 × 3.6 cm mass extending from the thyroid with features of increased vascularity and calcification extending from the thyroid (Figure 1). CT of the neck showed extension of the mass into the adjacent sternoclavicular junction with osteolysis of the middle third of the clavicle and the superior aspect of the sternum body (Figure 2). Due to suspicion of thyroid malignancy versus osteosarcoma, fine-needle aspiration of the mass was completed that showed a cohesive nest of neoplastic cells, and the nuclei were enlarged with pleomorphism. Focal calcification was noted, but there was no evidence of colloid or macrophages on multiple passes. Immunohistochemical stains were performed on the cell block, and the neoplastic cells were immunoreactive for TTF-1, PAX8, CK7, and thyroglobulin, and they were negative for CK20, calcitonin, synaptophysin, or chromogranin (Figure 3). The overall findings supported the diagnosis of papillary thyroid carcinoma. To assess the extent of the mass for total thyroidectomy, a chest CT scan with contrast confirmed marked enlargement of the right thyroid gland, measuring 5.3 × 7 × 4.9 cm, with invasion into the right proximal clavicle, adjacent strap muscles, and first rib as well as tracheal deviation and extension into the mediastinum.

The oral and maxillofacial surgery team performed a composite resection of the tumor, including a segmental osteotomy of approximately two-thirds of the medial clavicle. In continuity with the suprasternal and clavicular portion of the mass, the cardiothoracic surgery team performed a sternotomy to access and resect the substernal component, dissecting it off the first rib and manubrium without a segmental osteotomy. The great vessels were dissected and preserved with dissection of the mass off the superior mediastinum and thoracic inlet. The maxillofacial surgery team continued cephalad to perform a total thyroidectomy. Left levels 2–4, right levels 2–5, and bilateral central compartment selective neck dissections were completed. The mass was then delivered en bloc. The right sternocleidomastoid and strap muscles were sacrificed due to tumor involvement, but all other structures were dissected and preserved, including bilateral recurrent laryngeal nerves and the brachial plexus (Figure 4).

Postsurgically, the patient's serum calcium was low 7.9 mg/dL with simultaneously low PTH 9 pg/mL and low 25-hydroxyvitamin D 16.8 ng/mL. Thyroglobulin was markedly high at 15655.0 ng/mL (confirmed on dilution), and thyroglobulin antibody <1.0 IU/mL. Pathological examination of the right thyroid and clavicle showed PTC with extrathyroidal extension and clavicle involvement (staged pT4a pN0) with margins and lymph nodes negative for carcinoma (Figure 5). The tumor showed a predominantly solid pattern with areas of the follicular pattern, but there were no cribriform areas identified. Immunohistochemical stain for beta-catenin showed no evidence of nuclear staining, which is not compatible with the morular pattern of papillary thyroid carcinoma. Next-generation sequencing revealed KRAS Q61 R mutation, and the following mutations were not detected: BRAF, HRAS, TP53, PTEN, TERT, RET, NTRK, and PPARg. The left thyroid showed benign pathology. Due to the perceived need for treatment with radioiodine therapy, the patient was not discharged home on levothyroxine, but was given supplemental calcium and vitamin D with subsequent follow-up with endocrinology.

Postoperatively, the patient's course was complicated by a large expanding left neck hematoma that developed after a fall at home. The patient was readmitted and underwent an emergent hematoma evacuation without further incidence. He was able to follow up with endocrinology with laboratory studies at that time showing serum calcium was 8.6 mg/dL, TSH > 150.00 mIU/L, and free T4 0.2 ng/dL. He was started on calcitriol 0.5 mcg daily), vitamin D 50,000 units weekly, and calcium 1000 mg 4 times daily. Levothyroxine was held at this time with a plan for radioactive iodine treatment. On follow-up, an iodine-123 whole-body scan noted increased uptake over the lower lumbar spine that was suspicious for skeletal metastasis. A positron emission tomography (PET) scan confirmed a high fluorodeoxyglucose (FDG) avid lytic lesion along the posterior element of S2 with a maximum standardized uptake value (SUV) of 13.32. Magnetic resonance imaging (MRI) also revealed an enhancing sacral mass measuring 3.4 cm × 3.3 cm × 2.7 cm at the level of posterior elements of S1 extending to the sacral canal, causing severe sacral canal stenosis. There was a mass effect upon the traversing bilateral S2 nerve roots. These findings were consistent with metastatic disease.

3. Discussion

PTC is the most common form of thyroid cancer, accounting for approximately 80% of all thyroid cancers [10]. While bone metastases are rare, they can manifest as a complication of aggressive thyroid carcinoma [3]. Bone has been reported as the second most common metastasis site with well-differentiated thyroid cancer, with follicular

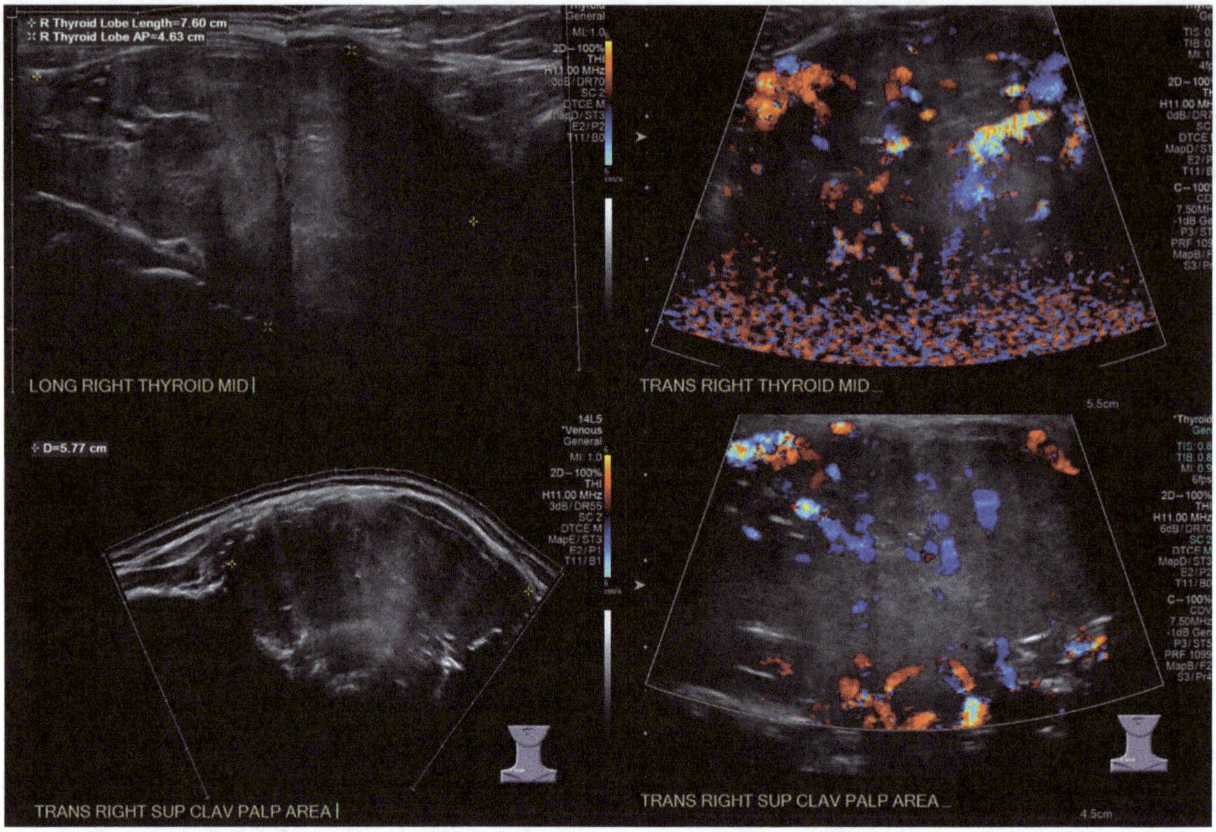

FIGURE 1: Ultrasound image demonstrating a diffuse mildly heterogeneous enlargement of the right thyroid lobe (a). The associated increased flow within the right thyroid lobe on the color Doppler image (b). A soft tissue mass also seen in the region of palpable concern in the right supraclavicular area, measuring 5.77 cm (c). The associated internal flow in the mass on the color Doppler image (d).

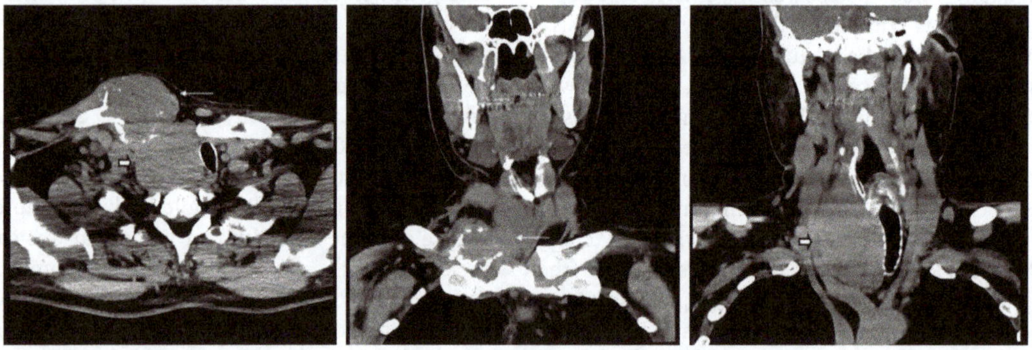

FIGURE 2: Axial CT image of the soft tissues of the neck (left image) demonstrating a heterogeneous mass within the right clavicular head, which is expansile with associated bony destruction (thin white arrow). There is also mass-like enlargement of the right thyroid lobe (short thick arrow). A coronal CT image of the soft tissues of the neck (middle image) also shows the destructive mass in the right clavicular head with soft tissue component (thin white arrow). A coronal CT image of the neck soft tissues more posterior in position (right image) demonstrates the mass-like enlargement of the right thyroid lobe (short thick arrow).

carcinoma more prevalent as an etiology (7–28%) than that of PTC origin (1.4–7%) [9, 11]. To this end, our case depicts a unique presentation of thyroidal tissue metastases to the bone due to being confirmed a papillary subtype of well-differentiated thyroid cancer, which typically has a very low propensity for bone metastasis.

Numerous factors contribute to the development of bone metastases. Increased blood flow in bone marrow serves as a powerful mechanism to favor the hematogenous spread of tumor cells [4, 11]. Malignant cells are also known to secrete angiogenesis compounds, which enhance bone resorption, creating an optimal environment for tumors to grow and develop [4]. Thyroid carcinoma is known as an osteolytic tumor. It can enhance the production of IL-1, IL-6, and receptor activator of nuclear factor-kB ligand (RANK-L), which ultimately leads to the resorptive activity of the bone and secondary bone formation as a response [12]. Furthermore, adhesive molecules synthesized by tumor cells allow them to attach to the bone matrix easily. Some studies have shown that bone

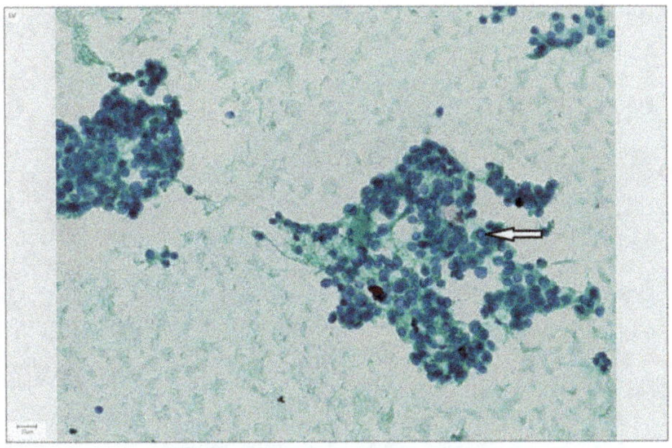

FIGURE 3: FNA of right neck mass shows cohesive nests of neoplastic thyroid tissue with overlapping nuclei and nuclear pleomorphism. The absence of colloid and macrophages is noted, and a subset of the cells shows nuclear pseudonuclear inclusions (arrow) supporting the diagnosis of papillary thyroid carcinoma (PAP stain, 200x).

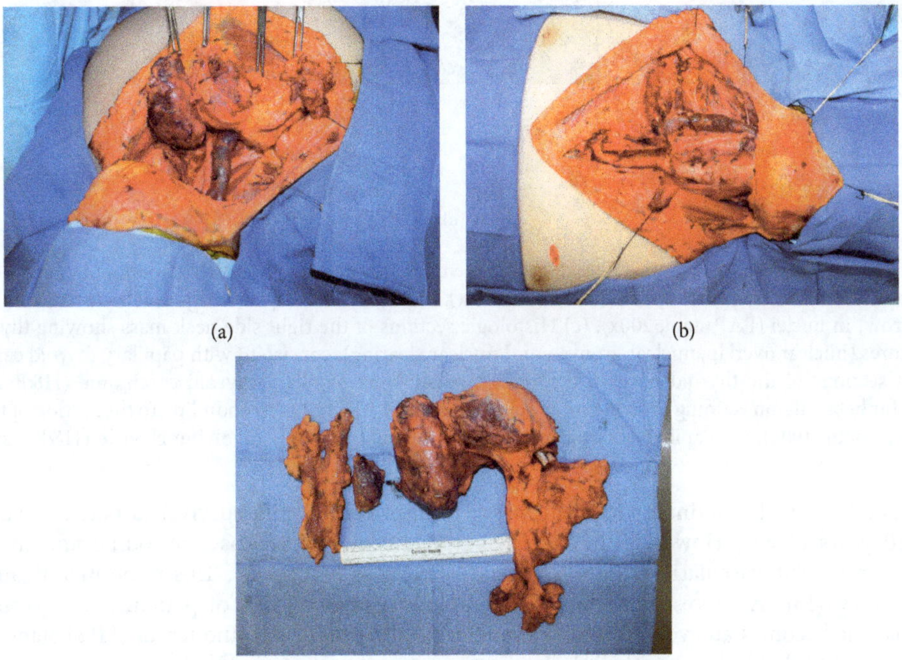

(a) (b) (c)

FIGURE 4: (a), (b) Retracted and removed gross pathology of the PTC mass. (c) Gross pathology of the resected neck mass.

involvement is more frequent in well-differentiated thyroid cancer than moderately or poorly differentiated thyroid cancer, but this is not conclusive [13, 14]. Typically, cancer cells that exchange biological information with bone environments can establish bone metastases. The "seed and soil" hypothesis is widely accepted [6]. Circulating cancer cells (seeds) have a propensity to metastasize to organs with the microenvironment (soil) advantageous for their growth. The ability of cells to survive, multiply, and recruit a blood supply gives rise to metastases. Bone is a large repository for immobilized growth factors, including transforming growth factors, insulin-like growth factors-I and II (IGF-I and II), fibroblast growth factors, platelet-derived growth factors, bone morphogenetic proteins, and calcium. Released and activated during bone resorption, these factors render the bone fertile for tumor growth [7]. More than 80% of bone metastases from all tumors, including DTC, are in axial skeleton red marrow where blood flow is high (vertebrae, ribs, and hips). In our patient, osseous metastasis to the sacrum is consistent with this finding. Tumor cell adhesive molecules bind the tumor cells to marrow stromal cells and bone matrix, allowing them to grow and produce angiogenic and bone-resorbing factors [11]. Most DTC patients have predominantly osteolytic lesions, with the secondary formation of the bone in response to bone destruction.

Moreover, with respect to metastatic bone lesions, our case is unique, in that it shows primary bone metastasis initially noted to the clavicle. The clavicle is a unique bone from a developmental standpoint. It is known to be the first

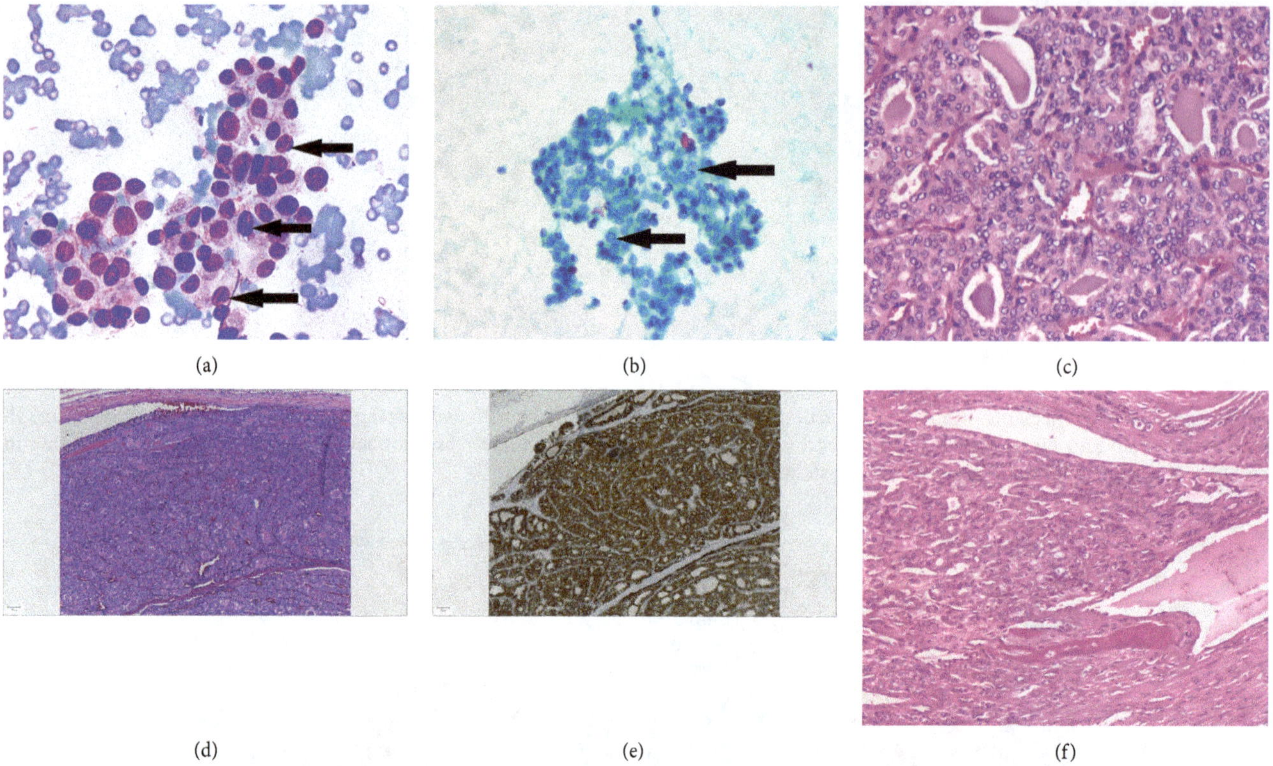

FIGURE 5: Papillary thyroid carcinoma. (a) Fine-needle aspirate of the right side neck mass showing abundant clusters of neoplastic thyroid tissue, and nuclear grooves (arrow) are present (Diff Quick stain, 200x). (b) Cluster of neoplastic thyroid tissue from the neck mass with focal pseudoinclusions (arrow) in nuclei (PAP stain, 200x). (c) Histologic sections of the right side neck mass showing thyroid carcinoma with papillary nuclear features (nuclear overlap, nuclear grooves, and nuclear clearing), consistent with papillary thyroid carcinoma (H&E stain, 200x). (d) Histologic sections of the thyroid mass in the right lobe showing papillary thyroid carcinoma (H&E stain, 100x). (e) Immunohistochemistry for beta-catenin staining showing no evidence of nuclear staining corresponding to the section of the thyroid mass in D (immunohistochemical stain, 100x). (f) Papillary thyroid carcinoma (follicular variant) involving clavicle (H&E stain, 100x).

bone to ossify in the embryo while continuing its ossification process until 18–20 years of age. However, the clavicle's scarce red marrow and scant vascularity make it a rare location for malignancy [15]. As a result, metastatic involvement of the clavicle becomes an even more rare event (0–15% of all known clavicular lesions) with little known about its management [9]. Most presentations of clavicular lesions are reported in small case studies with a broad spectrum of presentations [16]. Regarding the lesion location, the medial third of the clavicular is the most commonly affected location in the clavicular bone, with 60% of the lesions localized to this area [15]. In our case, the lesion encapsulated the medial third of the clavicle, consistent with the most common location of clavicular lesions.

Previous studies have investigated the various prognostic factors in patients with bone metastases from thyroid cancer. These factors, including age (greater than 45 years), poor differentiation, follicular thyroid carcinoma, and Hurthle cell variant, as well as extrapulmonary metastasis, have generally been associated with poorer cancer-specific survival [17]. A study by Durante et al. showed that the 10-year survival was reduced from 80% to 95% in patients with well-differentiated thyroid carcinoma to 14% in patients older than 40 years of age with macronodular lung metastases or multiple bone metastases [18]. Other studies have reported improved overall survival in patients who had lesions that concentrated radioactive iodine and those who had non-osseous lesions [3]. This same investigation reported bone metastasis in 47% of patients, with vertebra (29%), pelvis (22%), ribs (17%), and femur (11%) being the most common sites of metastasis [3]. In a more recent retrospective study that included 64 patients, improved long-term outcomes were associated with younger age, lower tumor stage, no extrathyroidal extension, and nonspinal metastases [5]. Not only was our patient below the age of 45 but his presentation of thyroid extension was also only limited to the clavicular bone with no known evidence of additional metastases. These factors would give our patient a more favorable outcome for his presentation.

While distant metastases from thyroid cancer can be challenging to identify, several imaging modalities are used in its evaluation. While post-I-131 therapy whole-body scans can be quite sensitive in detecting bone lesions, X-rays and bone scintigraphy are also used to evaluate bone metastases [4, 19]. However, the latter is sometimes only useful when more than half of an involved bone has been destroyed [19]. Also, these same modalities are limited by low specificity when pinpointing thyroid cancer as the primary etiology [4, 20]. An advantage of using bone scintigraphy is that it can detect skeletal metastasis much earlier than plain radiographs. But this approach may be of a limited value when evaluating from a thyroid cancer standpoint due to its osteolytic nature [19]. Furthermore, osteolysis can give rise to secondary bone formation in response to bone destruction and contribute to high false-negative and false-positive rates [20].

The biopsy's role in the diagnosis of bone metastasis depends on its clinical presentation and the site of metastasis. Generally, a bone biopsy is unnecessary for those with uptake localized to bone lesions on either diagnostic or posttherapy I-131 scans and in patients with multiple relapses who have previously undergone a biopsy documenting bone metastasis from thyroid cancer. However, a needle biopsy is recommended in the setting of suspected metastatic disease to the spine or pelvis. Biopsy samples should be examined for histological subtypes by utilizing special stains such as the thyroid transcription factor-1 (TTF-1), thyroglobulin (Tg), cytokeratin, and calcitonin [4]. For fine-needle aspirate of nonthyroidal masses with high suspicion of metastases from a thyroid origin, the detection of thyroglobulin levels in the aspirate sample washout can be utilized [21]. Studies of this diagnostic modality have evaluated lymph nodes of patients with PTC, demonstrating sensitivity and specificity close to 100% [22, 23]. While this method has not been extensively studied in bone metastasis cases of thyroid origin, the value of this technique in these specific cases would likely be similar. In our case, the extrathyroidal spread was limited to the right clavicle. Thus, only a biopsy of the neck mass itself was performed as the diagnostic modality. The diagnosis was later confirmed in surgical pathology as PTC.

4. Conclusion

We describe a case of PTC with its initial presentation as a neck mass involving the clavicle. While bone metastases from differentiated thyroid cancer are rare, the clavicular spread becomes an even more unique finding arising from PTC. Bone scintigraphy, X-ray, and fine-needle biopsy are some of the widely utilized methods employed in evaluating bone metastasis in the setting of thyroid malignancy. However, one should consider the benefits and limitations of these modalities. While the prospect of recovery is generally favorable, clinicians should be mindful of the various essential factors that determine prognosis in these cases.

Two specimens were received for pathologic evaluation. The first was a composite resection of the right thyroid with attached tissue, including a separate tumor mass, part of the clavicle, and left side neck dissection. The second specimen was an unremarkable left thyroid gland with attached left side neck dissection. The thyroid mass in the right lobe measured 7 cm in the greatest dimension, and the adjacent tissue mass was 10 cm in the greatest dimension. Both masses showed papillary thyroid carcinoma (solid variant and follicular variant). The adjacent tissue mass was separate from the thyroid gland, and the tissue in between the soft tissue mass and the gland was not involved by carcinoma. The adjacent tissue mass may represent either metastatic papillary carcinoma focus versus papillary thyroid carcinoma in aberrant thyroid tissue. However, there was no evidence of nonneoplastic thyroid tissue surrounding the adjacent tissue mass. Immunohistochemical stain for beta-catenin shows no evidence of nuclear staining, which argues against the possibility of a morular pattern of papillary thyroid carcinoma. Next-generation sequencing revealed KRAS Q61 R mutation, and the following mutations were not detected: BRAF, HRAS, TP53, PTEN, TERT, RET, NTRK, and PPARg.

Disclosure

Portions of this manuscript were presented as a poster at the Endocrine Society Annual Meeting (online) March 20–23, 2021, and published as an abstract [24].

References

[1] R. L. Siegel, K. D. Miller, and A. Jemal, "Cancer statistics, 2020," *CA: A Cancer Journal for Clinicians*, vol. 70, no. 1, pp. 7–30, 2020, In eng.

[2] D. S. A. McLeod, L. Zhang, C. Durante, and D. S. Cooper, "Contemporary debates in adult papillary thyroid cancer management," *Endocrine Reviews*, vol. 40, no. 6, pp. 1481–1499, 2019, In eng.

[3] A. G. Pittas, M. Adler, M. Fazzari et al., "Bone metastases from thyroid carcinoma: clinical characteristics and prognostic variables in one hundred forty-six patients," *Thyroid*, vol. 10, no. 3, pp. 261–268, 2000, In eng.

[4] J. A. Wexler, "Approach to the thyroid cancer patient with bone metastases," *Journal of Clinical Endocrinology & Metabolism*, vol. 96, no. 8, pp. 2296–2307, 2011, In eng.

[5] O. Slook, S. Levy, I. Slutzky-Shraga et al., "Long-term outcomes and prognostic factors in patients with differentiated thyroid carcinoma and bone metastases," *Endocrine Practice*, vol. 25, no. 5, pp. 427–437, 2019, In eng.

[6] L. A. Liotta and E. C. Kohn, "The microenvironment of the tumour-host interface," *Nature*, vol. 411, no. 6835, pp. 375–379, 2001, In eng.

[7] G. D. Roodman, "Mechanisms of bone metastasis," *New England Journal of Medicine*, vol. 350, no. 16, pp. 1655–1664, 2004, In eng.

[8] E. L. Mazzaferri, "Long-term outcome of patients with differentiated thyroid carcinoma: effect of therapy," *Endocrine Practice*, vol. 6, no. 6, pp. 469–476, 2000, In eng.

[9] A. Krishnamurthy, "Clavicle metastasis from carcinoma thyroid- an atypical skeletal event and a management dilemma," *Indian Journal of Surgical Oncology*, vol. 6, no. 3, pp. 267–270, 2015, In eng.

[10] M. I. Abdullah, S. M. Junit, K. L. Ng, J. J. Jayapalan, B. Karikalan, and O. H. Hashim, "Papillary thyroid cancer: genetic alterations and molecular biomarker investigations," *International Journal of Medical Sciences*, vol. 16, no. 3, pp. 450–460, 2019, In eng.

[11] M. M. Muresan, P. Olivier, J. Leclère et al., "Bone metastases from differentiated thyroid carcinoma," *Endocrine-Related Cancer*, vol. 15, no. 1, pp. 37–49, 2008, In eng.

[12] G. Mazziotti, A. M. Formenti, M. B. Panarotto et al., "Real-life management and outcome of thyroid carcinoma-related bone metastases: results from a nationwide multicenter experience," *Endocrine*, vol. 59, no. 1, pp. 90–101, 2018, In eng.

[13] C. Marcocci, F. Pacini, R. Elisei et al., "Clinical and biologic

behavior of bone metastases from differentiated thyroid carcinoma," *Surgery*, vol. 106, no. 6, pp. 960–966, 1989, In eng.
[14] G. V. Glinsky, O. Berezovska, and A. B. Glinskii, "Microarray analysis identifies a death-from-cancer signature predicting therapy failure in patients with multiple types of cancer," *Journal of Clinical Investigation*, vol. 115, no. 6, pp. 1503–1521, 2005, In eng.
[15] S. Suresh and A. Saifuddin, "Unveiling the "unique bone": a study of the distribution of focal clavicular lesions," *Skeletal Radiology*, vol. 37, no. 8, pp. 749–756, 2008, In eng.
[16] J. Smith, F. Yuppa, and R. C. Watson, "Primary tumors and tumor-like lesions of the clavicle," *Skeletal Radiology*, vol. 17, no. 4, pp. 235–246, 1988, In eng.
[17] B. H.-H. Lang, K. P. Wong, C. Y. Cheung, K. Y. Wan, and C.-Y. Lo, "Evaluating the prognostic factors associated with cancer-specific survival of differentiated thyroid carcinoma presenting with distant metastasis," *Annals of Surgical Oncology*, vol. 20, no. 4, pp. 1329–1335, 2013, In eng.
[18] C. Durante, N. Haddy, E. Baudin et al., "Long-term outcome of 444 patients with distant metastases from papillary and follicular thyroid carcinoma: benefits and limits of radioiodine therapy," *Journal of Clinical Endocrinology & Metabolism*, vol. 91, no. 8, pp. 2892–2899, 2006, In eng.
[19] S. Chua, G. Gnanasegaran, and G. J. R. Cook, "Miscellaneous cancers (lung, thyroid, renal cancer, myeloma, and neuroendocrine tumors): role of SPECT and PET in imaging bone metastases," *Seminars in Nuclear Medicine*, vol. 39, no. 6, pp. 416–430, 2009, In eng.
[20] S. Ito, K. Kato, M. Ikeda et al., "Comparison of 18F-FDG PET and bone scintigraphy in detection of bone metastases of thyroid cancer," *Journal of Nuclear Medicine*, vol. 48, no. 6, pp. 889–895, 2007, In eng.
[21] F. Pacini, L. Fugazzola, F. Lippi et al., "Detection of thyroglobulin in fine needle aspirates of nonthyroidal neck masses: a clue to the diagnosis of metastatic differentiated thyroid cancer," *Journal of Clinical Endocrinology & Metabolism*, vol. 74, no. 6, pp. 1401–1404, 1992, In eng.
[22] N. Cunha, F. Rodrigues, F. Curado et al., "Thyroglobulin detection in fine-needle aspirates of cervical lymph nodes: a technique for the diagnosis of metastatic differentiated thyroid cancer," *European Journal of Endocrinology*, vol. 157, no. 1, pp. 101–107, 2007, In eng.
[23] M. Cignarelli, A. Ambrosi, A. Marino et al., "Diagnostic utility of thyroglobulin detection in fine-needle aspiration of cervical cystic metastatic lymph nodes from papillary thyroid cancer with negative cytology," *Thyroid*, vol. 13, no. 12, pp. 1163–1167, 2003, In eng.
[24] R. K. Fung, M. Fasen, F. Warda et al., "Clavicular metastasis as an initial presentation of papillary thyroid cancer," *Journal of the Endocrine Society*, vol. 5, no. Supplement_1, pp. A885–A886, 2021, In eng.

22

Three Cases of Anaplastic Thyroid Carcinoma Transformation and Leukocytosis during Lenvatinib Treatment

Hiroyuki Iwasaki,[1] **Soji Toda**,[1] **Daisuke Murayama**,[1] **and Hiroyuki Takahashi**[2]

[1]*Department of Breast and Endocrine Surgery, Kanagawa Cancer Center, Yokohama, Japan*
[2]*Department of Oncology, Kanagawa Cancer Center, Yokohama, Japan*

Correspondence should be addressed to Hiroyuki Iwasaki; iwasaki.h@kcch.jp

Academic Editor: Mihail A. Boyanov

Since 2015, the cancer treatment lenvatinib has been used for patients with advanced radioactive iodine- (RAI-) refractory thyroid differentiated cancer; however, the drug's long-term effects have not been fully investigated. We report three cases in which lenvatinib treatment initially improved the patients' conditions, although they all died approximately 2 months after leukocytosis due to very aggressive disease progression with anaplastic thyroid carcinoma transformation. Serum interleukin-6 (IL-6) was elevated in all three cases, and granulocyte-colony stimulating factor (G-CSF) was elevated in two cases. The patients had a similar clinical course, with multiorgan metastasis and aggressive disease progression. Even with advanced cancer, lenvatinib has provided control of the disease. However, as long-term use of lenvatinib grows, it is possible that similar cases will increase, and we report our findings as an alert to other clinicians.

1. Introduction

Lenvatinib has been recognized to be effective against progressive radioactive iodine- (RAI-) refractory differentiated thyroid carcinoma (DTC) [1]. This targeted cancer drug has been used in Japan with documented effectiveness since 2015 [2]. We saw three patients who underwent lenvatinib treatment and died approximately 2 months after anaplastic transformation with leukocytosis. They initially saw good results and shrinkage of their tumors from the lenvatinib use, but they developed excessive leukocytosis and rare anaplastic thyroid cancer. There have been other cases where patients who were later diagnosed with anaplastic thyroid cancer (ATC) originally presented with excessive leukocytosis and high levels of granulocyte-colony stimulating factor (G-CSF) and interleukin-6 (IL-6) [3]. Very rarely, leukocyte hyperplasia and rapid disease progression have been reported as aggressive cancers in the lung or stomach [4, 5]. In addition to describing our patients' experience with this aggressive disease, we will caution other clinicians about the possible consequences of long-term lenvatinib treatment.

2. Case Presentation

The following three patients were initially diagnosed with DTC and treated at the Kanagawa Cancer Center, Japan. During the postoperative follow-up, disease progression with distant metastases was observed, followed by treatment with lenvatinib. Although the treatment process was satisfactory, anaplastic transformation developed unexpectedly with leukocytosis and aggressive disease progression. This study was approved by the Institutional Review Board of Kanagawa Cancer Center (IRB approval number 27–61 for DTC and 28–49 for ATC). All patients provided a comprehensive consent stating that their samples collected for medical examination can be utilized for investigation and clinical research.

Case 1 was a 58-year-old woman with an unexceptional medical history (height: 152 cm and weight: 42 kg). She had been diagnosed with thyroid cancer that metastasized to the lungs and pelvis; she had previously undergone total thyroidectomy in 2015. The pathology was follicular thyroid carcinoma containing poorly differentiated components, and she was treated postoperatively by external beam

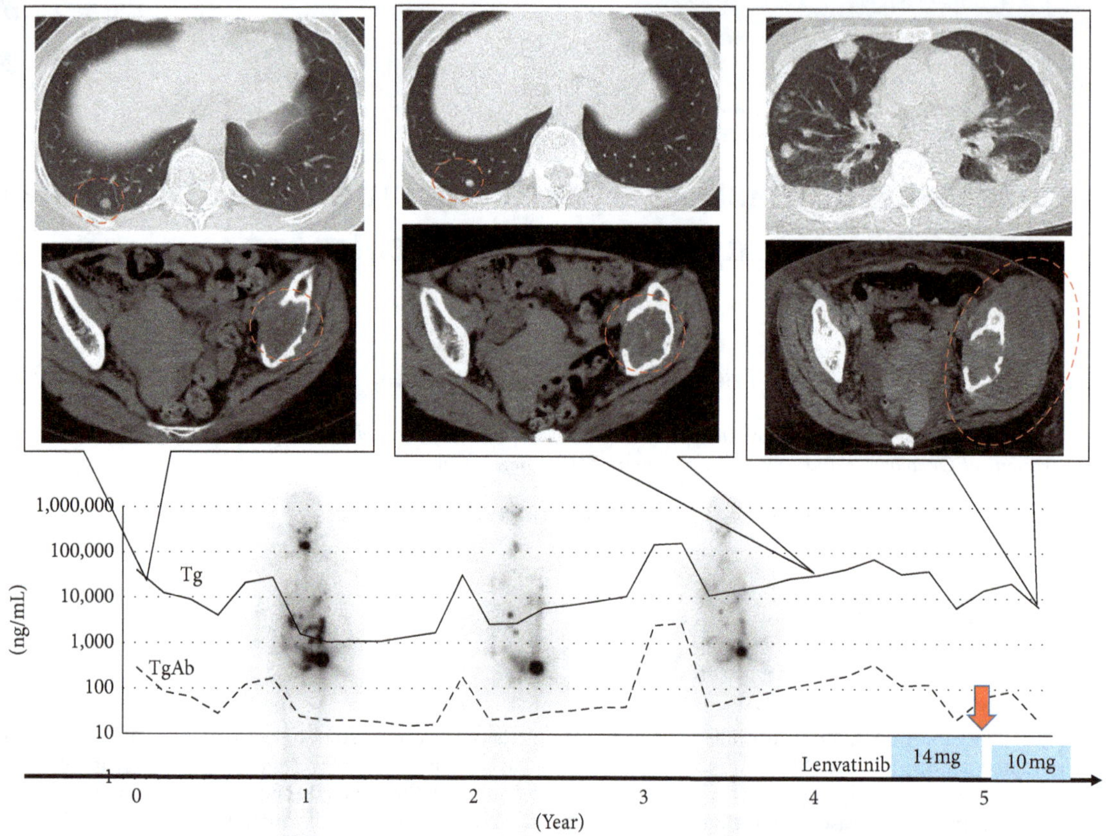

FIGURE 1: Clinical course of Case 1. The upper image is a chest computed tomography (CT) image. Although lung metastasis did not change after three courses of radioactive iodine (RAI) treatment, the patient's condition became progressive disease after anaplastic transformation and bilateral pleural effusion accumulated. The lower image is a CT image of the pelvis, and the left iliac metastasis increased rapidly after anaplastic transformation. The graph below the image shows the transition of thyroglobulin and antibodies, the timing of lenvatinib treatment and the dose. Whole body scintigraphy images after three RAI treatments are also shown in the background. RAI uptake is decaying. The red dotted circle indicates the lesion. The red arrow indicates the time of anaplastic transformation.

radiation to the left pelvis, denosumab, and three courses of RAI treatment. The pelvic metastasis remained unchanged, the pulmonary metastasis was exacerbated, and her serum thyroglobulin (Tg) level gradually increased in 5 years after the initial surgery. Then, we started treatment with lenvatinib at an initial dose of 14 mg, decreased to 10 mg after eight weeks, and the adverse events (AE) included grade 1 hypertension (HT) and grade 1 appetite loss. The pulmonary metastasis decreased slightly, but the pelvic metastasis remained unchanged; the efficacy according to the response evaluation criteria in solid tumors (RECIST) was stable disease [6]. Twelve weeks after commencing lenvatinib treatment, she developed a high fever with excessive leukocytosis (white blood cells (WBC) = 50300/μL).

When the lenvatinib treatment was discontinued, her WBC increased to 70,800 μL, followed by an increase in G-CSF to 748 pg/mL and IL-6 to 114 pg/mL; there was a continued progression of the pulmonary metastasis, pleural effusion, and a rapid increase in the necrosis of the left pelvic metastasis (Figure 1). Drainage was performed, and cytology was submitted twice, but it was negative. The patient transitioned to best supportive care (BSC) and died 51 days later. The duration of lenvatinib treatment was 5.1 months.

Case 2 was a 70-year-old woman with an unexceptional medical history (height: 157 cm and weight: 50 kg). She had surgery in 2004 previously for papillary thyroid carcinoma (PTC), and multiple pulmonary metastases were recognized in 2009. RAI treatment was performed twice but was ineffective for the pulmonary metastasis, which gradually increased. Active surveillance continued with thyroid stimulating hormone (TSH) suppression therapy, but the pulmonary tumor increased to 17 mm in 2015. We started lenvatinib treatment at the initial dose of 24 mg, which was reduced to 10 mg after 12 weeks. The AE induced by lenvatinib included grade 3 HT, grade 1 alopecia, and grade 2 arthralgia.

The tumor shrank upon treatment, from 17 to 9 mm in diameter, and the RECIST efficacy was categorized as a partial response. While the disease condition was stable for 56 months following lenvatinib treatment, her WBC unexpectedly increased to 19,700, and a computed tomography (CT) scan showed exacerbation of the pulmonary metastasis, left lung S3 atelectasis, and pleural effusion, which gave a negative cytology result; she was reclassified with progressive disease. Her WBC continued to increase to 33,700, G-CSF was 22.4 pg/mL, within a normal range, but IL-6 was

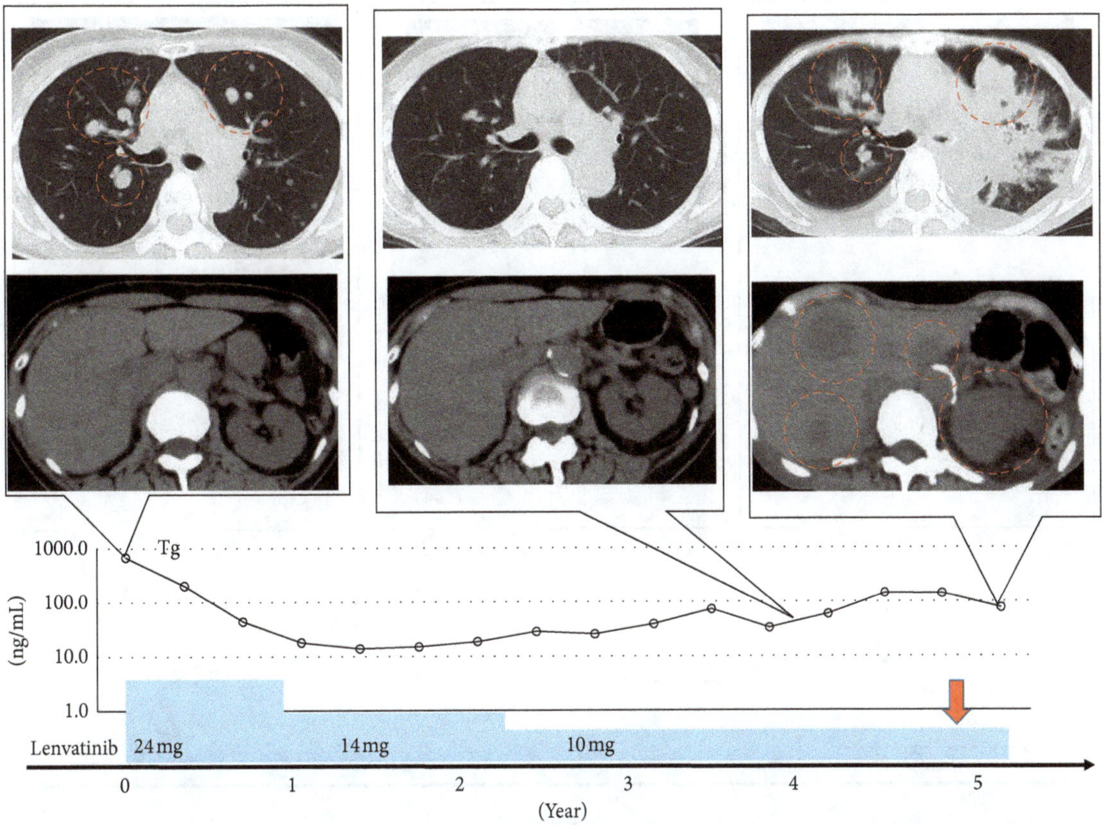

Figure 2: Clinical course of Case 2. The upper image is a chest computed tomography (CT) image. The patient was classified as partial response after treatment with lenvatinib, but then was reclassified as progressive disease after anaplastic transformation and became left atelectasis. The lower image is a CT image of the upper abdomen, and multiple liver metastases and metastases to the left adrenal gland and kidney appeared after anaplastic transformation. The graph below the image shows the transition of thyroglobulin, the timing of lenvatinib treatment and the dose. The red dotted circle indicates the lesion. The red arrow indicates the time of anaplastic transformation.

elevated to 22.8 pg/mL. When her physical condition began to deteriorate, with weight loss and an inability to walk, a CT scan revealed multiple metastases on the liver, left adrenal gland, and kidneys (Figure 2). She transitioned to BSC and died 50 days after the rise in WBC. The duration of lenvatinib treatment was 5.09 years.

Case 3 was a 71-year-old woman with a history of HT, hyperlipidemia, and chronic kidney disease (height: 154 cm and weight: 73 kg). She was diagnosed with PTC, and her initial surgery was performed in 2002. Multiple pulmonary metastases had been recognized in 2011, but RAI treatment was not effective. The maximum diameter of pulmonary metastasis was 6 mm, the serum Tg level remained stable at <1 ng/dL for 8 years after the diagnosis of pulmonary metastasis, and active surveillance was continued with TSH suppression; however, the size of the pulmonary tumor increased to 15 mm in 2019.

We started lenvatinib treatment at the initial dose of 14 mg, which was reduced to 10 mg after four weeks. The AE induced by lenvatinib included grade 2 HT and grade 1 stomatitis. The tumor shrank from 15 mm to 6 mm in diameter, and the efficacy was categorized as a partial response. Ten months after commencing lenvatinib treatment, her WBC increased to 19,700, and a CT scan showed multiple new lesions of 28 mm, changing her disease category to progressive disease (Figure 3). Her WBC increased to 33,700, G-CSF to 617 pg/mL, and IL-6 to 46.4 pg/mL. She developed low back pain, and an examination revealed progressive pulmonary and pelvic bone metastases. She was given 20 Gy external beam radiation to treat bone metastasis but suffered weight loss. She transitioned to BSC, and she died 66 days after the initial rise in WBC. The duration of lenvatinib treatment was 13.5 months.

3. Discussion

3.1. Characteristics of Anaplastic Thyroid Carcinoma Transformation. ATC is one of the most aggressive neoplasms. There have been several reports of leukocytosis due to the leukemoid paraneoplastic reaction resulting from G-CSF, granulocyte-macrophage (GM) CSF, and IL-6 production. Excessive WBC counts that continue to increase are linked to a poorer prognosis [7–11]. However, there are very few reports where leukocytosis is a primary marker in an ATC diagnosis. Since 1992, 17 cases diagnosed as ATC with leukocytosis have been reported worldwide, of which 13 cases have been in Japan [3]. It is significant that three patients in the same facility were diagnosed within 3 months for this disease. The clinical course of each case was similar,

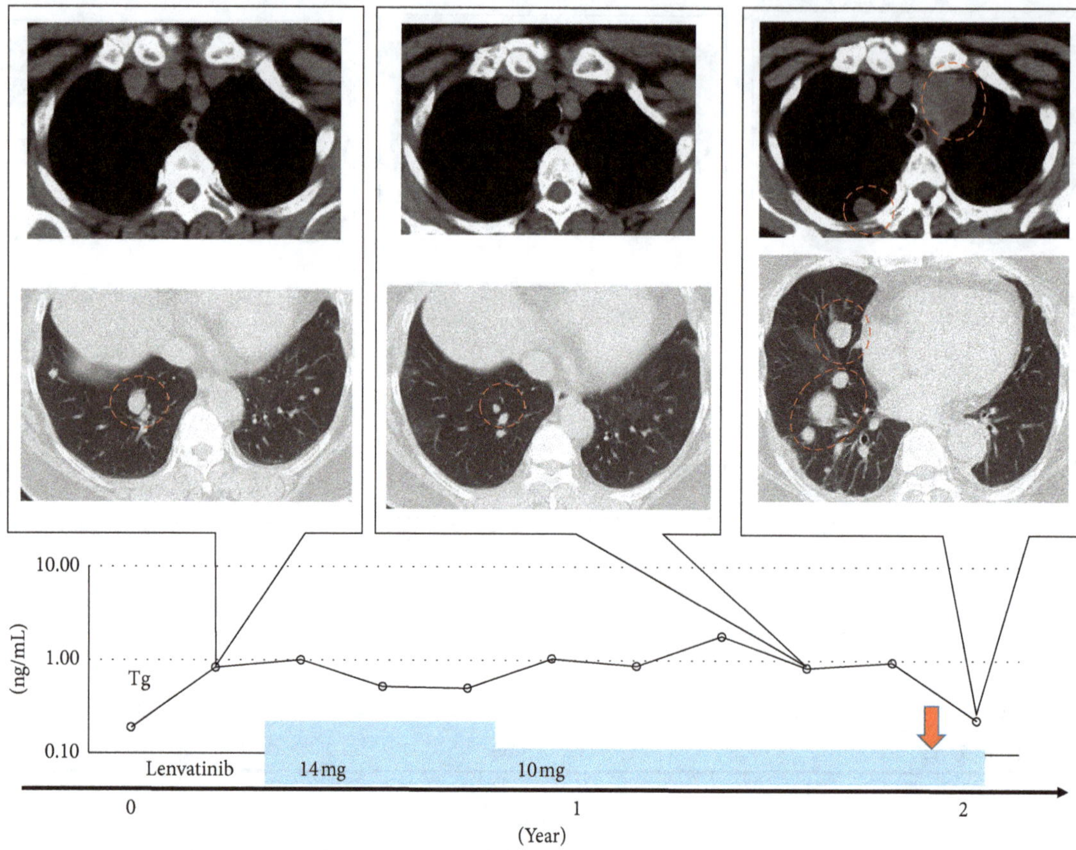

Figure 3: Clinical course of Case 3. The upper image is a chest computed tomography image of the mediastinal condition, and new lesions appeared in the mediastinal lymph nodes and pleura. In the lower image, the target lesion became partial response after lenvatinib treatment; then, it became progressive disease after anaplastic transformation. The graph below the image shows the transition of thyroglobulin, the timing of lenvatinib treatment, and the dose. The red dotted circle indicates the lesion. The red arrow indicates the time of anaplastic transformation.

and it is especially notable that each treatment course was controlled by the use of lenvatinib.

3.2. Blood Results. Table 1 shows inflammatory reactions demonstrated by increased WBCs, hemoglobin, platelet counts, neutrophil-lymphocyte ratio, C-reactive protein (CRP), G-CSF, and IL-6 in all cases. Figure 4 shows the WBC counts, which remained high in all patients, although the CRP did not decrease. The high fever observed in cases 1 and 2 was successfully treated with naproxen, but the leukocytosis did not subside. Lenvatinib was continued. After the WBC increased, the disease progressed rapidly, and all of them died approximately 2 months later. The serum Tg levels for each patient are shown in Figures 1–3, but Tg levels cannot be used as an indicator in ATC; so, the disease progression and the increase in Tg were not linked.

Table 1: Blood test findings in the three cases.

Case	1	2	3
WBC (/μL)	70800	36900	83500
Hb (g/dL)	8.4	11.5	10.6
Neutrophils (%)	86	95	92
Lymphocytes (%)	3	2	7
Eosinophils (%)	4		
Monocytes (%)	2	2	1
Myelocytes (%)	3		
NLR	28.7	47.5	13.1
PLT(104/μL)	31.6	17.8	29.4
CRP(mg/dL)	19.38	10.24	11.16
G-CSF(pg/mL)	748	22.4	617
IL-6 (pg/mL)	114	22.8	46.4

NLR, neutrophil/lymphocyte ratio; CRP, C-reactive protein; G-CSF, granulocyte-colony stimulating factor; IL-6, interleukin-6.The normal value of G-CSF is 5.78–27.5 pg/mL, and the normal value of IL-6 is 8 pg/mL or less.

3.3. Analysis of G-CSF and IL-6 and Cancer. G-CSF is a growth factor that is known to be a key regulator of hemopoiesis and for the proliferation and differentiation of neutrophils. G-CSF-producing tumors have aggressive characteristics that have been the subject of many Japanese investigations [4, 5, 12]. G-CSF-producing malignant tumors are sometimes accompanied by fever and high CRP levels, but G-CSF itself does not have the effect of inducing

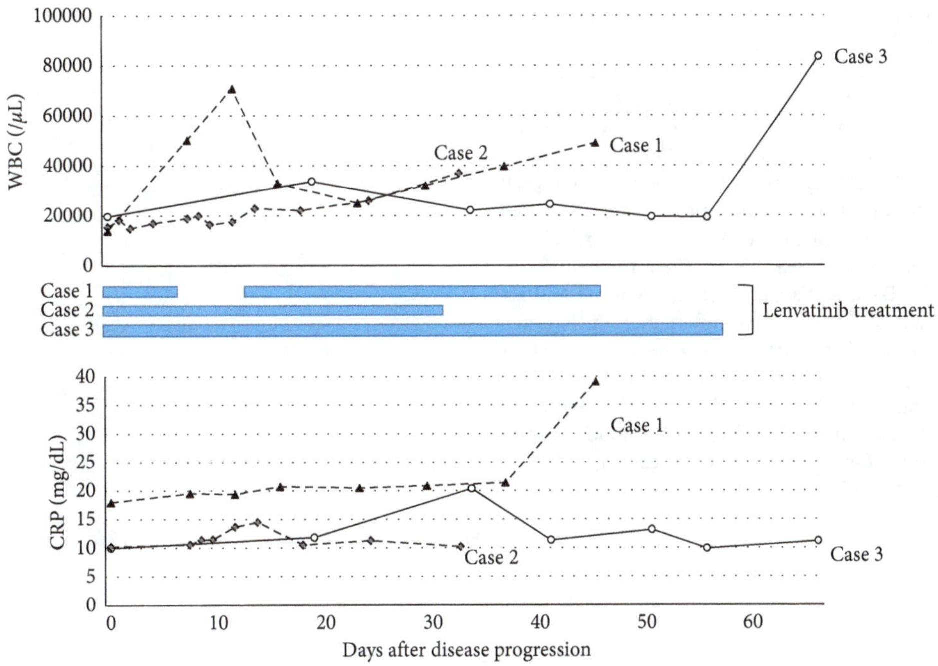

FIGURE 4: Changes in white blood cell counts and C-reactive protein. This figure shows changes after leukocytosis was observed in three cases. Leukocytes in Case 1 increased rapidly with a one-week washout of lenvatinib, decreased with resumption, but increased again. Patients in the second and third cases did not stop taking lenvatinib, based on the experience of Case 1. The broken line indicates Case 1, the dotted line indicates Case 2, and the solid line indicates Case 3.

these reactions, and an inflammatory cytokine such as IL-6 could be involved. IL-6 is secreted by T lymphocytes; it differentiates B lymphocytes into antibody-producing cells and is an acute phase response during inflammation [13].

3.4. Future Monitoring and Investigation. In the future, if a patient experiences progressive disease while being treated with lenvatinib, the clinician should investigate whether anaplastic transformation has developed. Since there are limited long-term results for lenvatinib treatment alone, genetic tests should be performed, and if indicated, BRAF inhibitors and PD-L1 inhibitors should be used in combination; however, these are not yet available for clinical use in Japan [14]. Until then, clinicians should monitor the clinical course and leukocyte levels of patients being treated with lenvatinib. The findings from our institution also warrant further research from other investigators whose patients have had a similar clinical course.

Acknowledgments

The authors would like to thank Enago (http://www.enago.com) for the English language review.

References

[1] M. Schlumberger, M. Tahara, L. J. Wirth et al., "Lenvatinib versus placebo in radioiodine-refractory thyroid cancer," *New England Journal of Medicine*, vol. 372, no. 7, pp. 621–630, 2015.

[2] H. Iwasaki, H. Yamazaki, H. Takasaki et al., "Treatment outcomes of differentiated thyroid cancer with distant metastasis improve by tyrosine kinase inhibitors," *Oncology Letters*, vol. 17, no. 6, pp. 5292–5300, 2019.

[3] A. Polymeris, C. Kogia, D. Ioannidis et al., "Excessive leukocytosis leading to a diagnosis of aggressive thyroid anaplastic carcinoma: a case report and relevant review," *European Thyroid Journal*, vol. 9, no. 3, pp. 162–168, 2020.

[4] T. Yokoyama, M. Hyodo, Y. Hosoya et al., "Aggressive G-CSF-producing gastric cancer complicated by lung and brain abscesses, mimicking metastases," *Gastric Cancer*, vol. 8, no. 3, pp. 198–201, 2005.

[5] Y. Matsui, T. Yamada, N. Masuzawa, S. Hamada, K. Takayama, and O. Hiranuma, "Advanced G-CSF-producing non-small cell lung cancer-not otherwise specified, with favourable response to pembrolizumab monotherapy," *Respirology Case Reports*, vol. 8, no. 7, Article ID e00625, 2020.

[6] Y. Tsuchida and P. Therasse, "Response evaluation criteria in solid tumors (RECIST): new guidelines," *Medical and Pediatric Oncology*, vol. 37, no. 1, pp. 1–3, 2001.

[7] K. Iwasa, M. Noguchi, K. Mori et al., "Anaplastic thyroid carcinoma producing the granulocyte colony stimulating factor (G-CSF): report of a case," *Surgery Today*, vol. 25, no. 2, pp. 158–160, 1995.

[8] S. Yazawa, H. Toshimori, K. Nakatsuru, H. Katakami, J. Takemura, and S. Matsukura, "Thyroid anaplastic carcinoma producing granulocyte-colony-stimulating factor and parathyroid hormone-related protein," *Internal Medicine*, vol. 34, no. 6, pp. 584–588, 1995.

[9] T. Nakada, H. Sato, F. Inoue, F. Mizorogi, K. Nagayama, and T. Tanaka, "The production of colony-stimulating factors by thyroid carcinoma is associated with marked neutrophilia and eosinophilia," *Internal Medicine*, vol. 35, no. 10, pp. 815–820, 1996.

[10] T. Sato, M. Omura, J. Saito et al., "Neutrophilia associated with anaplastic carcinoma of the thyroid: production of

macrophage colony-stimulating factor (M-CSF) and Interleukin-6," *Thyroid*, vol. 10, no. 12, pp. 1113–1118, 2000.

[11] T. Fujita, Y. Ogasawara, M. Naito, H. Doihara, and N. Shimizu, "Anaplastic thyroid carcinoma associated with granulocyte colony-stimulating factor: report of a case," *Surgery Today*, vol. 36, no. 1, pp. 63–67, 2006.

[12] A. Ogawa, G. Oda, T. Yasukawa et al., "A case of rapidly advancing G-CSF producing pleomorphic carcinoma of the breast appearing as an inflammatory breast cancer," *Cancer and Chemotherapy*, vol. 44, no. 12, pp. 1760–1762, 2017.

[13] T. Kishimoto, T. Taga, K. Yamasaki et al., "Normal and abnormal regulation of human B cell differentiation by a new cytokine, BSF2/IL-6," *Mechanisms of Lymphocyte Activation and Immune Regulation II*, vol. 254, pp. 135–143, 1989.

[14] A. V. Chintakuntlawar, J. Yin, R. L. Foote et al., "A phase 2 study of pembrolizumab combined with chemoradiotherapy as initial treatment for anaplastic thyroid cancer," *Thyroid*, vol. 29, no. 11, pp. 1615–1622, 2019.

Cardiogenic Shock and Guillain–Barré Syndrome as the First Manifestations of Pheochromocytoma

Maryam Heidarpour,[1] Nafiseh Sereshti,[1] Davood Shafie,[2] Bijan Iraj,[1] and Hassan Rezvanian[1]

[1]*Isfahan Endocrine and Metabolism Research Center, Isfahan University of Medical Sciences, Isfahan, Iran*
[2]*Heart Failure Research Center, Isfahan Cardiovascular Research Institute, Isfahan University of Medical Sciences, Isfahan, Iran*

Correspondence should be addressed to Davood Shafie; d.shafie87@gmail.com and Hassan Rezvanian; hasan.rezvanian@gmail.com

Academic Editor: Osamu Isozaki

Febrile congestive heart failure is a rare first manifestation of pheochromocytoma. Herein, the case of a 31-year-old female with febrile congestive heart failure and subsequent cardiogenic shock is presented. After intensive care unit (ICU) admission and further evaluating the right adrenal mass observed in abdominal ultrasonography, the diagnosis of pheochromocytoma was confirmed. Then, she was scheduled for the right adrenalectomy. Before surgery, she complained of acute-onset progressive muscle weakness in the lower limbs, followed by the upper limbs. After further investigation, she was diagnosed with Guillain–Barré syndrome and treated with intravenous immunoglobulin (IVIG). She recovered well after the right adrenalectomy, and during the subsequent 18 months, the follow-up did not reveal any complications, and left ventricular function recovered to normal.

1. Introduction

Pheochromocytoma is a rare neuroendocrine tumor with the ability to synthesize and overproduce catecholamines, developed in the adrenal medulla [1, 2]. Its clinical presentation is highly variable, but the classic triad is headache, sweating, and palpitation [3]. Less often, the tumor will cause severe cardiovascular complications such as myocardial infarction, arrhythmias, pericardial effusion, and congestive heart failure. Pheochromocytoma-induced cardiomyopathy is similar to Takotsubo cardiomyopathy and myocarditis [4, 5]. Diagnosis of pheochromocytoma-related cardiomyopathies is often delayed because of the atypical presentation. Given the potential reversibility of the cardiomyopathy, early diagnosis and resection of the pheochromocytoma are critical, while delayed diagnosis may lead to irreversible cardiac remodeling and death [6].

On the other hand, Guillain–Barré syndrome (GBS) is an acute immune-mediated polyradiculoneuropathy. Symmetrical limb weakness and hyporeflexia are typical manifestations of the GBS. However, half of these patients present with cranial nerve involvement. There have been few case reports of cardiovascular involvement in patients with GBS [7–10]. Here, we describe a case of pheochromocytoma presented as febrile congestive heart failure with subsequent cardiogenic shock and GBS. Finally, we discuss our diagnostic and management insights and report the patient's condition over 18-month follow-up period.

2. Case Presentation

A 31-year-old female presented to the emergency room with severe dyspnea, palpitation, acute generalized abdominal pain, and vomiting without blood or bile in February 2019. Upon reviewing systems and past medical and surgical history, she admitted to a 5 kg weight loss over the past month. She had a cesarean section 18 months ago without any complications. She had no history of hypertension (HTN), diabetes mellitus (DM), and cigarette smoking. Her drug history was negative, especially for illegal drugs, such as methamphetamines and cocaine. Her symptoms started 5-6 hours before admission. Initial vital signs included a blood pressure of 80/50 mmHg, heart rate of 130 beats per minute (bpm), respiratory rate of 30 per minute, O_2 saturation of 81% on room air, and temperature of 38.1°C. Physical examination revealed diffuse bilateral crackles but no decreased breath sounds at the base. Generally, the patient appeared confused and unstable. During the initial physical examination, she had a cardiac arrest, and cardiopulmonary resuscitation was done for 10 minutes, and it was successful. After that, she was sent to the intensive care unit (ICU). At this time, ECG showed sinus tachycardia, and transthoracic echocardiogram (TTE) demonstrated severe left ventricular (LV) systolic dysfunction with ejection fraction (EF) of 10%, normal LV size, mild to moderate mitral regurgitation, mild tricuspid regurgitation, and moderate pericardial effusion. Laboratory data are shown in Table 1. She received norepinephrine (starting infusion rates of 0.025 μg/kg/min), meropenem (500 mg IV every 8 hours), and ciprofloxacin (500 mg IV every 12 hours). On the fourth day, norepinephrine was discontinued, and hemodynamic stability was maintained even after discontinuation of vasopressor support. However, her fever continued to peak at 39°C. Tracheal aspirate, blood, and urine cultures were taken, and abdominal ultrasonography was performed due to non-specific abdominal discomfort. Ultrasonography showed a well-defined hypoechoic mass (44 × 57 mm) with internal vascularity in the right adrenal gland. In the next step, on the seventh day, abdominal computed tomography (CT) and catecholamine urine tests were requested for suspicion of an adrenal tumor. Abdominal CT showed a heterogeneous right adrenal mass measuring 47 × 54 mm (Figure 1). The adrenal mass on the unenhanced images had a density of 36 Hounsfield units. Laboratory values were notable for a 24-hour urine metanephrine of 2510 μg/day (normal <315 μg/day), normetanephrine of 8657 μg/day (normal <670 μg/day), adrenaline of 386 μg/day (normal < 20 μg/day), noradrenaline of 1044 μg/day (normal < 90 μg/day), and vanillylmandelic acid of 70 mg/day (normal < 13.6 mg/day). Indeed, all cultures were negative for infectious organisms. These findings were consistent with the diagnosis of pheochromocytoma. She was started on phenoxybenzamine 10 mg twice a day, and the dosage was increased by 10 mg every three days to a maximum dosage of 20 mg twice a day. On the tenth day, she complained of acute-onset progressive muscle weakness in the lower limbs, followed by the upper limbs. The muscle strength examination showed severe weakness in four limbs with a Medical Research Council (MRC) scale of 1/5 in proximal and 2/5 in distal of the upper extremities and 2/5 in proximal and 2/5 in distal of the lower limbs. She had no spine sensory level. Deep tendon reflexes were absent. Upper motor neuron disorders and meningeal irritation signs were absent. Lumbar puncture for cerebrospinal fluid (CSF) analysis was performed, and study results are shown in Table 2. Brain magnetic resonance imaging (MRI) was done and showed a normal finding except for a few foci of cortical and subcortical infarction. Electromyography (EMG) and nerve conduction velocity (NCV) showed acute predominantly motor axonal polyneuropathy. Therefore, the diagnosis of GBS was made, and the patient was treated with intravenous immunoglobulin (IVIG) 2 g/kg divided over five days. After that, muscle weakness gradually improved. On the fourteenth day, propranolol was prescribed with a dose of 10 mg every 8 hours. Then, the right adrenalectomy was performed without any surgical complications, and the postoperative histopathologic report was in agreement with a diagnosis of pheochromocytoma. No complications were reported in the postoperative period. Predischarge TTE showed LVEF of 40%, normal LV size, mild mitral regurgitation, mild tricuspid regurgitation, and no pericardial effusion. She was followed in an outpatient setting regularly. Two weeks after adrenalectomy, the patient had no evidence of the disease.

TABLE 1: Laboratory test results.

Test	Day 1	Day 10	Normal values
FBS	104	109	Up to 100 mg/dl
BUN	26	88	7–20 mg/dl
Cr	1.3	1.6	0.8–1.3 mg/dl
Na	138	152	135–145 mEq/L
K	3.7	3.3	3.5–5 mEq/L
Ca	8.4	7.8	8.5–10.5 mg/dl
Ph	4.6	3.9	3.4–4.5 mg/dl
Mg	2.2	1.7	1.7–2.2 mg/dl
Troponin	17.9	54	Up to 0.4 ng/ml
D-Dimer	5794	—	Up to 500 ng/ml
TSH	1.4	—	0.35–0.5 mIU/L
WBC	30.9	29.0	$4.5–11 \times 10^9$/L
Neut	82.4%	91%	55–70%
Lymph	7.6%	4%	20–40%
HB	10.1	9.8	12–15 g/dl
aPTT	43	35	30–40 msec
INR	1.2	1.5	Up to 1.1
AST	401	390	5–40 IU/L
ALT	535	912	7–56 IU/L
ALP	306	342	20–140 IU/L
ESR	1	2	Up to 29 mm/hr
CRP	13	47	Up to 10 mg/L
Alb	3.3	3.2	3.3–5.4 g/dl

BUN: blood urea nitrogen; Cr: creatinine; Na: sodium; K: potassium; Ca: calcium; Ph: phosphorus; Mg: magnesium; TSH: thyroid-stimulating hormone; WBC: white blood cell; Neut: neutrophil; Lymph; lymphocyte; HB: hemoglobin; aPTT: activated partial thromboplastin time; INR: international normalized ratio; AST: aspartate aminotransferase; ALT: alanine aminotransferase; ALP: alkaline phosphatase; ESR: erythrocyte sedimentation rate; CRP: C-reactive protein; Alb: albumin.

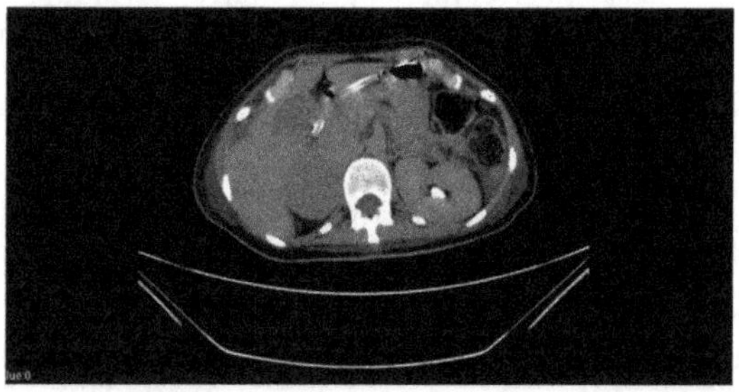

FIGURE 1: Abdominal CT scan of the patient shows heterogeneous right adrenal mass.

Table 2: CSF analysis results.

Test	Patient's values	Normal values
CSF glucose	68	>50% serum
Serum glucose	118	Up to 200 mg/dl(random sampling)
Protein	0.48	0.15–0.45 g/L
WBC	0	<5 (mm^3)
RBC	3	0 (mm^3)
Viral PCR (HSV 1 and 2, VZV, and Enterovirus)	Negative	Negative

CSF: cerebrospinal fluid; WBC: white blood cell; RBC: red blood cell; HSV: herpes simplex virus; VZV: varicella-zoster virus.

Laboratory values were notable for a 24-hour urine metanephrine of 107 μg/day (normal <315 μg/day), normetanephrine of 210 μg/day (normal <670 μg/day), adrenaline of 15 μg/day (normal < 20 μg/day), noradrenaline of 34 μg/day (normal < 90 μg/day), and vanillylmandelic acid of 7.1 mg/day (normal < 13.6 mg/day). Today, 18 months after hospital discharge, her general condition is good, and the catecholamine urine test results are negative for pheochromocytoma. The latest echocardiography demonstrates the LVEF to be 50%, and other echocardiographic measurements are within the normal values.

3. Discussion

This case report presented a young female with complicated pheochromocytoma having unusual presentations of hypotension, cardiac arrest, cardiomyopathy, and fever. Also, she was complicated with GBS in the course of hospitalization.

Pheochromocytoma exhibits variable characteristics with diverse presentations. Although it is rare, it is a fatal emergency, and diagnosis can be extremely challenging. Since our case presented predominantly with cardiac problems, it is mandatory to discuss cardiovascular complications of pheochromocytoma in detail. Pheochromocytoma usually manifests as severe hypertension, circulatory shock, arrhythmias, myocardial injury, and cardiomyopathy—the excessive catecholamine exposure of myocardium results in toxic effects like myocardial necrosis and cardiomyopathy [11]. The prevalence of cardiomyopathy in pheochromocytoma has been reported to be about 11% [12]. Of course, we must also consider cases of pheochromocytoma that have not been diagnosed and reported. In these patients, cardiomyopathy may be presented as a global or focal abnormality. Interestingly, a complete reversal of pheochromocytoma cardiomyopathy has been reported in a short period of as much as eight days, following the tumor's removal [13].

Approximately 50% of patients with pheochromocytoma have a hypertensive crisis; however, 5–15% are normotensive, and in rare instances, these patients have hypotension. Bergland et al. reported in a review of 539 cases of pheochromocytoma that 2% of the cases presented with hypotension and shock [14]. Possible hypotension mechanisms in pheochromocytoma are hypovolemia, desensitization of blood vessels to catecholamine, reduced vascular resistance due to high epinephrine release from the tumor, myocardial contractile dysfunction, and hemorrhagic necrosis of the tumor [14].

Fever is also an uncommon presentation in these patients. In a case series of 25 patients, 12% presented with fever [15]. The excessive release of epinephrine has been postulated as a cause of fever by combining hypermetabolism and cutaneous vasoconstriction [16]. Of course, infectious causes and inflammatory disease should always be considered in all patients with febrile pericarditis and it should be evaluated first.

The further exciting twist in our case is the co-occurrence of GBS and pheochromocytoma. Although this is not impossible, it rarely happens. The average annual incidence of GBS was 1 per 100 000 patient-years, while the incidence of pheochromocytoma are approximately 0.8 per 100 000 patient-years [5, 17]. Abdel-Salam et al. reported the case of GBS with subsequent pheochromocytoma [17].

Indeed, Ahmad et al. reported that urine and plasma catecholamine levels were elevated in patients with GBS who had autonomic instability [18]. However, in our case, the clinical manifestations of GBS occurred after the diagnosis of pheochromocytoma, and cardiac complications began to improve after adrenalectomy. Although the exact cause of GBS remains to be clearly understood, previous studies indicated an association between immunological stressors (such as viral infection and vaccination) and GBS. Our case denied any flu-like symptoms or vaccination in the preceding two weeks. Therefore, the question arises that can hypersecretion of catecholamine and pro-inflammatory states in pheochromocytoma provoke GBS?

In our case, considering the young age, female sex, fever and dyspnea as first manifestations, normal ECG except for sinus tachycardia, lack of traditional cardiovascular risk factors, and negative drug history for cocaine, coronary heart disease was less suspected.

Fortunately, the patient was diagnosed and treated at a referral center despite having a large tumor and catastrophic symptoms and signs. Finally, we emphasize that the clinical manifestations of pheochromocytoma depend on the various hormone secretion, and the diversity of this matter should be considered in any clinical scenario. However, whether there is a direct link between GBS and pheochromocytoma is a mystery that needs to be answered with more detailed studies.

References

[1] J. W. Lenders, G. Eisenhofer, M. Mannelli, and K. Pacak, "Phaeochromocytoma," *The Lancet*, vol. 366, no. 9486, pp. 665–675, 2005.

[2] R. Hodin, C. Lubitz, R. Phitayakorn, and A. Stephen, "Diagnosis and management of pheochromocytoma," *Current Problems in Surgery*, vol. 51, no. 4, pp. 151–187, 2014.

[3] J. T. Adler, G. Y. Meyer-Rochow, H. Chen et al., "Pheochromocytoma: current approaches and future directions," *The Oncologist*, vol. 13, no. 7, pp. 779–793, 2008.
[4] P. A. Marcovitz, P. Czako, S. Rosenblatt, and S. S. Billecke, "Pheochromocytoma presenting with Takotsubo syndrome," *Journal of Interventional Cardiology*, vol. 23, no. 5, pp. 437–442, 2010.
[5] M. Heidarpour, M. A. Haghighatpanah, H. Rezvanian et al., "Polyserositis: an extremely rare life-threatening manifestation of pheochromocytoma," *Case Reports in Endocrinology*, vol. 2020, Article ID 8814699, 3 pages, 2020.
[6] R. Zhang, D. Gupta, and S. G. Albert, "Pheochromocytoma as a reversible cause of cardiomyopathy: analysis and review of the literature," *International Journal of Cardiology*, vol. 249, pp. 319–323, 2017.
[7] J. S. Finkelstein and B. H. Melek, "Guillain-barré syndrome as a cause of reversible cardiomyopathy," *Texas Heart Institute Journal*, vol. 33, pp. 57–59, 2006.
[8] K. Iga, Y. Himura, C. Izumi et al., "Reversible left ventricular dysfunction associated with guillain-barre syndrome. An expression of catecholamine cardiotoxicity?" *Japanese Circulation Journal*, vol. 59, no. 4, pp. 236–240, 1995.
[9] A. Hiraga, K. Nagumo, K. Suzuki, Y. Sakakibara, and S. Kojima, "A patient with Guillain-Barre syndrome and recurrent episodes of ST elevation and left ventricular hypokinesis in the anterior wall [in Japanese]," *No To Shinkei*, vol. 55, pp. 517–520, 2003.
[10] M. Boon, P. J. Dennesen, and R. F. Veldkamp, "A rare stress cardiomyopathy in a patient with Guillain-Barré syndrome," *The Netherlands Journal of Medicine*, vol. 74, no. 2, pp. 86–88, 2016.
[11] P. Sethi and C. D. Peiris, "A review of catecholamine associated cardiomyopathies and channelopathies," *Cureus*, vol. 12, no. 2, p. e6957, 2020.
[12] A. Giavarini, A. Chedid, G. Bobrie, P.-F. Plouin, A. Hagège, and L. Amar, "Acute catecholamine cardiomyopathy in patients with phaeochromocytoma or functional paraganglioma," *Heart*, vol. 99, no. 19, pp. 1438–1444, 2013.
[13] M. Salathe, P. Weiss, and R. Ritz, "Rapid reversal of heart failure in a patient with phaeochromocytoma and catecholamine-induced cardiomyopathy who was treated with captopril," *Heart*, vol. 68, no. 11, pp. 527-528, 1992.
[14] B. E. Bergland, "Pheochromocytoma presenting as shock," *The American Journal of Emergency Medicine*, vol. 7, no. 1, pp. 44–48, 1989.
[15] W.-B. Liao, C.-F. Liu, C.-W. Chiang, C.-T. Kung, and C.-W. Lee, "Cardiovascular manifestations of pheochromocytoma," *The American Journal of Emergency Medicine*, vol. 18, no. 5, pp. 622–625, 2000.
[16] S. Fukumoto, T. Matsumoto, S.-I. Harada, J. Fujisaki, M. Kawano, and E. Ogata, "Pheochromocytoma with pyrexia and marked inflammatory signs: a paraneoplastic syndrome with possible relation to interleukin-6 production*," *The Journal of Clinical Endocrinology & Metabolism*, vol. 73, no. 4, pp. 877–881, 1991.
[17] F. Abdel-Salam, A. P. Basu, S. Johnson, and A. M. Devlin, "Suspected pheochromocytoma in a patient with guillain-barré syndrome," *Pediatrics*, vol. 191, no. 3, pp. 955–958, 2013.
[18] J. Ahmad, A. Kham, and M. Siddiqui, "Estimation of plasma and urinary catecholamines in Guillain-Barre syndrome," *Japanese Journal of Medicine*, vol. 24, no. 1, pp. 24–29, 1985.

24

Pheochromocytoma Presenting as Testicular Pain: An Unusual Case Report

Jinal K. Patel, Varun Reddy, Gauthier Stepman, Debra Angelo, and Johnathan Frunzi

Department of Internal Medicine, HCA Healthcare/USF Morsani College of Medicine GME: Medical Center of Trinity, Trinity, FL, USA

Correspondence should be addressed to Jinal K. Patel; jinal.patel@hcahealthcare.com

Academic Editor: Osamu Isozaki

Pheochromocytoma (PCC) is a rare catecholamine-secreting tumor that arises from chromaffin cells of the adrenal medulla which are derived from the neural crest. This report illustrates a 51-year-old Caucasian male with a history of hypertension diagnosed two years ago who presented to the hospital due to acute onset of right testicular pain of 3-day duration. Laboratory results and imaging revealed a presumptive diagnosis of PCC. The patient had undergone robot-assisted laparoscopic right adrenalectomy 14 days after being diagnosed with PCC due to perioperative management with phenoxybenzamine. The final pathology report revealed a PCC. At follow-up two weeks after discharge, the patient reported complete resolution of his testicular pain.

1. Introduction

Pheochromocytoma (PCC) is a rare catecholamine-secreting tumor that arises from chromaffin cells of the adrenal medulla [1–4]. Histologically, chromaffin cells are derived from the neural crest during development [1–4]. In 2017, the World Health Organization (WHO) classified PCC as an adrenal tumor and extraadrenal tumor as paraganglioma; since both types of tumor cannot be differentiated on histological findings [1–4]. The incidence of PCC and paraganglioma ranges between 2 and 8 per million, whereas the incidence of PCC is approximately 500–1600 cases per year [5]. PCC may occur at any age; however, it is more commonly seen in the 3rd to 5th decade of life [3]. Typically, patients present with a triad of severe headache, sweating, and palpitations which occur in waves as a result of excess hormone release [1–3]. Furthermore, half of the patients can have paroxysmal hypertension. Less common symptoms include flushing, tremor, chest pain, weight loss, constipation, diarrhea, and warmth or heat intolerance [2]. The diagnosis of PCC is a combination of urine and serum analysis showing excess catecholamines and localization of the tumor by computerized tomography (CT) and magnetic resonance imaging (MRI) [1–4, 6]. Here, we present a case of a 51-year-old Caucasian male with PCC presenting as testicular pain.

2. Case Presentation

A 51-year-old Caucasian male with a past medical history of hypertension (diagnosed two years ago, treated with lisinopril 10 mg daily), nephrolithiasis, presented to the hospital with a 3-day complaint of right testicular pain. The pain radiated to the right flank, was intermittent, sharp, 5/10 in severity, aggravated with movement, and alleviated with rest. The pain in the scrotum had not improved, which caused him to present to the emergency department. He denied having hypertensive episodes, headaches, sweating, flushing, and palpitations.

An initial evaluation in the emergency department revealed the following vitals: temperature of 98.6 F, heart rate of 81 beats per minute, blood pressure (BP) of 137/96 mmHg, and oxygen saturation of 97% on room air. Initial laboratory results revealed mild leukocytosis with a white blood cell (WBC) count of 12,900 cells/mL. Due to the patient having acute scrotal pain and elevated WBC count, testicular etiologies such as testicular torsion, epididymitis, varicocele, hydrocele, or chronic testicular pain were ruled out with a thorough physical examination and testicular ultrasound (US). A CT of the abdomen and pelvis without contrast revealed a large right suprarenal mass. A follow-up CT abdomen with adrenal protocol revealed a 5.1 cm enhancing right adrenal mass, which was further detailed with an MRI with contrast (Figure 1). With findings of an adrenal gland mass on imaging, urine and serum analyses (Tables 1 and 2) were obtained, which revealed elevated catecholamines consistent with possible PCC. The patient was discharged home as he required perioperative blood pressure management with phenoxybenzamine. The patient was brought back to the hospital 14 days later for transperitoneal robot-assisted laparoscopic right adrenalectomy due to having multiple back surgeries. He was transferred to the intensive care unit (ICU) postoperatively for close monitoring of hemodynamics. The final pathology report revealed a PCC, 6.2 cm in size, with no evidence of necrosis, capsular invasion, or extension into periadrenal adipose tissue. The patient was discharged home on postoperative day three and to follow-up with hematology and oncology for surveillance and possible adjuvant chemotherapy. At follow-up two weeks after discharge, the patient reported complete resolution of his testicular pain.

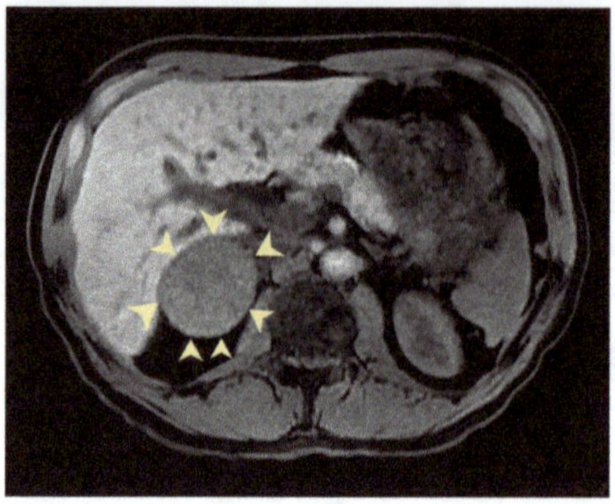

Figure 1: T2-Weighted MRI of the abdomen: slight increased T2 signal and heterogeneous enhancement of the right adrenal gland (arrows).

Table 1: Urine analysis.

Urine analysis	Results	Reference range
Epinephrine	24 ug/L	Undefined
Epinephrine in 24 hours	58	0–20 ug/24 hr
Norepinephrine	128 ug/L	Undefined
Norepinephrine in 24 hours	307	0–135 ug/24 hr
Metanephrine	562 ug/L	Undefined
Metanephrine in 24 hours	1345	45–290 ug/24 hr
Normetanephrine	4520 ug/L	Undefined
Normetanephrine in 24 hours	10848	82–500 ug/24 hr
Dopamine	112 ug/L	Undefined
Dopamine in 24 hours	269	0–510 ug/24 hr

Table 2: Serum analysis.

Serum analysis	Results	Reference range
Carcinoembryonic antigen	2.1	0.0–0.5 ng/mL
Renin activity	3.010	0.167–5.380 ng/mL/hr
Aldosterone	1.1	0.0–30.0 ng/dL
DHEA sulfate	151.0	80.0–560.0 ng/dL
AM cortisol	2.29	AM: 4.30–22.40 mcg/dL
PM: 3.09–16.66 mcg/dL		
ACTH	8.9	7.2–63.3 pg/mL
Plasma metanephrine	510	0–62 pg/mL
Plasma normetanephrine	5648	0–145 pg/mL

DHEA: dihydroepiandrosterone, ACTH: adrenocorticotropic hormone.

3. Discussion

Testicular pain with acute onset warrants emergent evaluation with a thorough history and physical examination as well as urinalysis and imaging [7, 8]. For example, testicular torsion is a medical emergency, which presents as a high-riding testicle, which is confirmed with a scrotal US and can result in loss of testes if there is a delay of care [7–9]. In our patient, we were able to rule out potential medical emergencies with examination, urinalysis, and imaging as stated above. While less common, extrascrotal etiologies can cause testicular pain due to common nerve root pathways (T10-T12, L1-L2, and S2-S4) [10]. Thus, pathologies such as ureteral calculi, back pain, aortic aneurysm, intervertebral disc prolapse, hernias, and other intrabdominal pathologies that share common nerve pathways may present as acute testicular pain [10], which was the case of our patient.

Our case is unique, as there have not been reported cases previously of PCC presenting as testicular pain. On the other hand, Cheungpasitporn et al. reported a case of adrenocortical carcinoma that presented as varicocele and renal vein thrombosis [11].

The majority of PCC are initially discovered as incidentalomas, while others are suspected in patients presenting with the typical symptoms as mentioned in the introduction or secondary cause of hypertension [12]. Our patient likely did not have the typical presentation of PCC as his hypertension was treated with lisinopril for the past 2 years, which likely masked his symptoms of catecholamine excess. In our case, the patient did not have evidence of acute testicular etiology as stated above, which warranted further investigation with a CT of the abdomen and pelvis as the patient had a history of renal calculi. There was no evidence of nephrolithiasis; however, there was an incidental finding of an adrenal mass. When an adrenal mass is found incidentally, the next step in management is to determine if it is malignant or functioning, which can be determined with laboratory tests and imaging studies [1–4]. PCC has increased attenuation on unenhanced CT scan revealing greater than 20 Hounsfield units (HU), with a delay in contrast medium washout [13, 14]. Our patient's CT scan measured 64 HU prior to contrast administration, which enhanced heterogeneously following contrast injection with delay in contrast medium washout. Also, PCC shows high signal intensity on T2-weighted MRI [13, 14]. Our patient's MRI demonstrated a slightly increased T2 signal and heterogeneous enhancement. Due to the imaging findings, PCC was higher on the differential and requires further investigation with biochemical assay [1–6, 15]. A 24-hour urinary metanephrine and plasma metanephrines were positive for excess catecholamines (Tables 1 and 2), further supporting the presumptive diagnosis of PCC. We later obtained a CT of the chest and MRI of the brain for staging, which was negative for metastatic disease. Once the diagnosis of PCC is confirmed, the next step in management is surgical resection [2, 16]. Our patient had undergone robot-assisted laparoscopic right adrenalectomy.

While surgical resection of the tumor is usually definitive, it is associated with high mortality risk if not managed medically first [15]. Physical manipulation of the adrenal gland during surgery can cause a sudden release of catecholamines and cause intraoperative hypertensive emergency [15–17]. Thus, in the perioperative period, it is important to start patients on adrenergic blocking agents 10–14 days prior to surgery to decrease intraoperative hypertensive crisis [15–17]. Initial treatment consists of alpha-blockade with medications like phenoxybenzamine [17]. Our patient in the perioperative period was treated with phenoxybenzamine beginning 14 days prior to surgery. Alpha-blockage prevents peripheral vascular constriction and subsequently causes reflexive tachycardia. Beta-blockers are initially avoided, as blocking this initial reflex can cause dangerous hypertension due to unopposed alpha blockade. Once an adequate alpha-blockade has been achieved, which can be indicated by postural hypotension, a beta-blocker can be added. Our patient did report postural hypotension but was not treated with a beta-blocker. On the other hand, increased salt and fluid intake can be recommended to expand the intravascular volume and maintain BP preoperatively, which was done in our patient. After appropriate perioperative management is achieved, the final step in management is adrenalectomy. A patient may have the option of undergoing an open approach, laparoscopic or robotic-assisted laparoscopy adrenalectomy [16, 18, 19]. Comparing the different surgical approaches, robotic-assisted approach has been shown to decrease blood loss and have shorter hospital course when compared to open and laparoscopic approach [19]. In robotic-assisted adrenalectomy, patients may undergo transperitoneal or retroperitoneal laparoscopic adrenalectomy [16, 18]. Ultimately, our patient had undergone transperitoneal robot-assisted laparoscopic right adrenalectomy as he had multiple previous back surgeries. After surgical removal of the adrenal gland, patients should be monitored closely in the ICU due to potential complications of abrupt decline in catecholamine levels after tumor resection [20]. Finally, patients should be followed up with an MRI for recurrence for at least 10 years even after complete resection [6].

4. Conclusion

Physicians should be aware that testicular tenderness needs further evaluation if a thorough history and physical exam do not reveal a cause. Furthermore, the combination of testicular pain and hypertension should raise suspicion for PCC, even in the absence of the typical symptoms for PCC.

Consent

The patient provided informed consent.

Acknowledgments

This research was supported in part by the HCA Healthcare and/or an HCA Healthcare affiliated entity.

References

[1] H. P. H. Neumann, W. F. Young, and C. Eng, "Pheochromocytoma and paraganglioma," *New England Journal of Medicine*, vol. 381, no. 6, pp. 552–565, 2019.

[2] N. Reisch, M. Peczkowska, A. Januszewicz, and H. P. Neumann, "Pheochromocytoma: presentation, diagnosis and treatment," *Journal of Hypertension*, vol. 24, no. 12, pp. 2331–2339, 2006.

[3] F.-A. Farrugia and A. charalampopoulos, "Pheochromocytoma," *Endocrine Regulations*, vol. 53, no. 3, pp. 191–212, 2019.

[4] E. Sbardella and A. B. Grossman, "Pheochromocytoma: an approach to diagnosis," *Best Practice & Research Clinical Endocrinology & Metabolism*, vol. 34, no. 2, p. 101346, 2020.

[5] N. Aygun, "Pheochromocytoma and paraganglioma: from epidemiology to clinical findings," *SiSli Etfal Hastanesi Tip Bulteni/The Medical Bulletin of Sisli Hospital*, vol. 54, 2020.

[6] S. Nölting, M. Ullrich, J. Pietzsch et al., "Current management of pheochromocytoma/paraganglioma: a guide for the practicing clinician in the era of precision medicine," *Cancers*, vol. 11, no. 10, pp. 1505–1527, 2019.

[7] C. G. Gordhan and H. Sadeghi-Nejad, "Scrotal pain: evaluation and management," *Korean Journal of Urology*, vol. 56, no. 1, pp. 3–11, 2015.

[8] S. Wright and B. Hoffmann, "Emergency ultrasound of acute scrotal pain," *European Journal of Emergency Medicine*, vol. 22, no. 1, pp. 2–9, 2015.

[9] V. J. Sharp, K. Kieran, and A. M. Arlen, "Testicular torsion: diagnosis, evaluation, and management," *American Family Physician*, vol. 88, no. 12, pp. 835–840, 2013.

[10] A. P. Patel, "Anatomy and physiology of chronic scrotal pain," *Translational Andrology and Urology*, vol. 6, no. S1, p. S51, 2017.

[11] W. Cheungpasitporn, J. M. Horne, and C. B. Howarth, "Adrenocortical carcinoma presenting as varicocele and renal vein thrombosis: a case report," *Journal of Medical Case Reports*, vol. 5, no. 1, pp. 1–5, 2011.

[12] P. K. Whelton, R. M. Carey, W. S. Aronow et al., "Detection, evaluation, and management of high blood pressure in adults a report of the american college of cardiology/American heart association task force on clinical Pratice guidelines," *Hypertension*, vol. 71, 2017.

[13] K. Leung, M. Stamm, A. Raja, and G. Low, "Pheochromocytoma: the range of appearances on ultrasound, CT, MRI, and functional imaging," *American Journal of Roentgenology*, vol. 200, no. 2, pp. 370–378, 2013.

[14] F. Wang, J. Liu, R. Zhang et al., "CT and MRI of adrenal gland pathologies," *Quantitative Imaging in Medicine and Surgery*, vol. 8, no. 8, p. 853, 2018.

[15] F. M. Brouwers, J. W. M. Lenders, G. Eisenhofer, and K. Pacak, "Pheochromocytoma as an endocrine emergency," *Reviews in Endocrine and Metabolic Disorders*, vol. 4, no. 2, pp. 121–128, 2003.

[16] D. Patel, "Surgical approach to patients with pheochromocytoma," *Gland Surgery*, vol. 9, no. 1, pp. 32–42, 2020.

[17] J. Naranjo, S. Dodd, and Y. N. Martin, "Perioperative management of pheochromocytoma," *Journal of Cardiothoracic and Vascular Anesthesia*, vol. 31, no. 4, pp. 1427–1439, 2017.

[18] A. Arezzo, A. Bullano, G. Cochetti et al., "Transperitoneal versus retroperitoneal laparoscopic adrenalectomy for adrenal tumours in adults," *Cochrane Database of Systematic Reviews*, vol. 12, no. 12, p. CD011668, 2018.

[19] J. Jayakumaran, S. D. Patel, B. K. Gangrade, D. M. Narasimhulu, S. R. Pandian, and C. Silva, "Robotic-assisted laparoscopy in reproductive surgery: a contemporary review," *Journal of Robotic Surgery*, vol. 11, no. 2, pp. 97–109, 2017.

[20] D. Mamilla, K. Araque, A. Brofferio et al., "Postoperative management in patients with pheochromocytoma and paraganglioma," *Cancers (Basel)*, vol. 11, 2019.

25

Biochemical and Clinical Features of Insulinoma in a Patient with Turner Syndrome

Darius A. Schneider,[1] M. Zare,[1] F. Behnia,[1] M. Matesan,[1] and T. Tylee[1,2]

[1]*University of Washington, Department of Medicine, Seattle, WA, USA*
[2]*Department of Radiology, Harborview Medical Center, Seattle, WA, USA*

Correspondence should be addressed to Darius A. Schneider; schndar@gmail.com

Academic Editor: Lucy Mastrandrea

Turner syndrome (TS), i.e., mosaic or nonmosaic states with only one normal X chromosome in females, is characterized by a wide spectrum of somatic, hormonal, and metabolic features. Here we report an unusual case of recurrent hypoglycemia in a 53-year-old woman with TS. Biochemical work-up following a 72h fast revealed detectable, inappropriate for low glucose insulin levels and elevated proinsulin and beta-hydroxybutyrate (BOHB) levels. MR and multiphase CT showed a solid 2.5 cm pancreatic tail mass with absent uptake in the ^{111}In-pentetreotide (Octreoscan) scan. Subsequent hepatic vein blood sampling after intra-arterial calcium stimulation showed sharp increase in insulin and modest increase in proinsulin levels. The patient underwent excision of the mass with resolution of symptoms. Histopathologic examination confirmed the neuroendocrine etiology of the tumor. This is, to our knowledge, the third report of TS and concomitant insulinoma. Impaired counterregulatory response to hypoglycemia in patients with TS may result in symptomatic hypoglycemia with only mild insulin elevation and elevated proinsulin in setting of hypoglycemia may be the only indication of insulinoma in these patients. BOHB levels should not be used for ruling out EHH in patients with TS.

1. Introduction

TS is a chromosomal abnormality, affecting one in 2,000 female live-births [1]. X-chromosome monosomy (45XO karyotype) accounts for >55% of Turner syndrome cases, while mosaicism, mainly 45XO/46XX or 45XO/47XXX, has been detected in the remaining cases.

Endocrinopathies associated with TS include growth hormone resistance, insulin resistance, and diabetes [1].

Insulinomas are neuroendocrine tumors arising from the pancreatic beta-cells and most common cause of endogenous hyperinsulinemic hypoglycemia (EHH) [2]. Their incidence is 2-4 cases per million individuals per year [2]. Prominent features are fasting hypoglycemia with elevated serum insulin and proinsulin levels. Recently, two cases of histologically confirmed insulinoma were described in women with TS [3, 4]. Here we present a third case of a pancreatic tail insulinoma in a patient with TS with interesting clinical/biochemical features: severe, symptomatic hypoglycemia despite rather low, yet inappropriately detectable insulin levels following 72h fast; sharp increase of insulin levels upon arterial calcium stimulation; and elevated BOHB levels.

2. Case Report

A 53-year-old woman with small stature and dysmorphic features consistent with TS, not previously diagnosed with diabetes, presented to the endocrinology clinic for evaluation of episodes of hypoglycemia <20mg/dl with transient loss of consciousness. She was admitted to the inpatient service and underwent a controlled 72h fast. After 64h, she developed hypoglycemia to the low 30s mg/dl with mild neuroglycopenic symptoms (emotional outbursts). Biochemical workup showed unsuppressed insulin levels (1.2mIU/L), markedly elevated proinsulin (30 pmol/L), and BOHB levels (6500μmol/L).

MR and multiphase CT (Figure 1) showed a solid, hyper-enhancing 2.5cm pancreatic tail mass with slow washout.

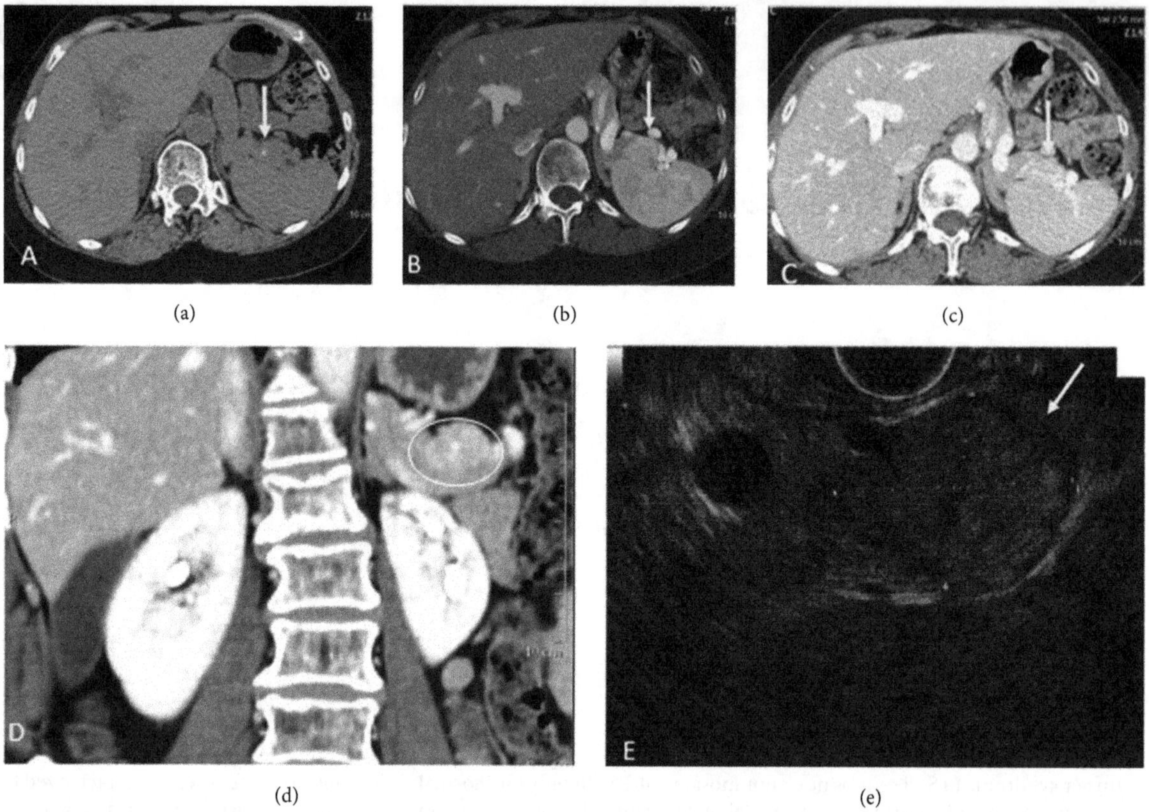

FIGURE 1: Axial noncontrast CT (a) shows a small calcification at the tail of the pancreas. Axial arterial phase CT (b) shows a 2.5 cm hyperenhancing pancreatic mass which on venous phase ((c) and (d)) shows slightly more heterogeneity compared to the spleen. Endoscopic ultrasound (e) showed heterogeneous hypoechoic 1.7 x 2.5 cm pancreatic tail mass with calcifications.

^{111}In-pentetreotide (Octreoscan) study (Figure 2) demonstrated absence of radiotracer uptake ruling out a splenule. CT guided fine needle biopsy of the mass confirmed neuroendocrine etiology. Since Octreoscan sensitivity is not high, hepatic vein blood sampling after intra-arterial calcium stimulation was further performed and showed robust increase of insulin (9.4 to 17.8mIU/L) and proinsulin (7pmol/L to 20pmol/L) and high c-peptide levels at the distal splenic artery, consistent with insulinoma of the tail of the pancreas.

Surgical excision of the mass resulted in complete resolution of symptoms up to 3 years postop. Histologic examination confirmed a well differentiated neuroendocrine tumor with immunostainings positive for chromogranin and synaptophysin and a KI index of <2%.

3. Discussion

Insulinomas are rare neuroendocrine tumors with estimated incidence of 1 case per 250,000 patient-years [2]. They are more common in women and usually occur in the fifth or sixth decade [2]. The tumor should be suspected in a patient presenting with spontaneous fasting hypoglycemia and represent the most prevalent cause of EHH [2].

Although a slightly increased incidence of solid tumors has been described in patients with TS, insulinoma prevalence is not generally thought to be increased in women with TS [5]. Thus far, there were two cases reported of insulinoma in a patient with 45X TS and in a patient with mosaic 45XO/47XXX TS [3, 4].

Here, we present a case of an insulinoma in a 53-year-old woman with TS and reoccurring episodes of severe, life-threatening hypoglycemia. A 72h fast test was positive, with hypoglycemia below 30mg/dl and mild neuroglycopenic symptoms. Biochemical analysis revealed low yet inappropriately detectable insulin and c-peptide levels, and high proinsulin levels. Beta-hydroxybutyrate (BHOB) levels were markedly elevated. Arterial calcium stimulation test confirmed both hyperinsulinemia and hyperproinsulinemia in the distal splenic artery, localizing the mass in the pancreatic tail, consistent with imaging studies. Surgical removal of the pancreatic mass led to complete and consistent resolution of symptoms.

Some aspects of this case were somewhat unusual and, hence, worth discussing: (i) hypoglycemia occurred relatively late during the 72h fast in our patient (normally after <48h of fasting for insulinomas [2]). This may be caused by underlying insulin resistance and/or increased hepatic glucose output in patients with TS and has not been described before; (ii) despite severe fasting hypoglycaemia with neuroglycopenic symptoms and clearly positive 72h fast test, measured insulin levels were only modest compared to previously described insulinoma cases [6], albeit inappropriately

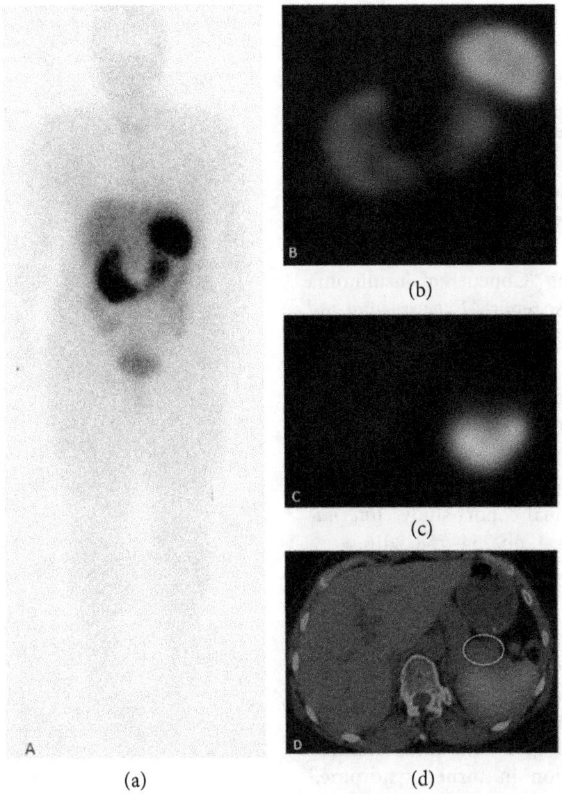

Figure 2: 24-hour ^{111}In-pentetreotide scan. Anterior whole body planar image (a), MIP reconstruction of SPECT acquisition (b), axial SPECT image (c), and fused axial SPECT/CT image (d) show normal biodistribution of the radiotracer and no uptake in the pancreatic tail mass, ruling out a splenule.

elevated relative to low glucose. This may be the result of an impaired hormonal (epinephrine, growth hormone, and glucagon) counterregulatory response to hypoglycemia in people with TS. While this exact mechanism has not been previously described in TS, it has been shown that catecholamine release [7] is diminished in adults with TS. Hence, low yet detectable insulin levels in TS patients with documented hypoglycemia should prompt evaluation for insulinoma, as impaired counterregulatory hormones may result in symptomatic hypoglycemia with only mild insulin elevation.

While insulin levels were only modestly increased, proinsulin levels in the 72h fast test were robustly elevated, consistent with previous literature [6]. Both insulin and proinsulin levels increased sharply upon arterial calcium stimulation. The discrepancy between insulin and proinsulin levels may be explained by insulin resistance and/or impaired beta-cellular processing of proinsulin to insulin in this patient with TS. Elevated proinsulin in the setting of hypoglycemia may be the only indication of insulinoma for TS patients.

Furthermore, we saw markedly elevated BOHB levels. This may seem surprising, since elevated BOHB levels are thought to rule out EHH with 100% sensitivity and specificity [8]; however, as in this case and consistent with previously described cases [9] their diagnostic specificity is much lower when plasma glucose levels drop below 45mg/dl. High BOHB levels may be explained by the combination of modest elevation in insulin levels and increased insulin resistance specific for TS, facilitating the escape of ketogenesis from the inhibitory effects of insulin, as previously described in setting of posthypoglycemia insulin resistance [10]. Hence, BOHB levels should not be used for ruling out EHH in patients with TS.

4. Conclusion

The development of insulinoma in patients with Turner syndrome has to be considered if there is clinical suspicion for hyperinsulinemic hypoglycemia. Due to impairments of insulin sensitivity and glycemic counterregulation inherent to patients with TS, symptomatic hypoglycemia may result with only mild insulin elevation and beta-hydroxybutyrate (BOHB) levels may be elevated and should not be used for ruling out EHH. Elevated proinsulin in the setting of hypoglycemia may be the only indication of insulinoma.

This is, thus far, the third case of TS presenting with insulinoma; considering the rarity of both TS and insulinoma, a potential underlying association may be worth exploring.

Disclosure

M. Matesan and T. Tylee shared senior authorship.

References

[1] M. D. C. Donaldson, E. J. Gault, K. W. Tan, and D. B. Dunger, "Optimising management in Turner syndrome: From infancy to adult transfer," *Archives of Disease in Childhood*, vol. 91, no. 6, pp. 513–520, 2006.

[2] F. J. Service, "Diagnostic approach to adults with hypoglycemic disorders," *Endocrinology and Metabolism Clinics of North America*, vol. 28, no. 3, pp. 519–532, 1999.

[3] S. Wang, L. Yang, J. Li, and Y. Mu, "Concurrent insulinoma with mosaic Turner syndrome: A case report," *Experimental and Therapeutic Medicine*, vol. 9, no. 3, pp. 801–804, 2015.

[4] M. Sirinart Sirinvaravong, M. D. Thirajit Boonsaen, and M. D. Kanokporn Sanpawithayakul, "Insulinoma in Unrecognized Turner Syndrome," in *Endo 2016*, Boston, Mass, USA, 2016.

[5] J. Ji, B. Zöller, J. Sundquist, and K. Sundquist, "Risk of solid tumors and hematological malignancy in persons with Turner and Klinefelter syndromes: A national cohort study," *International Journal of Cancer*, vol. 139, no. 4, pp. 754–758, 2016.

[6] J.-M. Guettier, A. Lungu, A. Goodling, C. Cochran, and P. Gorden, "The role of proinsulin and insulin in the diagnosis of insulinoma: A critical evaluation of the endocrine society clinical practice guideline," *The Journal of Clinical Endocrinology & Metabolism*, vol. 98, no. 12, pp. 4752–4758, 2013.

[7] N. Zuckerman-Levin, O. Zinder, A. Greenberg, M. Levin, G. Jacob, and Z. Hochberg, "Physiological and catecholamine response to sympathetic stimulation in turner syndrome," *Clinical Endocrinology*, vol. 64, no. 4, pp. 410–415, 2006.

[8] K. A. Placzkowski, A. Vella, G. B. Thompson et al., "Secular trends in the presentation and management of functioning insulinoma at the mayo clinic, 1987–2007," *The Journal of Clinical Endocrinology & Metabolism*, vol. 94, no. 4, pp. 1069–1073, 2009.

[9] A. Buffet, D. Vezzosi, J. C. Maiza, S. Grunenwald, A. Bennet, and P. Caron, "Increased plasma β-hydroxybutyrate levels during the fasting test in patients with endogenous hyperinsulinaemic hypoglycaemia," *European Journal of Endocrinology*, vol. 169, no. 1, pp. 91–97, 2013.

[10] P. Lucidi, P. Rossetti, F. Porcellati et al., "Mechanisms of insulin resistance after insulin-induced hypoglycemia in humans: the role of lipolysis," *Diabetes*, vol. 59, no. 6, pp. 1349–1357, 2010.

Current Approach of Functioning Head and Neck Paragangliomas: Case Report of a Young Patient with Multiple Asynchronous Tumors

Alejandro Terrones-Lozano,[1] Alan Hernández-Hernández,[2] Edgar Nathal Vera,[2] Gerardo Yoshiaki Guinto-Nishimura,[2] Jorge Luis Balderrama-Bañares,[3] Claudia Ramírez-Rentería,[4] Judith de la Serna-Soto,[5] Alfredo Adolfo Reza-Albarran,[6] and Lesly Portocarrero-Ortiz[1]

[1]*Instituto Nacional de Neurología y Neurocirugía Manuel Velasco Suárez (INNN) Neuroendocrinology, Mexico City, Mexico*
[2]*Neurosurgery (INNN), Mexico City, Mexico*
[3]*Endovascular Therapy (INNN), Mexico City, Mexico*
[4]*Unidad de Investigación en Endocrinología Experimental, Siglo XXI Instituto Mexicano del Seguro Social, Mexico City, Mexico*
[5]*Neuroanesthesia (INNN), Mexico City, Mexico*
[6]*Instituto Nacional de Ciencias Medicas y Nutrición, Mexico City, Mexico*

Correspondence should be addressed to Lesly Portocarrero-Ortiz; portocarrero.lesly@gmail.com

Academic Editor: Toshihiro Kita

Introduction. Pheochromocytomas (Pheo) and paragangliomas (PGL) are rare neuroendocrine tumors arising from chromaffin cells of the adrenal medulla and from the extra-adrenal autonomic paraganglia, respectively. Only 1–3% of head and neck PGL (HNPGL) show elevated catecholamines, and at least 30% of Pheo and PGL (PCPG) are associated with genetic syndromes caused by germline mutations in tumor suppressor genes and proto-oncogenes. *Clinical Case.* A 33-year-old man with a past medical history of resection of an abdominal PGL at the age of eleven underwent a CT scan after a mild traumatic brain injury revealing an incidental brain tumor. The diagnosis of a functioning PGL was made, and further testing was undertaken with a PET-CT with 68Ga-DOTATATE, SPECT-CT 131-MIBG, and genetic testing. *Discussion and Conclusion.* The usual clinical presentation of functioning PCPG includes paroxistic hypertension, headache, and diaphoresis, sometimes with a suggestive family history in 30–40% of cases. Only 20% of PGL are located in head and neck, of which only 1–3% will show elevated catecholamines. Metastatic disease is present in up to 50% of cases, usually associated with a hereditary germline mutation. However, different phenotypes can be observed depending on such germline mutations. Genetic testing is important in patients with PCPG since 31% will present a germline mutation. In this particular patient, an *SDHB* gene mutation was revealed, which can drastically influence the follow-up plan and the genetic counsel offered. A multidisciplinary approach is mandatory for every patient presenting with PCPG.

1. Introduction

Pheochromocytomas (Pheo) and paragangliomas (PGL) are rare neuroendocrine tumors arising from chromaffin cells of the adrenal medulla and from extra-adrenal autonomic paraganglia, respectively, with an estimated incidence of 0.8 cases per 100,000 person-years [1]. Pheo and sympathetic PGL are almost always functional (i.e., clinically active) while parasympathetic PGL are usually not [2], since only 1–3% of head and neck PGL (HNPG) show elevated catecholamines. At least 30% of Pheo and PGL (PCPG) are associated with germline mutations in certain susceptibility genes [2, 3]. However, different mutations may display different phenotypes, including tumor type, location, frequency, risk of malignancy, and heritability pattern. Since genetic testing is expensive and not widely available in most countries, prioritizing genetic testing requires a careful clinical and biochemical evaluation, which can significantly reduce costs and improve health care [4]. Functional imaging modalities may also be useful adjuncts for both diagnosis and workup for metastatic disease. Somatostatin receptor scintigraphy has been recently proposed as a useful method for localizing PGL, particularly in the head and neck [5]. We hereby present a case of head and neck catecholamine producing PGL, emphasizing on the importance of an individualized approach by a multidisciplinary team to guide diagnosis, treatment, and surveillance protocols based on current management recommendations.

2. Case Report

A 33-year-old man underwent a CT scan after a mild traumatic brain injury. The study revealed an incidental brain mass, which was initially considered to be a meningioma. The patient was referred to the National Institute of Neurology and Neurosurgery for surgical treatment. His family history was unremarkable for oncologic diseases. His past medical history as recalled by the patient included the resection of an abdominal para-aortic PGL at 11 years of age and a Pheo at 19 years of age. At that time, the patient was living abroad, where he was evaluated and treated, but his medical records were not available after request at the time of his referral to our center. During his childhood, he was initially evaluated because he had clinical symptoms of intermittent claudication, chest pain associated with exertion, severe hypertension, tachycardia, and excessive sweating. After a PGL was diagnosed, he was subject to a complete tumor resection and remained asymptomatic for 8 years, when the routine follow-up examination showed a marked elevation of catecholamines. A new imaging study was made, which revealed a right adrenal gland pheochromocytoma, which was also surgically removed, becoming once again asymptomatic for several years, after which he lost follow-up in that facility. During that time, he moved to Mexico, where he continued having an apparently normal life without any further medical evaluation for the next 14 years, up until the event of the head trauma.

During our initial evaluation, the patient was found to have right moderate hearing loss, right proptosis, optic nerve atrophy with right temporal hemianopsia, and face hyperesthesia in the area corresponding to the V2 and V3 branches of the trigeminal nerve. Blood pressure was reported to be intermittently high, between 130/90 and 140/100 mmHg. No weight changes, fatigue, nausea, hair loss, or other hormone deficiency-related symptoms were referred by the patient after purposely inquiring. The MRI was initially reported to be compatible with a meningioma vs. a hemangiopericytoma; however, the medical history called for additional diagnostic workup (Figure 1). Laboratory results showed normal metanephrines 208 μg (normal range 86–320 μg/24 H) and elevated normetanephrines 10,828 μg (normal range 120–400 μg/24 H; 27 times the upper limit of normal); the rest of the hormonal tests were normal. The diagnosis of a functioning PGL was then established, but the low incidence of functioning HNPG as well as the apparently aggressive behavior lead us to request a positron-emission tomography-computed tomography (PET-CT) with 68Ga-DOTATATE, which showed an increased expression of somatostatin receptors in the lesion (Figure 2). The single-photon emission computed tomography with meta-iodobenzylguanidine (SPECT-CT 131-MIBG) was also positive in the skull base lesion, related to an abnormal synthesis of catecholamines (Figure 2).

The patient was started on medical preoperative management with selective alpha-blockade (Prazosin) in a 3 mg three times a day dose and nifedipine 30 mg daily for two weeks, with the systolic blood pressure being lowered to 130/80 mmHg, when he was started on beta-blockers (Atenolol) 50 mg twice a day for an additional six weeks. In order to reduce excessive bleeding risk during open surgery, the decision was made to perform an endovascular preoperative embolization of the right maxillary artery using polyvinyl alcohol microspheres. Despite adequate preoperative medical treatment, the patient suffered from alternating episodes of bradycardia and supraventricular tachycardia, as well as hypertensive crisis during the procedure, when only 40% of the tumor been successfully embolized. The endovascular procedure was stopped, and an emergency MRI was performed. The image showed signs of increased intracranial pressure without any areas of hemorrhage or ischemia; however, since the patient had an altered mental status and bilateral pupillary dilation, a decompressive hemicraniectomy was emergently performed. After a successful intervention, he was transferred to the intensive care unit (ICU) for recovery.

After 20 days from the initial procedure, the patient was scheduled for a second embolization procedure and tumor resection surgery. After the second embolization, 95% of the tumor was successfully embolized without any complications, and 48 hours, later the patient underwent surgery achieving a subtotal tumor resection (Figure 3). He had an excellent postoperative recovery period with normalization of previously elevated catecholamines and improvement of his visual field, and was discharged home without further complications. He has now been followed-up for an additional 2 years. His blood pressure is normal without any medication, his urinary and serum catecholamines are normal, and the tumor remnant has not increased in follow-up MRI scans (Figure 3).

The genetic testing showed a heterozygous *SDHB* gene mutation, reference sequence; NM_003000.2: c.136C>T, NP_002991.2: p.Arg46* (clinvar: RCV000505277.1), which has been reported to be a pathogenic variant.

3. Discussion

PCPG are neuroendocrine tumors arising from chromaffin cells, which can produce catecholamines. The most common location is the adrenal glands (Pheo), while extra-adrenal tumors are called PGL [5]. The classical clinical presentation

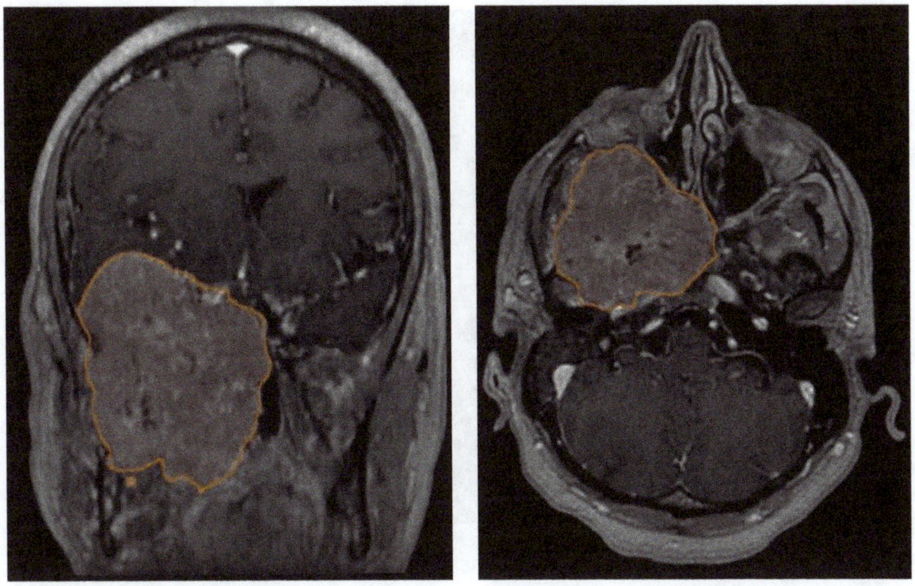

(a) (b)

Figure 1: T1 Enhanced-MRI: tumor lesion located at the right skull base with 163.2 cm^3 volume.

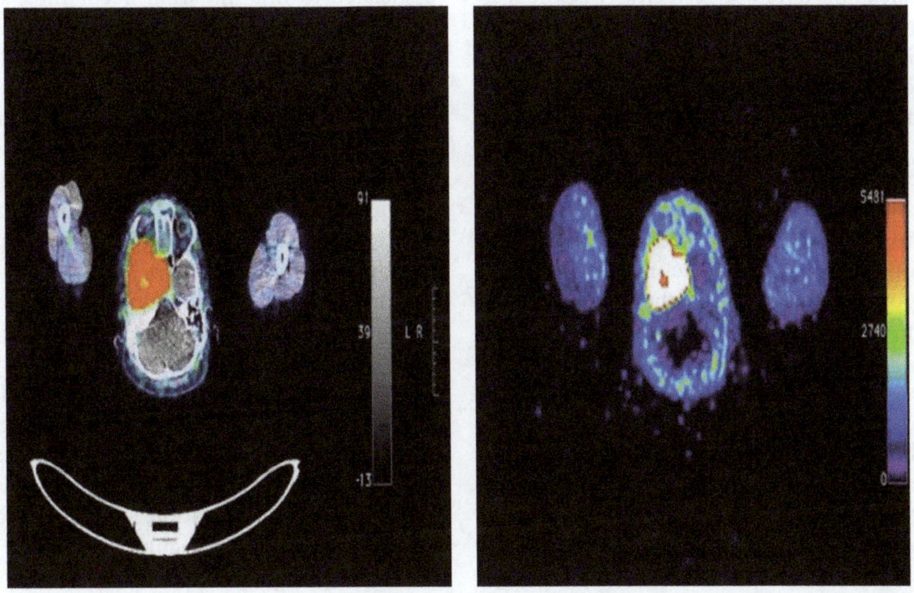

(a) (b)

Figure 2: Transversal image from the full body PET-CT scan with 68GA-DOTATATE (a) and 131-MIBG SPECT (b) showing intense uptake in the skull base tumor.

of functioning PCPG includes paroxistic hypertension, headache, and diaphoresis; a positive family history may be found in 30–40% of cases. These lesions can be found incidentally in 5% of cases [6]. Even though most HNPGs are clinically silent, some of them are actively synthesizing catecholamines but degrading them quickly inside the tumor tissue, without any biochemically or clinically significant secretion into the bloodstream under normal conditions. However, since these peptides may be released during surgical procedures or manipulation, planning an optimal preoperative medical management strategy with a multidisciplinary team is mandatory [7, 8]. The treatment of choice is a complete surgical resection, which may be difficult to achieve depending mainly on tumor size and location, as well as the team's surgical experience. For this reason, endovascular embolization has been extensively described in the management of several head and neck vascularized tumors including PGL [9]. Even though

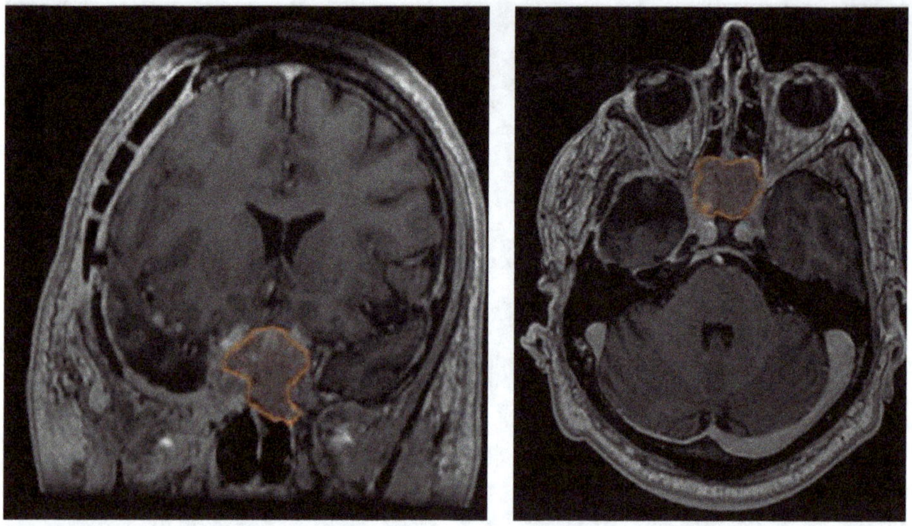

(a) (b)

FIGURE 3: Follow-up MRI with residual tumor lesion near the sellar region extending to nasal cavity with 11.9 cm^3 volume.

preoperative embolization has proven to reduce blood loss and operative time in the resection of most HNPG [10, 11], some particular indications have not been clearly defined, as in the case of carotid body tumors [12, 13]. However, in other types of PGL such as in this case, preoperative embolization has proven to be a useful adjunct to improve surgical conditions when performed appropriately by an experienced team [9, 14, 15]. Cranial base PGL may be an even stronger indication due to the relatively difficult access to this location [12]. It is important to consider the risk of cranial nerve palsies and other complications after preoperative embolization so that a correct decision can be made regarding the appropriate treatment for these patients.

Patients presenting at a young age, with multiple endocrine tumors, either synchronous or asynchronous, a positive family history, or other syndromic manifestations have an increased risk of having an underlying genetic mutation. Regardless, current recommendations suggest that all patients diagnosed with PCPG should be considered for genetic testing, since up to 30% of apparently sporadic cases may be associated to a germline mutation [16]. Different phenotypes, including location, size, risk of malignancy, and other associated tumors, have been linked to individual germline mutations. Based on these differences, particular management and surveillance guidelines have been proposed according to the genetic profile. [17] Approximately 20% of PGL are located in the head and neck, representing around 0.6% of all head and neck tumors and 0.03% of all tumors [7]. However, certain germline mutations may be associated with a significant predisposition for HNPG, with an estimated risk of 30% in cases of *SDHB* mutations but up to 79% in *SDHD* mutations [16–18]. Germline mutations in the *SDHB* gene are transmitted in an autosomal dominant pattern with an incomplete penetrance. The mean age at diagnosis is approximately 30 years, similar as in other germline mutations [19]. The penetrance of SDHB mutations varies widely but is generally lower than that of *SDHD* or *SDHAF2* mutations, with reported values of 20% at 50 years and 40% at 70 years of age [20, 21]. Tumors associated to this mutation occur most commonly at thoracic or abdominal extra-adrenal locations, but HNPG may be present in 20–30% of cases. Even though multifocal disease is not as frequent as in the case of other mutations (such as *SDHD*), *SDHB* mutations carry an increased risk for malignant transformation of PCPG as well as other malignant tumors such as renal cell carcinoma or thyroid carcinoma [16, 17, 19, 22]. In addition to the *SDHB* mutation status, several risk factors have been identified for malignant transformation of PGL as well as for overall survival in these patients, such as age at diagnosis, tumor size, and presence of synchronous metastases [1, 23–25]. In the present study, we describe the case of a patient with an initial diagnosis of a PGL during the pediatric age that developed other asynchronous and functioning tumors during the following 22 years. His initial age at diagnosis increases the chance of having a genetic mutation to >40%, while the biochemical profile and tumor location suggested that an *SDHB* gene mutation might be the culprit [22]. The clinical manifestations of parasympathetic-derived tumors arise mainly due to their large size and compressive effects such as hearing loss and cranial nerve palsy. Studies suggest that up to 41% of patients with functioning PGL have a germline mutation in one of the known common susceptibility genes (including *NF1*, *VHL*, *RET*, *SDHB*, *SDHD*, and *SDHC*). Up to fifty-three percent of patients coursing with at least one extra-adrenal PGL have an identified mutation [22, 26]. In this particular case, differential diagnosis must be established with an *SDHD* gene mutation, which is also associated with PCPG but present a rather different phenotype [27]. As in this case, the most commonly mutated gene is *SDHB*, which carries the highest risk of malignancy (up to 40%) and therefore present a poor prognosis [27]. The identification of a germline mutation in the *SDHB* gene demands close surveillance since these patients have a 4.7% risk of developing renal cell carcinoma by the age of 60 [26, 27]. A genetic test result will help us establish an adequate follow-up plan for the patient and his relatives to offer a more precise genetic counsel considering his prognosis and future quality of life.

At his age, he has already undergone four surgeries, and the cardiovascular and anesthetic risks have been increasing, not to mention the risk of malignancy or regrowth since the primary cranial tumor was not completely resected. Genetic counseling is also important in these patients in the long term due to the association of other endocrine and nonendocrine tumors [22, 27]. Close follow-up must be established in this patient in order to detect any tumor recurrence or other de novo neoplasms associated with his genetic condition. Current recommendations suggest that carriers of these mutations need to be screened for tumors beginning at age 5 at 6- to 12-months intervals. Biochemical testing (urinary or plasma metanephrines) is suggested annually, an anatomical imaging study (MRI or CT scan of the abdomen, thorax, and pelvis and skull base/neck) every 2 years, with further consideration of a functional imaging test (MIBG scintigraphy, PET-CT scan) [28]. Screening for renal cell carcinoma should also be considered [29]. However, follow-up must be individually tailored in every case, especially when malignant or remnant tumors are suspected or when clinical symptoms are present [30]. A successful transition from pediatric to adult care is mainstay for an adequate follow-up of these patients. In this case, the patient was lost to follow-up for several years without any medical evaluation, despite the fact that he had been closely monitored during his pediatric years. Apparently, neither the patient nor his family remember being told about the possibility of a new tumor later in life and they did not keep any documents from his consult visits, which would have increased our diagnostic suspicion and expedited the management. Given the cost of genetic testing, the family members have declined evaluation, which could also be a great limitation for an adequate treatment in many emerging economies.

4. Conclusion

The present case adequately highlights several important aspects to consider during the diagnostic workup and management of patients with PCPG. A complete family history and a detailed past medical history are necessary to raise suspicion about a certain disease pattern, while the appropriate laboratory and imaging studies are useful adjuncts to confirm the diagnosis. Preoperative management must be tailored to each patient and carefully considered since it may influence outcomes as much as the procedure itself. Even though there are risk factors associated to a germline mutation, genetic testing should be considered in all patients with PCPG in order to plan accordingly the appropriate follow-up plan and to offer adequate genetic counsel to the patients and their relatives. A multidisciplinary team must be actively involved in every aspect of the patient's care in order to enhance an adequate decision-making process.

References

[1] O. Hamidi, W. F. Young, N. M. Iñiguez-Ariza et al., "Pheochromocytoma and paraganglioma: 272 patients over 55 years," *The Journal of Clinical Endocrinology and Metabolism*, vol. 102, no. 9, pp. 3296–3305, 2017.

[2] J. Welander, P. Söderkvist, and O. Gimm, "Genetics and clinical characteristics of hereditary pheochromocytomas and paragangliomas," *Endocrine-Related Cancer*, vol. 18, no. 6, pp. R253–R276, 2011.

[3] C. Offergeld, C. Brase, S. Yaremchuk et al., "Head and neck paragangliomas: clinical and molecular genetic classification," *Clinics*, vol. 67, no. S1, pp. 19–28, 2012.

[4] H. P. H. Neumann, Z. Erlic, C. C. Boedeker et al., "Clinical predictors for germline mutations in head and neck paraganglioma patients: cost reduction strategy in genetic diagnostic process as fall-out," *Cancer Research*, vol. 69, no. 8, pp. 3650–3656, 2009.

[5] A. Hubalewska-Dydejczyk, H. J. L. M. Timmers, and M. Trofimiuk-Müldner, "The place of somatostatin receptor scintigraphy and other functional imaging modalities in the setting of pheochromocytoma and paraganglioma," *Somatostatin Analogues*, vol. 4, pp. 112–126, 2015.

[6] A. A. Kasperlik-Zaluska, E. Roslonowska, J. Slowinska-Srzednicka et al., "1,111 patients with adrenal incidentalomas observed at a single endocrinological center: incidence of chromaffin tumors," *Annals of the New York Academy of Sciences*, vol. 1073, no. 1, pp. 38–46, 2006.

[7] L. Fishbein, "Pheochromocytoma and paraganglioma," *Hematology/Oncology Clinics of North America*, vol. 30, no. 1, pp. 135–150, 2016.

[8] J. Li and C. H. Yang, "Improvement of preoperative management in patients with adrenal pheochromocytoma," *International Journal of Clinical and Experimental Medicine*, vol. 7, pp. 5541–5546, 2014.

[9] E. J. Duffis, C. D. Gandhi, C. J. Prestigiacomo et al., "Head, neck, and brain tumor embolization guidelines," *Journal of NeuroInterventional Surgery*, vol. 4, no. 4, pp. 251–255, 2012.

[10] J. B. White, M. J. Link, and H. J. Cloft, "Endovascular embolization of paragangliomas: a safe adjuvant to treatment," *Journal of Vascular and Interventional Neurology*, vol. 1, no. 1, pp. 37–41, 2008.

[11] R. S. Jackson, J. A. Myhill, T. A. Padhya, J. C. McCaffrey, T. V. McCaffrey, and R. S. Mhaskar, "The effects of preoperative embolization on carotid body paraganglioma surgery," *Otolaryngology-Head and Neck Surgery*, vol. 153, no. 6, pp. 943–950, 2015.

[12] C. Michelozzi, A. C. Januel, V. Cuvinciuc et al., "Arterial embolization with Onyx of head and neck paragangliomas," *Journal of NeuroInterventional Surgery*, vol. 8, no. 6, pp. 626–635, 2016.

[13] S. Abu-Ghanem, M. Yehuda, N. N. Carmel, A. Abergel, and D. M. Fliss, "Impact of preoperative embolization on the outcomes of carotid body tumor surgery: a meta-analysis and review of the literature," *Head & Neck*, vol. 38, no. S1, pp. E2386–E2394, 2016.

[14] M. S. Persky, A. Setton, Y. Niimi, J. Hartman, D. Frank, and A. Berenstein, "Combined endovascular and surgical treatment of head and neck paragangliomas? A team approach," *Head & Neck*, vol. 24, no. 5, pp. 423–431, 2002.

[15] M. G. Moore, J. L. Netterville, W. M. Mendenhall, B. Isaacson, and B. Nussenbaum, "Head and neck paragangliomas," *Otolaryngology-Head and Neck Surgery*, vol. 154, no. 4, pp. 597–605, 2016.

[16] A. Muth, J. Crona, O. Gimm et al., "Genetic testing and surveillance guidelines in hereditary pheochromocytoma and paraganglioma," *Journal of Internal Medicine*, vol. 285, no. 285, pp. 187–204, 2019.

[17] H. P. H. Neumann, C. Pawlu, M. Peczkowska et al., "Distinct clinical features of paraganglioma syndromes associated with SDHB and SDHD gene mutations," *JAMA*, vol. 292, no. 8, pp. 943–951, 2004.

[18] A. Guha, Z. Musil, A. Vicha et al., "A systematic review on the genetic analysis of paragangliomas: primarily focused on head and neck paragangliomas," *Neoplasma*, vol. 66, no. 5, pp. 671–680, 2019.

[19] H. P. Neumann, W. F. Young Jr., T. Krauss et al., "65 years of the double helix: genetics informs precision practice in the diagnosis and management of pheochromocytoma," *Endocrine-Related Cancer*, vol. 25, no. 8, pp. T201–T219, 2018.

[20] J. A. Rijken, N. D. Niemeijer, M. A. Jonker et al., "The penetrance of paraganglioma and pheochromocytoma in SDHB germline mutation carriers," *Clinical Genetics*, vol. 93, no. 1, pp. 60–66, 2018.

[21] E. F. Hensen, E. S. Jordanova, I. J. van Minderhout et al., "Somatic loss of maternal chromosome 11 causes parent-of-origin-dependent inheritance in SDHB-linked paraganglioma and pheochromocytoma families," *Oncogene*, vol. 23, no. 23, pp. 4076–4083, 2004.

[22] K. A. Andrews, D. B. Ascher, D. E. V. Pires et al., "Tumor risks and genotype-phenotype correlations associated with germline variants in succinate dehydrogenase subunit genes SDHB, SDHC and SDHD," *Journal of Medical Genetics*, vol. 55, no. 6, pp. 384–394, 2018.

[23] M. G. Sutton, S. G. Sheps, and J. T. Lie, "Prevalence of clinically unsuspected pheochromocytoma. Review of a 50-year autopsy series," *Mayo Clinic Proceedings*, vol. 56, no. 6, pp. 354–360, 1981.

[24] G. Eisenhofer, J. W. Lenders, G. Siegert et al., "Plasma methoxytyramine: a novel biomarker of metastatic pheochromocytoma and paraganglioma in relation to established risk factors of tumour size, location and SDHB mutation status," *European Journal of Cancer*, vol. 48, pp. 1739–1749, 2012.

[25] J. Schovanek, V. Martucci, R. Wesley et al., "The size of the primary tumor and age at initial diagnosis are independent predictors of the metastatic behavior and survival of patients with SDHB-related pheochromocytoma and paraganglioma: a retrospective cohort study," *BMC Cancer*, vol. 14, no. 1, p. 523, 2014.

[26] L. Fishbein, S. Merrill, D. L. Fraker, D. L. Cohen, and K. L. Nathanson, "Inherited mutations in pheochromocytoma and paraganglioma: why all patients should be offered genetic testing," *Annals of Surgical Oncology*, vol. 20, no. 5, pp. 1444–1450, 2013.

[27] I. Jochmanova, K. I. Wolf, K. S. King et al., "SDHB-related pheochromocytoma and paraganglioma penetrance and genotype-phenotype correlations," *Journal of Cancer Research and Clinical Oncology*, vol. 143, no. 8, pp. 1421–1435, 2017.

[28] K. Eijkelenkamp, T. E. Osinga, M. M. de Jong et al., "Calculating the optimal surveillance for head and neck paraganglioma in SDHB-mutation carriers," *Familial Cancer*, vol. 16, no. 1, pp. 123–130, 2017.

[29] C. J. Ricketts, J. R. Forman, E. Rattenberry et al., "Tumor risks and genotype-phenotype-proteotype analysis in 358 patients with germline mutations in SDHB and SDHD," *Human Mutation*, vol. 31, no. 1, pp. 41–51, 2010.

[30] M. Lerebvre and W. D. Foulkes, "Pheochromocytoma and paraganglioma syndromes: genetics and management update," *Current Oncology*, vol. 21, no. 1, pp. e8–e17, 2014.

27

Lenvatinib Administered via Nasogastric Tube in Poorly Differentiated Thyroid Cancer

Eleonora Molinaro,[1] David Viola,[1] Nicola Viola,[1] Pierpaolo Falcetta,[1] Francesca Orsolini,[1] Liborio Torregrossa,[2] Paola Vagli,[3] Alessandro Ribechini,[4] Gabriele Materazzi,[5] Paolo Vitti,[1] and Rossella Elisei[1]

[1]*Unit of Endocrinology, Department of Clinical and Experimental Medicine, University Hospital of Pisa, Pisa 56124, Italy*
[2]*Unit of Pathology, Department of Surgical, Medical, and Molecular Pathology and Critical Care Medicine, University Hospital of Pisa, Pisa 56124, Italy*
[3]*Diagnostic and Interventional Radiology, University Hospital of Pisa, Pisa 56124, Italy*
[4]*Endoscopic Section of Pneumology, University Hospital of Pisa, Pisa 56124, Italy*
[5]*Unit of Surgery, Department of Surgical, Medical, and Molecular Pathology and Critical Care Medicine, University Hospital of Pisa, Pisa 56124, Italy*

Correspondence should be addressed to Eleonora Molinaro; elemoli@hotmail.com

Academic Editor: Toshihiro Kita

Background. The tyrosine kinase inhibitors (TKIs) are indicated for the treatment of locally advanced or metastatic progressive thyroid carcinoma (CDT), refractory to radioactive iodine. The following report describes the efficacy of lenvatinib administered through a nose-gastric tube (SNG) in a patient affected with a poorly differentiated thyroid carcinoma (PDTC) which determined a stenosis of the esophagus. *Material and Methods.* A patient was followed up for papillary thyroid carcinoma follicular variant (T3NxMx), subjected to total thyroidectomy and treated with iodine-131 radio metabolic therapy. Two years after surgery, following the onset of dysphonia and dysphagia, patient was submitted to a computed tomography (CT) scan of the neck that showed the presence of a lesion of $6 \times 2.5 \times 3.5$ cm, which determined trachea deviation and cervical esophagus compression. The biopsy indicated the presence of PDTC, triggering tracheal lumen reduction and sub-stenosis of the cervical esophagus for an ab-extrinsic compression. A nose-gastric tube (SNG) was placed and lenvatinib was started at a dose of 20 mg/day, administered via this probe after opening the capsules and diluting the drug in 10 ml of saline solution. *Results.* One month later, CT showed a significant cervical lesion reduction. Bronchoscopy confirmed tracheal infiltration, but the residual caliber was improved from 50% to 75%. At the esophagogastroduodenoscopy (EGDS), the sub stenosis of the cervical esophagus was no longer appreciated; however, a double perforation of the esophagus was found, without fistula. *Conclusion.* Lenvatinib therapy is effective also when administered via SNG. Our result is of particular relevance in the management of thyroid cancer patients, especially in the presence of subjects unable to swallow. Further studies are needed to validate the administration of lenvatinib by SNG, in order to extend the indications to this alternative administration way, beside the oral one.

1. Introduction

Poorly differentiated thyroid cancer (PDTC) is a rare aggressive endocrine neoplasm accounting for about 5% of all thyroid tumours. It was first described, independently, by Sakamoto et al. [1] and Carcangiu et al. [2], in 1983 and 1984, respectively. It shows morphological and behavioral features between those of well differentiated thyroid cancer (WDTC) and anaplastic thyroid cancer (ATC) and it may arise, de novo, in a thyroid gland, or from pre-existing well-differentiated follicular and papillary carcinomas. Several studies showed a poorer prognosis for patients with PDTC compared to those with DTC, with a 10-year recurrence rate near 30% [3, 4]. Extra-thyroidal extension has negative impact on prognosis, with 10-year overall survival rates of 45% [5]. The incidence of extra-thyroidal extension varies, with a range from 6% to

13%. Trachea and esophagus were involved in 37% and 21% of patients with invasive thyroid cancer, respectively, as reported by McCaffrey et al. [6].

Surgery remains the mainstay for locally advanced thyroid cancer. However, the resection of vital neck structures can be associated with significant morbidity. For patients with advanced PDTC who are not suitable for surgical resection or radioiodine therapy, there are only few therapeutic strategies available. These patients could benefit of the new treatments, like the tyrosine-kinase inhibitors (TKI) [7, 8].

Lenvatinib, an oral multi-kinase inhibitor, has shown improvement in the progression-free survival and response rate among patients with iodine-131 (131-I) refractory (RAI refractory) thyroid cancer, including PDTC, compared to those receiving placebo [9]. Moreover, the drug was also able to reduce the tumoral lesions size as demonstrated by the significantly better objective response rate (ORR) in respect to patients treated with placebo [9].

We report a case of a PDTC showing an extremely aggressive behavior with tracheal and esophageal invasion, treated lenvatinib mesilate (Lenvima, Eisai Inc.), diluted in saline solution and administered via nasogastric feeding tube. The interest of this case report is that, although the company does not provide any indication for this administration route, the drug was effective in reducing the tumoral mass.

2. Patient

In December 2015, a 62-year-old female patient, underwent to a total thyroidectomy, following the finding of malignant cytology (TIR5) on thyroid nodule of the right lobe, and most likely malignant cytology (TIR4) on the nodule of the left lobe. Histological examination showed a papillary thyroid carcinoma (1.7 cm), multifocal, follicular variant with focal oxyphilous differentiation with involvement of the posterior peri-thyroid adipose tissue (pT3NxMx). In March 2016, 80 mCi of 131-I was administered for ablative purpose, with a whole body scan (WBS) documenting anterior cervical uptake; serum thyroglobulin was 0.25 ng/ml with AbTg 169 UI/ml. In December 2017, two years after the intervention, the patient came to our attention for the development of dysphagia and dysphonia, and underwent to an otorhinolaryngoiatric examination that documented the vocal cord paralysis, in the para-median position. Bronchoscopy also showed circumferential infiltration of the trachea, with 50% lumen reduction.

The esophagogastroduodenoscopy (EGDS) showed the sub-stenosis of the cervical esophagus due to an ab-extrinsic compression. A 4.9 mm nose-gastric tube (SNG) placement was performed and set, by endoscopic guidance. The neck CT documented a local recurrence of the disease, at the lower portion of the left thyroid loggia, which appeared as a fluid-air collection with necrotic evolution of 6 × 2.5 × 3.5 cm and which determined deviation and compression of the trachea and the proximal portion of the esophagus and showing no cleavage planes from cricoid cartilage, first tracheal rings and esophagus (Figure 1(a)). A biopsy was performed and histological examination documented morphological findings consistent

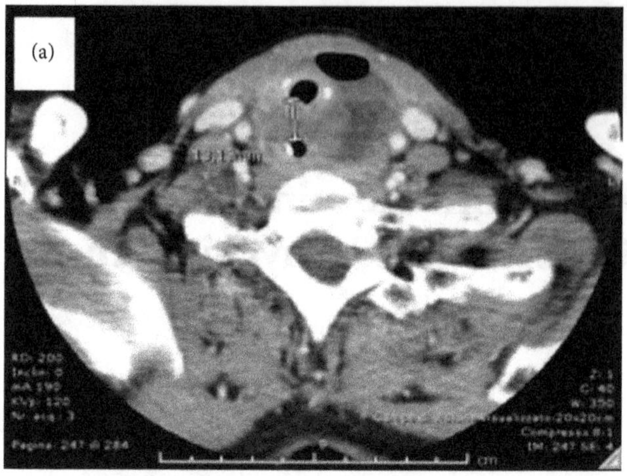

(a)

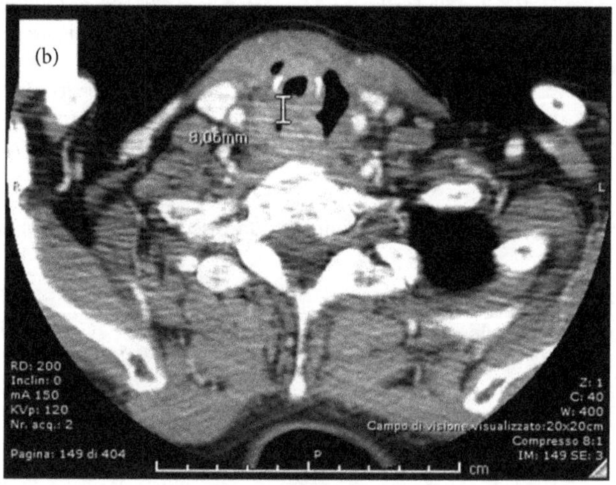

(b)

Figure 1

with PDTC with squamous cells (Figure 2(a)–2(g)). The immunohistochemistry was positive for CK7, p40, and p63, focally positive for PAX-8 and negative for Tg and TTF-1. The proliferation index Ki-67 (MIB-1) was 30% and V600E mutation of BRAF was found. Radiotherapy was excluded due to the necrotic appearance of the lesion.

Lenvatinib therapy was immediately started and administered at a dose of 20 mg/day, via SNG, to our inpatient, opening the drug capsule and diluting the inside powder in 10 ml of saline solution; no special washes were made after the drug was administered. After one month from the start of therapy, the patient was re-evaluated. Neck CT showed the reduction of the fluid component, volume, and compressive effects of the cervical necrotic pathology (Figure 1(b)).

The bronchoscopy confirmed the paralysis of the left vocal cord, but the residual caliber in the most stenotic tracheal tract was increased from 50% up to 75%. The EGDS no longer documented the sub stenosis of the cervical esophagus, which was now traversed with the 6.5 mm instrument. However, a double esophageal perforation was reported at about 21 cm from the nostrils (without fistulous tract with the trachea).

In light of this finding, the drug was discontinued for a week, and the following control with EGDS showed the

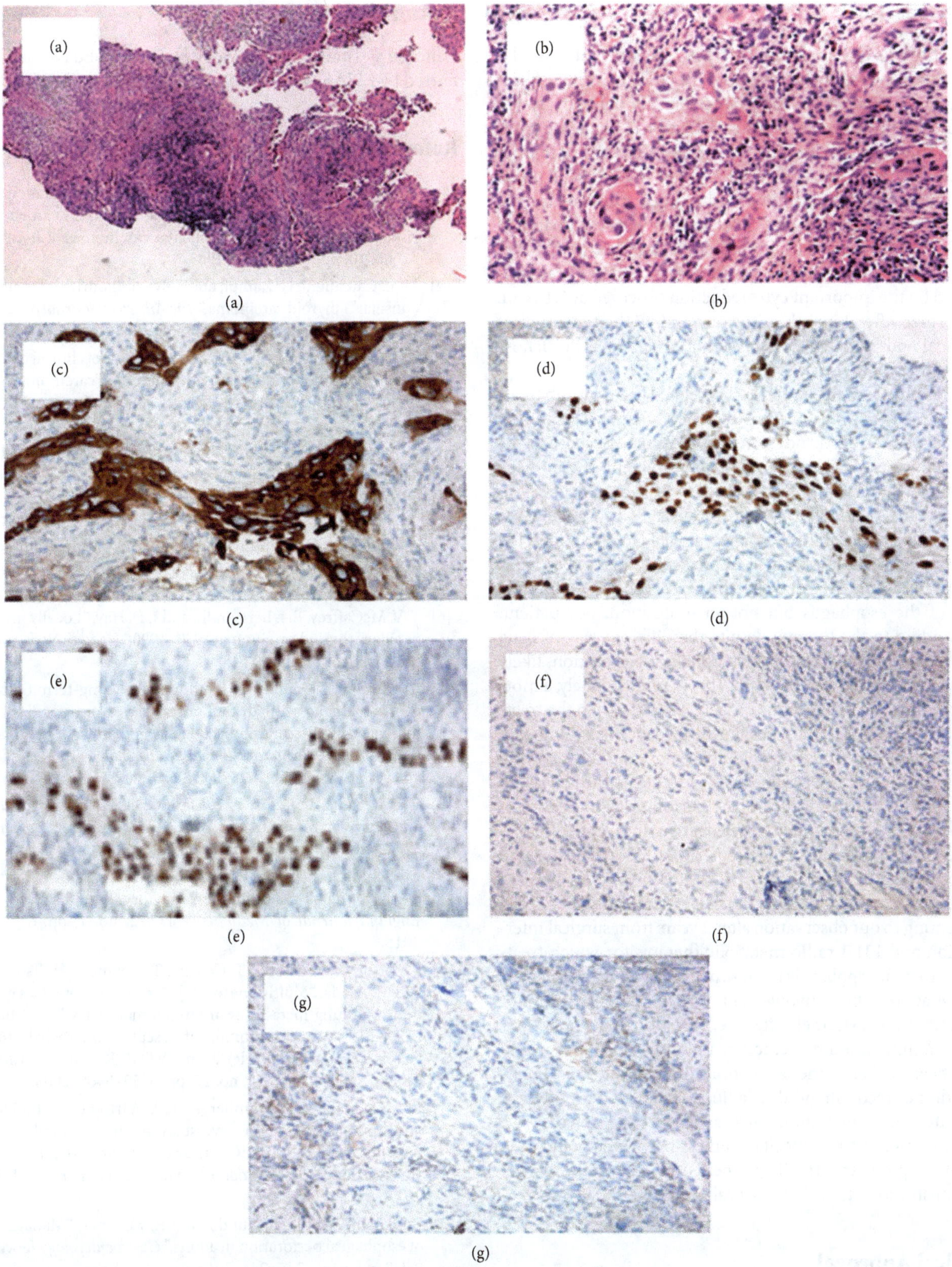

FIGURE 2

presence of a single perforation. Lenvatinib was restarted at a lower dose of 10 mg/day and the SNG was kept in place to continue the enteral nutrition. After one month, the second perforation appeared to be reduced but still present. Unfortunately, the patient died one month later for pulmonary embolism.

3. Discussion

Lenvatinib is an oral, multi-target, inhibitor of vascular endothelial growth factor receptors (VEGFR) 1, 2, and 3, fibroblast growth factor receptors 1–4, platelet-derived growth factor receptor alpha, and of the RET and KIT signaling pathways [10]. Its anti-tumoral activity in RAI-refractory thyroid cancer has been clearly demonstrated in the SELECT phase III clinical trial [9] and the drug has been approved for the treatment of these patients. Since our patient was unable to swallow, it was decided to administer the drug, lenvatinib, after capsules opening, via SNG. The treatment efficacy was confirmed by the important cyto-reduction observed at CT scan, performed after 1 month of therapy and by the reduction of tracheal and esophageal involvement observed at bronchoscopy and EGDS, respectively.

Common adverse events (AEs) related to lenvatinib treatment include hypertension, diarrhea, fatigue, rash, and palmar-plantar erythrodysestesia syndrome. Because of its strong anti-VEGFR activity, if the involvement of vital neck structures like trachea and esophagus by the tumor mass is of severe entity, the extensive necrosis caused by anti-angiogenic tyrosine kinase inhibitor therapy could lead to potentially, life threatening, AEs, like tracheoesophageal fistula and esophageal perforation [11]. Although the EGDS showed a compression of the esophagus but not an infiltration, our patient, responding to the therapy despite the different way of drug administration, developed the esophageal perforation, likely due to a microscopic infiltration. This is, unfortunately, a morbid condition with a mortality rate of 40–60% when the treatment is delayed [12], thus, despite the evidence of a significant reduction of the stenosis, we did not remove the SNG to avoid mediastinitis and, at the same time, we reduced the lenvatinib daily dose with the aim to let the perforations to heal. This strategy was demonstrated to be effective since, at the following EGDS control, one of the two perforations was healed and the other one reduced.

In our experience, this is the first reported case of PDTC, presenting to our observation after 2 years from surgical intervention and 131-I radio metabolic therapy, for which treatments were not applicable because of the disease aggressiveness and vital structures involvement. The multikinase inhibitor lenvatinib was extremely effective, even utilizing a not established administration method at the same dose that would have been chosen in the case of oral administration; we therefore do not recommend dose adjustments based on the type of route of administration. This case report has a pivotal role to encourage further specific studies in a wider population able to demonstrate the helpfulness of an alternative way of administration other than the oral one.

Ethical Approval

The study has been conducted in accordance with the rules of the local Ethics Committee and the Declaration of Helsinki. Patient provided a written consent for the use of her clinical data.

Acknowledgments

Editorial assistance was provided by Content Ed Net and supported by EISAI, with an unrestricted grant.

References

[1] A. Sakamoto, N. Kasai, and H. Sugano, "Poorly differentiated carcinoma of the thyroid. A clinicopathologic entity for a high-risk group of papillary and follicular carcinomas," *Cancer*, vol. 52, no. 10, pp. 1849–1855, 1983.

[2] M. L. Carcangiu, G. Zampi, and J. Rosai, "Poorly differentiated ("insular") thyroid carcinoma," *The American Journal of Surgical Pathology*, vol. 8, no. 9, pp. 655–668, 1984.

[3] K. Tanaka, H. Sonoo, W. Saito et al., "Analysis of clinical outcome of patients with poorly differentiated thyroid carcinoma," *ISRN Endocrinology*, vol. 2011, Article ID 308029, 5 pages, 2011.

[4] Y. Ito, I. Hirokawa, M. Fukushima et al., "Prevalence and prognostic significance of poor differentiation and tall cell variant in papillary carcinoma in Japan," *World Journal of Surgery*, vol. 32, no. 7, pp. 1535–1543, 2008.

[5] P. E. Andersen, J. Kinsella, T. R. Loree, A. R. Shaha, and J. P. Shah, "Differentiated carcinoma of the thyroid with extrathyroidal extension," *The American Journal of Surgery*, vol. 170, no. 5, pp. 467–470, 1995.

[6] T. V. McCaffrey, E. J. Bergstralh, and I. D. Hay, "Locally invasive papillary thyroid carcinoma: 1940–1990," *Head & Neck*, vol. 16, no. 2, pp. 165–172, 1994.

[7] C. Durante, N. Haddy, E. Baudin et al., "Long-term outcome of 444 patients with distant metastases from papillary and follicular thyroid carcinoma: benefits and limits of radioiodine therapy," *The Journal of Clinical Endocrinology & Metabolism*, vol. 91, no. 8, pp. 2892–2899, 2006.

[8] C. E. DeSantis, C. C. Lin, A. B. Mariotto et al., "Cancer treatment and survivorship statistics, 2014," *CA: A Cancer Journal for Clinicians*, vol. 64, no. 4, pp. 252–271, 2014.

[9] M. Schlumberger, M. Tahara, L. J. Wirth et al., "Lenvatinib versus placebo in radioiodine-refractory thyroid cancer," *New England Journal of Medicine*, vol. 372, no. 7, pp. 621–630, 2015.

[10] J. Matsui, Y. Funahashi, T. Uenaka, T. Watanabe, A. Tsuruoka, and M. Asada, "Multi-kinase inhibitor E7080 suppresses lymph node and lung metastases of human mammary breast tumor MDA-MB-231 via inhibition of vascular endothelial growth factor-receptor (VEGF-R) 2 and VEGF-R3 kinase," *Clinical Cancer Research*, vol. 14, no. 17, pp. 5459–5465, 2008.

[11] R. I. Haddad, M. Schlumberger, L. J. Wirth et al., "Incidence and timing of common adverse events in lenvatinib-treated patients from the SELECT trial and their association with survival outcomes," *Endocrine*, vol. 56, no. 1, pp. 121–128, 2017.

[12] L. Kaman, J. Iqbal, B. Kundil, and R. Kochhar, "Management of esophageal perforation in adults," *Gastroenterology Research*, vol. 3, no. 6, pp. 235–244, 2010.

28

Rare Presentation of Hypoglycemia in a Patient with Anaplastic Large-Cell Lymphoma

Raed Aldahash

Department of Medicine, Ministry of National Guard Health Affairs, King Abdullah International Medical Research Center (KAIMRC), King Saud Bin Abdulaziz for Health Science, Riyadh, Saudi Arabia

Correspondence should be addressed to Raed Aldahash; dr.raaed@hotmail.com

Academic Editor: Mihail A. Boyanov

Anaplastic large-cell lymphoma is a rare type of aggressive non-Hodgkin's lymphoma, and arriving at a final diagnosis for this tumor is a challenge for the healthcare providers. Usually, it involves the lymph nodes and extranodal tissues such as the lungs, skin, and other soft tissues. Its presentation by extending into different organs such as the liver, lungs, bones, spleen, and thyroid is rare. Thus, involvement of other organs is very rare as we found in a 54-year-old male patient, a known case of hypertension and end-stage renal disease who was on hemodialysis, who presented to the emergency department with a history of generalized weakness and weight loss of about 20 kg for two months. The tumor cells are positive for CD45, CD30, CD15, MUMi, and Ki-67 (80%) and negative for CD20, PAX-5, CD79a, CD3, CD5, CD10, BCL6, BCL2, EMA, ALK-1, and CD138. The patient was hypoglycemic and hypercalcemic and was managed accordingly. The patient was evaluated, and the third assessment showed that hypoglycemia was resolved due to dexamethasone. The patient's glucose storage was depleted most likely due to liver involvement plus poor general condition. It was asserted that the patient's hypoglycemia could be related to his underlying malignancy. Also, the patient was advised to start tablet diazoxide 45 mg three times a day (3 mg/kg/day TID) in addition to levothyroxine tablet 50 mcg once a day. Tablet diazoxide was stopped, and nutritional support was recommended. This case reveals a rare systematic ALK-1-negative anaplastic large-cell lymphoma that involves multiple organs. The main learning point from this report is that these tumors can present atypically even in adults and can be ALK-1 negative, which is contrary to the typical systematic anaplastic large-cell lymphomas that are positive for ALK.

1. Introduction

Lymphomas are the typical heterogeneous category of malignancies primarily of lymph nodes and are considered as a very rare type of aggressive non-Hodgkin's lymphomas [1]. More specifically, anaplastic large-cell lymphoma constitutes 5% of all cases of non-Hodgkin's lymphomas [2]. The unique property or feature of anaplastic large-cell lymphoma is the proliferation of pleomorphic cells that carry CD30, which are constantly expressed on almost all neoplastic cells [3]. This tumor is most commonly found in children and constitutes about 40% of all non-Hodgkin's lymphomas among children with a greater percentage found among males than females [2]. There is no definitive etiology of anaplastic large-cell lymphoma; however, Epstein–Barr virus has been reported to play an important role in the pathogenesis of this disease, mainly in immunocompromised patients and among cases that occur in Asian countries [4]. Two clinical types have been recognized including localized cutaneous tumors or systematic neoplasms [5]. The former category mainly constitutes CD30-positive proliferative cells including lymphoproliferative skin disorders, and these types are ALK-negative [6]. The survival rate for cutaneous neoplasms is more than 90%, while the systematic type is more aggressive that may involve the skin and other extranodal organs [7]. In contrast to these types, systematic anaplastic large-cell lymphomas are typically ALK positive [8,9]. Both types of anaplastic large-cell lymphoma, ALK positive and ALK negative, are made up of lymphoid cells having a huge cytoplasm and pleomorphic characteristics along with horseshoe-shaped nuclei [10]. It has been found that systematic anaplastic large-cell lymphomas that are ALK positive show a better prognosis than ALK-negative tumors [7]. Through the following case report, we aim to communicate our experience with healthcare providers and to discuss the management plan necessary for patients with similar presentations.

2. Case Report

2.1. Investigation

2.1.1. Description of the Case. This was a 54-year-old man, a known case of hypertension and end-stage renal disease who was on hemodialysis, who presented to the emergency department with a history of generalized weakness and weight loss of about 20 kg for two months. He had been managed and treated in an external healthcare system where he was diagnosed with a case of anaplastic large-cell lymphoma. The PAN-CT revealed extensive and innumerable lesions in different organs such as the liver, lungs, bones, spleen, and thyroid. On liver biopsy, an infiltrated high-grade/undifferentiated malignant neoplasm was found. Furthermore, his serum calcium levels were very high [11], which were managed by adequate hydration and denosumab injections [12]. His family history was not remarkable.

2.1.2. Clinical Findings on Examination and Laboratory Investigations at the Time of Admission. On arrival at the emergency department, the patient was found conscious, alert, oriented, looking ill, and cachexic. However, he was hemodynamically stable and on auscultation, and the chest was found to be clear with S1 and S2 being audible on auscultating the heart with no added third sound or murmur. His initial blood pressure was 101/65 mmHg, his heart rate was 65 beats per minute with an oxygen saturation of 99% on room air, and he was breathing spontaneously. Table 1 shows the laboratory values of the patient at the time of admission.

2.1.3. Assessment by the Team of the Hospital. During the hospital course, the patient was admitted as a case of tumor lysis syndrome and was evaluated by a team of specialists including specialists from hematology/oncology, nephrology, and mental health. During the hospital stay, the patient was given a reduced dose of the 1st cycle of CVP (chemotherapy protocol) due to poor performance status and very poor nutrition without significant complications. The patient was monitored during the hospital stay, and his necessary laboratory investigations were sent to assess the progress and response to treatment.

2.2. Diagnosis

2.2.1. Results and Conclusion Based on CT Performed outside the Hospital. A right apical micronodule, measuring 5 mm, was found. There was bilateral mild-to-moderate pleural effusion with adjacent atelectasis. However, no mediastinal, hilar, or axillary lymphadenomegaly was noticed. There were diffuse osteosclerotic and osteolytic changes throughout the sternum, vertebrae, and ribs. Based on these results, a conclusion was made about the right apical parenchymal micronodule, likely metastatic within the context.

Based on the findings of the CT scan, an impression of diffuse metastatic bony disease was given by the radiologist and team (Figure 1).

2.2.2. Results of a Blood Smear, Biopsy, and Doppler Ultrasound. The blood smear of the patient shows normocytic normochromic red cells with mild anisocytosis. Furthermore, occasional polychromatophilic cells were seen with no significant schistocytes (less than 1%). Rare left-shifted granulocytes with mild toxic changes in neutrophils were noted. No definite circulating blasts were seen. Platelets were essentially unremarkable. Liver lesion needle core biopsy (outside materials- H 2342–20, File No. 1051463) showed anaplastic large-cell lymphoma, ALK negative. Cores of hepatic tissue were found to be infiltrated by a high-grade or undifferentiated malignant neoplasm. Poorly differentiated hepatocellular carcinoma is included in the differential diagnosis. On immunostaining, the tumor cells are positive for CD45, CD30, CD15, MUMi, and Ki-67 (80%) and negative for CD20, PAX-5, CD79a, CD3, CD5, CD10, BCL6, BCL2, EMA, ALK-1, and CD138. Findings on upper extremity venous doppler ultrasound showed patent left internal jugular, innominate, subclavian, axillary, brachial, basilic, and forearm veins. However, the left arteriovenous (AV) fistula was thrombosed. The final impression of negative study for left upper limb deep vein thrombosis (DVT) was made with thrombosed AV fistula.

2.2.3. PET/CT Oncology. The study is in keeping with known lymphoma involving the skeleton extensively, liver, right posterior chest wall, left lung hilar lymph node, and possibly left upper lung lobe. Also, a suspicion of peritoneal disease was made based on the PET/CT scan (Figure 2).

2.3. Treatment

2.3.1. Two Weeks after Admission. After two weeks of admission, the endocrinology team received a consultation regarding a hypoglycemic attack while the patient was undergoing a PET scan that was treated with 50 mL dextrose 50% in water injection with an intravenous (IV) push. The patient was seen and evaluated by the endocrinology team. After reviewing lab investigations, the patient was found to have had a low glucose profile since admission that ranges between 1.7 and 5.1 mmol/L. Hence, the patient was labeled as a case of hypoglycemia for investigations with a differential diagnosis of [1] anaplastic lymphoma with infiltration to adrenal glands, [2] end-stage renal disease (ESRD) causing hypoglycemia, [3] or nutritional inadequacy.

2.3.2. Management Plan. The hospital specialists' team advised getting his serum insulin level, C-peptide, proinsulin, B-hydroxybutyrate, cortisol, and thyroid profile

Table 1: Clinical findings on admission to the Emergency Department (ED) of the hospital.

Assessment on arrival by ED staff	Normal value	Clinical findings and labs of the patient
Blood pressure, mmHg	120/80	101/65
Heart rate (beats per minute)	60–100	65
Oxygen saturation, (Spo2), %	≥ 95	99
Sodium, mmol/L	136–145	136
Potassium, millimoles per liter (mmol/L)	3.5–5.1	3.1
Serum chloride, milliequivalents per liter (mEq/L)	98–107	102
Random glucose	2.9–7.8	5.6
Blood urea nitrogen (BUN), mg/dL	3.0–9.2	18.5
Creatinine, umol/L	64–110	243
CO2, mmol/L	22–29	17
AGAP, mmol/L	7–15	20
Calcium, mmol/L	2.10–2.5	1.88, 1.74
eGFR	>= 60 mL/min/1.73 m^2	26
Phosphorus, mmol/L	0.74–1.52	0.97
Magnesium, mmol/L	0.66–1.07	0.74
Uric acid, umol/L	210–420	153
Adj Ca, mmol/L	2.10–2.55	2.06
Hgb, gm/L	135–180	90
Hct, L/L	0.420–0.540	0.273
MCV, fL	76.0–96.0	89.2
MCH, pg	27.0–32.0	29.3
Platelet	150–400 x 10^9/L	98
MPV, fL	7.4–10.4	5.9
PT, second (s)	9.38–12.34	12.2
INR	0.80–1.20	1.1
PT, second (s)	24.84–32.96	26.5
GGT	12–64 U/L	505
LDH	125–220 U/L	2944
Alk Phos	40–150 U/L	332
Bili T	3.4–20.5 umol/L	8.3
AST	5–34 U/L	31
ALT	5–55 U/L	21
Total protein	60–83 g/L	55

including TSH and free T4 at the time of hypoglycemia (blood glucose level < 2.8 mmol/L).

After taking labs, the patient was started on dextrose-infused fluids (and was watched for overload). The patient needed nutritional support and was advised to have adequate nutritional support.

2.4. Follow-Up and Outcomes

2.4.1. Labs after Two Weeks (Second Assessment). The patient's labs were repeated after two weeks, and the insulin was found to be < 11.50 (22.96–116.95 pmol/L), while his TSH was 21.57 (0.35–4.94 mIU/L), free T4 was 6.15 (9.00–19.00 pmol/L), IGF-1_RY was 25 (61–200 ng/mL) and 0.36 (.26–1.72 nmol/L), random glucose level was 1.7, and eGFR was 11, which further deteriorated over two weeks. However, sodium (136 mmol/L), potassium (3.1 mmol/L), chloride (102 mmol/L), BUN (18.5 mmol/L), and creatinine (243 umol/L) levels remained the same as they were at the baseline.

2.4.2. Impression or Plan. It was asserted that the patient's hypoglycemia could be related to his underlying malignancy [13]. Also, the patient was advised to start tablet diazoxide 45 mg three times a day (3 mg/kg/day TID) in addition to levothyroxine tablet 50 mcg once a day. A clinical nutritional referral was made to plan proper nutritional support for him. Unfortunately, the patient was not improved on diazoxide. As planned by the hematology team, the patient was started on dexamethasone injection 40 mg IV for 5 days regarding his lymphoma situation.

2.4.3. Third Assessment. The patient was evaluated, and the third assessment showed that hypoglycemia was resolved due to dexamethasone. The patient's glucose storage was depleted most likely due to liver involvement plus poor general condition. Tablet diazoxide was stopped, and nutritional support was highly recommended.

3. Discussion

A case of anaplastic large-cell lymphoma is presented in this case report that encroached multiple vital organs including the liver, spleen, and thyroid. The tumor cells were found to be positive for CD30, but negative for ALK-1. Both morphological and phenotypic features of systematic anaplastic large-cell lymphoma (negative for ALK-1) mimic mucosal CD30 positive T-cell lymphoproliferative

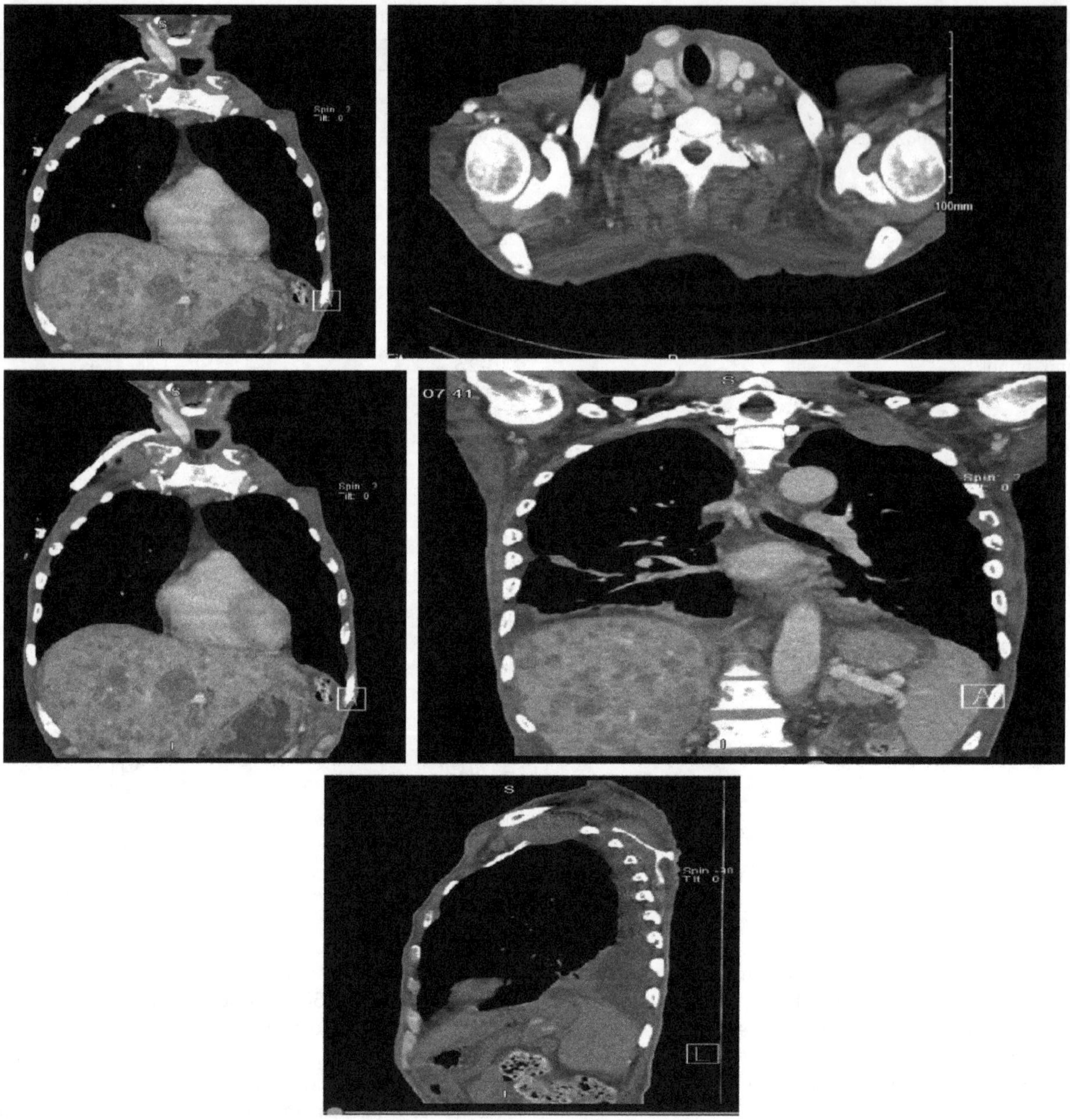

Figure 1: Images of the chest CT scan showing metastasis to the liver and chest wall.

disorders [14]. It is important to distinguish between ALK-positive and ALK-negative types of anaplastic large-cell lymphomas because there are differences between their clinical presentation and prognosis [15]. These tumors may be initially misdiagnosed and need a vigilant assessment plan with reasonable imaging and other investigations to diagnose correctly.

We found hypercalcemia and hypoglycemia in this case, which were associated with the tumor. The existing literature demonstrates that hypercalcemia due to neoplasms is a commonly found sign and it is the humoral hypercalcemia rather than Vit-D3-mediated hypercalcemia that is usually found in malignancies [11]. However, findings related to hypoglycemia in tumors that are the outside the pancreas, such as this anaplastic large-cell lymphoma, are rare and hardly ever reported in similar case reports. Glucose is a necessary fuel for the function of the brain, and complex neural, cellular, and hormonal controls try to maintain the glucose levels within a reasonably narrow range. Usually, we find hypoglycemia rarely in nondiabetic patients, and therefore, one may need to be ruled out for potential malignancies as we found in our case.

After evaluating the patient, we also concluded that hypoglycemia is more likely due to lymphoma and it was resolved by giving dexamethasone to the patient. The patient's glucose storage was depleted most likely due to liver involvement plus poor general condition. Although we did not obtain bone marrow biopsy or insulin-like growth factors in the blood, we presumed that this hypoglycemia is most likely due to the anaplastic large-cell lymphoma because we did not find other alternative mechanisms of severe hypoglycemia in the patient such as sepsis, adrenal

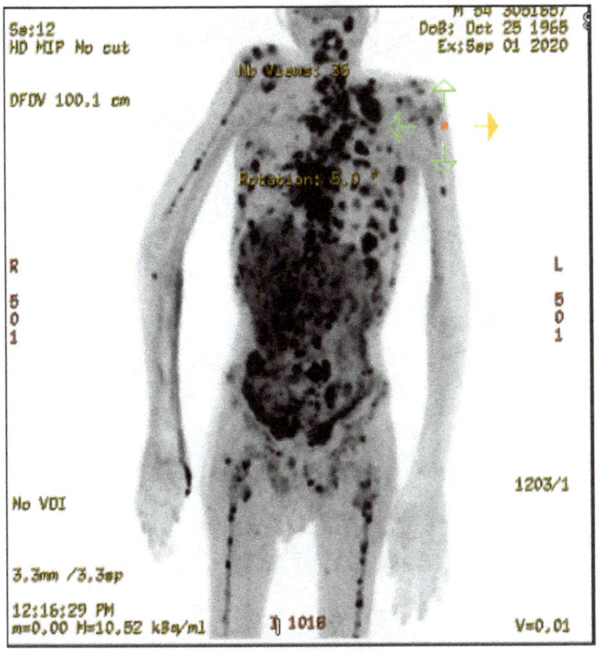

FIGURE 2: PET/CT scan of the patient admitted to the emergency department.

insufficiency, or insulinoma [13]. Furthermore, it is likely that such hypoglycemia may also be due to overproduction of insulin-like growth factor (IGF)-2 precursor protein, which is commonly known as "big insulin-like growth factor- (IGF-) 2" [16]. This is also supported by the literature whereby large neoplasms sometimes may produce IGF-2 that can circulate in the blood followed by binding to insulin and IGF receptors. This will result in increased uptake of glucose in the tissues and reduced glucose in the blood; thereby, the liver reduces the release of glucose to the blood. This provokes the feedback mechanism and suppresses insulin, insulin-like growth factor 1, and the production of growth hormone. Thus, it is unique to find IGF-2-related lower blood glucose levels in tumors such as anaplastic large-cell lymphomas [17]. This case of a middle-aged gentleman revealed that although rare, sometimes hypoglycemia may be due to the release of IGF-2 in nonsolid neoplasms such as anaplastic large-cell lymphomas. Because most literature has shown that hypoglycemia may be associated with the uncommon tumors of the pancreas such as insulinomas, however, hypoglycemia can also be found in non-islet cell tumors outside the pancreas by following both insulin-dependent and -independent mechanisms [18].

Furthermore, the existing study by Gorden et al. who investigated 7 patients with hypoglycemia and lymphoma found low levels of insulin-like growth factor in the blood. They found these levels lower than the normal population [19]. On the other hand, some patients with hypoglycemia with Hodgkin's disease showed reduced plasma insulin levels and proinsulin. However, these patients' levels for C-peptide and insulin-like growth factor 1 were found lower, which may indicate a reasonable relationship between non-islet cell tumors such as anaplastic large-cell lymphomas and IGF-2-associated hypoglycemia.

To recapitulate, it may be easy to pay attention to hypoglycemia in diabetic patients or patients diagnosed with islet cell tumors. However, it is important to pay attention to the history of the patient, histological features, and other investigations that may help to reach the cause of severe hypoglycemia in patients not suspected of islet cell tumors. A holistic approach should be made to make a connection between hypoglycemia non-islet cell tumors such as anaplastic large-cell lymphomas to avoid missing such cases. One may tend to miss these tumors when a patient presents with hypoglycemia because it is not a common finding in such patients with nonsolid tumors who may be either missed or diagnosed late with anaplastic large-cell lymphomas. Therefore, keeping hypoglycemia in mind as a possible finding in such patients, such patients presenting with severe hypoglycemia should be ruled out for nonsolid tumors or hematological diseases to manage them on time and save their lives. For example, one may plan to conduct an initial evaluation to determine the cause of hypoglycemia by taking a detailed history to find out the nature of symptoms and how these are related to time, for example, is it related to a meal or not [20]. Furthermore, the physician should also evaluate the patient for any signs and symptoms of the tumor as well as medications taken by the patient. This can be followed by laboratory work-up of insulin-like growth factors, insulin, C-peptide, and plasma glucose.

3.1. Learning Points. Hypoglycemia is a rare finding among patients diagnosed with anaplastic large-cell lymphomas. One should suspect hypoglycemia in patients diagnosed with nonsolid tumors such as anaplastic large-cell lymphomas. Patients presenting with severe hypoglycemia should be ruled out for nonsolid tumors or hematological disease.

Consent

Informed consent was taken from the patient.

Authors' Contributions

Dr. Raeed, the primary author, is the only author of this study who contributed to this work and is the sole author of this manuscript.

References

[1] O. Kamel, L. Rozen, S. Lecomte, P. Heimann, and A. Demulder, "Pleural effusion as a rare sign of anaplastic large-cell lymphoma in a COVID-19 patient: a case report and literature review," *The International Journal of Literary Humanities*, vol. 43, no. 4, pp. O211–O213, 2021.

[2] O. Fatusi, O. Gbolahan, F. Owotade, O. Rotimi, S. Edward, and K. Adelusola, "Anaplastic large cell lymphoma: case report and literature review," *Journal of Oral and Maxillofacial Surgery*, vol. 68, no. 4, pp. 884–888, 2010.

[3] M. Agnihotri, K. Kothari, L. Naik, and S. Patil, "Anaplastic large cell lymphoma: a great mimic on cytology," *Journal of Cytology*, vol. 34, no. 3, Article ID 165, 2017.

[4] A. Kreuter, I. Pantelaki, A. L. Michalowitz et al., "CD30-positive primary cutaneous anaplastic large cell lymphoma with coexistent pseudocarcinomatous hyperplasia," *Clinical Experimental Dermatology*, vol. 43, no. 5, pp. 585–588, 2018.
[5] N. Moodley, P. Nombona, and A. Mosam, "Primary cutaneous anaplastic large-cell lymphoma," *Dermatopathology*, vol. 6, no. 2, pp. 163–169, 2019.
[6] E. Y. Kao, S. K. R. Mukkamalla, and D. T. Lynch, *ALK Negative Anaplastic Large Cell Lymphoma*, StatPearls, Treasure Island, FL, USA, 2021.
[7] N. Mahajan, I. Gupta, A. Sharma, and K. Gupta, "A rare case of anaplastic large cell lymphoma," *Indian Journal of Pathology*, vol. 4, no. 3, pp. 473–475, 2017.
[8] A. Shustov and L. Soma, "Anaplastic large cell lymphoma: contemporary concepts and optimal management," *Cancer Treatment and Research*, vol. 176, pp. 127–144, 2019.
[9] X. Yu, J. Zhang, K. Xu, M. Li, and Z. Yao, "Skin involvement as the first symptom of rapidly progressive ALK-positive systemic anaplastic large cell lymphoma," *Clinical Experimental Dermatology*, vol. 42, no. 5, pp. 539–542, 2017.
[10] V. Leventaki, S. Bhattacharyya, and M. S. Lim, "Pathology and genetics of anaplastic large cell lymphoma," *Seminars in Diagnostic Pathology*, vol. 37, no. 1, pp. 57–71, 2020.
[11] M. Mitobe, K. Kawamoto, T. Suzuki et al., "Anaplastic large cell lymphoma, with 1, 25 (OH) 2D3-mediated hypercalcemia: a case report," *Journal of Clinical Experimental Hematopathology*, vol. 59, no. 1, pp. 22–28, 2019.
[12] K. L. Feldenzer and J. Sarno, "Hypercalcemia of malignancy," *Journal of the advanced practitioner in oncology*, vol. 9, no. 5, p. 496, 2018.
[13] L. Akavia and I. Krause, "Extreme hypoglycaemia in anaplastic large cell lymphoma," *European journal of case reports in internal medicine*, vol. 4, no. 2, Article ID 000510, 2017.
[14] A. P. Sciallis, M. E. Law, D. J. Inwards et al., "Mucosal CD30-positive T-cell lymphoproliferations of the head and neck show a clinicopathologic spectrum similar to cutaneous CD30-positive T-cell lymphoproliferative disorders," *Modern Pathology*, vol. 25, no. 7, pp. 983–992, 2012.
[15] S. Huang, T. S. C. Ng, X. Xu, and H. Chen, "A case report of primary anaplastic large cell lymphoma arising from the trachea," *Translational Cancer Research*, vol. 8, no. 2, pp. 699–704, 2019.
[16] S. Noguchi, Y. Kubo, M. Araki et al., "Big insulin-like growth factor 2-producing tumor in a hypoglycemic dog," *Veterinary pathology*, vol. 57, no. 3, pp. 432–436, 2020.
[17] J. Schovanek, L. Cibickova, F. Ctvrtlik et al., "Hypoglycemia as a symptom of neoplastic disease, with a focus on insulin-like growth factors producing tumors," *Journal of Cancer*, vol. 10, no. 26, pp. 6475–6480, 2019.
[18] J. W. B. De Groot, B. Rikhof, J. van Doorn et al., "Non-islet cell tumour-induced hypoglycaemia: a review of the literature including two new cases," *Endocrine-Related Cancer*, vol. 14, no. 4, pp. 979–993, 2007.
[19] P. Gorden, C. M. Hendricks, C. R. Kahn, K. Megyesi, and J. Roth, "Hypoglycemia associated with non-islet-cell tumor and insulin-like growth factors," *New England Journal of Medicine*, vol. 305, no. 24, pp. 1452–1455, 1981.
[20] B. Abdulhadi, C. Anastasopoulou, and P. Lekprasert, "Tumor-Induced hypoglycemia: an unusual case report and review of literature," *AACE Clinical Case Reports*, vol. 7, no. 1, pp. 80–83, 2021.

29

Was it an Adrenocortical Adenoma or an Adrenocortical Carcinoma? Limitation of the Weiss Scoring System in Determining the Malignant Potential of Adrenocortical Tumor: Report on Two Cases

Cheuk-Lik Wong,[1] Chun-Kit Fok,[1] Yuk-Kit Chan,[2] Vicki Ho-Kee Tam,[1] and Lai-Ming Fung[1]

[1]*Department of Medicine and Geriatrics, Caritas Medical Centre, Shamshuipo, Kowloon, Hong Kong*
[2]*Department of Medicine and Geriatrics, Pok Oi Hospital, Yuen Long, The New Territories, Hong Kong*

Correspondence should be addressed to Cheuk-Lik Wong; cl.wong@qualigenics.com

Academic Editor: Toshihiro Kita

Background. Adrenocortical carcinoma (ACC) is a rare endocrine malignancy. An accurate diagnosis of ACC is of paramount importance as it greatly impacts the management and prognosis of a patient. However, the differentiation between early stage, low-grade ACC and adrenocortical adenoma (ACA) may not always be straightforward. The recommended classification system, namely, the Weiss scoring system, is not without flaws. We herein report two cases of ACC which were initially diagnosed as ACA according to the Weiss scoring system but developed distant metastases in subsequent years. *Case Presentation.* Case 1: A 60-year-old Chinese woman presented with a recent onset of worsening of blood pressure control and clinical features of Cushing's syndrome. Investigations confirmed ACTH-independent endogenous hypercortisolism, and a CT abdomen showed a 6 cm right adrenal mass. Twenty-four-hour urine steroid profiling revealed co-secretion of adrenal androgens and atypical steroid metabolites. Laparoscopic right adrenalectomy was performed, and pathology of the tumor was classified as an ACA by the Weiss scoring system. Four years later, the patient presented with an abrupt onset of severe hypercortisolism and was found to have a metastatic recurrence in the liver and peritoneum. The patient received a combination of mitotane, systemic chemotherapy, and palliative debulking surgery and succumbed 8.5 years after the initial presentation due to respiratory failure with extensive pulmonary metastases. *Case 2*: A 68-year-old Chinese woman presented with acute bilateral pulmonary embolism and was found to have a 3 cm left adrenal mass. Hormonal workup confirmed ACTH-independent endogenous hypercortisolism, and laparoscopic left adrenalectomy revealed an ACA according to the Weiss scoring system. Five years later, she presented with recurrent hypercortisolism due to hepatic and peritoneal metastases. The patient had progressive disease despite mitotane therapy and succumbed 7 years after initial presentation. *Conclusions.* Although the Weiss scoring system is recommended as the reference pathological classification system to diagnose adrenocortical carcinoma, there remain tumors of borderline malignant potential which may escape accurate classification. Various alternative classification systems and algorithms exist but none are proven to be perfect. Clinicians should recognize the potential limitation of these histological criteria and scoring systems and incorporate other clinical parameters, such as the pattern of hormonal secretion, urinary steroid profiling, and radiographic features, to improve the prognostication and surveillance strategy of these tumors.

1. Background

Adrenocortical carcinoma (ACC) is a rare, highly aggressive malignancy with a reported annual incidence of 0.7–2 per one million people, while adrenocortical adenoma (ACA) is one of the commonest adrenal tumors and is benign [1, 2]. An accurate diagnosis of ACC is of paramount importance as it greatly impacts the management, prognosis, and surveillance strategy of a patient. Although ACC can be readily diagnosed in the presence of metastases, the differentiation between early stage ACC and ACA could be challenging histologically, especially in the setting of a well-differentiated low-grade ACC [3–5]. The Weiss scoring system, first proposed in 1984 and subsequently modified in 2002, is the most widely employed pathology classification system in adrenocortical tumors and is recommended as the gold standard for the diagnosis of ACC by international guidelines [2, 6, 7]. Nine histological criteria, which are based on the morphological assessment of tumor structure, cytological features, and invasive tumor properties under light microscopy, are graded by the pathologist, and a diagnosis of malignancy is made if three or more criteria are present [6]. Despite a very high diagnostic performance, 100% sensitivity and specificity could not be achieved. Factors affecting its diagnostic performance include tumors of borderline malignant potential with only one or two fitting criteria, interobserver reproducibility, adequacy of tumor sampling, low applicability among nonexpert pathologists, and ACC variants [8–11]. Other histopathological algorithm and scoring system, namely, the reticulin algorithm and Helsinki score, are recently developed and validated [12, 13]. They are shown to be highly accurate in differentiating between benign and malignant adrenocortical tumors with almost 100% or nearly 100% sensitivity and specificity, but their routine use is yet to be widely adopted [14]. Nevertheless, certain clinical, biochemical, and radiological features may provide physicians with important complementary information to predict the malignant potential of an adrenocortical tumor. We therein report two cases with presumable ACA years ago and several years later presented with Cushing's syndrome and metastatic ACC, highlighting the limitation of the Weiss scoring system and the importance of integrating clinical, biochemical, radiological, and histological information to accurately determine the malignant potential of an adrenocortical tumor.

2. Case Presentation

2.1. Case 1. Patient A, a 60-year-old Chinese lady, who had a history of gastroesophageal reflux disease, hypertension, and hyperlipidemia, presented with insidious onset of right loin pain for 3 months in June 2012. She also had worsening of blood pressure control over the past few months and occasional palpitations. Physical examination was notable for moon face and buffalo hump suggesting Cushing's syndrome. Computed tomography (CT) of the abdomen performed for suspected urinary tract pathology showed a 6 cm right adrenal mass (Figure 1). Subsequent hormonal investigations (Table 1) confirmed the diagnosis of ACTH-independent Cushing's syndrome, which was likely due to a cortisol-secreting adrenal tumor. There was also co-secretion of adrenal androgens and atypical steroid metabolites.

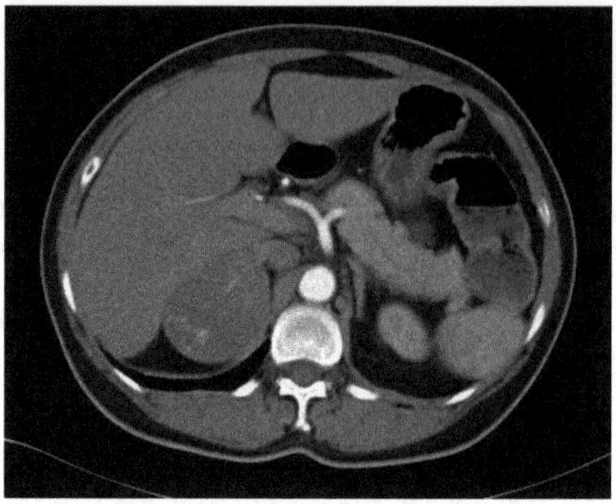

Figure 1: CT abdomen of Patient A on 9 August 2012. A $6.4 \times 5.2 \times 5.8$ cm heterogeneously enhancing mass in the right adrenal gland with pre-contrast HU 35.4 (red arrow).

The patient underwent laparoscopic right adrenalectomy in August 2012. The pathology of the resected tumor was reported to be ACA. Postoperatively, hypertension was cured and antihypertensives were stopped. A follow-up CT at 9 months after the operation did not show any evidence of recurrence, and urine steroid profiling (USP) at 1.5 years postoperatively showed normalization of the previously abnormal steroid metabolites together with normal free cortisol and androgens. She also developed adrenal insufficiency and was maintained on hydrocortisone replacement postoperatively until 2015.

In May 2016, the patient presented to us with a relatively acute onset of ACTH-independent hypercortisolism with marked hypertension and fluid overload in addition to clinical (hirsutism) and biochemical hyperandrogenism (Table 1). ^{18}F-fluorodeoxyglucose positron emission tomography/computed tomography (^{18}FDG-PET/CT) scan showed a large solid mass at the right lobe of the liver (maximum standardized uptake value [SUV_{max}] 8.4), a small nodule around the previous right adrenalectomy bed (SUV_{max} 2.1), and multiple foci of hypermetabolic peritoneal lesions in both sides of the abdominal cavity (highest SUV_{max} 4.6) (Figure 2). A laparoscopic peritoneal biopsy was performed. Histologically, the biopsy showed a metastatic carcinoma composed of large polygonal cells with abundant pink cytoplasm arranged in trabeculae infiltrating a fibromyxoid stroma. Nuclear hyperchromatism and prominent nucleoli were evident in the carcinoma cells. Immunohistochemical studies showed positivity towards synaptophysin, Melan A, and inhibin. Ki-67 proliferative index was 50% (Figure 3). A pathological diagnosis of metastatic adrenocortical carcinoma was made.

We retrospectively reviewed the histology of the right adrenal tumor which was removed in August 2012 and compared it with that of the peritoneal nodule. The

TABLE 1: Biochemical investigations of Patient A in 2012 and 2016.

Test	Date		Reference Range
	8/2012	5/2016	
Serum			
Renin	0.45	2.91	0.15–2.33 ng/mL/hr
Aldosterone	267	<80	28–444 pmol/L
Estradiol	83	222	<147 pmol/L
Testosterone	3.8	4.2	0.28–1.2 nmol/L
DHEA-S	29.1	33.0	0.5–5.6 umol/L
1 mg overnight dexamethasone suppression test (Cortisol)	518	666	<50 nmol/L
ACTH	11	<5	10- 46 pg/ml
Urine			
24-h urinary free cortisol	188	2798	24–140 nmol/ day
24-hr urine adrenaline	26	—	<110 nmol/day
24-hr urine noradrenaline	181	—	<440 nmol/day
24-hr urine metanephrine	105	—	<275 nmol/day
24-hr urine normetanephrine	120	—	<240 nmol/day
Urinary steroid profiling	Markedly increased free cortisol, cortisol metabolites, and androgen. Also, elevated levels of THS, 3-α, 16-α, 20-α-pregnenetriol, 3-β,16-α, 20-α-pregnenetriol, and 17-β androstenediol	—	
Low dose dexamethasone suppression test			
	Day 0 / Day 2		
Cortisol	469 / 450	—	<50

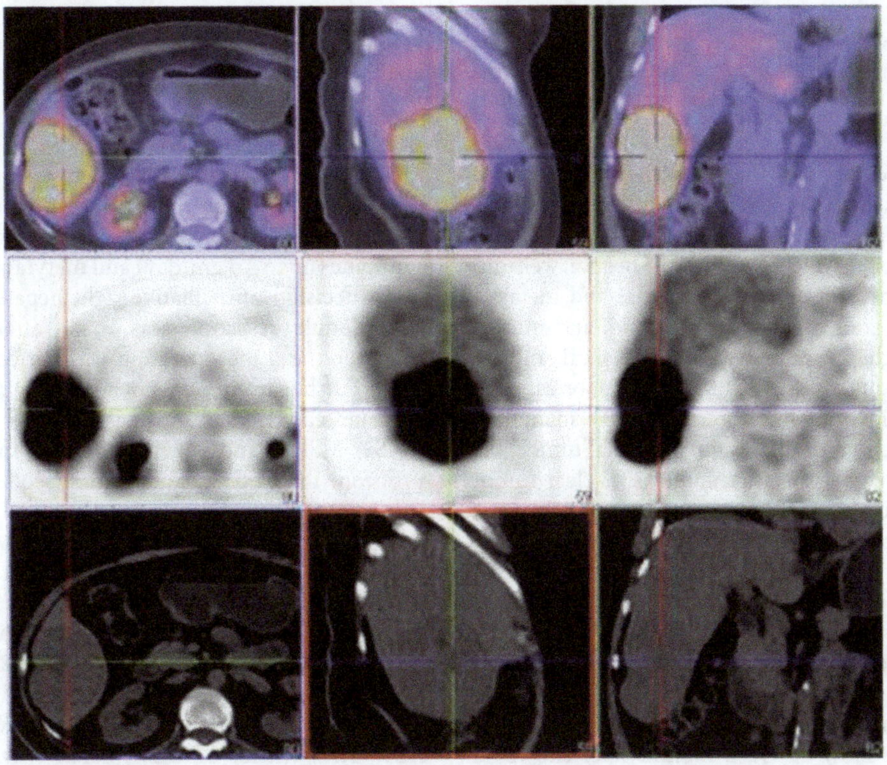

FIGURE 2: ^{18}FDG-PET-CT scan of Patient A on 6 July 2016. CT abdomen of Madam F on 9 August 2012. An 8 cm liver mass (SUVmax 8.4) was found at segment 8.

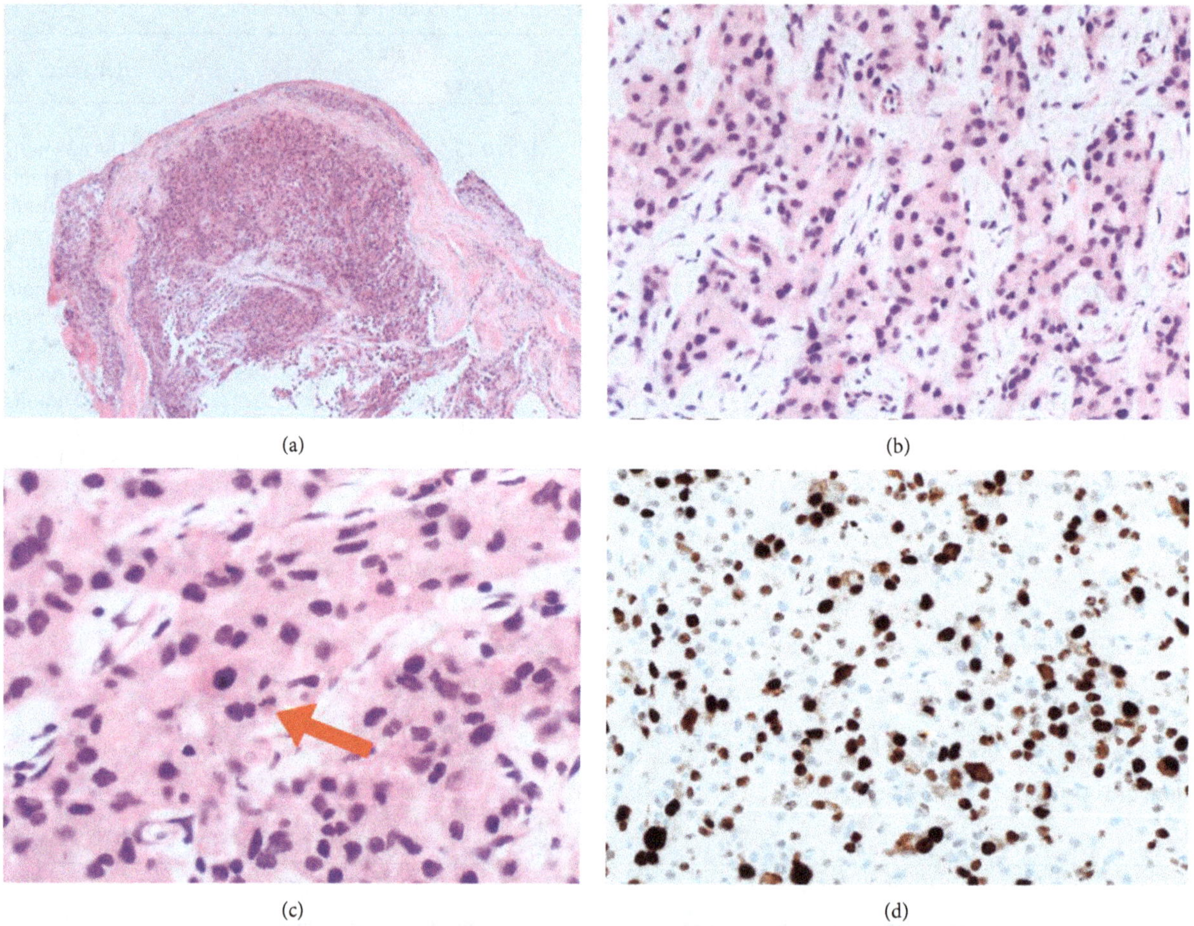

Figure 3: Photomicrographs of peritoneal nodule biopsy of Patient A. (a) Peritoneal nodule section (H&E × 40). (b) Tumor cells arranged in the cords and trabeculae (H&E × 200). (c) Hyperchromatic nuclei of tumor cells. The presence of mitosis was noted in a tumor cell (red arrow) (H&E × 400). (d) Ki-67 proliferative index was 50% (IHC × 400).

morphological appearance of the previous adrenal tumor shared a focal resemblance with that of the peritoneal nodule, suggesting that the current tumor might be arising from the original one, which would have been a well-differentiated ACC and had presently recurred and metastasized. The focal myxoid change was observed, and mitosis was up to 4/50 high power field (HPF). Atypical mitosis, necrosis, broad fibrous bands, vascular invasion, or capsular invasion was not identified. Although frankly malignant features were not present in the original adrenal tumor, the presence of a diffuse growth pattern and <25% clear tumor cells (Figure 4), which were not mentioned previously, were suspicious of malignancy.

Mitotane was initiated once the diagnosis was made in July 2016 with the dose titrated to maintain a target mitotane level of 14–20 micrograms/ml. A follow-up CT abdomen 4 months later showed progressive disease with enlarging liver metastasis (up to ~10 cm) and peritoneal nodules. Chemotherapy with etoposide (EP) and cisplatin was added in January 2017, and follow-up CT 2 months later showed a reduction of peritoneal metastases and stable liver metastasis. EP was continued for five cycles until May 2017, but in July 2017, progressive disease was noted again on interval imaging with enlarging liver metastasis. At the same time, the patient became highly symptomatic with marked hypercortisolism which was uncontrolled despite high-dose mitotane (up to 4.5 gm/day) and metyrapone (up to 6 g/day).

A decision on palliative right hepatectomy and peritoneal nodule resection was made after multidisciplinary discussion and the operation was performed in September 2017. Further immunohistochemical studies showed intact immunoreactivity of mismatch repair proteins (MLH1, PMS2, MSH2, and MSH6) and less than 1% PD-L1 expression. Targeted next-generation sequencing on extracted tumor cell DNA did not reveal any variants or small insertion/deletion in the following genes: *AKT1, AKT3, ALK, ARAF, AURKA, BAP1, BRAF, BRCA1, BRCA2, CBFB, CCND1, CCND2, CCND3, CCNE1, CD79A, CD79B, CDH1, CDK4, CDK6, CDKN2A, CSF1R, CTNNB1, DDR2, EGFR, ERBB2, ERBB3, ERBB4, ESR1, EZH2, FGFR1, FGFR2, FGFR3, FLT1, FLT3, FLT4, GNA11, GNAQ, HGF, HIF1A, HRAS, IDH1, IDH2, IGF1R, JAK1, JAK2, JAK3, KDM6A, KDR, KIT, KRAS, LRRK2, MAP2K1, MAP2K2, MAP2K4, MAP3K1, MAP3K9, MAPK1, MAPK3, MET, MPL, MST1R, MTOR, MYD88, NF1, NOTCH1, NOTCH2, NOTCH3, NRAS, NRG1, NTRK1, NTRK2, NTRK3, PAK6, PDGFRA,*

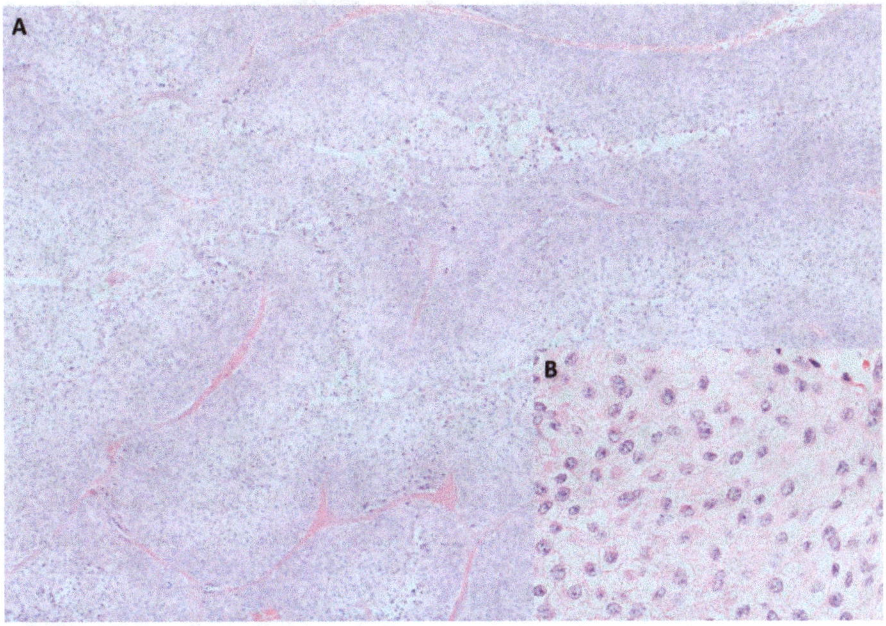

FIGURE 4: Photomicrographs of right adrenal tumor of Patient A on pathology review. (a) Diffuse growth pattern (H&E × 40). (b) Regular nuclei and eosinophilic cytoplasm of tumor cells (H&E × 400).

PIK3CA, PIK3R1, PTCH1, PTEN, PTK2, PTK2B, RAF1, RET, RHOA, ROS1, SMO, SRC, STK11, SYK, TOP1, TSC1, and *TSC2*. The postoperative course was complicated with bilateral subphrenic collection, left pleural effusion, pulmonary embolism, and steroid withdrawal syndrome which necessitated several drainage procedures, anticoagulation, and prolonged hospitalization for 3 months. After extended rehabilitation, the patient gradually regained independent self-care and functional ability.

In April 2018 (about 7 months after palliative debulking surgery), Patient A was found to have bilateral lung metastases. Chemotherapy was resumed with EP and subsequently the addition of doxorubicin (i.e., EDP) in view of progression in October 2018. She completed 6 cycles of EDP in May 2019 and enjoyed stable disease until August 2019, when she had disease progression with increasing pulmonary and peritoneal metastases. Gemcitabine and carboplatin were initiated as second-line palliative chemotherapy in September 2019. However, disease progression was again noted after 3 cycles, and chemotherapy was stopped. Patient A was then offered palliative care and she subsequently passed away due to respiratory failure with extensive pulmonary metastases in January 2021, almost 5 years after the relapse of the disease and 9 years after her initial presentation.

2.2. Case 2. Patient B, a 68-year-old Chinese lady, whose past medical history was remarkable for hypertension, presented to us in August 2011 for acute shortness of breath, chest discomfort, and transient loss of consciousness. She was later found to have extensive bilateral acute pulmonary embolism and was treated with intravenous thrombolysis followed by anticoagulation (Figure 5(a)). After stabilization, an abdominal US examination done for malignancy screening showed a 3 cm left suprarenal which was later confirmed to be a left adrenal mass on a CT scan (Figure 5(b)). Further examination of the patient showed clinical features of Cushing's syndrome which was confirmed with hormonal testing (Table 2). ACTH was suppressed, pointing to a diagnosis of a cortisol-producing adrenal tumor, and USP only showed elevated free cortisol and cortisol metabolites.

Laparoscopic left adrenalectomy was performed in May 2012. Intraoperatively, a 5 cm left adrenal tumor was found and removed. Histologically, the lesion consisted of nests and trabeculae of medium-sized tumor cells and a rich capillary network. The tumor cells were polygonal, with pale to amphophilic cytoplasm, as well as round, deeply stained nuclei with nuclear pleomorphism (Figure 6). The maximal mitotic count was 5 in 50 HPFs. One fibrous septum thicker than 1 HPF was noted. There were also some areas of myxoid change and a large area of old hemorrhage while necrosis was not seen. A pathological diagnosis of an adrenocortical tumor was made, and the tumor was classified as an adenoma (ACA) according to the Weiss system. The patient was put on hydrocortisone 10 mg twice a day for postoperative adrenal insufficiency and morning cortisol remained low at 156 nmol/L in August 2016.

However, in November 2016, the patient was noted to have the reappearance of Cushing's syndrome with central obesity and buffalo hump. Repeat hormonal testing showed relapse of endogenous ACTH-independent Cushing's syndrome as well as the presence of markedly elevated 17-hydroxyprogesterone (17-OHP) metabolites that were not seen in the previous urinary steroid profiling. An abdominal CT showed local recurrence of a 2 cm nodule at the left adrenal bed, a 4 cm liver mass, multiple peritoneal nodules,

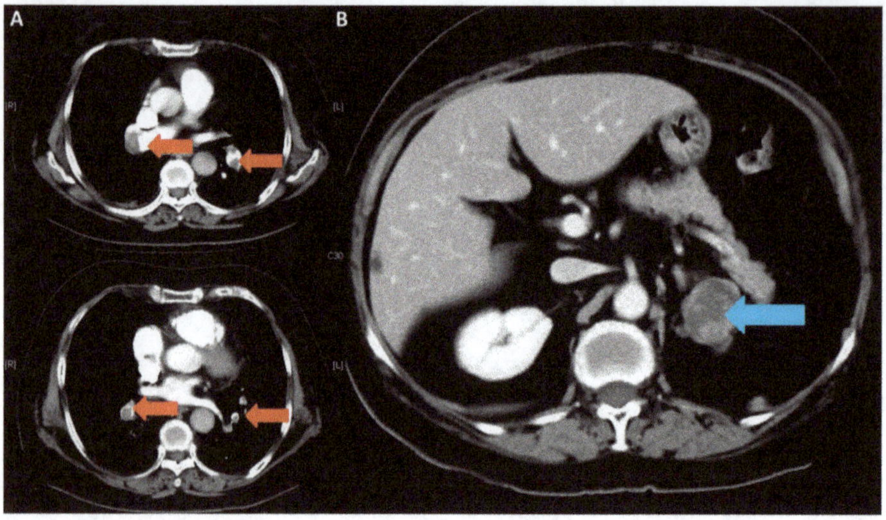

Figure 5: (a) CT pulmonary artery of Patient B on 25 August 2011 showing extensive bilateral pulmonary embolism (red arrow). (b) CT abdomen of Patient B on 13 October 2011. A 3.6 × 3.5 cm lobulated heterogeneously enhancing lesion with a focal calcified spot at the lateral limb of left adrenal with 30HU in pre-contrast scan (blue arrow).

Table 2: Biochemical investigations of Patient B in 2011 and 2016.

Test	Date		Reference Range
	11/2011	12/2016	
Serum			
Renin	0.75	—	0.15–2.33 ng/mL/hr
Aldosterone	81	—	28–444 pmol/L
Estradiol	—	<133	<147 pmol/L
Testosterone	—	0.6	0.28–1.2 nmol/L
DHEA-S	—	33.0	0.5–5.6 umol/L
1 mg overnight dexamethasone suppression test (Cortisol)	612	666	<50 nmol/L
ACTH	13	<5	10–46 pg/ml
Urine			
24 h	722	689	24–140 nmol/ day
24-hr urine adrenaline	32	—	<110 nmol/day
24-hr urine noradrenaline	298	—	<440 nmol/day
24-hr urine metanephrine	36	—	<275 nmol/day
24-hr urine normetanephrine	106	—	<240 nmol/day
Urinary steroid profiling	Free cortisol and cortisol intermediates and metabolites were grossly elevated	Moderate to large increases in free cortisol and cortisol metabolites. 17-OHP metabolites were grossly elevated	
Low-dose dexamethasone suppression test			
	Day 0 Day 2	Day 0 Day 2	
Cortisol	632	558 348 338	<50

and recurrent pulmonary embolism (Figure 7). Apixaban was started for the treatment of pulmonary embolism, and US-guided fine needle aspiration of the liver mass in February 2017 showed tumor cells with round nuclei and finely vacuolated cytoplasm that were arranged in anastomosing cords with delicate vasculature, resembling the previous left adrenal tumor (Figure 8). Immunohistochemical studies revealed strong and diffuse staining for Melan A and weak staining for inhibin in the tumor cells, which were consistent with an adrenocortical origin, confirming the diagnosis of metastatic adrenocortical carcinoma.

Patient B declined surgical debulking of the metastases due to old age (73 years old at that time) and risk of open surgery, while percutaneous radiofrequency ablation was deemed not feasible anatomically. Mitotane was thus started as monotherapy in February 2017 and titrated gradually to 3 g daily, which was the maximally tolerated dose to achieve a mitotane level of approximately 11 micrograms/ml. Follow-up ^{18}FDG-PET/CT 8 months later (in October 2017) showed a mild interval reduction of liver metastasis (Figure 9(a)) together with stable disease in the left adrenal bed and peritoneal metastases.

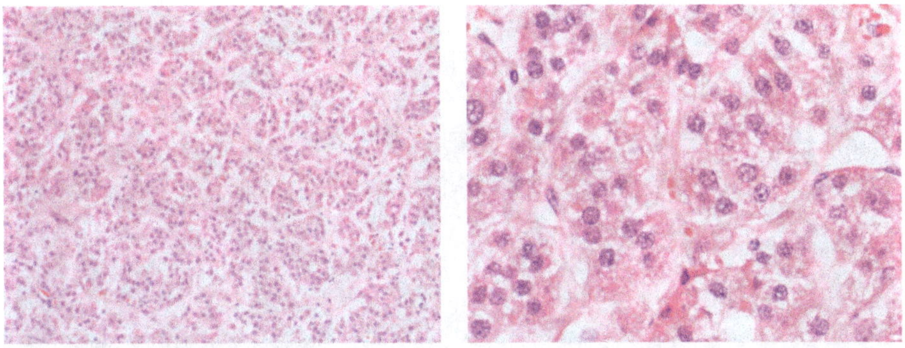

(a) (b)

FIGURE 6: Photomicrograph of left adrenal tumor of Patient B. (a) Tumor cells in trabecular pattern (H&E × 100). (b) Tumor cells demonstrate nuclei of variable size and eosinophilic granular cytoplasm (H&E × 400).

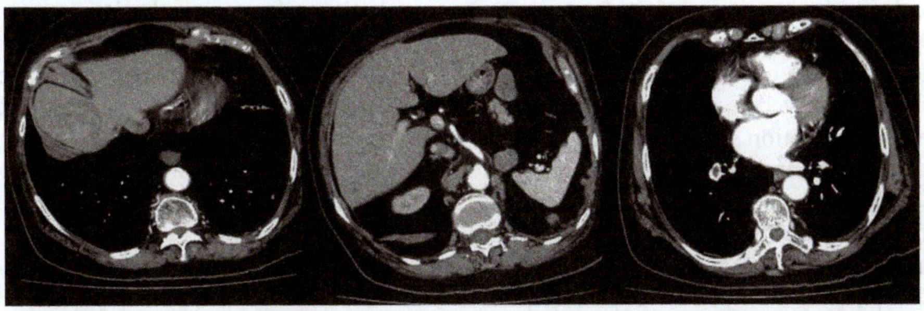

FIGURE 7: CT abdomen of Patient B on 30 December 2016. (a) Presence of liver metastasis. (b) Nodule at left adrenal bed and peritoneal nodule posterior to spleen. (c) Right descending pulmonary artery embolism.

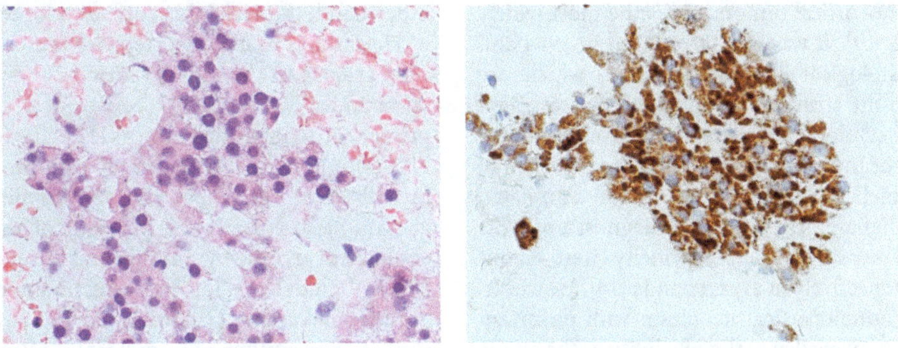

(a) (b)

FIGURE 8: Photomicrograph of liver mass biopsy of Patient B. (a) Tumor cells with round nuclei and finely vacuolated cytoplasm that were arranged in anastomosing cords with delicate vasculature, resembling the previous left adrenal tumor (Figure 6) (H&E × 400). (b) Immunohistochemical staining showed diffuse positivity for Melan A.

Despite the initial response, Patient B experienced significant progression of the disease since April 2018 with the growth of liver metastasis up to about 8 cm (Figure 9(b)). Systemic chemotherapy was also declined by the patient and she was managed medically with palliative intent. Patient B subsequently ran a downhill course and passed away in October 2018, 2 years after the recurrence of her disease and 7 years after her initial presentation.

3. Discussion

Histopathology remains the gold standard for diagnosing ACC and should be obtained in all patients [2]. Despite the fact that ACC often manifests clinical aggressiveness, its histological differentiation from benign ACA is not always straightforward, especially in a patient with early stage, low-grade disease which may behave more indolently [3, 15]. About 10% of ACC may be misdiagnosed according to two

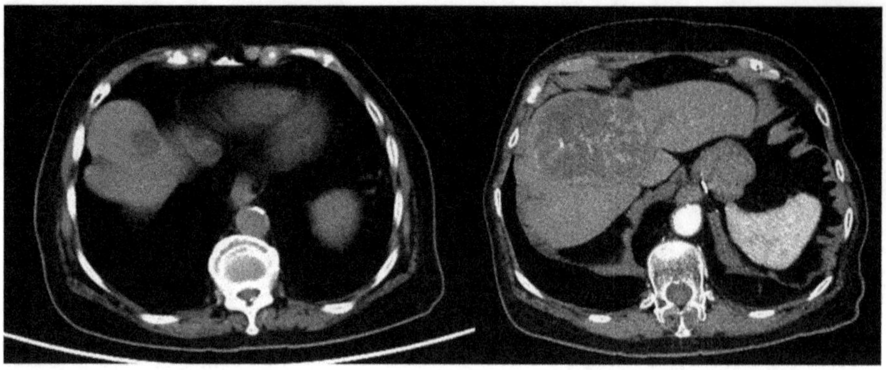

Figure 9: (a) Non-contrast CT abdomen of Patient B in October 2017 showing reduction of liver metastasis 8 months after mitotane (compared with Figure 7). (b) Contrast CT abdomen of Patient B in April 2018 showing the progression of liver metastasis 14 months after mitotane.

large observational cohorts. In the German ACC Registry, 21 of 161 patients (13%) had the diagnosis of ACC revised by the reference pathologist, while a misdiagnosis rate of 9% (26 out of 300 patients) was observed in another large Italian series [10, 16]. Several classification systems (Table 3) have been proposed for distinguishing between benign and malignant adrenocortical tumors, with varying sets of histological criteria with or without additional clinical/biochemical parameters but none were proved to be perfect [6, 7, 12, 13, 17, 18]. Importantly, no single histopathological parameter is pathognomonic of ACC. In the latest clinical guidelines co-authored by the European Society of Endocrinology (ESE) and the European Network for the Study of Adrenal Tumors (ENS@T), the Weiss scoring system is recommended as the preferred system for classifying benign and malignant adrenocortical tumors and is the most widely employed system [2, 19]. It was first introduced in 1984 and comprises nine histological criteria (Table 3), which are graded according to the stringent morphological assessment of tumor structure, cytological features, and invasive tumor properties under light microscopy [2, 8, 20]. The presence of three or more of which was reported to be highly correlated with subsequent malignant behavior and is diagnostic of ACC [10]. The reported sensitivity and specificity were about 86–95% and 90%, respectively in expert hands [14]. However, borderline cases of adrenocortical neoplasm with uncertain malignant potential may challenge the reliability of the Weiss system, and these tumors often have a Weiss score of 1–3 [2, 8, 11]. It has been observed that adrenocortical tumors with a Weiss score of 3 or less could eventually turn out to be malignant ACC, posing particular challenges in the postoperative surveillance in these patients [3, 8, 11, 21]. Interobserver reproducibility is another factor affecting the accuracy of the Weiss scoring system as some features, namely diffuse growth, necrosis, sinusoidal, vascular and capsular invasion, and nuclear atypia, are determined subjectively [3, 8, 22]. Other factors potentially undermining the diagnostic performance of the Weiss scoring system include the inadequacy of tumor sampling, increasing prevalence of incidentally detected small ACC, low applicability among nonexpert pathologists, and ACC variants [8, 11].

The imperfection of the Weiss scoring system has instigated the development of a more unequivocal pathological classification system over the past three decades. In 2002, Aubert et al. modified the Weiss scoring system to include only five of the original nine items with a maximum score of 7. Being easier to use in clinical practice and more reproducible, the modified Weiss score has a reported specificity of 96.9% (vs. 90.2% in the original score) [7]. More recently, the reticulin algorithm and the Helsinki score (Table 3) have been validated and are shown to be highly accurate in differentiating between benign and malignant adrenocortical tumors with 100% or nearly 100% sensitivity and specificity [3, 4, 14]. The rationale of the reticulin algorithm relies on the histochemical assessment of the reticulin network, which is commonly disrupted in ACC [12]. On the other hand, the Helsinki score, developed by the University of Helsinki, is based on a stepwise regression analysis of the nine criteria in the Weiss scoring system and the proliferation index Ki-67 in 177 consecutive adult patients with primary adrenocortical tumors [13]. The final model consists of 3 criteria only and correlates with prognosis [23]. While interobserver agreement and applicability among pathologists remain a drawback for both of these systems, these could be overcome by training and are endorsed by the ESE/ENS@T guidelines for the assessment of tumors of borderline malignant potential [2, 14, 24]. However, these systems were either not applicable (reticulin algorithm) or not available (Helsinki score) at the time when our patients received their first operation. Latest effort and research have been put into the development of novel immunohistochemical (e.g., insulin-like growth factor-2 [IGF-2], MAD2L1, CNNB1, and markers for cell proliferation, mitotic spindle regulation [p53, BUB1Bm HURP, and NEK2], and DNA damage repair [PBK and y-H2Ax]) and genomic markers (e.g., aberrations in methylome and transcriptome, micro-RNA expression, chromosomal aberrations, and DNA mutation profile) that can improve the distinction between ACA and ACC [14]. Although these might be valuable in diagnosing ACC, especially when the diagnosis cannot be made definitively on histopathological and/or clinical grounds, protocol standardization, availability, cost,

Table 3: Summary of published classification systems for adrenocortical tumors and their diagnostic threshold for adrenocortical carcinoma.

Criteria	Weiss [6]	Hough [16]	Van Slooten [17]	Modified Weiss [7]	Reticulin algorithm [12]	Helsinki score [13]
Nuclear atypia (Fuhrman grade III or IV)	1	0.39	2.1			
Nuclear hyperchromatism			2.6			
Abnormal nucleoli			4.1			
Atypical mitoses	1			1		
Mitoses > 5/50 HPF >10/100 HPF > 2/10 HPF	1	0.60	9.0	2	Optional	3
Clear cells < 25% of total tumor volume	1			2		
Architecture diffuse loss of normal structure	1	0.92	1.6			
Venous invasion	1	0.92				
Capsular invasion	1	0.37		1		
Sinusoidal invasion	1					
Vascular invasion					Optional	
Capsular or vascular invasion	1		3.3			
Necrosis	1	0.69		1	Optional	5
Regressive changes (necrosis, hemorrhage, fibrosis, or calcification)			5.7			
Thick fibrous band		1.00				
Response to ACTH (17-hydroxysteroids increased two times after 50 mcg of IV ACTH)		0.42				
Urinary 17-ketosteroids (10 mg/1 g creatinine 24 h)		0.50				
Cushing's syndrome with virilism, virilism alone, or no clinical manifestations		0.42				
Weight loss (>10 Ib/3 months)		2.00				
Tumor mass (>100 g)		0.60				
Disruption of reticulin network					Mandatory	
Proliferative index (Ki-67) in the most proliferative area of tumor						1-100
Diagnostic threshold of ACC	≥3	>2	≥8	≥3	Mandatory criteria + any 1 optional	3 × mitoses + 5 necrosis + PI in % by Ki-67 > 8.5

and large genetic diversity of ACC are the main hindrances of their routine incorporation in clinical practice.

The diagnostic difficulty of ACC is well exemplified in the present two cases where the features of overt malignancy were not evident pathologically. The presence of only a diffuse growth pattern and <25% clear cells of the tumor volume in Patient A, and the presence of borderline mitosis of 5/50 HPF and regressive changes (fibrosis and hemorrhage) in Patient B would not be sufficient to classify either tumor as ACC under the Weiss scoring system or other systems (Tables 4 and 5). Only the Van Slooten system would classify Patient B's tumor as ACC retrospectively (Table 5). Laparoscopic surgery may have further complicated the diagnostic challenge during which the tumor was fragmented upon surgical manipulation, thus affecting the integrity of the tissue specimens to be examined and making a detailed assessment of capsular and stromal invasion difficult. Laparoscopic adrenalectomy for ACC has been linked to inferior survival and higher recurrence rates, where rupture of the tumor capsule and peritoneal seeding are recognized as major factors for recurrence [9, 19]. Nevertheless, the identification of the above histopathological features, either individually or in combination, should alert the clinician of the malignant potential of the tumor. Furthermore, the presence of focal myxoid change, which is not incorporated in any of the abovementioned systems, has been reported to be associated with ACC having a low Weiss score [3, 8, 25].

Apart from the above histopathological clues that speak for the potential malignant behavior of an adrenocortical tumor, several clinical, radiological, and biochemical features in our present cases should have been recognized as incongruent with a simple benign ACA in retrospect. These included the large size of the tumor on presentation, an imaging phenotype inconsistent with adenoma, and co-secretion of adrenal cortisol and androgens and their precursors. The presence of both having a diameter greater than 4 cm and a CT tumor attenuation >10 HU are shown to be highly sensitive to adrenal malignancy [26–28]. A more recent prospective study published in 2020 by Bancos et al.

TABLE 4: Suggested pathological diagnosis of the adrenocortical tumor at the first operation of Patient A based on different classification systems on retrospective pathology review. The tumor would have been classified as ACA by the majority of systems.

Clinical features	Weiss	Hough	Van Slooten	Modified Weiss	Reticulin algorithm	Helsinki score
Case 1	Diffuse growth clear cells < 25%	Diffuse growth (0.92). Cushing's syndrome with virilism (0.42). Insufficient data on ACTH response, 24-hr urinary 17-ketosteroids, and tumor mass	Loss of normal architecture (1.6)	Clear cells <25% (2)	Mandatory criteria not available but optional criteria not met	Criteria on mitoses and necrosis not met and PI not available
Score	2	At least 1.34	1.6	2	—	—
Classification based on system	ACA	Not clear	ACA	ACA	ACA	Not clear

TABLE 5: Suggested pathological diagnosis of the adrenocortical tumor at the first operation of Patient B based on different classification systems on retrospective pathology review. Only the Van Slooten system would have classified the tumor as ACC unequivocally.

Clinical features	Weiss	Hough	Van Slooten	Modified Weiss	Reticulin algorithm	Helsinki score
Case 2	No matching criteria	Thick fibrous band (1.00). Insufficient data on ACTH response, 24-hr urinary 17-ketosteroids, and tumor mass	Nuclear hyperchromatism (2.6). Regressive changes (5.7)	No matching criteria	Mandatory criteria not available and optional criteria not met	Criteria on mitoses and necrosis not met and PI not available
Score	0	At least 1.00	8.3	0	—	—
Classification based on system	ACA	Not clear	ACC	ACA	ACA	Not clear

suggested that a tumor diameter of 4 cm and unenhanced CT tumor attenuation of 20 HU may be more appropriate threshold values for the consideration of an ACC. In their study of 2169 participants from 14 specialist centers in 11 countries involving 98 (4.9%) patients with ACC, increasing the unenhanced CT tumor attenuation threshold from the recommended 10HU to 20 HU (and keeping a diameter threshold of 4 cm) increased the specificity for the detection of ACC (64% vs. 80·0%) while maintaining sensitivity (100% vs. 99%) in patients with newly identified adrenal masses more than 1 cm after exclusion of phaeochromocytoma and patients with a history of cancer [29]. Other radiological features suggestive of ACC include inhomogeneous appearance, presence of calcification, central low attenuation with a thin enhancing rim (representing tumor necrosis), and contrast washout characteristics concordant with non-adenoma (i.e., absolute washout <60% and relative washout <40%) [1, 30–32]. The latest ESE guideline on adrenal incidentaloma stated that further washout CT characterization for inhomogeneous lesions should not be performed and recommended surgical resection in unilateral adrenal masses with radiological suspicion of malignancy, recognizing the potential of ACC in these lesions [27].

The pattern of steroid secretion may also indicate if an adrenal lesion is an ACC as disorganized steroidogenesis is almost always observed in ACC. Co-secretion of androgens and cortisol, secretion of immature steroid precursors, or secretion of estradiol in males are highly suspicious for ACC [14]. In recent decades, USP has emerged as an important diagnostic and surveillance tool in the evaluation of adrenal tumors. Specifically, USP can reveal the specific fingerprints of ACC coinciding with immature and disorganized early stage steroidogenesis and has been shown to differentiate malignant from benign adrenocortical tumors with high sensitivity and specificity [33, 34]. The adrenal steroid precursor, tetrahydro-11-deoxycortisol (THS), a 11-deoxycortisol metabolite, was found to be the most discriminative steroid in differentiating ACC from ACAs in a study supported by ENS@T [33]. Another Dutch study also showed that urinary THS excretion at a cut-off value of 2.35umol/24 hr differentiated ACC from other adrenal disorders with a sensitivity of 100% and specificity of 99% [35]. Of note, USP can detect significantly increased steroid precursor excretion in those ACCs that would have been classified as endocrinologically inactive based on routine endocrine workup and can serve as a surveillance marker. Similarly, urine steroid metabolomics has lately been shown to improve the diagnostic accuracy of ACC in patients with newly found adrenal masses in addition to CT tumor attenuation values and tumor diameter by virtue of the specific biological secretory signature of ACC [29]. Apart from USP, different groups have started to explore the use of plasma steroid metabolome profiling by LS-MS/MS in discriminating between ACA and ACC. Their findings found an increase in 11-deoxycortisol, 11-deoxycorticosterone, androstenedione, and 17-OHP levels in patients with ACC compared to those with ACA and suggested that plasma steroid profiling may emerge as a potential diagnostic tool for ACC [36, 37]. However, as the method is not widely available at present and its diagnostic value on top of USP is still unknown, further evaluation should be performed before its routine clinical use.

In Hong Kong, USP using gas chromatography-mass spectrometry (GC-MS) identified 3α, 16α, 20α-pregnenetriol and 3β, 16α, 20α-pregnenetriol to be highly specific for ACCs in addition to THS and these steroid metabolites were also observed in Patient A. USP can identify residual or recurrent ACCs even before the disease becomes radiologically apparent and is useful in the surveillance and monitoring of recurrent disease [34, 38]. Chortis et al. suggested that the appearance of abnormal metabolites may predate imaging abnormality by 2 months based on their analysis of 135 patients with ACCs after R0 resection. They also proposed that the availability of preoperative urine samples considerably improved the ability of USP to detect ACC recurrence [39].

In terms of treatment, complete surgical removal is the only curative therapy for localized ACC. In patients with unresectable tumors or incomplete tumor resection, the prognosis is significantly worse [1, 9, 40]. However, despite complete surgical removal, the recurrence rate can be as high as 50–80% [40, 41]. Predictors for recurrence include advanced disease stage, incomplete surgical resection, hypercortisolism, laparoscopic adrenalectomy, and high proliferation rate (Ki-67 proliferation index) [9, 41]. Molecular markers such as somatic gene mutations (*TP53, ZNFR3, CTNNB1, PRKAR1A, CCNE1, TERF2, TERT, CDK*s, and genes involved in histone modification [*MLL, MLL2, MLL4*] and chromatin remodeling [*ATRX, DAXX*]), alterations in methylome and transcriptome, miRNAome, and chromosomal aberrations are emerging tools for further prognostication of ACC but yet to be incorporated into clinical practice due to the resource-intensive nature of pangenomic bioinformatic analysis [14, 40–44]. The use of adjuvant mitotane is controversial as there is much uncertainty regarding its efficacy in preventing recurrence and improving mortality. A meta-analysis in 2018 including 5 retrospective studies and 1249 patients found that adjuvant mitotane was associated with longer recurrence-free survival (HR 0.62; 95% CI 0.42–0.94) and overall survival (HR 0.69; 95% CI 0.55–0.88). In another meta-analysis by ESE and ENS@T in 2018, favorable effects were also observed on recurrence (HR 0.7; 95% CI 0.5–1.1) and mortality 0.7 (95% CI 0.5–0.9) in patients receiving adjuvant mitotane, while acknowledging the fact that all six studies included in the meta-analysis were non-randomized with the potential of a confounding effect [2, 41]. Despite the absence of completely convincing evidence, the ESE and ENS@T guidelines recommended that adjuvant mitotane should be offered to patients at high risk of recurrence (Stage III or IV, R1 resection, or Ki67 > 10%), and the duration of treatment should last for at least 2 years but not longer than 5 years. For patients at low to intermediate risk of recurrence (Stage I/II, R0 resection, and Ki-67 </ = 10%), adjuvant mitotane should be individualized, while for patients with adrenocortical tumors of uncertain malignant potential, adjuvant therapy should not be started [2, 24].

For patients who develop recurrent disease at least 12 months beyond the initial surgery, complete surgical removal of the recurrence is still recommended if it is achievable [1, 2, 19, 45]. At the same time, mitotane should be commenced as soon as possible if it has not been given before as in our patients, while acknowledging the fact that the objective response rate to mitotane in metastatic ACC is at best 24% [2, 9, 45]. In our patients, there seemed to be initial stabilization of tumor growth for the first few months after mitotane in Patient B, while a response was not observed in Patient A. In selected patients (e.g., patients with severe hormone excess), debulking surgery may be offered as palliation if >80% of the tumor can be removed, the hormonal excess remains uncontrolled despite maximally tolerated medical therapy, and the patient is deemed a surgical candidate [2, 45]. In line with the recommendation, our first patient did enjoy an extended period of survival with good quality of life after palliative surgery. Further localized therapy and systemic therapy should be individualized and discussed in a multidisciplinary team. In patients with progressive metastatic ACC not amenable to surgery or mitotane monotherapy, systemic chemotherapy with EDP combined with mitotane represents the current standard of care as supported by the FIRM-ACT trial, the largest randomized controlled trial in ACC to date. However, the response rate remained dismal with only a modest improvement in progression-free survival of 5 vs. 2.1 months (HR 0.55, $p < 0.001$) and no effect on overall survival as compared to streptozocin plus mitotane (14.8 vs. 12 months, HR 0.79, $p = 0.07$) [46]. EP combined with mitotane might have modest activity against ACC with an objective response rate of 11% [47]. This regime was employed as the initial palliative chemotherapy in Patient A after balancing her fair performance status at that juncture and risk of toxicity with EDP. The combination of gemcitabine and capecitabine has been proposed as second- or third-line therapy in heavily pretreated patients with metastatic ACC and has been reported to achieve a 4 months' non-progression rate of 46%. The lack of a control arm is a major limitation of the study [48]. Other systemic therapies involving IGF2/IGF-I receptor inhibition (linsitinib, cixutumumab), mTOR inhibition (everolimus, sirolimus, temsirolimus), selective or multi-tyrosine kinase inhibition including EGFR, VEGF/VEGFR2, RET, and FGFR inhibition (gefinitib, erlotinib, sorafenib, sunitinib, lenvatinib, dovitinib, axitinib, nilotinib, cabozantinib), sterol O-acyltransferase-1 (SOAT) inhibition (nevanimibe) and immunotherapy (avelumab), either alone and in combination, were ineffective in achieving clinically meaningful outcomes [19, 40, 49, 50]. A recent phase II study with pembrolizumab may hold a sign of promise for immune checkpoint inhibitor for advanced ACC, in which an objective response rate of 23% and s disease control rate of 23% were observed in 39 patients over a median follow-up of 17.8 months [51]. Other potential emerging therapies or therapeutic targets under investigation include peptide receptor radionuclide therapy (PRRT), cyclin-dependent kinase (CDK) inhibition, Notch inhibition, Ras/Raf/MARK/

ERK pathway inhibition, murine double minute (MDM2) inhibition, and Poly-ADP-ribose polymerase (PARP) inhibition [45, 50, 52].

4. Conclusion

Adrenocortical carcinoma is an aggressive endocrine cancer in which therapeutic options are often limited and prognosis becomes gloomy once metastatic disease is manifested. It is also a heterogeneous disease with varying clinical behavior, where a small subset of patients harboring low-grade well-differentiated tumors may demonstrate a more indolent clinical course [52]. It should not be overstated that histology can be deceptive in these patients and clinicians should be aware of the potential limitation of and overreliance on the Weiss scoring system in the differentiation of benign and malignant adrenocortical tumors. Other clinical parameters, particularly the pattern of hormonal secretion, urinary steroid profiling, and imaging features, should be incorporated into the prediction of the malignant potential of these "borderline" tumors, thus assisting the subsequent surveillance strategies. Mitotane therapy forms the cornerstone of treatment in metastatic ACC, and in combination with etoposide, doxorubicin, and cisplatin represents the currently best evidence-based treatment in patients with advanced ACC.

Abbreviations

17-OHP: 17-hydroxyprogesterone
ACA: Adrenocortical adenoma
ACC: Adrenocortical carcinoma
CDK: Cyclin-dependent kinase
CT: Computed tomography
EDP: Chemotherapy regime containing a combination of etoposide, doxorubicin, and cisplatin
EGFR: Epidermal growth factor receptor
ENS@T: European Network for the Study of Adrenal Tumors
EP: Chemotherapy regime containing a combination of etoposide and cisplatin
ESE: European Society of Endocrinology
^{18}FDG-PET-CT: ^{18}F-fluorodeoxyglucose positron emission tomography/ computed tomography FGFR:
FIRM-ACT: First International Randomized Trial in Locally Advanced and Metastatic Adrenocortical Carcinoma Treatment
GC-MS: Gas chromatography-mass spectrometry
HPF: High power field
HU: Hounsfield unit
IGF-1: Insulin-like growth factor 1
IGF-2: Insulin-like growth factor 2
MDM2: Mouse double minute 2 homolog
mTOR: Mammalian target of rapamycin
PARP: Poly-adenosine diphosphate-ribose polymerase
PD-L1: Programmed-death ligand 1
PRRT: Peptide receptor radionuclide therapy
RET: Rearranged during transfection
SOAT: Sterol O-acyltransferase-1
SUVmax: Maximum standardized uptake value
THS: Tetrahydro-11-deoxycortisol
US: Ultrasound
USP: Urinary steroid profiling
VEGF1: Vascular endothelial growth factor 1
VEGFR2: Vascular endothelial growth factor receptor 2.

Ethical Approval

Not applicable.

Consent

Written consent for publication was obtained from the patients' next-of-kin mentioned in the case report.

Authors' Contributions

CLW analyzed and interpreted the patient data including clinical, biochemical, radiological, and histological data; prepared figures and tables; and was a major contributor in writing the manuscript. CKF, YKC, VHKT, and LMF analyzed and interpreted the patients' clinical, biochemical, and radiological data. All authors had major participation in the direct care of the patients and read and approved the final manuscript.

References

[1] T. Else, A. C. Kim, A. Sabolch et al., "Adrenocortical carcinoma," *Endocrine Reviews*, vol. 35, no. 2, pp. 282–326, 2014 Apr.

[2] M. Fassnacht, O. M. Dekkers, T. Else et al., "European society of Endocrinology clinical practice guidelines on the management of adrenocortical carcinoma in adults, in collaboration with the European network for the study of adrenal tumors," *European Journal of Endocrinology*, vol. 179, no. 4, pp. G1–G46, 2018 Oct.

[3] L. A. Erickson, "Challenges in surgical pathology of adrenocortical tumours," *Histopathology*, vol. 72, no. 1, pp. 82–96, 2018 Jan.

[4] R. C. Oliveira, M. J. Martins, C. Moreno et al., "Histological scores and tumor size on stage II in adrenocortical carcinomas," *Rare Tumors*, vol. 13, Article ID 20363613211026494, 2021 Jun.

[5] L. M. Weiss, L. J. Medeiros, and A. L. Vickery, "Pathologic features of prognostic significance in adrenocortical carcinoma," *The American Journal of Surgical Pathology*, vol. 13, no. 3, pp. 202–206, 1989 Mar.

[6] L. M. Weiss, "Comparative histologic study of 43 metastasizing and nonmetastasizing adrenocortical tumors," *The American Journal of Surgical Pathology*, vol. 8, no. 3, pp. 163–170, 1984 Mar.

[7] S. Aubert, A. Wacrenier, X. Leroy et al., "Weiss system revisited: a clinicopathologic and immunohistochemical study of 49 adrenocortical tumors," *The American Journal of Surgical Pathology*, vol. 26, no. 12, pp. 1612–1619, 2002 Dec.

[8] M. Papotti, R. Libè, E. Duregon, M. Volante, J. Bertherat, and F. Tissier, "The Weiss score and beyond--histopathology for

adrenocortical carcinoma," *Hormones and Cancer*, vol. 2, no. 6, pp. 333–340, 2011 Dec.

[9] R. Libé, "Adrenocortical carcinoma (ACC): diagnosis, prognosis, and treatment," *Frontiers in Cell and Developmental Biology*, vol. 3, p. 45, 2015 Jul.

[10] E. Duregon, M. Volante, E. Bollito et al., "Pitfalls in the diagnosis of adrenocortical tumors: a lesson from 300 consultation cases," *Human Pathology*, vol. 46, no. 12, pp. 1799–1807, 2015 Dec.

[11] F. Tissier, "Classification of adrenal cortical tumors: what limits for the pathological approach?" *Best Practice & Research Clinical Endocrinology & Metabolism*, vol. 24, no. 6, pp. 877–885, 2010 Dec.

[12] M. Volante, E. Bollito, P. Sperone et al., "Clinicopathological study of a series of 92 adrenocortical carcinomas: from a proposal of simplified diagnostic algorithm to prognostic stratification," *Histopathology*, vol. 55, no. 5, pp. 535–543, 2009 Nov.

[13] M. Pennanen, I. Heiskanen, T. Sane et al., "Helsinki score-a novel model for prediction of metastases in adrenocortical carcinomas," *Human Pathology*, vol. 46, no. 3, pp. 404–410, 2015 Mar.

[14] C. L. Viëtor, S. G. Creemers, F. J. van Kemenade, T. M. van Ginhoven, L. J. Hofland, and R. A. Feelders, "How to differentiate benign from malignant adrenocortical tumors?" *Cancers*, vol. 13, no. 17, p. 4383, 2021 Aug.

[15] T. M. Nogueira, R. Lirov, E. M. Caoili et al., "Radiographic characteristics of adrenal masses preceding the diagnosis of adrenocortical cancer," *Hormones and Cancer*, vol. 6, no. 4, pp. 176–181, 2015 Aug.

[16] S. Johanssen, S. Hahner, W. Saeger et al., "Deficits in the management of patients with adrenocortical carcinoma in Germany," *Deutsches Arzteblatt International*, vol. 107, no. 50, pp. 885–891, 2010 Dec.

[17] A. J. Hough, J. W. Hollifield, D. L. Page, and W. H. Hartmann, "Prognostic factors in adrenal cortical tumors. A mathematical analysis of clinical and morphologic data," *American Journal of Clinical Pathology*, vol. 72, no. 3, pp. 390–399, 1979 Sep.

[18] H. V. Slooten, A. Schaberg, D. Smeenk, and A. J. Moolenaar, "Morphologic characteristics of benign and malignant adrenocortical tumors," *Cancer*, vol. 55, no. 4, pp. 766–773, 1985 Feb.

[19] B. Kiesewetter, P. Riss, C. Scheuba et al., "Management of adrenocortical carcinoma: are we making progress?" *Therapeutics Advanced Medical Oncolology*, vol. 13, Article ID 17588359211038409, 2021 Aug.

[20] A. K. Lam, "Adrenocortical carcinoma: updates of clinical and pathological features after renewed World Health Organisation classification and pathology staging," *Biomedicines*, vol. 9, no. 2, p. 175, 2021 Feb 10.

[21] C. Pohlink, A. Tannapfel, U. Eichfeld et al., "Does tumor heterogeneity limit the use of the Weiss criteria in the evaluation of adrenocortical tumors?" *Journal of Endocrinological Investigation*, vol. 27, no. 6, pp. 565–569, 2004 Jun.

[22] M. Papotti, E. Duregon, M. Volante, and A. M. McNicol, "Pathology of the adrenal cortex: a reappraisal of the past 25 years focusing on adrenal cortical tumors," *Endocrine Pathology*, vol. 25, no. 1, pp. 35–48, 2014 Mar.

[23] E. Duregon, R. Cappellesso, V. Maffeis et al., "Validation of the prognostic role of the Helsinki Score in 225 cases of adrenocortical carcinoma," *Human Pathology*, vol. 62, pp. 1–7, 2017 Apr.

[24] E. Duregon, A. Fassina, M. Volante et al., "The reticulin algorithm for adrenocortical tumor diagnosis: a multicentric validation study on 245 unpublished cases," *The American Journal of Surgical Pathology*, vol. 37, no. 9, pp. 1433–1440, 2013 Sep.

[25] M. Papotti, M. Volante, E. Duregon et al., "Adrenocortical tumors with myxoid features: a distinct morphologic and phenotypical variant exhibiting malignant behavior," *The American Journal of Surgical Pathology*, vol. 34, no. 7, pp. 973–983, 2010 Jul.

[26] E. Kebebew, "Adrenal incidentaloma," *New England Journal of Medicine*, vol. 384, no. 16, pp. 1542–1551, 2021 Apr.

[27] A. H. Hamrahian, A. G. Ioachimescu, E. M. Remer et al., "Clinical utility of noncontrast computed tomography attenuation value (Hounsfield units) to differentiate adrenal adenomas/hyperplasias from nonadenomas: Cleveland Clinic experience," *Journal of Clinical Endocrinology and Metabolism*, vol. 90, no. 2, pp. 871–877, 2005 Feb.

[28] M. Fassnacht, W. Arlt, I. Bancos et al., "Management of adrenal incidentalomas: European society of Endocrinology clinical practice guideline in collaboration with the European network for the study of adrenal tumors," *European Journal of Endocrinology*, vol. 175, no. 2, pp. G1–G34, 2016 Aug.

[29] I. Bancos, A. E. Taylor, V. Chortis et al., "Urine steroid metabolomics for the differential diagnosis of adrenal incidentalomas in the EURINE-ACT study: a prospective test validation study," *Lancet Diabetes & Endocrinology*, vol. 8, no. 9, pp. 773–781, 2020 Sep.

[30] C. S. Peña, G. W. Boland, P. F. Hahn, M. J. Lee, and P. R. Mueller, "Characterization of indeterminate (lipid-poor) adrenal masses: use of washout characteristics at contrast-enhanced CT," *Radiology*, vol. 217, no. 3, pp. 798–802, 2000 Dec.

[31] H. M. Zhang, N. D. Perrier, E. G. Grubbs et al., "CT features and quantification of the characteristics of adrenocortical carcinomas on unenhanced and contrast-enhanced studies," *Clinical Radiology*, vol. 67, no. 1, pp. 38–46, 2012 Jan.

[32] D. H. Szolar, M. Korobkin, P. Reittner et al., "Adrenocortical carcinomas and adrenal pheochromocytomas: mass and enhancement loss evaluation at delayed contrast-enhanced CT," *Radiology*, vol. 234, no. 2, pp. 479–485, 2005 Feb.

[33] W. Arlt, M. Biehl, A. E. Taylor et al., "Urine steroid metabolomics as a biomarker tool for detecting malignancy in adrenal tumors," *Journal of Clinical Endocrinology and Metabolism*, vol. 96, no. 12, pp. 3775–3784, 2011 Dec.

[34] C. Rossi, I. Cicalini, S. Verrocchio, G. Di Dalmazi, L. Federici, and I. Bucci, "The potential of steroid profiling by mass spectrometry in the management of adrenocortical carcinoma," *Biomedicines*, vol. 8, no. 9, p. 314, 2020 Aug.

[35] T. M. A. Kerkhofs, M. N. Kerstens, I. P. Kema, T. P. Willems, and H. R. Haak, "Diagnostic value of urinary steroid profiling in the evaluation of adrenal tumors," *Hormones and Cancer*, vol. 6, no. 4, pp. 168–175, 2015 Aug.

[36] D. R. Taylor, L. Ghataore, L. Couchman et al., "A 13-steroid serum panel based on LC-MS/MS: use in detection of adrenocortical carcinoma," *Clinical Chemistry*, vol. 63, no. 12, pp. 1836–1846, 2017 Dec.

[37] S. Schweitzer, M. Kunz, M. Kurlbaum et al., "Plasma steroid metabolome profiling for the diagnosis of adrenocortical carcinoma," *European Journal of Endocrinology*, vol. 180, no. 2, pp. 117–125, 2019 Feb.

[38] S. C. Tiu, A. O. K. Chan, N. F. Taylor et al., "Use of urinary steroid profiling for diagnosing and monitoring adrenocor-

tical tumours," *Hong Kong Medical Journal*, vol. 15, no. 6, pp. 463–470, 2009 Dec.

[39] V. Chortis, I. Bancos, T. Nijman et al., "Urine steroid metabolomics as a novel tool for detection of recurrent adrenocortical carcinoma," *The Journal of Cinical Endocrinology and Metabolism*, vol. 105, no. 3, pp. e307–18, 2020 Mar.

[40] G. Alyateem and N. Nilubol, *Frontiers in Endocrinology*, vol. 12, 2021 Mar.

[41] S. Bedrose, M. Daher, L. Altameemi, and M. A. Habra, "Adjuvant therapy in adrenocortical carcinoma: reflections and future directions," *Cancers*, vol. 12, no. 2, p. 508, 2020 Feb.

[42] G. Assié, E. Letouzé, M. Fassnacht et al., "Integrated genomic characterization of adrenocortical carcinoma," *Nature Genetics*, vol. 46, no. 6, pp. 607–612, 2014 Jun.

[43] S. Zheng, A. D. Cherniack, N. Dewal et al., "Comprehensive pan-genomic characterization of adrenocortical carcinoma," *Cancer Cell*, vol. 29, no. 5, pp. 723–736, 2016 May.

[44] J. Lippert, S. Appenzeller, R. Liang et al., "Targeted molecular analysis in adrenocortical carcinomas: a strategy toward improved personalized prognostication," *Journal of Clinical Endocrinology and Metabolism*, vol. 103, no. 12, pp. 4511–4523, 2018 Dec.

[45] M. Fassnacht, M. Kroiss, and B. Allolio, "Update in adrenocortical carcinoma," *Journal of Clinical Endocrinology and Metabolism*, vol. 98, no. 12, pp. 4551–4564, 2013 Dec.

[46] M. Fassnacht, M. Terzolo, B. Allolio et al., "Combination chemotherapy in advanced adrenocortical carcinoma," *New England Journal of Medicine*, vol. 366, no. 23, pp. 2189–2197, 2012 Jun.

[47] S. K. Williamson, D. Lew, G. J. Miller, S. P. Balcerzak, L. H. Baker, and E. D. Crawford, "Phase II evaluation of cisplatin and etoposide followed by mitotane at disease progression in patients with locally advanced or metastatic adrenocortical carcinoma: a Southwest Oncology Group Study," *Cancer*, vol. 88, no. 5, pp. 1159–1165, 2000 Mar.

[48] P. Sperone, A. Ferrero, F. Daffara et al., "Gemcitabine plus metronomic 5-fluorouracil or capecitabine as a second-/third-line chemotherapy in advanced adrenocortical carcinoma: a multicenter phase II study," *Endocrine-Related Cancer*, vol. 17, no. 2, pp. 445–453, 2010 Apr.

[49] D. R. Mohan, A. M. Lerario, and G. D. Hammer, "Therapeutic targets for adrenocortical carcinoma in the genomics era," *Journal of Endocrine Soceity*, vol. 2, no. 11, pp. 1259–1274, 2018 Sep 26.

[50] B. Altieri, C. L. Ronchi, M. Kroiss, and M. Fassnacht, "Next-generation therapies for adrenocortical carcinoma," *Best Practice & Research Clinical Endocrinology & Metabolism*, vol. 34, no. 3, Article ID 101434, 2020 May.

[51] N. Raj, Y. Zheng, V. Kelly et al., "PD-1 blockade in advanced adrenocortical carcinoma," *Journal of Clinical Oncology*, vol. 38, no. 1, pp. 71–80, 2020 Jan.

[52] O. A. Shariq and T. J. McKenzie, "Adrenocortical carcinoma: current state of the art, ongoing controversies, and future directions in diagnosis and treatment," *Ther Advanced Chronic Disease*, vol. 12, Article ID 20406223211033103, 2021 Jul.

30

Recurrent Macroprolactinoma with Malignant Conversion to Carcinoma with Spinal Metastasis

Madeline Mori,[1] Amanda Frugoli,[2,3] Udesh Shah,[2,3] Brad Barrows,[4] Tricia Westhoff,[2,5] and David Westra[2,6]

[1]*Western University of Health Sciences, Pomona, CA 91766, USA*
[2]*Department of Graduate Medical Education, Community Memorial Hospital, Ventura, CA 93003, USA*
[3]*Department of Internal Medicine, Community Memorial Hospital, Ventura, CA 93003, USA*
[4]*Department of Pathology, Community Memorial Hospital, Ventura, CA 93003, USA*
[5]*Department of Endocrinology, Community Memorial Hospital, Ventura, CA 93003, USA*
[6]*Department of Neurosurgery, Community Memorial Hospital, Ventura, CA 93003, USA*

Correspondence should be addressed to Amanda Frugoli; afrugoli@cmhshealth.org

Academic Editor: Wayne V. Moore

In contrast to pituitary adenomas, pituitary carcinomas represent a rare malignant neoplasm with a remarkable high mortality. Pituitary carcinomas can arise from any pituitary tumor cell line and are determined to be carcinomas when there is distant metastasis or central nervous system dissemination. In this case vignette, we describe a rare case of malignant prolactinoma with intraspinal metastasis, and we also provide a review of relevant literature and treatment.

1. Introduction

Anterior pituitary adenomas/tumors (pituitary tumors) are not uncommon [1, 2]. In a meta-analysis of postmortem studies by Ezzat et al., pituitary tumors were incidentally found to have an estimated prevalence of 14.4% [1]. These tumors can also be incidentally detected by neuroimaging studies in up to 22.5% of the general population [1]. Pituitary tumors have traditionally been classified as adenomas (macroadenoma >1 cm; microadenoma <1 cm) but represent a diverse group of histologic subtypes [3]. To address the variability in clinical outcomes for these neoplasms, a new terminology, pituitary neuroendocrine tumors (PitNETs), has recently been proposed [4]. This proposal is based on the similar absence of specific histologic characteristics that could be used to reliably predict tumor behavior and is similar to the classification utilized in gastrointestinal neuroendocrine tumors. The current classification of pituitary tumors is primarily based on clinical findings (radiology, hormone-associated symptoms, and mass effect), histomorphology, and immunohistochemistry, with additional tools including ultrastructure analysis by electron microscopy and in difficult cases molecular studies [4, 5]. Nonfunctioning adenomas cause disease by slow growth and encroachment with displacement of brain structures (mass effect), while functioning adenomas produce symptoms related to hormone production [3, 6]. Despite the relatively high prevalence of pituitary tumors, only a small fraction (~0.2%) undergoes malignant transformation to pituitary carcinoma, which has a remarkably high mortality [3, 4, 6]. Pituitary carcinomas can arise from any anterior pituitary tumor cell line and are defined when there is distant metastasis or central nervous dissemination [6–8]. Current limitations in the diagnosis and management of pituitary carcinomas arise from an inability to distinguish the potential for a pituitary adenoma to transform into a pituitary carcinoma based on histologic characteristics alone in most cases. It is only after metastasis is confirmed that a pituitary tumor can be classified as a pituitary carcinoma [9]. Pituitary carcinoma metastasis is commonly found in both intracranial (cerebral cortex, cerebellum, cerebellopontine, angle, and dura) and extracranial (lymph nodes, bones, lungs, and liver) locations [10–15]. Metastatic foci are typically identified by either manifestation of symptoms or as an incidental finding on imaging [11, 16].

Pituitary carcinomas comprise 0.2% of all pituitary tumors [17, 18]. Of the limited cases described, a large majority are hormonally active, with estimates approaching 88% [17, 19]. In Ragel and Couldwell's literature review, they were able to estimate that the majority of hormonally active carcinomas included ACTH at about 42% followed by prolactin producing 33%, followed by growth hormone, LF/FSH, and finally TSH producing [17]. Curiously, pituitary carcinomas have displayed a greater tendency toward systemic metastasis than craniospinal metastasis [3, 4, 19]. Despite the higher prevalence of ACTH hormone producing pituitary carcinomas, the rate of systemic metastasis is seen more commonly with prolactin producing tumors at 71% [19]. In a comprehensive review of 72 cases of pituitary carcinoma by Yoo et al., they found an average age of diagnosis of pituitary carcinoma to be 46.3 years, with a range from 9 to 75 years [20]. Diagnosis of pituitary carcinoma is "extremely rare" in children [21]. Of the 72 cases of pituitary carcinoma described by Yoo et al., there was only one pediatric case, a 9-year-old female with spinal and intracranial metastasis [20, 22].

Pituitary carcinomas are difficult to treat, with patients having an average of 2-3 surgeries in addition to radiation or chemotherapy treatment [20]. These carcinomas account for a striking mortality rate between 43% and 54.8% with a median survival of 10 months after diagnosis [13, 20]. In this case vignette, we describe a rare case of metastatic prolactinoma, and we also provide relevant literature review.

2. Case Report

The patient is a 71-year-old right-handed and physically active female with an extensive history of pituitary macroprolactinoma first diagnosed in 2006. Her treatment course has been complicated with recurrence and has required two resections. Initial treatment for her macroprolactinoma included a debulking procedure in September 2006, followed by partial transnasal transsphenoidal surgery in November 2012, and gamma knife external beam radiation treatment localized to the cavernous sinus in January 2014. She underwent radiographic and hormonal surveillance with MRI in August 2014 and July 2019. She concurrently underwent hormonal treatment with cabergoline. Pituitary MRI on August 2014 showed resolution of the tumor in the cavernous sinus. Pituitary MRI on November 2019 showed no evidence of tumor. She had normal prolactin levels between November 2014 and August 2017, with a steady increase from November 2017–July 2020 from 21.74 ng/ml to 656.60 ng/ml despite increasing the dose of cabergoline to 2 mg oral daily and a repeat course of gamma knife external beam radiation to the cavernous sinus in 2019.

She presented in August 2020 with constant sharp, burning 9/10 low back pain, and left lower extremity pain worsening for the past 2 months. She described her presenting pain as most intense in the left buttock, posterior thigh, and calf. Pain was aggravated by motion initially, with only slight relief by taking naproxen or ibuprofen. She denied weakness, numbness, bowel, or bladder difficulties. She was treated with physical therapy, with only slight benefit, and had otherwise not had any other treatment for her pain. On her neurologic exam, her sensation was intact to light touch and pinprick in all dermatomes except a slight decrease in pinprick sensation to both modalities at the lateral aspect of her left foot. Her reflexes were 2+ throughout except for absent left Achilles' jerk. No evidence of Hoffmann sign, Babinski sign, or clonus. Positive straight leg raise on the left side. She had an antalgic gait, but was able to walk with her heels, toes, and heel-to-toe. She was sent for neuroimaging of the lumbar spine (Figures 1 and 2).

In August 2020, she was admitted to the hospital for surgical resection of an intradural tumor causing severe debilitating spinal stenosis (Figure 2). She underwent posterior lumbar laminectomy, facetectomy, and foraminotomy from L4 to S1 with instrumentation arthrodesis from L4 to S1. In addition to resection of the intradural tumor, she required posterolateral fusion of L4 and L5 with a partial reduction of L4-5 spondylolisthesis and use of an autograft. Intraoperatively, she was found to have a 3 cm friable tumor with nerve roots in the tumor capsule, which was highly suspicious for pituitary carcinoma given her history. Intraoperative frozen section pathology showed histologic features compatible with pituitary neoplasm (Figure 3). Permanent pathology showed minimal nuclear pleomorphism of tumor cells and overall histomorphology similar to a typical pituitary adenoma (Figure 4). Immunohistochemistry confirmed the presence of prolactin in tumor cells (Figure 5) and showed a moderately increased Ki-67 (Figure 6) proliferation index (18%; pituitary adenoma usually <3%). Given the location within the lumbar spine, the tumor met criteria for the final diagnosis of pituitary carcinoma, a lactotroph subtype associated with intradural, extramedullary drop metastasis. Postoperative imaging showed gross total resection of the tumor. Patient noted improved lower back pain and was evaluated by physical therapy and occupational therapy and was stable on discharge home hospital day 6. She had close follow-up labs in September 2020, November 2020, and March 2021 with reduced prolactin levels of 3.00, 1.23, and 1.17, respectively. She underwent 29 days of radiation therapy to the lumbosacral spine, which she completed in April 2021. She continues on cabergoline 2.0 mg daily and clinically is doing well.

3. Discussion

Pituitary tumors are characterized as functional or nonfunctional, i.e., hormone producing or nonhormone producing. Prolactinomas (prolactin secreting pituitary tumors) are the most commonly diagnosed hormone-producing pituitary adenomas, comprising about 40% of all functional pituitary tumors [2, 5]. Though pituitary adenomas are generally rare in children, of the pituitary adenomas, prolactinomas are the most common adenoma in children [21]. Many prolactinomas are asymptomatic and found

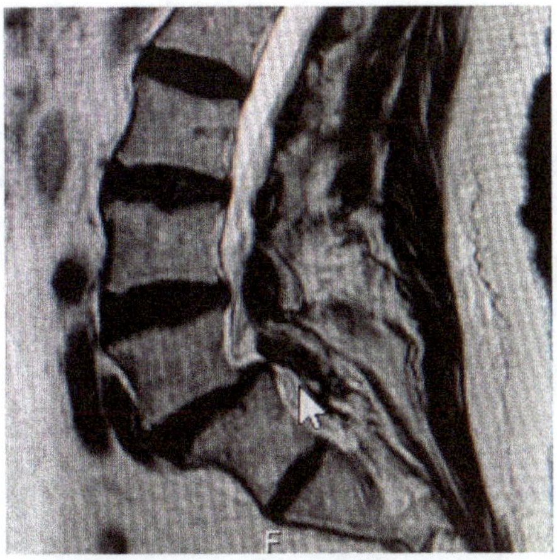

FIGURE 1: MRI lumbar spine with contrast showing grade 1 spondylolisthesis at L5–S1 with S1-S2 disk space causing severe spinal stenosis. There is a large object extending inferiorly from L5–S1 disk space.

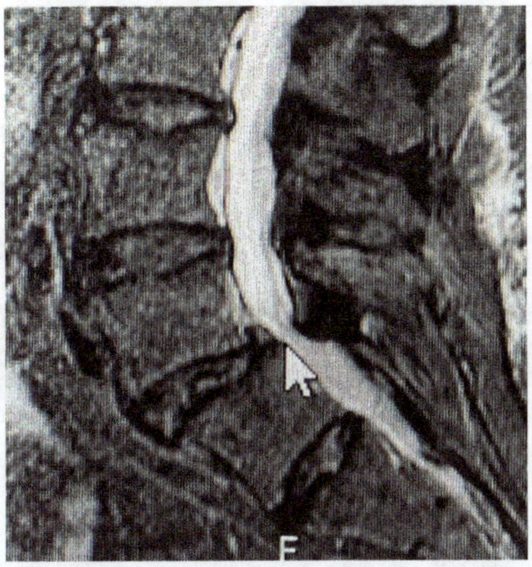

FIGURE 2: MRI lumbar spine with contrast showing an intradural and enhancing mass in the L5–S1 disc space causing severe stenosis within the intradural space. This object is an intradural enhancing mass causing severe stenosis within the intradural space.

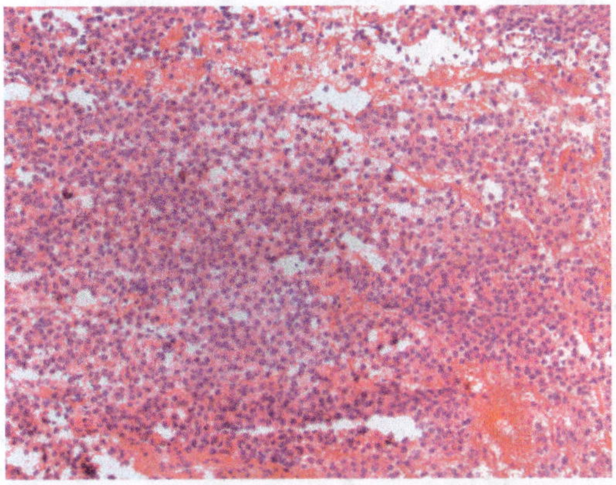

FIGURE 3: Intraoperative frozen section evaluation showing a homogeneous population of tumor cells with round nuclei, indistinct nucleoli, and cytoplasmic granules (200x magnification).

incidentally on imaging or during autopsy [1, 2, 23]. Due to the inhibitory effect that prolactin has on follicle stimulating hormone and luteinizing hormone secretion, patients with functional prolactinomas may complain of symptoms typical of hypogonadism including decreased libido and fertility issues [2, 5]. Prolactinomas can also be classified based on size: <1 cm considered microprolactinoma and >1 cm considered macroprolactinoma [23]. Most

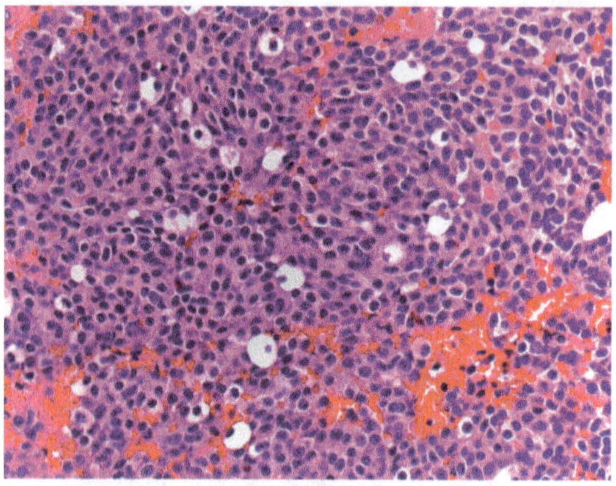

Figure 4: Permanent pathology demonstrating minimal nuclear pleomorphism and only rare mitotic figures (400x magnification).

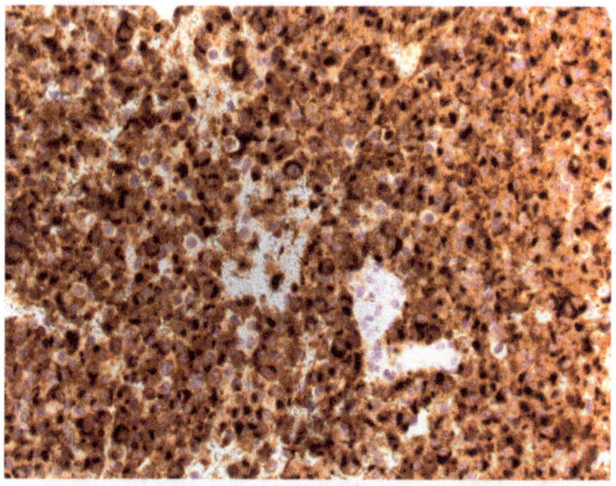

Figure 5: Immunohistochemical stain for prolactin showing prominent granular cytoplasmic staining with perinuclear Golgi pattern accentuation (400x magnification).

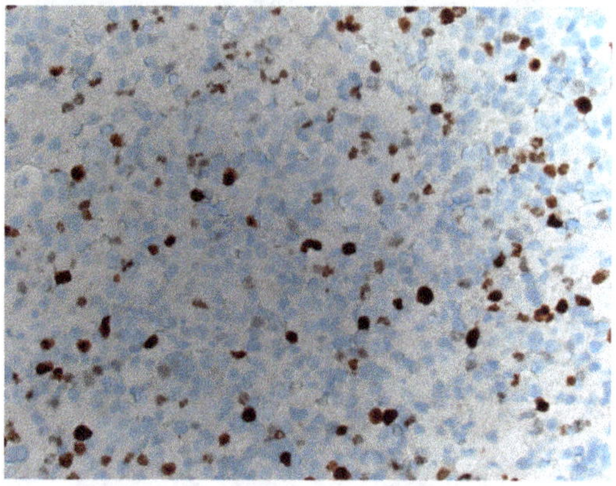

Figure 6: Immunohistochemical stain for Ki-67 showing a proliferation index of 18% by 1000 tumor cell count (400x magnification).

prolactinomas (90%) are small and stay within the suprasellar space [5]. However, macroprolactinomas, defined as being more than 1 cm in size, often cause symptoms due to mass effect, commonly causing symptoms of visual field defects due to compression of the optic chiasm and headaches [5]. Depending on their size and functionality, they can be successfully treated with dopamine agonists, cabergoline or bromocriptine, or with resection [3].

A small subset of pituitary adenomas, 5%, show aggressive features, which are more difficult to manage, leading to increased mortality and morbidity [4, 6, 14]. Unlike other pituitary adenomas, aggressive adenomas tend to have multiple local recurrences or are found to be resistant to treatment [11, 17, 18]. Although there is no clear definition for an aggressive adenoma, Ilie et al. suggest thinking about those tumors that show clinically relevant tumor growth, for example, those causing signs and symptoms [6]. Although many aggressive adenomas have nuclear atypia and cellular pleomorphism, many studies have shown that histomorphology and/or immunostaining alone is not a good predictor of aggressive adenoma or potential for metastasis [8, 19, 20]. Weirinckz et al. specifically tried to evaluate diagnostic markers for prolactin pituitary tumors. In their review of proliferation markers, no marker could distinguish between noninvasive and invasive tumors. They were able to notice a small difference in mitosis and Ki-67 labeling, and they suggested using a combination of markers to reclassify adenomas as "atypical" [24]. This was introduced into the 2004 WHO classification of tumors, adding this focus of molecular biology and pathogenesis. However, it is not overwhelmingly supported as many authors have been able to demonstrate a lack of reliable histological markers to determine atypia (aggressive local behavior) or risk of developing carcinoma [16, 24]. These markers are likely limited in usefulness as more information is needed to determine the complex function that regulates pituitary plasticity and the role in normal physiological function vs. tumor behavior [24]. This is also limited by the multiple cell lines within the anterior pituitary and numerous possible combinations of histomorphology and immunostaining that may be unique to each cell line. Even more rarely, pituitary carcinomas consist of 0.2% of all pituitary tumors [18, 25]. Most authors believe that pituitary carcinomas evolve through malignant transformation from a preexisting adenoma rather than developing de novo, as both aggressive adenomas and pituitary carcinomas often show increased proliferation of Ki-67, increased mitosis, and/or p53 overexpression [7, 13, 24]. Most pituitary carcinomas are diagnosed between 4.7 and 9.04 years after initial pituitary tumor detection [7, 20].

Clinicians must have a high index of suspicion when managing a patient that has multiple occurrences after initial pituitary surgery [7, 20]. On average, patients with pituitary carcinoma had 2.77 surgical interventions before the diagnosis was confirmed [14]. Pituitary carcinoma with metastasis must be suspected in patients when there is a discrepancy between prolactin levels and MRI neuroimaging [5, 7]. Dedicated endocrine tumor imaging may be more helpful in these cases than standard 18F-FDG PET/CT and enhanced magnetic resonance imaging (MRI). Utilization of gallium-68 (68 Ga)-DOTATATE positron emission tomography (PET)/computer tomography (CT) may be more useful for evaluating metastatic CNS involvement [4, 11].

The European Society of Endocrinology (ESE) recently published clinical practice guidelines for the management of these forms of pituitary lesions, including aggressive pituitary tumors and carcinomas. They outline that optimal conventional medical and surgical treatment should be utilized as the primary treatment, but useful adjuvant therapies in aggressive prolactinomas can include radiation therapy and radiation therapy combined with temozolomide (TMZ) [25, 26]. Unfortunately, the efficacy of such regiments is variable, and significant side effects or complications may arise. Radiotherapy is recommended in clinically relevant tumor growth despite surgical resection in nonfunctioning tumors and after failed standard medical and surgical treatment in functioning tumors [25]. Additionally, adjuvant radiotherapy should be considered in the setting of a clinically relevant invasive tumor remnant with pathological markers (Ki-67 index, mitotic count, and p53 immunodetection) that strongly suggest aggressive behavior. All radiotherapy planning and discussion should occur under expert guidance with specific consideration for size, location, and prior radiotherapy dose. For patients with isolated metastases, consideration of loco-regional therapy should be considered independent of decisions regarding the need for systemic treatment [25]. The ESE is also recommended for patients with rapid tumor growth combining temozolomide with radiotherapy using the Stupp protocol. Overall management of these tumors requires a multidisciplinary approach.

4. Conclusion

Pituitary tumors are not uncommon. They represent a highly heterogeneous group varying histologically and in clinical relevance. They are routinely considered benign, but a surprising number can be locally invasive and up to 15% can be clinically aggressive. Pituitary tumors are classified as carcinomas when any anterior pituitary tumor cell line demonstrates distant metastasis or central nervous dissemination. Due to the rare incidence, the management of pituitary carcinoma is still very challenging and needs further investigation. Clinicians should suspect pituitary carcinoma with metastasis when there is a discrepancy between prolactin levels and MRI neuroimaging.

Consent

Consent for this publication has been granted by the patient.

References

[1] S. Ezzat, S. L. Asa, W. T. Couldwell et al., "The prevalence of pituitary adenomas," *Cancer*, vol. 101, no. 3, pp. 613–619, 2004.

[2] A. F. Daly and A. Beckers, "The epidemiology of pituitary adenomas," *Endocrinology and Metabolism Clinics of North America*, vol. 49, no. 3, pp. 347–355, 2020.

[3] G. A. Kaltsas, P. Nomikos, G. Kontogeorgos, M. Buchfelder, and A. B. Grossman, "Diagnosis and management of pituitary carcinomas," *Journal of Clinical Endocrinology & Metabolism*, vol. 90, no. 5, pp. 3089–3099, 2005.

[4] N. C. Olarescu, L. G. Perez-Rivas, F. Gatto et al., "Aggressive and malignant prolactinomas," *Neuroendocrinology*, vol. 109, no. 1, pp. 57–69, 2019.

[5] F. F. Casanueva, M. E. Molitch, J. A. Schlechte et al., "Guidelines of the Pituitary Society for the diagnosis and management of prolactinomas," *Clinical Endocrinology*, vol. 65, no. 2, pp. 265–273, 2006.

[6] M. D. Ilie, E. Jouanneau, and G. Raverot, "Aggressive pituitary adenomas and carcinomas," *Endocrinology and Metabolism Clinics of North America*, vol. 49, no. 3, pp. 505–515, 2020.

[7] A. R. Hong, J. H. Yoon, H. K. Kim, and H.-C. Kang, "Malignant prolactinoma with liver metastases masquerading as metastatic gastrointestinal stromal tumor: a case report and literature review," *Frontiers in Endocrinology*, vol. 11, Article ID 451, 2020.

[8] J. Phillips, H. East, S. French et al., "What causes a prolactinoma to be aggressive or to become a pituitary carcinoma?" *Hormones*, vol. 11, no. 4, pp. 477–482, 2012.

[9] A. P. Heaney, "Pituitary carcinoma: difficult diagnosis and treatment," *Journal of Clinical Endocrinology & Metabolism*, vol. 96, no. 12, pp. 3649–3660, 2011.

[10] M. Kars, F. Roelfsema, J. A. Romijn, and A. M. Pereira, "Malignant prolactinoma: case report and review of the literature," *European Journal of Endocrinology*, vol. 155, no. 4, pp. 523–534, 2006.

[11] J. Seltzer, J. D. Carmichael, D. Commins et al., "Prolactin-secreting pituitary carcinoma with dural metastasis: diagnosis, treatment, and future directions," *World Neurosurgery*, vol. 91, pp. e23–676, 2016.

[12] Y. Q. Wang, T. Fan, X. G. Zhao, C. Liang, X. L. Qi, and J. Y. Li, "Pituitary carcinoma with intraspinal metastasis: report of two cases and review of the literature," *International Journal of Clinical and Experimental Pathology*, vol. 8, no. 8, pp. 9712–9717, 2015.

[13] J. Trouillas, P. Roy, P. Roy et al., "A new prognostic clinicopathological classification of pituitary adenomas: a multicentric case-control study of 410 patients with 8 years post-operative follow-up," *Acta Neuropathologica*, vol. 126, no. 1, pp. 123–135, 2013.

[14] G. A. Kaltsas, P. Nomikos, G. Kontogeorgos, M. Buchfelder, and A. B. Grossman, "Diagnosis and management of pituitary carcinomas," *Journal of Clinical Endocrinology & Metabolism*, vol. 90, no. 5, pp. 3089–3099, 2005.

[15] D. Lübke and W. Saeger, "Carcinomas of the pituitary: definition and review of the literature," *General & Diagnostic Pathology*, vol. 141, no. 2, pp. 81–92, Article ID 8548598, 1995.

[16] A. D. Elster, "Modern imaging of the pituitary," *Radiology*, vol. 187, no. 1, pp. 1–14, 1993.

[17] B. T. Ragel and W. T. Couldwell, "Pituitary carcinoma: a review of the literature," *Neurosurgical Focus*, vol. 16, no. 4, pp. 1–9, 2004.

[18] G. Raverot, P. Burman, A. McCormack et al., "European Society of Endocrinology Clinical Practice Guidelines for the management of aggressive pituitary tumours and carcinomas," *European Journal of Endocrinology*, vol. 178, no. 1, pp. G1–G24, 2018.

[19] P. J. Pernicone, B. W. Scheithauer, T. J. Sebo et al., "Pituitary carcinoma," *Cancer*, vol. 79, no. 4, pp. 804–812, 1997.

[20] F. Yoo, E. C. Kuan, A. P. Heaney, M. Bergsneider, and M. B. Wang, "Corticotrophic pituitary carcinoma with cervical metastases: case series and literature review," *Pituitary*, vol. 21, no. 3, pp. 290–301, 2018.

[21] A. R. Lafferty and G. P. Chrousos, "Pituitary tumors in children and adolescents," *Journal of Clinical Endocrinology & Metabolism*, vol. 84, no. 12, pp. 4317–4323, 1999.

[22] A. Guzel, M. Tatli, S. Senturk, E. Guzel, S. R. Cayli, and A. Sav, "Pituitary carcinoma presenting with multiple metastases: case report," *Journal of Child Neurology*, vol. 23, no. 12, pp. 1467–1471, 2008.

[23] M. E. Molitch, "Pituitary incidentalomas," *Best Practice & Research Clinical Endocrinology & Metabolism*, vol. 23, no. 5, pp. 667–675, 2009.

[24] A. Wierinckx, C. Auger, P. Devauchelle et al., "A diagnostic marker set for invasion, proliferation, and aggressiveness of prolactin pituitary tumors," *Endocrine-Related Cancer*, vol. 14, no. 3, pp. 887–900, Article ID 17914117, 2007 Sep.

[25] G. Raverot, P. Burman, A. McCormack et al., "European Society of Endocrinology Clinical Practice Guidelines for the management of aggressive pituitary tumours and carcinomas," *European Journal of Endocrinology*, vol. 178, no. 1, pp. G1–G24, 2018.

[26] C. Hagen, H. D. Schroeder, S. Hansen, C. Hagen, and M. Andersen, "Temozolomide treatment of a pituitary carcinoma and two pituitary macroadenomas resistant to conventional therapy," *European Journal of Endocrinology*, vol. 161, no. 4, pp. 631–637, 2009.

A Glucagonoma Presenting as Cerebral Vein Thrombosis and Diabetes

Marina Delli Colli,[1] Bader N. Alamri,[1] Laura Palma,[2] and Juan Rivera[1]

[1]*Division of Endocrinology and Metabolism, Department of Medicine, McGill University, Montreal, Quebec, Canada*
[2]*Division of Medical Genetics, Department of Specialized Medicine, McGill University, Montreal, Quebec, Canada*

Correspondence should be addressed to Marina Delli Colli; marina.dellicolli@mail.mcgill.ca

Academic Editor: Toshihiro Kita

Glucagonomas are rare pancreatic neuroendocrine tumors (pNETs), malignant in 80% of cases, thus highlighting the importance of early diagnosis and treatment. Primary manifestations are diabetes, dermatosis, depression, weight loss, and deep vein thrombosis. Unlike other pNETs, glucagonomas are associated with a higher incidence of thromboembolic events, often resulting in death. We present the case of a glucagonoma patient whose primary manifestation was cerebral sinus venous thrombosis (CS-VT). Early diagnosis enabled curative resection. The purpose of this paper is to review the underlying mechanisms associated with increased coagulopathy in glucagonomas.

1. Background

Glucagonoma is a rare, functional, pancreatic neuroendocrine tumor (pNET) in which the islet alpha cells of the pancreas oversecrete glucagon [1]. Accounting for only 4% of all pNETs, glucagonomas have a malignancy rate of 80% and therefore require early detection and treatment [2]. Their typical presentation, glucagonoma syndrome, is a paraneoplastic syndrome characterized by diabetes, dermatosis, and weight loss. Additionally, patients often present with anemia, malnutrition, diarrhea, glossitis, cheilitis, depression, and other psychiatric manifestations, and deep vein thrombosis [3, 4]. Herein, we present the case of a patient with a glucagonoma whose primary manifestation was cerebral sinus venous thrombosis (CS-VT), which to our knowledge has not been reported before.

2. Case Report

A 68-year-old man with a history of psoriasis and benign prostate hyperplasia experienced severe headaches, insomnia, and dizziness for three consecutive days. On the fourth day post symptom onset, he presented to the emergency department due to a worsening right-sided headache, along with new-onset vomiting and left-sided weakness/discoordination. A brain CT scan showed multicompartmental right parietal hemorrhage adjacent to the superior sagittal sinus with a surrounding meningioma. A CTA scan revealed an extensive superior sagittal sinus thrombosis extending into the right transverse and right sigmoid sinus. Treatment with intravenous heparin was initiated. During his hospitalization, the patient's headache improved, and his left-sided weakness resolved within one week. Left sensory ataxia remained. Workup for occult malignancy revealed, on a CT abdomen, an exophytic hyperdense enhancing lesion, measuring 1.1×2.2 cm, in the posterior aspect of the tail of the pancreas, suggestive of a neuroendocrine tumor. There was no evidence of primary malignancy or metastatic disease involving the chest, liver, or prostate. During this admission, a new diagnosis of hypertension and type 2 DM were made as he remained hyperglycemic, and his HbA1C was 11.8%. The patient denied a history of diarrhea, flushing, or abdominal pain but endorsed night sweats and weight loss. His family history was significant for a brother with a pancreatic neuroendocrine tumor (pNET) and sister with multiple meningiomas. Endocrinology was consulted, and a pertinent workup for pNET was ordered. Chromogranin A (CgA) was elevated at 439.9 ng/ml (≤82); however, the patient was already on proton pump inhibitors (PPIs). The urinary cortisol was normal. PTH, serum calcium, and the pituitary hormonal panel were all normal. hCG and CEA were also normal. Factor V Leiden and prothrombin were normal. Given the combination of new-onset DM, DVT, and pNET, serum glucagon was requested and reported as increased at 202 pg/ml and 174 pg/ml (reference range <80 pg/ml). A pancreatic MRI identified a well-defined round, T2 iso/hypointense lesion, measuring 10 x 11 × 10 mm in keeping with a pNET. A Ga68-DOTATATE PET scan identified the pancreatic lesion as DOTATATE-avid. Additional lesions were identified in the cranial cavity, compatible with meningiomas.

Based on the unusual presentation of pNET in two siblings, the patient was assessed in medical genetics and underwent germline testing for an 86-gene panel through a commercial laboratory (Invitae). No pathogenic/likely pathogenic variant was identified by next-generation sequencing, including all possible candidate genes known to be associated with hereditary predisposition to neuroendocrine tumors (i.e., *MEN1, VHL, NF1, NF2, TSC1, TSC2, PRKAR1A, PTEN, TP53, SMARCB1,* and *SMARCE1*). Two heterozygous variants of uncertain significance not thought to be associated with the patient's phenotype were detected, namely, *TSC2* (c.1952C > T) and *NBN* (c.806G > A). To date, the patient's brother with pNET has not been assessed in genetics.

The patient underwent laparoscopic distal pancreatectomy and splenectomy, with no complications. Pathology described a well-demarcated, white appearing, firm, homogenous nodule, measuring 13 x 10 × 9 mm, pT1N0M0, with a Ki-67 index of 2% (G1). The tumor cells showed moderate and diffuse glucagon staining with patchy insulin staining. Plasma glucagon decreased from 202 pg/ml to 47 pg/ml post surgical resection. Although measured while on an anti-factor *X* inhibitor (DOACs), LMWH anti-factor *X* was low at 0.37 U/mL (0.50–1.00 U/mL) presurgical resection, and factor *X* level was normal at 0.78 U/mL (N = 0.50–1.50 U/mL) post surgical resection.

3. Discussion

Glucagonomas are estimated to have an incidence rate of 1 case in 20 million people per year [5, 6]. Cases are reported either equally in both sexes, or in some series, with a male predominance of 70% [7]. While most cases are sporadic, 3% of glucagonomas are associated with genetic disorders such as MEN 1 or von Hippel–Lindau syndrome, the latter being less prevalent [8]. Most patients present in the fifth to sixth decade of life, and over 80% have metastatic disease at the time of diagnosis, often invading lymph nodes, liver, and bones. They tend to be large at the time of diagnosis (2–30 cm), with circulating glucagon levels from 120 to over 20,000 pg/mL [7, 9]. The classical manifestations of the glucagonoma syndrome include diabetes or prediabetes, dermatosis (necrolytic migratory erythema), diarrhea, dementia-like manifestations, deep vein thrombosis, anemia, and weight loss (often cachexia). The case discussed here was unusual in that it was diagnosed early while measuring under 2 cm, it had no metastases, and only some of the classical clinical manifestations.

Although glucagonomas are associated with a high incidence of thromboembolic events and cerebral sinus venous thrombosis (CS-VT) as the presenting manifestations, as seen in our case, are novel and merit recognition. Thromboembolic events have been reported in 30–80% of glucagonoma patients, particularly DVT of lower limbs and pulmonary embolism (PE). Over 50% of deaths in patients with glucagonoma are directly attributed to thromboembolic events [10]. However, glucagonomas do not seem to be typically associated with other signs of disseminated coagulopathy, and glucagon is not known to influence the coagulation cascade [11]. Therefore, the mechanism for this coagulopathy, aside from prothrombotic factors which are common to all malignancies is unclear [12]. Increased production of factor *X* by the tumor alpha cells of the pancreas has been a suggested mechanism [10]. It is more likely that the prothrombotic state associated with glucagonomas is multifactorial which contributing factors include zinc depletion [13], a potential direct effect of glucagon on fibrinolysis [14], imbalanced reduction of prothrombotic and fibrinolytic factors associated with impaired liver protein synthesis capacity, hyperhomocysteinemia, and endothelial dysfunction from B12 deficiency related to malabsorption and malnutrition [15].

In 70 to 90% of patients, CS-VT presents as acute or subacute headache lasting 1–3 days. Focal neurological deficits (mono- or paraparesis or hemiparesis) occur in about half of patients, hours or days after headache onset [16]. Glucagonomas, on the other hand, are also associated with neurological disturbances, occurring in 20% of patients [17]. These manifestations are highly diverse, including muscle weakness, hyperreflexia, insomnia, psychosis, depression, and overt dementia [17]. Our patient reported dizziness and insomnia prior to his admission to the hospital. Left hemiparesis was also present.

While literature suggests varying severities of glucose intolerance associated with glucagonoma, DM remains a cardinal sign of glucagonoma [17]. Glucagon's role in glucose homeostasis is mediated by its catabolic effects from stimulations of gluconeogenesis, glycogenolysis, ketogenesis, and lipolysis [10]. In addition to hepatic phosphorylase activation, glucagon stimulates insulin secretion and inhibits pancreatic enzymes excretion. The overall result is hyperglycemia [10]. Persistent hyperglucagonemia leads to the reduction of plasma amino acid concentrations, with amplification of essential amino acid catabolism [15]. Consequently, DM develops in 80% of glucagonoma patients along with muscle, fat mass, and glycogen store depletion [10, 15].

Weight loss is a very common finding in the initial presentation of glucagonomas, occurring in 56% to 91% of cases [17]. The catabolic action of glucagon directly causes nutritional and metabolic deficiencies of zinc, essential fatty acids, and amino acids [18]. Subsequent weight loss occurs as the hormone diverts dietary amino acids into glucose by the liver and away from protein synthesis by other tissues [11].

In link, glucagon induction of inflammatory mediators, such as arachidonic acid derivatives, contributes to generalized malabsorption and malnutrition [18]. Malnutrition is also worsened due to diarrhea, another common clinical feature of glucagonoma [19]. Diarrhea not only results from the increased glucagon levels but also from the cosecretion of gastrin, VIP, serotonin, or calcitonin [5]. This patient did not experience diarrhea, however, validated significant weight loss.

Such nutritional deficiency influences the integumentary system, causing cutaneous lesions characteristic of the glucagonoma syndrome [10]. Occurring in 70% of patients, necrolytic migratory erythema (NME) consists of erythematous scaling and crusting, often appearing in the groin and perineal areas [10]. Hypoaminoacidemia, vitamins B, and zinc deficiency are recognized causes [10]. As NME is most likely a late manifestation of years of tumor growth, early recognition of these lesions is crucial in preventing further risk of metastases [10]. Our patient's small tumor, with only mild elevation of plasma glucagon, was not associated with NME.

In summary, the case described here is a reminder to clinicians to keep alert for clues pointing in the direction of a treatable common denominator in a patient with an atypical constellation of symptoms or atypical presentation of common conditions. In reference to glucagonomas, we would like to highlight the fact that staying alert to concurrent clinical manifestation in the case of PNETs may lead to early recognition of this deadly tumor. At such early stage of the evaluation, surgical resection can potentially lead to a cure.

Consent

Informed consent was obtained from the patient.

References

[1] R. Eldor, B. Glaser, M. Fraenkel, V. Doviner, A. Salmon, and D. J. Gross, "Glucagonoma and the glucagonoma syndrome - cumulative experience with an elusive endocrine tumour," *Clinical Endocrinology*, vol. 74, no. 5, pp. 593–598, 2011.

[2] T. Karaaslan and C. Karatoprak, "New diagnosis diabetes and deep venous thrombosis with glucagonoma cases; case report," *Bezmialem Science*, vol. 7, no. 4, pp. 348–351, 2019.

[3] M. Cunha-Silva, J. G. d Costa, G. A. S. Faria et al., "Diarrhea: a missed D in the 4D glucagonoma syndrome," *Autopsy Case Reports*, vol. 9, no. 4, Article ID e2019129, 2019.

[4] X. Han, D. Wang, T. Kuang, Y. Rong, and W. Lou, "Glucagonoma syndrome: report of one case," *Translational Gastroenterology and Hepatology*, vol. 1, p. 70, 2016.

[5] S. Sandhu and I. Jialal, "Glucagonoma syndrome," in *StatPearls. 2021*, StatPearls Publishing, Treasure Island, FL, USA, 2021.

[6] A. M. John and R. A. Schwartz, "Glucagonoma syndrome: a review and update on treatment," *Journal of the European Academy of Dermatology and Venereology*, vol. 30, no. 12, pp. 2016–2022, 2016.

[7] H. Kindmark, A. Sundin, D. Granberg et al., "Endocrine pancreatic tumors with glucagon hypersecretion: a retrospective study of 23 cases during 20 years," *Medical Oncology*, vol. 24, no. 3, pp. 330–337, 2007.

[8] M. Alvarez, A. Almanzar, F. Sanabria, G. Meneses, L. Velasquez, and L. Zarate, "Manifestations of glucagonoma syndrome," *AACE clinical case reports*, vol. 6, no. 1, pp. e46–e49, 2020.

[9] R. A. Wermers, V. Fatourechi, A. G. Wynne, L. K. Kvols, and R. V. Lloyd, "The glucagonoma syndrome. clinical and pathologic features in 21 patients," *Medicine*, vol. 75, no. 2, pp. 53–63, 1996.

[10] P. G. Castro, A. M. de Leon, J. G. Trancon et al., "Glucagonoma syndrome: a case report," *Journal of Medical Case Reports*, vol. 5, no. 1, p. 402, 2011.

[11] P. W. Stacpoole, "The glucagonoma syndrome: clinical features, diagnosis, and treatment," *Endocrine Reviews*, vol. 2, no. 3, pp. 347–361, 1981.

[12] A. Falanga, L. Russo, V. Milesi, and A. Vignoli, "Mechanisms and risk factors of thrombosis in cancer," *Critical Reviews in Oncology*, vol. 118, pp. 79–83, 2017.

[13] T. T. Vu, J. C. Fredenburgh, and J. I. Weitz, "Zinc: an important cofactor in haemostasis and thrombosis," *Thromb Haemost*, vol. 109, no. 03, pp. 421–430, 2013.

[14] E. Henkel, S. Gallo, G. Siegert, C. Koehler, and M. Hanefeld, "Glucagon as a determinant of fibrinolytic activity in men with different stages of glucose tolerance: impact of glucagon on fibrinolysis," *Blood Coagulation & Fibrinolysis*, vol. 18, no. 4, pp. 327–334, 2007.

[15] A. P. van Beek, E. R. M. de Haas, W. A. van Vloten, C. J. M. Lips, J. F. M. Roijers, and M. R. Canninga-van Dijk, "The glucagonoma syndrome and necrolytic migratory erythema: a clinical review," *European Journal of Endocrinology*, vol. 151, no. 5, pp. 531–537, 2004.

[16] A. H. Ropper and J. P. Klein, "Cerebral venous thrombosis," *New England Journal of Medicine*, vol. 385, no. 1, pp. 59–64, 2021.

[17] M. A. Chastain, "The glucagonoma syndrome: a review of its features and discussion of new perspectives," *The American Journal of the Medical Sciences*, vol. 321, no. 5, pp. 306–320, 2001.

[18] E. P. Tierney and J. Badger, "Etiology and pathogenesis of necrolytic migratory erythema: review of the literature," *MedGenMed:Medscape General Medicine*, vol. 6, no. 3, p. 4, 2004.

[19] W. T. Zandee, J. Hofland, and W. W. de Herder, *Glucagonoma Syndrome*, MDText.com, Inc., South Dartmouth, MA, USA, 2000.

32

Unusual Case of Malignant Struma Ovarii and Cervical Thyroid Cancer Preceded by Ovarian Teratoma: Case Report and Review of the Literature

Elias G. Tzelepis,[1] **Elena Barengolts**,[1] **Steven Garzon**,[2] **Joseph Shulan**,[1] **and Yuval Eisenberg**[1]

[1]*Division of Endocrinology, Diabetes & Metabolism, University of Illinois at Chicago, Chicago, IL, USA*
[2]*Department of Pathology, University of Illinois at Chicago, Chicago, IL, USA*

Correspondence should be addressed to Elias G. Tzelepis; etzelepis@gmail.com

Academic Editor: Antonio S. Laganà

Objective. To present a rare case of malignant struma ovarii (MSO) and synchronous thyroid cancer, review the medical literature, and present the latest trends in management. *Methods*. The case of a woman with MSO and concomitant thyroid cancer is presented, including clinical presentation, treatment, and follow-up care. A search of the English-language literature was conducted using MEDLINE and Google Scholar data bases. *Results*. We found 10 publications (one abstract) describing 10 patients with MSO and concomitant thyroid cancer. Six additional patients were reported by a study that analyzed the SEER (cancer registry) database. The median age of women was 42 years, with the majority of them presenting with abdominal symptoms. Histologically, most tumors were papillary carcinomas in both organs. In 5 patients, there was extrathyroidal tumor extension at time of surgery. *Conclusion*. MSO can occasionally coexist with highly aggressive eutopic thyroid cancer. Although this concurrence is even rarer than MSO, clinicians should routinely investigate for possible synchronous thyroid cancer in all cases of MSO and also consider aggressive postoperative treatment including thyroidectomy and radioiodine ablation therapy in cases of MSO.

1. Introduction

Struma ovarii refers to a germ cell tumor that is composed of at least 50% thyroid tissue [1, 2]. These tumors account for about 2-3% of all ovarian tumors [1–3]. They are relatively rare, with no more than 200 cases reported in the literature [4].

Most struma ovarii are benign, with malignant transformation occurring in only 5% of these tumors [5, 6]. Malignant struma ovarii (MSO) coexisting with primary thyroid carcinoma is extremely rare, with only a handful of cases reported in the literature [2, 7, 8]. The synchronous development of primary thyroid carcinoma and MSO is not fully understood. Investigations including morphological, immunohistochemical, and molecular analysis suggest that synchronous, albeit distinct, primary tumors in the ovary and cervical thyroid may occur [8, 9]. A hypothesized "field cancerization" and early genomic instability may explain multifocality in all thyroid-type tissue. Some experts, therefore, recommend routine imaging of the thyroid gland for coexisting carcinoma in all patients with high risk MSO [8]. Supporting evidence for this approach also comes from a population-level analysis reporting an approximately 9% prevalence of synchronous or metachronous aggressive thyroid cancers in a series of 68 patients with MSO [10].

Given the overall rarity of MSO and its possible concurrence with thyroid cancer, the optimal management of MSO is controversial, especially when the tumor is not metastatic [11–13]. Areas of contention include aggressiveness of therapy, prophylactic thyroidectomy, and radioactive iodine (RAI) [7, 8, 13, 14]. Here, we present the case of a woman with MSO and concomitant thyroid carcinoma, along with a literature

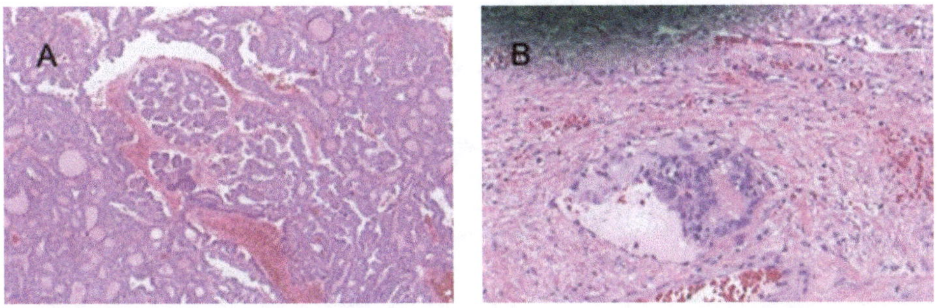

(a) (b)

FIGURE 1: (a) Papillary thyroid carcinoma arising in struma ovarii. (b) Vascular invasion of malignant struma ovarii.

review of similar cases reported in the English literature highlighting the current trends in management of this rare malignancy.

2. Clinical Case

A 32-year-old nulliparous female presented to the endocrinology clinic for further evaluation and treatment of a recently diagnosed MSO. Five years prior to this evaluation, she underwent bilateral ovarian cystectomy for complex ovarian masses which were histologically consistent with mature teratomas. Over the ensuing four years, serial ultrasonography showed progressive interval growth of the bilateral cystic masses, especially of the left adnexal mass growing from 4.3 cm to 12.9 cm in approximately 4 years.

Five months prior to her endocrinology evaluation, she underwent exploratory laparotomy with left salpingo-oophorectomy, right ovarian cystectomy, lysis of adhesions, and partial omentectomy. Pathology showed a 6.0 cm malignant struma ovarii, with predominantly follicular variant papillary thyroid carcinoma in the left ovary (Figure 1(a)). The tumor, classified as pT1a pNx; FIGO IA, was organ confined but with lymphatic/vascular invasion (Figure 1(b)). The omentum was free of tumor, and in the right ovary a hemorrhagic corpus luteum cyst was identified. Postoperatively she underwent an I-123 whole body scan which did not identify any metastatic disease. Specifically, there was no abnormal uptake in the adnexae or the abdomen, although this was likely of limited utility given the intact thyroid gland.

When seen in the endocrinology clinic, she had no abdominal complaints. Physical exam was unremarkable, including a normal neck exam without palpable thyroid enlargement or nodularity and with a soft abdomen without palpable masses or ascites. Family history was significant for cervical and lung cancer in her mother as well as the maternal grandmother with breast and bone malignancies.

Laboratory testing showed TSH 2.98 mcIU/ml (0.35-4.0), FT4 16.7 pmol/L [1.3 ng/dL (0.6-1.7)], FT3 49.1 pmol/L [3.2 ng/dL (87-178)], thyroglobulin antibody negative, (<1.0) thyroglobulin 108.5 ng/mL (1.3-31.8). A thyroid ultrasound showed a mixed hypo- and isoechoic 0.8 x 0.4 x0.7 cm nodule with several echogenic punctate foci consistent with microcalcifications. Fine needle aspiration biopsy of the nodule was interpreted as atypia of undetermined significance (Bethesda III). Given the clinical history of MSO, indeterminate cytopathology, and patient preference, the decision was made to perform total thyroidectomy. Pathology revealed a 0.6cm papillary thyroid carcinoma with no lymphovascular invasion (Figure 2). There was, however, a single focus of extra thyroidal extension (pT3). Her postoperative course was complicated by hypoparathyroidism with symptomatic hypocalcemia which resolved with aggressive replacement of calcitriol and elemental calcium. Thyroglobulin levels were 9.5 ng/ml with negative thyroglobulin antibodies at two months after thyroidectomy. She was discharged on calcitriol 0.25mcg BID and calcium carbonate 2500mg TID (3000mg elemental calcium). She was started on liothyronine 25mcg PO daily, in anticipation of planned RAI therapy.

Three months later, I-123 WBS/SPECT/CT revealed multiple avid foci in the neck suggestive of lymph node metastasis and residual thyroid tissue, as well as one faint focus in the mid-abdomen possibly representing a metastatic mesenteric lymph node. Ultrasonography failed to reveal abnormal cervical lymph nodes. Considering these findings in total, it was decided to proceed with radioactive iodine therapy and she received 184.3 mCi of I-131 therapy. Post-therapy whole body scan revealed successful targeting of radioiodine therapy to thyroid tissue in the neck, and no convincing abnormal focal uptake in abdomen or pelvis to suggest radioiodine avid metastatic disease. Thyroglobulin levels post-RAI ablation decreased to 0.5ng/ml and subsequently to 0.1ng/ml upon later testing. BRAF mutational analysis testing for the V600E mutation was negative for both ovarian and thyroid papillary carcinomas. Patient also had testing for TERT promoter mutations, which were negative. Post-RAI ablation, patient was switched to levothyroxine 200mcg daily with subsequent titration to 225 mcg daily to achieve suppressed TSH. Hypocalcemia eventually resolved, and she was transitioned off calcitriol and calcium carbonate supplementation. A year after RAI ablation, the patient underwent rhTSH stimulated WBS which did not show any evidence of thyroid cancer recurrence. The most recent thyroid ultrasound (12/2017) showed stable benign appearing lymph nodes, and no evidence of residual or recurrent thyroid tissue (thyroglobulin level of 0.1 ng/ml). A pelvic surveillance MRI showed benign appearing cystic lesions at the right adnexa, but no evidence of metastatic disease. The patient provided written informed consent to publish her case.

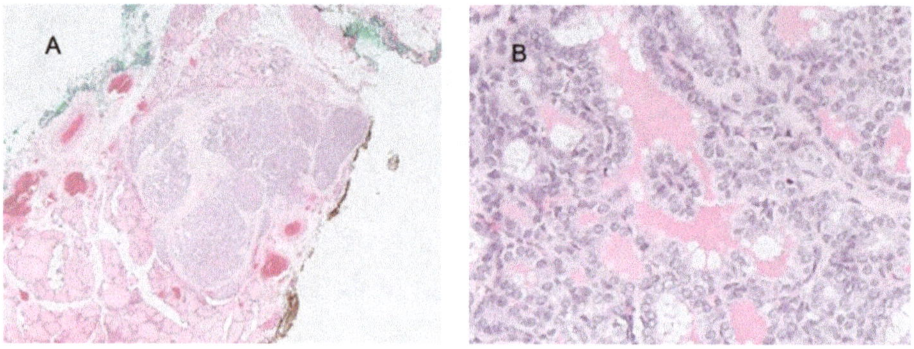

(a) (b)

FIGURE 2: (a) Well circumscribed nodule composed of papillary thyroid carcinoma with solid, follicular, and papillary architecture surrounded by fibrosis. (b). Areas with papillary architecture with cytologically enlarged nuclei with grooves and open chromatin.

3. Discussion

Malignant transformation of struma ovarii occurs in less than 5% of these ovarian tumors [5, 13]. Patients with MSO typically present with abdominal pain or an incidental ovarian mass, vaginal bleeding, menstrual cycle abnormalities, and symptoms of hyperthyroidism or rarely with ascites [13, 20–22]. Patients may occasionally present with symptoms of hyperthyroidism (5-8% of cases) [13] or elevated ovarian cancer markers (CA-125) [23]. Following diagnosis of differentiated thyroid cancer arising in struma ovarii, further work-up should include thyroid evaluation to exclude synchronous thyroid carcinoma.

Concurrence of MSO and intrathyroidal cancer is quite rare. In reviewing the literature, we found 10 publications, 9 case reports [2, 7–9, 14–16, 18], and one abstract [17], describing 10 patients with synchronous MSO and thyroid carcinoma (Table 1). Not shown in Table 1 are additional patients reported by two retrospective analyses of the Surveillance, Epidemiology, and End Results (SEER) database from 1973 to 2011 by Goffredo et al. [10] and Sisti et al. [24]. Goffredo et al. analyzed the entire database (SEER 18 Registries) whereas Sistri et al. only part of it (SEER 9 Registries). Although an overlap of the reported patients between the two analyses cannot be excluded, Goffredo et al. identified 6 patients (median age 36) with concomitant thyroid cancer out of 68 patients with MSO and Sisti et al. one patient with synchronous and one with metachronous thyroid cancer out of 21 patients with MSO. As most patients reported are from institutions outside the US (unlikely overlap with those reported by Goffredo et al.), the total number of reported MSO patients with coexisting thyroid cancer in the English literature is not greater than 17.

The median age of women described with concomitant MSO and intrathyroidal was 42 years (range 30-55), with the majority of them having ovarian masses larger than 5 cm. With exception of two patients [16, 19] who sought advice for cervical thyroid nodules (MSO diagnosed after thyroidectomy with radioiodine), the remaining patients had manifestations related to the abdomen. Size of thyroid tumors ranged from 0.2 to 1.7 cm. There were two patients with MSO size less than 1.0 cm. Histologically, most tumors were papillary thyroid carcinomas in both sites, with only one discordant case of a follicular thyroid cancer in MSO and papillary thyroid cancer in the cervical thyroid [7]. There were five patients with extrathyroidal tumor extension or metastasis to regional lymph nodes at time of thyroidectomy. Our patient had evidence of extrathyroidal tumor extension on thyroid pathology. She was also believed to have metastatic disease to cervical lymph nodes three months after thyroidectomy, based on thyroglobulin measures and nuclear imaging. Similarly, Goffredo et al. reported that the majority (two-thirds) of the patients with synchronous MSO and thyroid carcinoma had evidence of cancer extension outside the gland.

The relatively high prevalence (about 9%) of MSO coexisting with thyroid cancer reported by Goffredo et al. may support the notion for a true association and common pathogenic mechanism [10]. Evidence for a common pathogenesis for all papillary thyroid carcinomas was also provided by Schmidt et al. who found BRAF gene mutations in 4 out of 6 patients with MSO and in none of 9 patients with benign struma ovarii [25]. These data indicate that the development of MSO is associated with *BRAF* mutations of the type commonly seen in cervical thyroid papillary carcinoma. Although BRAF mutations in MSO were additionally found in other case reports [26] or small series of patients [27], we could not find any literature reports of BRAF mutations in both MSO and cervical thyroid cancer. Reporting differences in tumor expression of CK-19 in a patient with synchronous MSO and cervical thyroid cancer, Leong et al. [8] supported the notion of an autonomous existence of the two cancers and postulated an early genetic instability to explain the multifocal oncogenesis.

Concomitant MSO and thyroid cancer should be differentiated from papillary carcinoma of the cervical thyroid with ovarian metastasis, which is extremely rare [28]. Presence of teratomatous elements and normal thyroid epithelial tissue in the ovary is suggestive of MSO rather than metastatic thyroid cancer [8]. In this respect, ovarian MRI may help distinguish the two by revealing multiloculated ovarian cystic mass with a solid component and a variable signal intensity between

Table 1: Reported cases of synchronous malignant struma ovarii and thyroid carcinoma.

Reference	Patient Age (yrs)	Ovarian Mass Size (cm)	MSO Size (cm)	MSO Pathology	MSO Stage	Thyroid Carcinoma Size (cm), Type	ONCOGENIC EXPRESSION
Boyd et al [15]	30	8.5x5x4	----	Papillary	No surface involvement, No LV invasion	1.0, Papillary, NO ETE	-------
Brusca et al. [14]	30	7.3x3	0.9	Papillary	------	0.2, Papillary, No ETE	--------
Janszen et al. [7]	52	10x8	----	Follicular	-------	0.3, Papillary, No ETE	------
Catalina et al. [9]	33	9.5x7.5x3.5	2.5	Papillary	No surface involvement, No LV invasion	1.4, Papillary With ETE, Metastatic to lymph nodes	-----
Leong et al. [8]	42	13.5	----	Papillary	No surface involvement, No LV invasion	0.6-0.8, Papillary, bilateral multifocal, with ETE, mets to lymph nodes	BRAF – K-RAS – RET/PTC -
Marti et al. [2]	44	2.4	-----	Papillary	--------	0.5, Papillary with ETE, mets to lymph nodes	BRAF -
Middelbeek et al [16]	55		1.5	Papillary	No surface involvement, No LV invasion	1.2, Papillary, No ETE	BRAF -
Capitato et al. [17]	35	8.2x7x6		Papillary	No surface involvement	1.7, Papillary, No ETE	BRAF -
Krishnamurthy et al. [18]	51	13x7.6	0.8	Papillary		0.4, papillary follicular variant	----
Lim et al. [19]	63	3x2.5x1.5	-----	Papillary	No surface involvment, No LV invasion	Papillary, mets to lymph nodes	----
Present case	30	12.9	6.0	Papillary	No surface involvment, LV invasion	0.6, Papillary, with ETE, mets to lymph nodes	BRAF – RET/PTC – TERT -

Abbreviations: MSO, malignant struma ovarii; LV, lymphovascular; ETE, extrathyroid extension.

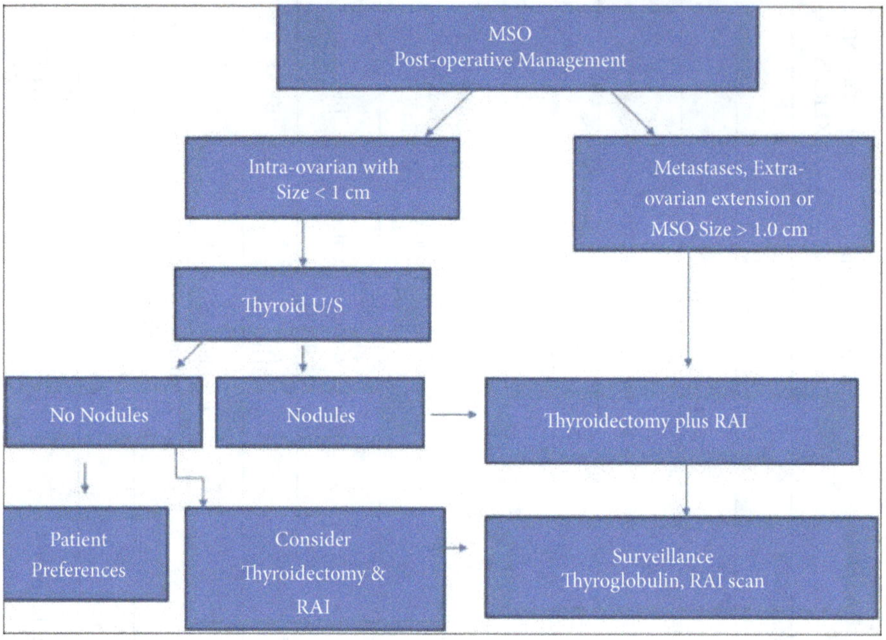

FIGURE 3: Algorithm summarizing current trends in postoperative management of malignant struma ovarii.

locules ("stained glass imaging") [29]. Our patient had known history of mature ovarian teratoma and the MRI was also consistent with multiloculated cysts.

The optimal management of MSO remains controversial [11–13]. As with most rare diseases, the natural history of MSO is not fully defined and there is a paucity of evidence-based clinical practice guidelines. The extent of ovarian surgery can be a subject of debate [30], especially when preservation of fertility is an issue. Preoperative ultrasonography may help differentiate benign from malignant pathologies and allow for ovarian sparing surgical planning if appropriate [31]. The most contentious aspects of MSO treatment include need for thyroidectomy and postoperative RAI in patients with no evidence of metastases [2]. Presence of metastases poses no therapeutic dilemma and all patients should be treated with thyroidectomy followed by RAI [2, 5, 32]. Given the possible coexistence of synchronous thyroid cancer, total thyroidectomy will exclude thyroid cancer, permit RAI for micrometastasis, and increase reliability of thyroglobulin as a marker for follow-up [7]. In six patients treated with thyroidectomy and RAI after resection of MSO, DeSimone et al. [13] reported no recurrence. In contrast, Jean et al. [33] reported a 21 % recurrence in 42 MSO patients treated only surgically.

Most authors [5, 13–15, 34–37] endorse an aggressive postoperative treatment with thyroidectomy followed by RAI therapy on the basis that RAI may reduce recurrence and possibly mortality [32, 33, 38] especially in cases of uncertainty about surgery completeness, in an analogy used to treat cervical thyroid cancer [1]. In two separate analyses of MSO patients reported in the literature, Devaney et al. [1] and DeSimone et al. [13] noted that more recurrences occurred in patients who were conservatively treated with surgery only than in those who received primary adjuvant therapy.

Risk stratification in MSO has been proposed as a means to help choose the appropriate treatment postoperatively in patients with no evidence of metastases at time of surgery [6]. Yassa et al. [6] suggested that MSO measuring over 2 cm, or with extraovarian extension, or aggressive histological features should be treated with thyroidectomy and RAI. However, tumor size criteria are not unanimously agreed upon by all authors, with some using cutoff tumor size of 1 cm [7]. Furthermore, measuring tumor size can be extremely difficult in cases in which the tumor is intermixed with teratomatous tissue [2]. Likewise, histological features of MSO were not found to correlate with clinical outcome in 26 patients with MSO followed up for a period ranging from 5 to 20 years [39]. Extraovarian tumor extension is generally considered an indication for aggressive treatment with thyroidectomy and RAI [2]. In our patient, the choice of postoperative treatment was indisputable as she had extraovarian tumor extension.

Given the rarity of the disease, the postoperative management of MSO will likely continue to be controversial and be based on results of small observational studies, rather than controlled studies. The present literature review provided a description of the coexistence of MSO and thyroid cancer, highlighting the relatively aggressive cervical thyroid cancer found in 45 % of reported cases (Table 1) which is in agreement with the findings of Goffredo et al. Considering the relatively high prevalence of these synchronous tumors in the SEER database and the generally increasing incidence of thyroid cancer [40], the clinician should be aware of the possible association and further investigate it in all patients with MSO. Despite the significant uncertainty and many unsettled issues about treatment, we propose an algorithm (Figure 3) for the postoperative management of MSO. Again, this algorithm summarizes the current trend of recommendations in the literature, which are based on small retrospective observational studies and are by no means firm and indisputable. As most authors [5, 13–15, 34–37], we endorse an aggressive postoperative management that should include thyroidectomy and RAI in all patients with MSO. Patient preferences might only be considered in cases in which the tumor is small and confined to ovary and there is no evidence of thyroid nodules. Ultrasonographic detection of thyroid nodules postoperatively will simply reinforce and justify this aggressive approach.

4. Conclusion

MSO, a rare malignant tumor arising from struma ovarii, can occasionally coexist with thyroid cancer. The present literature review supports the notion that the concurrent cervical thyroid tumors are usually aggressive cancers. Clinicians should be aware of this association and routinely investigate for thyroid nodules in all cases of MSO. In view of this association, we endorse an aggressive postoperative management of all MSO cases that includes thyroidectomy and RAI.

Abbreviations

MSO:	Malignant struma ovarii
RAI:	Radioactive iodine
TSH:	Thyroid stimulating hormone
FT4:	Free thyroxine
FT3:	Free triiodothyronine
WBS:	Whole body scan
SPECT/CT:	Single-photon emission computer tomography/computer tomography
LV:	Lymphovascular
ETE:	Extrathyroid extension.

Acknowledgments

We thank Dr. M. Xing, Johns Hopkins Hospital, for help with TERT promoter mutation testing.

References

[1] K. Devaney, R. Snyder, H. J. Norris, and F. A. Tavassoli, "Proliferative and histologically malignant struma ovarii: a clinicopathologic study of 54 cases," *International Journal of Gynecological Pathology*, vol. 12, no. 4, pp. 333–343, 1993.

[2] J. L. Marti, V. E. Clark, H. Harper, D. C. Chhieng, J. A. Sosa, and S. A. Roman, "Optimal surgical management of well-differentiated thyroid cancer arising in struma ovarii: a series of 4 patients and a review of 53 reported cases," *Thyroid*, vol. 22, no. 4, pp. 400–406, 2012.

[3] E. D. Wirtz, N. Bothwell, and C. Klem, "Role of the otolaryngologist in the treatment of struma ovarii," *The Laryngoscope*, vol. 120, no. 2, pp. 259-260, 2009.

[4] P. Marcy, J. Thariat, D. Benisvy, and P. Azuar, "Lethal, malignant, metastatic struma ovarii," *Thyroid*, vol. 20, no. 9, pp. 1037–1040, 2010.

[5] J. McGill, C. Sturgeon, and P. Angelos, "Metastatic struma ovarii treated with total thyroidectomy and radioiodine ablation," *Endocrine Practice - American Association of Clinical Endocrinologists*, vol. 15, no. 2, pp. 167–173, 2009.

[6] L. Yassa, P. Sadow, and E. Marqusee, "Malignant struma ovarii," *Nature Clinical Practice Endocrinology & Metabolism*, vol. 4, no. 8, pp. 469–472, 2008.

[7] E. W. Janszen, H. C. Van Doorn, P. C. Ewing et al., "Malignant struma ovarii: good response after thyroidectomy and I ablation therapy," *Clinical Medicine: Oncology*, vol. 2, pp. 147–152, 2008.

[8] A. Leong, P. J. Roche, M. Paliouras, L. Rochon, M. Trifiro, and M. Tamilia, "Coexistence of malignant struma ovarii and cervical papillary thyroid carcinoma," *The Journal of Clinical Endocrinology & Metabolism*, vol. 98, no. 12, pp. 4599–4605, 2013.

[9] P. F. Catalina, A. R. Iraeta, M. L. Solar, and P. S. Sobrino, "Sincronous malignant struma ovarii and papillary thyroid carcinoma," *Endocrinol Y Nutr Organo La Soc Esp Endocrinol Y Nutr*, vol. 63, no. 7, pp. 366-367, 2016.

[10] P. Goffredo, A. M. Sawka, J. Pura, M. A. Adam, S. A. Roman, and J. A. Sosa, "Malignant struma ovarii: a population-level analysis of a large series of 68 patients," *Thyroid*, vol. 25, no. 2, pp. 211–215, 2015.

[11] S. Gunasekaran, E. Kopecka, K. H. Maung, and R. J. England, "Struma ovarii and the thyroid surgeon," *The Journal of Laryngology & Otology*, vol. 126, no. 08, pp. 858–860, 2012.

[12] J. Luo, C. Xie, and Z. Li, "Treatment for malignant struma ovarii in the eyes of thyroid surgeons: a case report and study of Chinese cases reported in the literature," *Medicine*, vol. 93, no. 26, p. e147, 2014.

[13] C. P. DeSimone, S. M. Lele, and S. C. Modesitt, "Malignant struma ovarii: a case report and analysis of cases reported in the literature with focus on survival and I131 therapy," *Gynecologic Oncology*, vol. 89, no. 3, pp. 543–548, 2003.

[14] N. Brusca, S. C. Del Duca, R. Salvatori et al., "A case report of thyroid carcinoma confined to ovary and concurrently occult in the thyroid: is conservative treatment always advised?" *International Journal of Endocrinology and Metabolism*, vol. 13, no. 1, 2014.

[15] J. C. Boyd, B. A. Williams, M. H. Rigby et al., "Malignant Struma ovarii in a 30-year old nulliparous patient," *Thyroid Research*, vol. 10, no. 1, 2017.

[16] R. J. Middelbeek, B. T. O'Neill, M. Nishino, and J. A. Pallotta, "Concurrent intrathyroidal thyroid cancer and thyroid cancer in struma ovarii: a case report and literature review," *Journal of the Endocrine Society*, vol. 1, no. 5, pp. 396–400, 2017.

[17] R. Capitao, C. Saraiva, F. Santos et al., "Malignant struma ovarii and synchronous tumour of thyroid gland in the same patient: a single pathway for two different tumours?" *Endocrine Abstracts*, vol. 13, p. S9, 2007.

[18] A. Krishnamurthy, V. Ramshankar, V. Vaidyalingam, and U. Majhi, "Synchronous papillary carcinoma thyroid with malignant struma ovarii: a management dilemma," *Indian Journal of Nuclear Medicine*, vol. 28, no. 4, pp. 243–245, 2013.

[19] S. T. Lim, H. Jeong, M. Chung, C. Yim, and M. Sohn, "Malignant struma ovarii demonstrated on post-therapy radioiodine scan after total thyroidectomy for papillary thyroid cancer," *Clinical Nuclear Medicine*, vol. 33, no. 6, pp. 429–431, 2008.

[20] S. Makani, W. Kim, and A. R. Gaba, "Struma Ovarii with a focus of papillary thyroid cancer: a case report and review of the literature," *Gynecologic Oncology*, vol. 94, no. 3, pp. 835–839, 2004.

[21] M. Hatami, D. Breining, R. L. Owers, G. Del Priore, and G. L. Goldberg, "Malignant struma ovarii – a case report and review

of the literature," *Gynecologic and Obstetric Investigation*, vol. 65, no. 2, pp. 104–107, 2008.

[22] S. K. Sussman, S. A. Kho, E. Cersosimo, and A. Heimann, "Coexistence of malignant struma ovarii and graves' disease," *Endocrine Practice - American Association of Clinical Endocrinologists*, vol. 8, no. 5, pp. 378–380, 2002.

[23] S. Menon, K. Deodhar, B. Rekhi, A. John, and A. Maheshwari, "Unilateral malignant struma ovarii in a case of bilateral ovarian teratoma with raised CA-125 level: A rare case with treatment dilemmas," *Indian Journal of Pathology and Microbiology*, vol. 54, no. 3, p. 578, 2011.

[24] A. Sisti, J. Tassinari, G. Nisi et al., "Synchronous and metachronous malignancies after malignant struma ovarii in the seer database," *In Vivo*, vol. 30, no. 5, pp. 713–716, 2016.

[25] J. Schmidt, V. Derr, M. C. Heinrich et al., "BRAF in papillary thyroid carcinoma of ovary (struma ovarii)," *The American Journal of Surgical Pathology*, vol. 31, no. 9, pp. 1337–1343, 2007.

[26] R. Flavin, P. Smyth, P. Crotty et al., "BRAF T1799A mutation occurring in a case of malignant struma ovarii," *International Journal of Surgical Pathology*, vol. 15, no. 2, pp. 116–120, 2016.

[27] A. Tan, C. J. Stewart, K. L. Garrett, M. Rye, and P. A. Cohen, "Novel BRAF and KRAS mutations in papillary thyroid carcinoma arising in struma ovarii," *Endocrine Pathology*, vol. 26, no. 4, pp. 296–301, 2015.

[28] G. Corrado, G. Pomati, A. Russo et al., "Ovarian metastasis from thyroid carcinoma: a case report and literature review," *Diagnostic Pathology*, vol. 9, no. 1, 2014.

[29] I. T. Leite, T. M. Cunha, J. P. Figueiredo, and A. Felix, "Papillary carcinoma arising in struma ovarii versus ovarian metastasis from primary thyroid carcinoma: a case report and review of the literature," *Journal of Radiology Case Reports*, vol. 7, no. 10, pp. 24–33, 2013.

[30] A. Llueca, Y. Maazouzi, J. L. Herraiz et al., "Treatment and follow-up in an asymptomatic malignant struma ovarii: A case report," *International Journal of Surgery Case Reports*, vol. 40, pp. 113–115, 2017.

[31] J. S. Abramowicz and D. Timmerman, "Clinical opinion ovarian mass e differentiating benign from malignant: the value of the international ovarian tumor analysis ultrasound rules," *American Journal of Obstetrics & Gynecology*, vol. 217, no. 6, pp. 652–660, 2017.

[32] X. Zhang and C. Axiotis, "Thyroid-type carcinoma of struma ovarii," *Archives of Pathology & Laboratory Medicine*, vol. 134, no. 5, pp. 786–791, 2010.

[33] S. Jean, J. L. Tanyi, K. Montone, C. McGrath, M. M. Lage-Alvarez, and C. S. Chu, "Papillary thyroid cancer arising in struma ovarii," *Journal of Obstetrics & Gynaecology*, vol. 32, no. 3, pp. 222–226, 2012.

[34] M. L. Mattucci, A. Dellera, A. Guerriero, F. Barbieri, L. Minnelli, and L. Furlani, "Malignant struma ovarii: A case report and review of the literature," *Journal of Endocrinological Investigation*, vol. 30, no. 6, pp. 517–520, 2007.

[35] A. Oudoux, E. Leblanc, J. Beaujot, and H. Gauthier-Kolesnikov, "Treatment and follow-up of malignant struma ovarii: Regarding two cases," *Gynecologic Oncology Reports*, vol. 17, pp. 56–59, 2016.

[36] E. Monti, L. Mortara, S. Zupo et al., "Papillary thyroid cancer in a struma ovarii: a report of a rare case," *Hormones*, vol. 14, no. 1, pp. 154–159, 2014.

[37] B. Kraemer, E. Grischke, A. Staebler, P. Hirides, and R. Rothmund, "Laparoscopic excision of malignant struma ovarii and 1 year follow-up without further treatment," *Fertility and Sterility*, vol. 95, no. 6, pp. 2124.e9–2124.e12, 2011.

[38] F. Pacini, M. Schlumberger, C. Harmer et al., "Post-surgical use of radioiodine (^{131}I) in patients with papillary and follicular thyroid cancer and the issue of remnant ablation: a consensus report," *European Journal of Endocrinology*, vol. 153, no. 5, pp. 651–659, 2005.

[39] R. Shaco-Levy, R. Y. Peng, M. J. Snyder et al., "Malignant struma ovarii: a blinded study of 86 cases assessing which histologic features correlate with aggressive clinical behavior," *Archives of Pathology & Laboratory Medicine*, vol. 136, no. 2, pp. 172–178, 2012.

[40] H. Lim, S. S. Devesa, J. A. Sosa, D. Check, and C. M. Kitahara, "Trends in thyroid cancer incidence and mortality in the United States, 1974–2013," *Journal of the American Medical Association*, vol. 317, no. 13, pp. 1338–1348, 2017.

Factitiously Elevated Total Triiodothyronine in a Euthyroid Patient with Multiple Myeloma

Kaushik Mandal, Damilola Ashorobi, Alice Lee, Huijuan Liao, Salini C. Kumar, and David S. Rosenthal

Division of Endocrinology, Nassau University Medical Center, 2201 Hempstead Turnpike, East Meadow, NY 11554, USA

Correspondence should be addressed to David S. Rosenthal; drosenth@numc.edu

Academic Editor: Mihail A. Boyanov

Sporadic reports of factitious elevations of thyroid hormones related to laboratory interference from autoantibodies and multiple myeloma paraproteins have appeared in the literature. Such clinically confusing laboratory results can lead to erroneous diagnoses and inappropriate treatments. We report an additional case of a patient with multiple myeloma and an IgG paraproteinemia who had such a spurious elevation of total T3 complicating her levothyroxine management of hypothyroidism. In addition, we alert clinicians that differences in performance characteristics between various manufacturers' test platforms may also cause spurious reports.

1. Introduction

More than 99% of both total T3 (TT3) and total T4 (TT4) are bound for transport to either thyroxine-binding globulin (TBG), transthyretin (TTR), or albumin [1]. Anomalous hormone binding, such as that, may be, caused by interfering autoantibodies including Human Anti-Mouse Antibody (HAMA), or paraproteins such as those found in coexisting Multiple Myeloma (MM) may yield factitious and clinically inconsistent reports possibly leading to inappropriate diagnoses and treatments. Susceptibility to such spurious reports may also vary between test platforms used by the clinical laboratory. We report such a case to alert clinicians to this issue.

2. Case Report

A 72-year-old woman presented to our medical center with an altered mental status having suffered a fall. She had a history of primary hypothyroidism for many years treated with a stable dose of levothyroxine 0.075 mg/d. She was clinically euthyroid without tremors, palpitations, tachycardia, or other findings suggesting thyrotoxicosis. A pathologic fracture of her right humerus eight years before had led to a diagnosis of multiple myeloma with an IgG kappa M spike paraprotein. She received chemotherapy and went into remission. However, a recent reexacerbation had occurred, and she was being considered for further therapy. Routine admission labs revealed hematocrit 20.9% (normal 38–47%), sodium 132 mmol/L (136–145), potassium 4.0 mmol/L (3.5–5.1), chloride 104 mmol/L (98–107), urea nitrogen 45 mmol/L (20–31), and creatinine 2.8 mg/dL (0.6–1.0). Oncologic studies were consistent with multiple myeloma with an M spike kappa IgG paraprotein: total protein 10.1 g/dL (5.7–8.2), albumin 1.8 g/dL (3.4–5.0), and serum albumin: globulin ratio: 0.22 (0.60–1.50). Serum protein electrophoresis revealed gamma globulin 5.8 g/dL (0.8–1.7), kappa chain 9270 mg/L (3.3–19.4), Lambda chain 9.3 mg/dL (5.7–26.3), K/L ratio 996.7 (0.26–1.65), and B2—macroglobulin: 17.9 mg/L (<or = 2.51).

Thyroid biochemistry (Table 1) on presentation performed with the Siemens Atellica chemiluminescent immunoassay kit reported a slightly high TSH of 6.27 uIU/mL (normal 0.55–4.78) with normal total T4 of 4.5 μg/dL (3.2–12.6) and free T4 1.22 ng/dL (0.89–1.76). However, total T3 was markedly elevated at >600 ng/dL (60–181). Tests for

Table 1: Summary of laboratory results.

TFTs	Roche Cobas kit, 08/28/19	Siemens Atellica kit, 10/25/20	Siemens Atellica kit, 10/26/20	Roche Cobas kit 11/17/20
TSH	0.750 (0.27–4.2 uIU/mL)	6.27 (0.55–4.78 uIU/mL)	4.84 (0.55–4.78 uIU/mL)	1.82 (0.27–4.2 IU/mL)
FT4		1.22 (0.89–1.76 ng/dL)	1.28 (0.89–1.76 ng/dL)	
TT4	7.6 (4.5–12.0 μg/dL)	4.5 (3.2–12.6 μg/dL)	4.7 (3.2–12.6 μg/dL)	
TT3	82 (80–200 ng/dL)	>600 (60–181 ng/dL)	>600 (60–181 ng/dL)	47.4 (80–200 ng/dL)
HAMA			<56 (<74 ng/mL)	
TPO ab			<1 (<9 IU/mL)	
TG ab			<1 (<1 IU/mL)	
TSI			<89 (<140%)	
T3 antibody			Negative (Quest/Nichols proprietary test)	
Free T3			1.7 (2.3–4.2 pg/mL) (Siemens Advia kit)	
Reverse T3			21 (8–25 ng/dL) (Thermo Aria kit)	

anti-ThyroPerOxidase (AntiTPO), anti-ThyroGlobulin (antiTG), Thyroid-Stimulating Immunoglobulin (TSI), and Human Anti-Mouse Antibodies (HAMA) were within normal limits at <1 IU/mL (<9), <1 IU/mL (<1), <89% (<140), and <56 ng/mL (<74), respectively. Assay for anti-T3 antibodies was negative using a proprietary chemiluminescent competitive immunoassay procedure performed by Quest/Nichols Laboratories. Repeat testing on the Siemens Atellica platform again reported an elevated TT3 >600 ng/dL. Reverse T3 (Thermo Aria platform) was normal at 21 ng/dL (8–25), while results for TSH, total T4, and free T4 were similar to those reported previously. Free T3 was low at 1.7 (2.3–4.2 pg/ml (Siemens Advia kit) consistent with Euthyroid Sick Syndrome. 14 months earlier, her thyroid biochemistry was reported to be normal using the Roche Cobas chemiluminescent immunoassay kit with total T3 82 ng/dL (80–200). Thyroid Hormone-Binding Protein (THBP) electrophoresis was normal: TBG 14.3 mcg T4/dL (10.3–24.9), albumin 16.6 mcg T4/dL (11.5–34.1), and transthyretin (prealbumin) 69 mg T4/dL (48.8–70.4). Follow-up testing on the Roche Cobas platform again reported normal total T3 47.4 ng/dL (Table 1). Polyethylene glycol (PEG) precipitation was planned, but the patient expired before it could be accomplished.

We conclude that the factitious elevation in TT3 was most likely due to assay interference from the documented multiple myeloma paraprotein as well as differences between the test platforms used.

3. Discussion

We report a case of a clinically euthyroid patient with longstanding hypothyroidism treated with a stable dose of levothyroxine who was reported to have a factitiously elevated TT3 during an exacerbation of multiple myeloma with an IgG kappa M spike paraprotein having been identified. More than 99% of both TT3 and TT4 are bound to either thyroxine-binding globulin (TBG), transthyretin (TTR), or albumin [1]. In our case, Thyroid Hormone-Binding Protein (THBP) electrophoresis was normal. Test interference from Human Mouse Antibodies (HAMAs), anti-T3 antibodies, or antibodies to TPO or TG was ruled out. Thyroid biochemistry 14 months earlier using the Roche Cobas platform had reported a normal TT3, while both initial and follow-up tests at our institution using the Siemens Atellica kit reported spuriously elevated TT3 values. Once again, repeat analysis on the Roche Cobas system documented a normal TT3 level. Varying susceptibility to such spurious results between different manufacturers' platforms has been previously reported [2] and may in part be related to differences in antigen capture characteristics between the monoclonal antibodies used by each test kit manufacturer involving either TT3, TT4, or both.

Interfering substances such as autoantibodies and paraproteins can be removed by polyethylene glycol (PEG) precipitation followed by reanalysis. Sadly, our patient expired from her multiple myeloma before that could be carried out. We conclude that the most likely scenario in this case is interference in the assay caused by the patient's myeloma IgG paraprotein immunoglobulin identified on serum protein electrophoresis. Such immunoglobulins can bind with high affinity to T3 and/or T4 capture antibodies used in the laboratory assay which may result in falsely high values for T3 (as in this case) or T4.

Cissewski et al. [3] first described a case of factitious hyperthyroxinemia in multiple myeloma. IgA monoclonal antibody was bound to both T4 and T3 producing euthyroid hyperthyroxinemia with elevations of both TT3 and TT4.

Antonopoulou and Silverberg [4] reported a case of spurious T3 thyrotoxicosis unmasking multiple myeloma. In this report, a 54-year-old clinically euthyroid woman with normal TSH and TT4 was evaluated for isolated elevation of TT3 >800 ng/dL (60–181). Laboratory studies confirmed the diagnosis of multiple myeloma, and the authors ascribed the abnormal immunoglobulin as the cause of the assay interference yielding a spurious result.

Ram et al. [5] reported another case of factitious isolated TT3 elevation. Here, a 56-year-old man was investigated for a TT3 reported to be extremely high at 800 ng/dL (39–181) while TT4 and free T3 (FT3) were normal. Thyroid function tests had been performed on the Siemens Advia Centaur chemiluminescent analyzer. Repeat assay using the Abbot Architect immunoassay also reported very high TT3 at 519 ng/d. He was ultimately diagnosed with multiple myeloma. Polyethylene glycol (PEG) precipitation of the sample yielded a normal value for TT3 of 53.25 ng/dL on the Siemens platform. The interference was considered to be due to the paraprotein immunoglobulin.

Veechika and Chitra [6] described a 52-year-old male with an isolated abnormal TT3: >456 ng/dL (62–154) (Beckman Access one-step immunoassay). He was also subsequently diagnosed with an IgG kappa monoclonal gammopathy due to multiple myeloma. The interference was resolved by analyzing the sample using the Abbott Architect two-step immunoassay.

Recently, Pan et al. [7] analyzed thyroid function tests using the Siemens Advia Centaur platform in 105 clinically euthyroid patients newly diagnosed with multiple myeloma. They found that 13 (12.38%) had isolated strikingly elevated TT3 levels >8 ng/mL (0.6–1.81). 12 had paraprotein IgG immunoglobulins, and 1 had a light-chain kappa protein. Assay results normalized upon PEG precipitation and stayed so after myeloma chemotherapy. The abnormal paraprotein immunoglobulins were felt to be the cause of the spurious TT3 reports.

Favresse et al. [8] have reviewed pitfalls in the laboratory automated immunoanalysis of Thyroid Function Tests (TFTs) and pointed out that paraproteins may have antibody-like activity binding to analytes or reagents and, thus, may behave as heterophilic antibodies. Varying susceptibility to these types of interference between different manufacturers' platforms was also emphasized. This was evident in our case using the Siemens Atellica platform but not on the Roche Cobas platform. Both are chemiluminescent competitive immunoassays and use biotinylated T3 as a reagent. However, Siemens uses anti-mouse antibodies while Roche uses anti-sheep antibodies. Our patient was HAMA negative, suggesting other interference on the Siemens platform most likely due to the presence of multiple myeloma IgG paraprotein. When interference is suspected as in this case with the Siemens platform, a polyethylene glycol (PEG) precipitation study may help to clarify.

4. Conclusions

The cases reported to date have shown factitious elevation of either or both TT4 and TT3 caused by multiple myeloma paraproteins. In our case, the factitious elevation was limited to TT3 in the presence of an IgG kappa M spike paraprotein. Such spurious reports of TT3 or TT4 may be the initial presentation to the clinician and can lead to misdiagnosis and inappropriate management. Awareness of this issue is essential. Therefore, when clinically inconsistent results are encountered, one should consider the presence of such paraproteins and consider PEG precipitation and repeat testing with another test platform.

Abbreviations

TT3: Total T3
TT4: Total T4
TBG: Thyroxine-binding globulin
TTR: Transthyretin
HAMA: Human anti-mouse antibody
MM: Multiple myeloma
AntiTPO: Antithyroperoxidase
AntiTG: Antithyroglobulin
TSI: Thyroid-stimulating immunoglobulin
THBP: Thyroid hormone-binding protein.

Acknowledgments

The authors would like to thank Rachel Robbins, MD, Chair, Department of Pathology, Nassau University Medical Center, and Erica M Fatica, PhD, Mayo Clinic Laboratories, for their assistance and Mr. Matthew R Oswald for his assistance in the preparation of this manuscript.

References

[1] L. Bartalena and J. Robbins, "Variations in thyroid hormone transport proteins and their clinical implications," *Thyroid*, vol. 2, no. 3, pp. 237–245, 1992.

[2] P. Srichomkwun, N. H. Scherberg, J. Jakšić, and S. Refetoff, "Diagnostic dilemma in discordant thyroid function tests due to thyroid hormone autoantibodies," *AACE Clinical Case Reports*, vol. 3, no. 1, pp. e22–e25, 2017.

[3] K. Cissewski, J. D. Faix, D. Reinwein, and A. C. Moses, "Factitious hyperthyroxinemia due to a monoclonal IgA in a case of multiple myeloma," *Clinical Chemistry*, vol. 39, no. 8, pp. 1739–1742, 1993.

[4] M. Antonopoulou and A. Silverberg, "Spurious T3 thyrotoxicosis unmasking multiple myeloma," *Case Reports in Endocrinology*, vol. 2013, Article ID 739302, 3 pages, 2013.

[5] N. Ram, S. Furqan, and S. Ahmed, "Is it T3 thyrotoxicosis? a case of falsely elevated tri-iodothyronine (T3) levels leading to a diagnosis of multiple myeloma," *Case Reports in Endocrinology*, vol. 2019, Article ID 5028534, 3 pages, 2019.

[6] P. Veechika and S. Chitra, "Multiple myeloma masquerading as T3 toxicosis," *Thyroid Research and Practice*, vol. 17, pp. 152–154, 2020.

[7] Q. Pan, Y. Zhang, W. Zhang et al., "The prevalence of euthyroid hypertriiodothyroninemia in newly diagnosed multiple myeloma and its clinical characteristics," *Endocrine Practice*, vol. 27, no. 3, pp. 236–240, 2021.

[8] J. Favresse, M.-C. Burlacu, D. Maiter, and D. Gruson, "Interferences with thyroid function immunoassays: clinical implications and detection algorithm," *Endocrine Reviews*, vol. 39, no. 5, pp. 830–850, 2018.

34

Polyserositis: An Extremely Rare Life-Threatening Manifestation of Pheochromocytoma

Maryam Heidarpour,[1] **Mohammad Ali Haghighatpanah**,[2] **Hassan Rezvanian**,[1] **Motahare Yadegarfar**,[3] **Amir Mohammad Mozafari**,[4] **Mehrbod Vakhshoori**,[5] **and Davood Shafie**[5]

[1]*Isfahan Endocrine and Metabolism Research Center, Isfahan University of Medical Sciences, Isfahan, Iran*
[2]*Isfahan University of Medical Sciences, Isfahan, Iran*
[3]*University Hospitals of Leicester NHS Foundation Trust, LE1 5WW Leicester, UK*
[4]*Medical Library and Information Sciences Department, Health Information Technology Research Center, School of Management and Medical Information Sciences, Isfahan University of Medical Sciences, Isfahan, Iran*
[5]*Heart Failure Research Center, Cardiovascular Research Institute, Isfahan University of Medical Sciences, Isfahan, Iran*

Correspondence should be addressed to Davood Shafie; d.shafie87@gmail.com

Academic Editor: Suat Simsek

The pericardium is an uncommon site for manifestation of pheochromocytoma. Herein, the case of a 57-year-old man with cardiac tamponade is presented. Pericardiocentesis was performed, and the vital signs were stabilized afterwards. An abdominal computed tomography (CT) scan illustrated a nonhomogeneous right adrenal mass suspicious of pheochromocytoma, planned for right adrenalectomy. He recovered well after surgery, and his subsequent follow-ups did not reveal any complications.

1. Introduction

Pheochromocytoma is a rare catecholamine-secreting tumor originating from adrenal chromaffin cells. The incidence of this tumor is approximately 0.8 per 100,000 people per year [1]. The classic triad of this tumor includes headache, palpitations, and sweating; however, it can present with a wide range of clinical symptoms; therefore, it is also referred as a great masquerader [2]. Pheochromocytoma increases morbidity and mortality by causing cardiovascular complications, but due to the rareness of this tumor, most cardiovascular complications related to the aforementioned disease are limited to case reports or series [3]. In this study, we presented a patient who initially referred with severe shortness of breath, caused by cardiac tamponade, in which further investigations revealed the presence of one of the rarest complication of pheochromocytoma.

2. Case Presentation

A 57-year-old man with a remote history of hypertension (HTN) presented to the emergency department with the chief complaint of shortness of breath. His medical history did not reveal any positive findings attributed to the probable occurrence of coronary artery diseases. He had no previous history of a sudden increase in blood pressure, palpitations, sweating, and headache. Initial vital signs included blood pressure 90/70 mmHg, a heart rate of 109 beats per minute (bpm), respiratory rate of 19 per minute, O_2 saturation of 97% on room air, and temperature of 37.1°C. On examination, he was found to have distended neck veins, tachycardia, and muffled heart sounds. The result of electrocardiogram (ECG) was not indicative of ischemic heart diseases. Echocardiography showed a normal left ventricular ejection fraction (LVEF) and massive pericardial effusion with diastolic right ventricular collapse without any regional

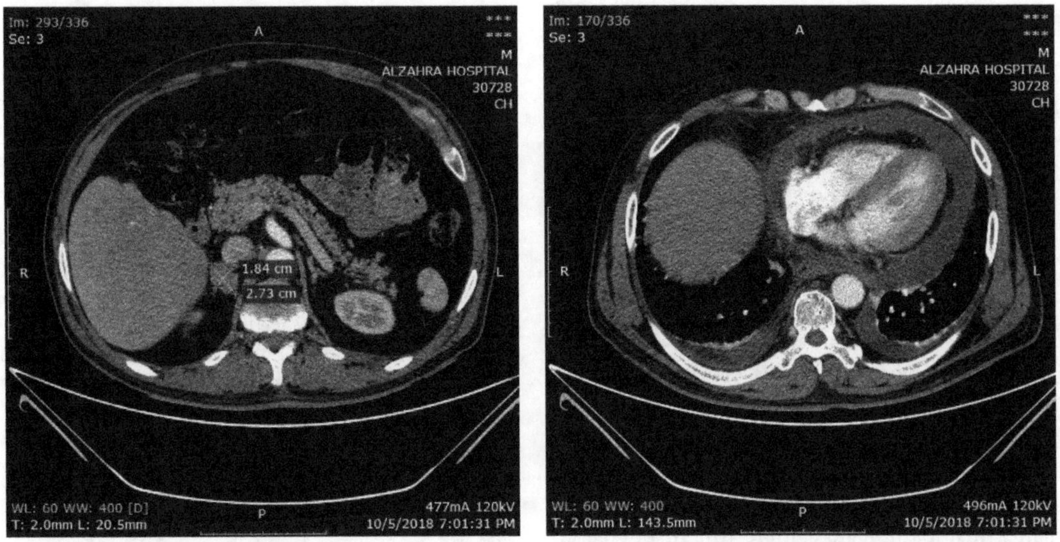

(a) (b)

FIGURE 1: Chest and abdominal CT scan of the patient shows heterogeneous right adrenal mass (a) and pericardial and bilateral pleural effusion (b).

wall motion abnormalities as well as positive findings in regards to takotsubo cardiomyopathy. Chest X-ray demonstrated large bilateral pleural effusion. He was scheduled for urgent pericardiocentesis by the subxiphoid approach, and 600 milliliters of serous pericardial fluid was drained; his symptoms were relieved. Chest tubes were also inserted, and approximately 750 milliliters of nonbloody fluid was drained. As of suspicion to pericarditis, colchicine and ibuprofen were prescribed for the patient. On the fifth day of admission, the pericardial effusion reaccumulated in spite of prolonged pericardial drainage. Therefore, a subxiphoid pericardial window with pericardial biopsy was performed. Pericardial cytology was nonhemorrhagic, and the microbiology test was negative. The histological study showed reactive mesothelial hyperplasia.

On day 7, chest and abdominal computed tomography (CT) scan was performed for further evaluation, which showed a heterogeneous right adrenal mass measuring 27 * 18 mm. The adrenal mass on the unenhanced images had a density of 70 Hounsfield units (Figure 1). Given these findings, pheochromocytoma and adrenocortical carcinoma were considered to be the most probable differential diagnoses for this adrenal mass. Laboratory values were notable for a 24-hour urine metanephrine of 260 μg/day (normal < 315 μg/day), normetanephrine of 510 μg/day (normal < 670 μg/day), adrenaline of 6.89 μg/day (normal < 20 μg/day), noradrenaline of 171 μg/day (normal < 90 μg/day), free cortisol of 23 μg/day (normal: 3.5–45 μg/day), serum aldosterone of 8 ng/dl (normal: 2–9 ng/dl), plasma renin activity of 1.15 ng/ml/h (normal: 1.1–1.28 ng/ml/h), and 17-OH progesterone of 125 ng/dl (normal: less than 200 ng/dL). All other hematological and biochemical tests were in normal ranges. These findings were consistent with the diagnosis of pheochromocytoma. He was started on phenoxybenzamine 10 mg twice a day, and the dosage was increased by 10 mg every three days to a maximum dosage of 20 mg twice a day. One week afterwards, propranolol with a dose of 10 mg every 8 hours was prescribed. Then, right adrenalectomy was performed without any complications, and the postoperative histopathologic report was in agreement with a diagnosis of pheochromocytoma (Figure 2). No complications were reported in the postoperative period. He was followed in an outpatient setting on a regular basis. Three months after adrenalectomy, the patient had no evidence of the disease. The latest echocardiography showed the LVEF to be 55%. Other echocardiographic measurements were within the normal values.

3. Discussion

The presented case was a middle-aged patient with a history of HTN who presented with pleural and pericardial effusions and highlights the point that the clinical presentation of pheochromocytoma could be varied significantly. Therefore, clinical suspicion of this disease is the key to a timely diagnosis [2]. Pheochromocytoma is a neoplasm of adrenal chromaffin cells producing excess catecholamines. It is estimated that at least 25% of the patients has never being diagnosed during their lifetimes [4]. Furthermore, pheochromocytoma has various cardiovascular manifestations, in which hypertension is categorized as the most common one. Other possible cardiovascular presentations include myocardial infarction, cardiac hypertrophy, systolic and diastolic heart failure, arrhythmia, myocarditis, and pericardial effusion [1]. The pericardium is a rare site for primary tumors or the metastasis of malignant neoplasms. Few studies revealed that pericardial effusion is a very rare manifestation of pheochromocytoma [4–6]. It is postulated that the elevated levels of catecholamines increase the level of inflammatory factors leading to inflammatory symptoms such as fever, weight loss, and polyserositis [7–11]. Westfried et al. reported a case of malignant pheochromocytoma presented

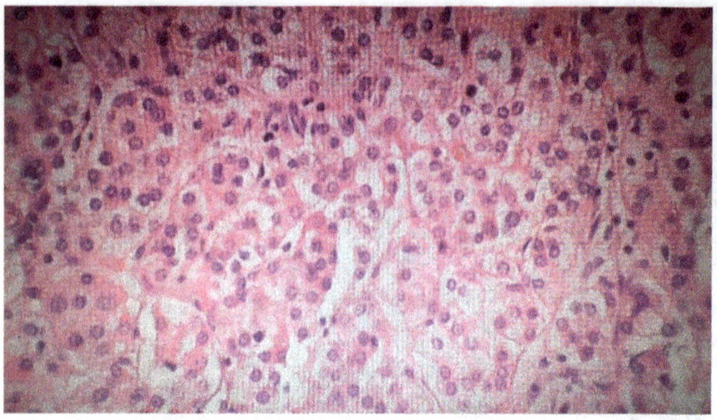

FIGURE 2: Histopathology of the adrenal mass. Polygonal cells with abundant granular amphophilic cytoplasm arranged in well-defined nests (zellbalen appearance).

with shortness of breath with demonstration of metastasis to pericardium in a histopathologic sample [6]. In our case, however, catecholamine-induced pericardial and pleural effusions were the first manifestation leading to further evaluation and prompt diagnosis of pheochromocytoma. As mentioned above, the histopathologic review showed only an inflammatory reaction. To our best knowledge, there is no published case report, in which pheochromocytoma would be presented with reactive pericardial and pleural effusion as the first manifestation, bearing in mind that pheochromocytoma can manifest with unusual presentations. Therefore, it is expected that only a small percentage of severe cases of pheochromocytoma would be diagnosed or reported [4]. Ferreira et al. designed a study in order to characterize cardiac involvement in sixty patients suffering from pheochromocytoma using cardiac magnetic resonance (CMR). They found that cardiac involvement, including impaired systolic and diastolic function, pericardial effusion, myocarditis, and markers for focal and diffuse fibrosis are common among these patients [1]. Indeed, some abnormalities such as subclinical systolic and dysfunction and markers for fibrosis might be persisted for a long time in spite of the curative surgery of the pheochromocytoma without any evidence of underlying disease. Thus, it seems that although pheochromocytoma is a rare disease, delayed diagnosis could be life-threatening [3].

In conclusion, it should be considered that clinical suspicion of pheochromocytoma is a key for a timely diagnosis, and more extensive studies are required to determine the actual rate of cardiovascular involvement in the acute phase of pheochromocytoma and after the curative surgery.

Ethical Approval

Ethical approval is not necessary for retrospective studies and case presentations in our institutional policies. However, informed consent had been obtained from the patient to publish this material.

Acknowledgments

This research did not receive any specific grant from any funding agency in the public, commercial, or not-for-profit sector.

References

[1] V. M. Ferreira, M. Marcelino, S. K. Piechnik et al., "Pheochromocytoma is characterized by catecholamine-mediated myocarditis, focal and diffuse myocardial fibrosis, and myocardial dysfunction," *Journal of the American College of Cardiology*, vol. 67, no. 20, pp. 2364–2374, 2016.

[2] H. A. Reyes, J. J. Paquin, and D. M. Harris, "Pheochromocytoma, "the great masquerader," presenting as severe acute decompensated heart failure in a young patient," *Case Reports in Cardiology*, vol. 2018, Article ID 8767801, 5 pages, 2018.

[3] L. R. Leite, P. G. Macedo, S. N. Santos, L. Quaglia, C. E. Mesas, and A. De Paola, "Life-threatening cardiac manifestations of pheochromocytoma," *Case Reports in Medicine*, vol. 2010, Article ID 976120, 4 pages, 2010.

[4] H. Falhammar, M. Kjellman, and J. Calissendorff, "Initial clinical presentation and spectrum of pheochromocytoma: a study of 94 cases from a single center," *Endocrine Connections*, vol. 7, no. 1, pp. 186–192, 2018.

[5] W. P. Skelton, D. Mahtta, S. Welniak, A. J. Franke, and L. H. Dang, "Pericardial effusion as an atypical initial presentation of extragonadal nonseminomatous germ cell tumor: a case report and literature review," *Oxford Medical Case Reports*, vol. 2018, no. 2, Article ID omx097, 2018.

[6] M. Westfried, D. Mandel, M. N. Alderete, J. Groopman, and S. Minkowitz, "Sipple's syndrome with a malignant pheochromocytoma presenting as a pericardial effusion," *Cardiology*, vol. 63, no. 5, pp. 305–311, 1978.

[7] S. Yarman, O. Soyluk, E. Altunoglu, and R. Tanakol, "Interleukin-6-producing pheochromocytoma presenting with fever of unknown origin," *Clinics*, vol. 66, no. 10, pp. 1843–1845, 2011.

[8] M. Ciacciarelli, D. Bellini, A. Laghi et al., "IL-6-producing, noncatecholamines secreting pheochromocytoma presenting as fever of unknown origin," *Case Reports in Medicine*, vol. 2016, Article ID 3489046, 5 pages, 2016.

[9] X. Cheng, M. Zhang, Y. Xiao, H. Li, Y. Zhang, and Z. Ji, "Interleukin-6-producing pheochromocytoma as a new reason for fever of unknown origin: a retrospective study," *Endocrine Practice*, vol. 24, no. 6, pp. 507–511, 2018.

[10] Y. Kawahara, A. Morimoto, A. Onoue, Y. Kashii, N. Fukushima, and Y. Gunji, "Persistent fever and weight loss due to an interleukin-6-producing adrenocortical oncocytoma in a girl: review of the literature," *European Journal of Pediatrics*, vol. 173, no. 8, pp. 1107–1110, 2014.

[11] T. Zelinka, O. Petrák, B. Štrauch et al., "Elevated inflammation markers in pheochromocytoma compared to other forms of hypertension," *Neuroimmunomodulation*, vol. 14, no. 1, pp. 57–64, 2007.

Surgical Treatment of Advanced Thyroid Cancer with Tracheal Invasion

Hau Xuan Nguyen,[1,2] **Huy Le Trinh**,[1,2] **Hien Xuan Nguyen**,[1] **Hung Van Nguyen**,[1] **and Quang Van Le**[1,2,3]

[1]*Department of Oncology, Hanoi Medical University, Hanoi, Vietnam*
[2]*Department of Oncology and Palliative Care, Hanoi Medical University Hospital, Hanoi, Vietnam*
[3]*Department of Head and Neck Surgery, National Cancer Hospital, Hanoi, Vietnam*

Correspondence should be addressed to Hien Xuan Nguyen; dr.nguyenxuanhien@gmail.com

Academic Editor: Wei Wu

Introduction. Tracheal invasion in thyroid cancer occurs in one-third of locally advanced cases and is the third most common site of infiltration following strap muscles and recurrent laryngeal nerves. Surgical resection plays an important role in the management strategy followed by either radioactive iodine or external beam radiotherapy. Nonetheless, there has been still controversy about the optimal extension of the surgery. *Case Presentation.* Total thyroidectomy, airway resection and bilateral neck dissection were performed in two cases diagnosed as advanced thyroid cancer with tracheal invasion (stage IV according to McCaffrey). The first case underwent partial tracheal resection and direct anastomosis by the V-shape technique, while the latter one required tracheal resection and permanent tracheotomy. After one-year follow-up, no evidence of tumor recurrence or any postoperative complications were found. *Conclusion.* Surgical resection still remains the mainstay of management for advanced thyroid cancer in general and for tracheal invasion cases in particular. The decision of surgical resection and tracheal reconstruction methods mostly depends on the extent of tracheal invasion.

1. Introduction

Thyroid cancer is the original from of follicular derived cells or neuroendocrine C-cell-derived types [1]. It is classified into three different histological groups: differentiated thyroid cancer, anaplastic carcinoma, and others (i.e., medullary thyroid cancer). Generally, differentiated thyroid carcinoma (DTC), which accounts for approximately 95% of all thyroid cancers [2], has slow expansion and favorable outcome with 10-year survival over 80% after curative treatment [3]. However, DTC can invade surrounding structures, for instance, strap muscle, recurrent laryngeal nerve (RLN), trachea, and esophagus. Thus, locally advanced DTC is associated with high risks of local recurrence, distal metastasis, and mortality.

The standard treatment of DTC with tracheal invasion is still under controversy. In previous studies, some authors reported that total thyroidectomy and involved structure resection with negative margins could improve survival rates [4–6]. However, others showed that combination therapy including limited operation and radioactive iodine (RAI) therapy or external beam radiotherapy (EBRT) may have similar long-term outcomes and lower risks of surgical complications, compared with aggressive treatment [5, 7]. In addition, some authors have described classification systems for DTC to assess the degree of tracheal invasion [8] and to determine surgical strategy.

In this paper, we reported two cases of DTC invading the trachea with different surgical approaches and favorable outcomes.

2. Case Presentation

2.1. Case 1. A 54-year-old man with normal previous medical history was admitted to our department because of a mass in his left neck. The patient reported that the tumor had appeared before one year. However, he did not receive any treatment because this tumor did not affect his daily activities. As a result, for the last few months, the tumor had gradually increased in size, and the patient had experienced increasing hoarseness. On examination, there was a 3 × 4 cm, hard and fixed tumor in his left neck without any palpable neck lymph nodes.

Ultrasound suggested a highly suspicious malignant lesion in the left lobe of the thyroid gland, categorized as TI-RADS 5 (according to Thyroid Imaging Reporting and Data System (TI-RADS) 2017). Neck CT scan (as per Figure 1) demonstrated a thyroid tumor with a size of 30 × 37 mm, infiltrating the tracheal wall and compressing the tracheal lumen as well. There were also several small lymph nodes found in the cervical central compartment with the largest diameter below 10 mm. Otorhinolaryngoscopy indicated left vocal cord paralysis, and bronchoscopy showed that tumor is covered by the normal mucosa and narrowing tracheal lumen. Finally, fine needle aspiration concluded papillary thyroid cancer (PTC).

Based on the above findings, the patient was diagnosed as left lobe PTC cT4aN0M0, stage I (according to AJCC, 8th edition, 2017) and stage IV (according to McCaffrey). Intraoperative evaluation reported a hard tumor in the size of 30 × 40 mm at the left thyroid lobe, invading the left recurrent laryngeal nerve and the anterior wall of trachea with 30 mm in length. There were multiple lymph nodes in the central compartment and the bilateral neck compartments. The patient underwent total thyroidectomy, central and bilateral cervical lymph nodes dissection, partial tracheal resection, and reconstruction by direct suturing with the V-shape technique (as per Figure 2). The final diagnosis was PTC of the left thyroid lobe staged as pT4aN1bM0. To protect the tracheal anastomosis, the S-head was fixed continuously in the folding position for 6 days. This patient was discharged after 14 days without any complications, and he had his normal neck movement after 1 month. RAI was indicated afterward. During one-year follow-up, there was no evidence of tumor recurrence and postoperative complication.

In addition, the immunohistochemical analysis was performed and revealed that the tumor was positive with CK19, TTF1, CEA (slightly), HBME1, Claudin1, and Ki67 (2%) and negative with CD 56 and p63.

2.2. Case 2. A 55-year-old man presented to our hospital with a hard mass in his neck. He noticed that the mass had been gradually increasing in size for six months. In the last month, he reported of having experience of hoarseness and dyspnea. In addition, his previous medical history was unremarkable. Clinical examination showed not only the hard mass with a size of 3 × 4 cm and limited movement but also bilateral cervical lymph nodes.

Neck ultrasound and 128-slice computed tomography scan (as per Figure 3) revealed a diffusely enlarged thyroid gland, whereas the right lobe size was approximately 16 × 29 mm and the left lobe size was about 28 × 25 mm. The tumor was found to infiltrate the tracheal wall and narrow the tracheal lumen by 90%. Besides, there were suspected metastatic lymph nodes in levels II, III, and IV in both sides with the largest dimension roughly 14 × 10 mm. Flexible fiberoptic laryngoscopy demonstrated limited movement of bilateral vocal cords. Tracheobronchoscopy indicated that the mass invaded the upper part of the trachea but still was covered by normal tracheal mucosa. This mass caused the difficulty in the evaluation of the lower part of the trachea. Other examinations were not particular.

The clinical stage was classified as cT4aN1bM0, stage III (according to AJCC, 8th edition, 2017) and stage IV (according to the classification of McCaffrey et al.). Because endotracheal intubation was not applicable due to constricted trachea, tracheostomy was performed for anesthesia. Intraoperative evaluation has shown that (i) the tumor invaded the trachea in the length of approximately 7 cm and (ii) reconstruction of the remaining parts of the trachea after resection was impractical. Eventually, total thyroidectomy, resection of the involving part of the trachea, and permanent tracheotomy (as per Figure 4) were performed. This patient was discharged after 14 days. Subsequently, RAI ablation was administered. During one-year follow-up, evidence of tumor recurrence and complication was not found.

3. Discussion

Generally, diagnosis of thyroid cancer is based on the combination of clinical examination, neck ultrasound, and fine-needle aspiration (FNA). However, in patients with advanced thyroid cancer, it is necessary to perform laryngoscopy, neck CT scan, or neck MRI and sometimes tracheobronchoscopy [9]. Laryngoscopy can detect paralyzed vocal cord cases without voice change. Neck CT scan is used to evaluate the invasion of surrounding structures when tracheobronchoscopy is applied to access the invasive extent of airway lumen. According to Young Lan Seo, CT criteria for trachea invasion include tumor in contact with 180° or more of the tracheal circumferences (grades 3 and 4); deformity of the tracheal lumen at the level of the mass; and focal irregularity, thickening, or bulging in the mucosal portion adjacent to the mass. Based on these criteria, the basis of our criteria, the specificity and accuracy of CT, for tracheal invasion in this study were 91.4% and 83.2%, respectively [10]. However, MRI is more effective than CT in the assessment of invading soft tissue [10]. Most of authors consent to using CT scan for evaluating the tracheal invasion in advanced thyroid cancer [10, 11]. Previous studies showed a significant correlation between superficial lesions in tracheobronchoscopy and the classification of the extent of tracheal invasion [12, 13]. The signs, which suggest the tracheal invasion, include mucosal redness, telangiectasia, mucosal elevation, and mucosal erosion [12]. In our center, three main examinations including laryngoscopy, neck CT scan, and tracheobronchoscopy are regularly applied in case of thyroid carcinoma invading trachea.

The most common staging system applied to evaluate the extent of tracheal invasion in aggressive thyroid cancer is the classification described by Shin and McCaffrey (Table 1).

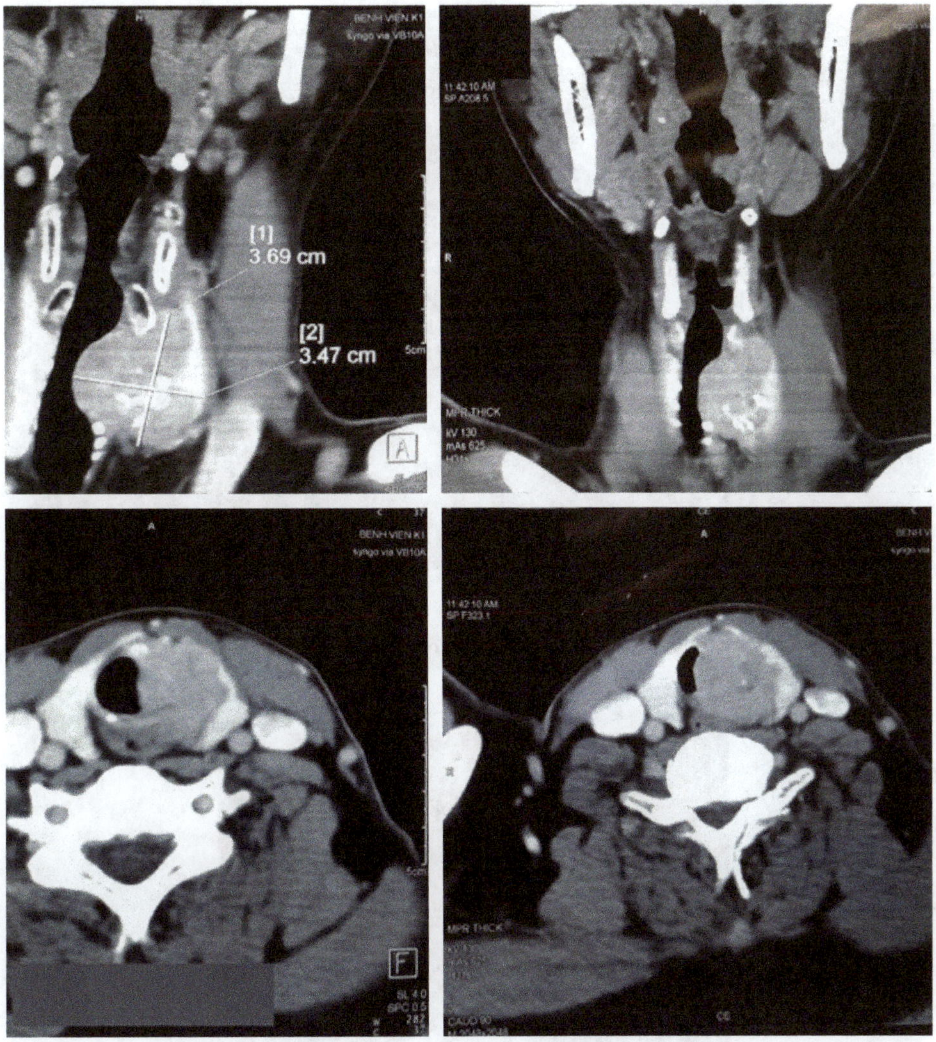

FIGURE 1: The thyroid tumor compressing the trachea.

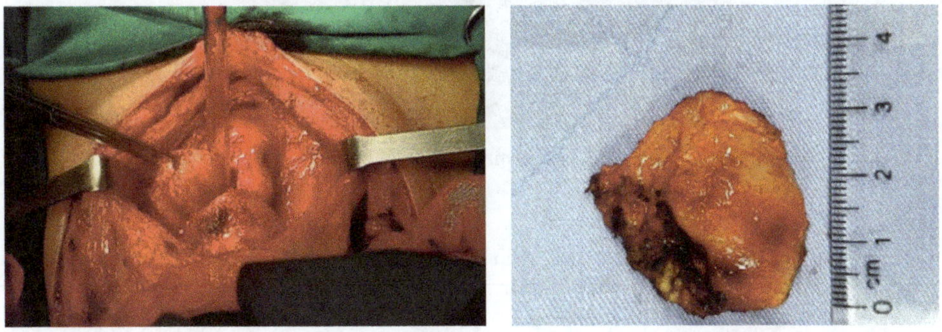

(a) (b)

FIGURE 2: Surgical procedure of partially tracheal resection and end-to-end anastomosis.

According to McCaffrey, the treatment options of tracheal resection depend on various stages, including total thyroidectomy for stage I, complete gross removal by "shave excision" and total thyroidectomy for stages II and III, and complete tracheal resection for stages III, IV.

Regarding thyroid cancer, tracheal resection could be repaired by the following procedures: (1) shave procedures, (2) segmental/partial resection and direct closure, (3) partial resection together with reconstruction of musculocutaneous flap or cartilage graft or materials, and (4) total laryngectomy

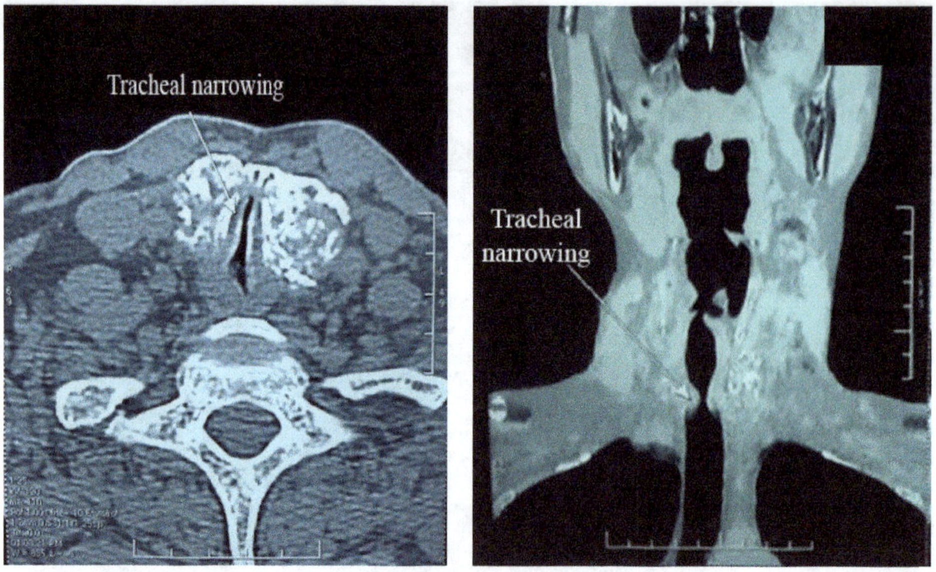

(a) (b)

FIGURE 3: The thyroid tumor compressing the trachea.

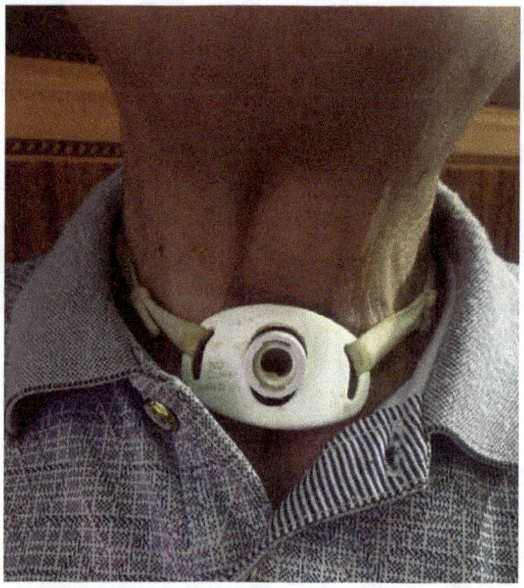

FIGURE 4: Permanent tracheotomy.

TABLE 1: Classification of the extent of tracheal invasion in thyroid cancer.

	Shin et al. [8]	McCaffrey [14]
I	Extension through the capsule of the thyroid gland and abutting the external perichondrium	Tumor locates entirely intrathyroidal gland without airway or surrounding muscle invasion
II	Invasion into the cartilage or the cartilaginous layer or destruction of the cartilage	Tumor invades the perichondrium of the aerodigestive tract or firmly abuts the muscle but does not invade into the cartilage or deeply into muscle
III	Extension into the lamina propria of the tracheal mucosa without epithelial invasion	Tumor invades through the airway perichondrium and into the cartilage or deeply into muscle but not into the submucosa
IV	Invasion into or beyond the trachea	Tumor invades through the perichondrium and cartilage or through the muscle and deforms the submucosa but does not penetrate the mucosa
V		Tumor is gross transmucosal involvement

and permanent tracheotomy. For stages II and III according to McCaffrey, the resection of all gross tumors can be performed by "shave procedures" meaning the removal of a partial thickness of the airway tract wall. Several retrospective studies comparing radical resection and shave procedures combined with RAI showed no survival benefit in the patients undergoing radical resection [15–18]. Similarly, Segal et al. also reported no difference in 5-year survival between two methods. However, Avenia et al. showed that the overall survival of the completely resected group is better than the positive margins group [6]. For stages IV and V according to McCaffrey, the surgery can be performed by either window resection or circumferential tracheal resection. The first method is appropriate for limited involvement of only anterior or lateral wall of trachea. The defect can be reconstructed by primary closure, with strap muscles, sternocleidomastoid muscle, or latissimus dorsi musculocutaneous flap [19]. Tumor invading extensively the anterolateral tracheal wall can be removed by segmental resection and primary end-to-end anastomosis. The maximum length of segmental tracheal resection is 5-6 cm, which is considered to be adequate for primary anastomosis without tracheal or laryngeal mobilization. In cases that both anastomosis and reconstruction could not be implemented, permanent tracheotomy is inevitable. In our first patient, due to the anterior invasion of the tumor, we decided to remove the anterior wall of 3 tracheal rings and reconstruct the trachea by V-shape. In the second patient, because of the extremely long tracheal segment, we chose the tracheal removal and permanent tracheotomy.

In several previous studies, postoperative complication rate after tracheal resection with direct closure ranges from 15% to 39%, and postoperative mortality rate is roughly 1.2% [20, 21]. The common complications after advanced thyroid carcinoma treatment include anastomotic dehiscence, airway stenosis, infection, and bleeding. The anastomotic dehiscence is one of the most serious complications, which can be life-threatening. This complication is related to the length of the tracheal segment resected over 5-6 cm. To reduce the tension of the anastomotic trachea, the neck of patient is fixed either in a "chin-to-chest" position during the 6th to 7th postoperative day [22–25] or by a C-collar.

4. Conclusion

In conclusion, *en bloc* resection of involved trachea is the standard treatment in advanced thyroid carcinoma. The surgical methods are based on the extent of airway wall invasion. The procedure of tracheal resection is safe with low rate of mortality.

Abbreviations

DTC: Differentiated thyroid carcinoma
RLN: Recurrent laryngeal nerve
RAI: Radioactive iodine
EBRT: External beam radiotherapy
TI-RADS: Thyroid imaging reporting and data system
PTC: Papillary thyroid cancer
AJCC: American joint committee on cancer
FNA: Fine-needle aspiration
MRI: Magnetic resonance imaging.

Ethical Approval

The study was approved by our research committee in Hanoi Medical University Hospital.

Consent

The authors are committed to that that both patients provided written informed consent for the case details and accompanying images to be published.

Disclosure

Hau Xuan Nguyen and Huy Le Trinh are co-first authors.

Acknowledgments

The authors really appreciate the help of their colleagues in Hanoi Medical University Hospital with their project.

References

[1] M. E. Cabanillas, D. G. McFadden, and C. Durante, "Thyroid cancer," *The Lancet*, vol. 388, no. 10061, pp. 2783–2795, 2016.

[2] N. Howlader, A. M. Noone, M. Krapcho et al., *SEER Cancer Statistics Review, 1975–2014*, National Cancer Institute, Bethesda, MD, USA, 2017, https://seer.cancer.gov/csr/1975_2014/.

[3] O. H. Beahrs, P. D. Kiernan, and J. P. Hubert Jr., "Cancer of the thyroid gland," in *Cancer of the Head and Neck*, J. Y. Suen and E. N. Meyers, Eds., pp. 599–632, Churchill Livingstone, New York, NY, USA, 1981.

[4] D. J. Mellière, N. E. Ben Yahia, J. P. Becquemin, F. Lange, and H. Boulahdour, "Thyroid carcinoma with tracheal or esophageal involvement: limited or maximal surgery?" *Surgery*, vol. 113, no. 2, pp. 166–172, 1993.

[5] E. Britto, S. S. Mbbs, D. M. Parikh, and R. S. Rao, "Laryngotracheal invasion by well-differentiated thyroid cancer: diagnosis and management," *Journal of Surgical Oncology*, vol. 44, no. 1, pp. 25–31, 1990.

[6] N. Avenia, J. Vannucci, M. Monacelli et al., "Thyroid cancer invading the airway: diagnosis and management," *International Journal of Surgery*, vol. 28, pp. S75–S78, 2016.

[7] A. J. Ballantyne, "Resections of the upper aerodigestive tract for locally invasive thyroid cancer," *The American Journal of Surgery*, vol. 168, no. 6, pp. 636–639, 1994.

[8] D.-H. Shin, E. J. Mark, H. C. Suen, and H. C. Grillo, "Pathologic staging of papillary carcinoma of the thyroid with airway invasion based on the anatomic manner of extension to the trachea: a clinicopathologic study based on 22 patients who underwent thyroidectomy and airway resection," *Human Pathology*, vol. 24, no. 8, pp. 866–870, 1993.

[9] Z. T. Hammoud and D. J. Mathisen, "Surgical management of thyroid carcinoma invading the trachea," *Chest Surgery Clinics of North America*, vol. 13, no. 2, pp. 359–367, 2003.

[10] Y. L. Seo, D. Y. Yoon, K. J. Lim et al., "Locally advanced thyroid cancer: can CT help in prediction of extrathyroidal invasion to adjacent structures?" *American Journal of Roentgenology*, vol. 195, no. 3, pp. W240–W244, 2010.

[11] K. H. Kwon, D. G. Lee, S. H. Koo, M. S. Jo, H. Shin, and J. H. Seul, "Usefulness of V-Y advancement flap for defects after skin tumor excision," *Archives of Plastic Surgery*, vol. 39, no. 6, pp. 619–625, 2012.

[12] E. Koike, "Bronchoscopic diagnosis of thyroid cancer with laryngotracheal invasion," *Archives of Surgery*, vol. 136, no. 10, p. 1185, 2001.

[13] H. Koshiishi, K. Toriya, O. Ozaki, K. Ito, C. Konaka, and H. Kato, "Fiberoptic bronchoscopy in thyroid carcinoma with tracheal invasion," *Diagnostic and Therapeutic Endoscopy*, vol. 4, no. 3, pp. 113–118, 1998.

[14] J. C. McCaffrey, "Aerodigestive tract invasion by well-differentiated thyroid carcinoma: diagnosis, management, prognosis, and biology," *The Laryngoscope*, vol. 116, no. 1, pp. 1–11, 2006.

[15] T. V. McCaffrey, E. J. Bergstralh, and I. D. Hay, "Locally invasive papillary thyroid carcinoma: 1940–1990," *Head Neck*, vol. 16, no. 2, pp. 165–172, 1994.

[16] T. V. McCaffrey and R. J. Lipton, "Thyroid carcinoma invading the upper aerodigestive system," *The Laryngoscope*, vol. 100, no. 8, pp. 824–830, 1990.

[17] J. M. Czaja and T. V. McCaffrey, "The surgical management of laryngotracheal invasion by well-differentiated papillary thyroid carcinoma," *Archives of Otolaryngology-Head and Neck Surgery*, vol. 123, no. 5, pp. 484–490, 1997.

[18] K. Segal, T. Shpitzer, A. Hazan, G. Bachar, G. Marshak, and A. Popovtzer, "Invasive well-differentiated thyroid carcinoma: effect of treatment modalities on outcome," *Otolaryngology—Head and Neck Surgery*, vol. 134, no. 5, pp. 819–822, 2006.

[19] K. Shigemitsu, "A case of thyroid cancer involving the trachea: treatment by partial tracheal resection and repair with a latissimus dorsi musculocutaneous flap," *Japanese Journal of Clinical Oncology*, vol. 30, no. 5, pp. 235–238, 2000.

[20] N. Rotolo, M. Cattoni, and A. Imperatori, "Complications from tracheal resection for thyroid carcinoma," *Gland Surgery*, vol. 6, no. 5, p. 5, 2017.

[21] S. Lin, H. Huang, X. Liu et al., "Treatments for complications of tracheal sleeve resection for papillary thyroid carcinoma with tracheal invasion," *European Journal of Surgical Oncology (EJSO)*, vol. 40, no. 2, pp. 176–181, 2014.

[22] K. Nakao, K. Kurozumi, M. Nakahara, and T. Kido, "Resection and reconstruction of the airway in patients with advanced thyroid cancer," *World Journal of Surgery*, vol. 28, no. 12, pp. 1204–1206, 2004.

[23] Y.-F. Tsai, Y.-L. Tseng, M.-H. Wu, C.-J. Hung, W.-W. Lai, and M.-Y. Lin, "Aggressive resection of the airway invaded by thyroid carcinoma," *British Journal of Surgery*, vol. 92, no. 11, pp. 1382–1387, 2005.

[24] C. Mossetti, N. Palestini, M. C. Bruna et al., "Segmental tracheal resection for invasive differentiated thyroid carcinoma. Our experience in eight cases," *Langenbeck's Archives of Surgery*, vol. 398, no. 8, pp. 1075–1082, 2013.

[25] G. Conzo, A. Polistena, P. G. Calò et al., "Efficacy of combined treatment for anaplastic thyroid carcinoma: results of a multinstitutional retrospective analysis," *International Journal of Surgery*, vol. 12, no. 1, pp. S178–S182, 2014.

36

Aggressive Differentiated Thyroid Cancer due to EML4e13-ALKe20 Fusion: A Case Presentation and Review of the Literature

Rodhan Khthir,[1] **Zainab Shaheen**,[1] **Prasanna Santhanam**,[2] **and Saroj Sigdel**[1]

[1]*Marshall University, School of Medicine, Huntington, WV, USA*
[2]*Johns Hopkins University, School of Medicine, Baltimore, MD, USA*

Correspondence should be addressed to Rodhan Khthir; rodhan.khthir@sanfordhealth.org

Academic Editor: Toshihiro Kita

Background. Differentiated thyroid cancer (DTC) is an indolent malignancy. It rarely presents with aggressive local invasion and/or distant metastatic disease. *Patient findings.* We describe a case of a 30-year-old man with a locally aggressive form of papillary thyroid cancer with *EML4e13-ALKe20* fusion (*EML4*: echinoderm microtubule-associated protein-like 4; *ALK*: anaplastic lymphoma kinase). He presented with right-side cervical lymphadenopathy with a highly suspicious right-side thyroid nodule. Total thyroidectomy and level IV lymph node resection showed extensive bilateral disease, with extrathyroidal and extranodal extension. FDG-PET CT scan following surgery confirmed the presence of significant residual disease in the neck area. He underwent bilateral lateral lymph node dissection followed by radioactive iodine treatment. Somatic mutation testing showed *EML4e13-ALKe20* fusion. *Summary.* This case represents an aggressive form of DTC with *EML4e13-ALKe20* fusion. The rapid progression of clinical signs and symptoms and the local extension beyond the thyroid and lymph nodes with the persistence of high-volume local disease after thyroidectomy highlight the aggressive nature of this mutation and the importance of performing genetic analysis to guide future treatments and determine prognosis. *Conclusion.* This case highlights the importance of using molecular diagnostics in patient care, especially if the presentation is unusual for DTC. A thorough evaluation of the tumor pathology and the somatic mutational profile analysis are important for obtaining vital therapeutic and prognostic guidance.

1. Introduction

Over the last several years, significant progress has been made in understanding the genetic mechanisms behind thyroid cancer and creating molecular tests for diagnosing cancer in thyroid nodules.

ALK-associated fusions and point mutations are found in various tumors, including anaplastic large cell lymphoma, non-small-cell cancers (NSCLCs), inflammatory myofibroblastic tumor, diffuse large B-cell lymphoma, esophageal squamous cell carcinoma, renal medullary carcinoma, renal cell carcinoma, breast cancer, colon cancer, and neuroblastoma [1], and serve as diagnostic markers and therapeutic targets. Their role in thyroid cancer is less well established.

We present a case of DTC with *EML4e13-ALKe20* fusion with atypical presentation. We conducted a literature review on this rare mutation to better understand its clinical characteristics and potential treatment options.

2. Case Presentation

A 30-year-old male with no significant past medical history presented to his primary care physician in early 2019, with a painless right neck swelling in addition to multiple palpable masses in the area. A neck ultrasound showed multiple irregular and enlarged lymph nodes on the right side of the neck (Figures 1 and 2) along with a calcified right thyroid nodule measuring $17 \times 20 \times 13$ mm. The left lobe of the thyroid was normal. The TSH value was

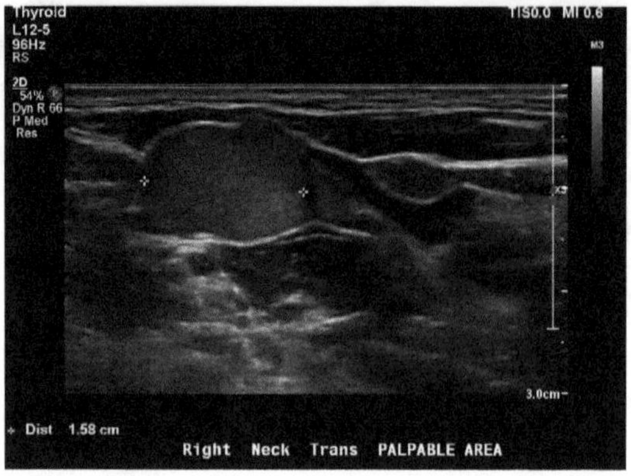

FIGURE 1: Ultrasound transverse image of the right palpable swelling showing abnormal cervical lymph node with localized invasion.

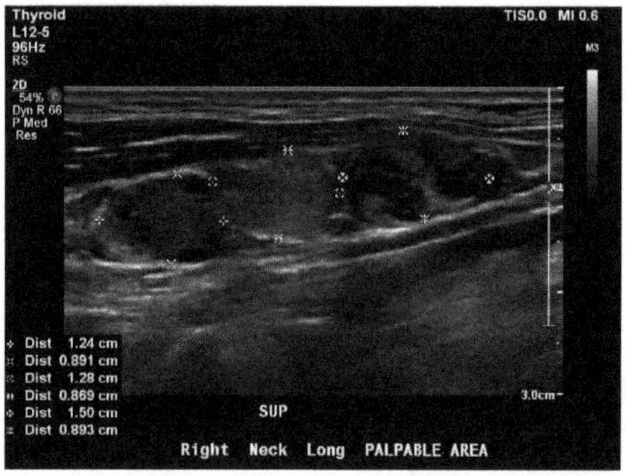

FIGURE 2: Ultrasound transverse image of lymphadenopathy in the right cervical area with distortion of normal morphology and cystic necrosis.

1.04 mIU/ml, confirming a euthyroid status. The patient reported no history of ionizing radiation exposure and no family history of thyroid cancer or other familial cancer syndromes.

Fine-needle aspiration (FNA) from the palpable lymph node revealed rare atypical epithelial cells and histocytes. Fine-needle aspiration from the right thyroid nodule was performed at an outside facility before referral, and the results were benign (presumably Bethesda class 2). We suspected a sampling error.

Because of the high index of suspicion for thyroid cancer, he underwent total thyroidectomy with central neck dissection and right lateral lymph node dissection at the end of July 2019.

Intraoperative findings showed the presence of extensively involved cervical lymphadenopathy at multiple levels (IV–VI), mainly on the right side. The right cervical level IV and V lymph nodes were tightly adherent to the internal jugular vein and the other large blood vessels. Abnormal paratracheal lymph nodes were dissected from both sides. Postoperatively, the patient developed right recurrent laryngeal nerve paralysis as there was local invasion around the nerve. However, there was no evidence of postsurgical hypocalcemia.

The histopathology of the resected thyroidectomy specimen showed multifocal follicular variant papillary thyroid cancer (FV-PTC) infiltrating both lobes and the isthmus with angioinvasion, lymphatic invasion, and microscopic extrathyroidal extension (Figure 3). The right superior and left superior lobe margins were also positive for the tumor. The largest tumor sizes were 3.5 and 1.5 cm in the most significant dimension, and the smallest tumor size was 0.1 cm. The Delphian lymph node and 4/4 right level VI lymph nodes had tumor involvement. Left paratracheal nodes (4/4) also had tumor involvement. A total of 5/9 lymph nodes from the right lymph node dissection at levels IV and V had metastatic tumor involvement. The largest metastatic tumor size was 4.0 cm, and this tumor showed an extranodal extension (Figure 4).

On the initial visit to the endocrine clinic four weeks after surgery, a physical exam was remarkable only to develop hoarseness of voice. No palpable lymphadenopathy was noted. The patient was not on thyroid replacement therapy. The thyroglobulin level was 294 ng/ml (TSH 52.9 mIU/ml). Antithyroglobulin antibodies were undetectable.

Because of the patient's DTC's aggressive nature, next-generation sequencing was performed on the tumor tissue (OmniSeq; Integrated Oncology Lab) using multiplexed PCR-based DNA and RNA sequencing. The results showed *EML4e13-ALKe20* fusion, a relatively common fusion described in non-small-cell lung cancer, which creates a more tumorigenic *ALK* kinase domain receptor by partnering with echinoderm microtubule-associated protein-like 4 (*EML4*) [1]. No other molecular alteration was found. Because of the high thyroglobulin level (294 ng/ml; TSH 52.9 mIU/ml), which was suggestive of persistent structural disease or distant metastasis, an FDG-PET/CT scan was performed. It showed two hypermetabolic lymph nodes in the upper cervical chain posterior to the internal carotid artery (SUV of 4.9 and 4.4). There was another hypermetabolic lymph node in the left supraclavicular area (SUV of 3.9). There was no significant uptake in the thyroid bed and no evidence of distant metastasis (Figure 5).

The patient underwent a second surgery (bilateral neck dissection for residual disease), and as per the surgeon's description, there was no macroscopic disease left in the explored area. Pathology showed metastatic papillary thyroid cancer in 2 out of 12 right level II lymph nodes and 6 out of 13 left level III lymph nodes. The size of the largest metastatic tumor was 1.3 cm on both sides. There was evidence of extranodal extension on both sides.

The thyroglobulin level was reduced to 28 ng/ml 10 weeks after the second neck dissection (TSH 83.70 mIU/ml). The patient received 150 mCi I-131 therapy for the treatment of remnant tissue and residual disease.

The posttreatment scan showed localized uptake in the neck area (Figure 6).

Four months after posttreatment with radioactive iodine, the thyroglobulin level decreased to 0.19 ng/ml with undetectable antithyroglobulin antibodies (TSH 0.261 mIU/ml). There was no evidence of local recurrence by physical examination.

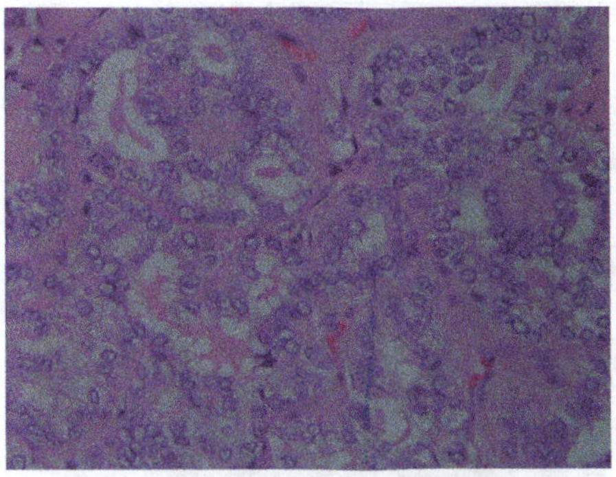

Figure 3: Microscopic examination showing infiltrative tumor with follicular architecture and eosinophilic scalloped colloid. There is overlapping and crowding of tumor cells with cytologic atypia. Numerous pseudoinclusions, nuclear grooves, and ground glass nuclei are also noted.

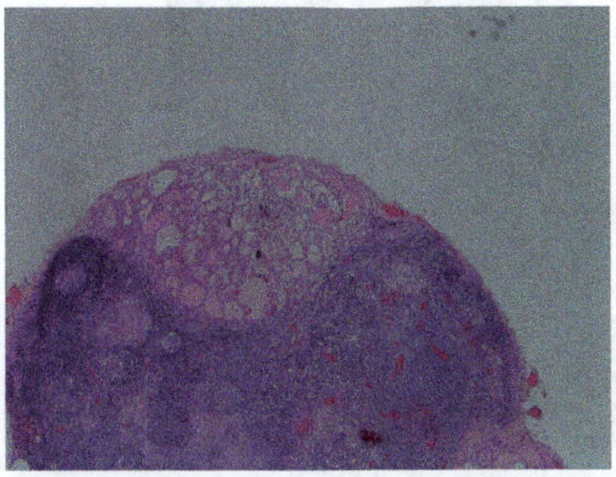

Figure 4: Positive lymph node: the image shows lymph node partially replaced by tumor cells.

3. Discussion

The above case represents a highly aggressive form of DTC with an unusual somatic mutation.

Classical molecular abnormalities involving the *MAPK* (mitogen-activated protein kinase) and *PI3K* (phosphoinositide 3-kinase) pathways that play a crucial role in follicular-derived thyroid cancer have been previously described [2]. Point mutations in the gene encoding *BRAF* are the most common genetic alterations in papillary thyroid cancer [3, 4]. Such mutations are found in 40–60% of classic papillary thyroid cancers with or without tall cell features, 20–40% of poorly differentiated thyroid cancers (PDTCs), and 30–40% of anaplastic thyroid cancers (ATCs). Point mutations in the gene encoding *RAS* are found in 40–50% of follicular thyroid cancers and 20–40% of PDTCs and ATCs [5].

Papillary thyroid cancers are also associated with gene fusion and rearrangements involving receptor tyrosine kinases (RTKs), such as ALK, RET, MET, NTRK, FGFR, and ROS1. The activation of most RTK requires molecular dimerization. Rearrangements of RTK-encoding genes lead to ligand-independent dimerization, which results in the constitutive tyrosine kinase activity and signal transduction to the RAS/RAF/MAPK, PI3K/AKT/mTOR, and JAK-STAT pathways [6]. The chimeric genes resulting from RET rearrangements are referred to as RET/PTC and those resulting from NTRK1 rearrangements as RTK. These gene fusions are prevalent in up to 40% of sporadic papillary thyroid cancers [7].

Our patient has an aggressive DTC with a less common gene fusion involving the *ALK* gene (*EML4e13-ALKe20* fusion). ALK fusion proteins have been shown to activate various signaling pathways, among which are the phosphtidylinositol 3-kinase (PI3K)/Akt pathway and the Ras ⟶ Raf ⟶ MEK ⟶ ERK (MAP kinase) pathway with multiple interaction points to mediate the ALK signaling. Such fusion promotes ligand-independent signaling and increases growth and cell invasion [1].

EML4 is a member of the echinoderm microtubule-associated protein-like family. The gene encodes a WD-repeat-containing protein that may be involved in microtubule formation. An abnormal fusion of parts of this gene with portions of the anaplastic lymphoma receptor tyrosine kinase gene generates EML4-ALK fusion transcripts.

The *ALK* gene encodes a receptor tyrosine kinase that belongs to the insulin receptor superfamily (https://www.genecards.org/Search/Keyword?queryString=ALK%20EML). This protein comprises an extracellular domain, a hydrophobic stretch corresponding to the single-pass transmembrane region, and an intracellular kinase domain. It appears to play an important role in the development of the brain and exerts its effects on specific neurons in the nervous system. Chromosomal rearrangements are the most common genetic alterations in this gene and result in the creation of multiple fusion genes which act as oncogenes, leading to constitutive autophosphorylation and activation of ALK tyrosine kinase. For reasons that are not currently understood, it seems that ALK locus is prone for translocation. Nearly 30 different *ALK* gene rearrangements have been described, few of which have been extensively studied like *NPM1* (5q35)/*ALK* (2p23), which was the first identified *ALK* fusion to nucleophosmin (*NPM1*) in anaplastic large cell lymphoma [8] and *EML4* (2p21)/*ALK* (2p23) in non-small-cell lung cancer [9, 10]. *EML4-ALK* in non-small-cell lung cancer (NSCLC) serves as a diagnostic marker and therapeutic target. Advanced NSCLC associated with the *ALK* fusion oncogene is highly sensitive to ALK tyrosine kinase inhibitors (TKIs), such as ceritinib, alectinib, and brigatinib [11, 12].

Other described fusion genes are *RANBP2*(2q12)/*ALK(2p23)* associated with inflammatory myofibroblastic tumors; *ATIC(2q35)/ALK(2p23)*, *TFG(3q12)/ALK(2p23)*, and *MSN(Xq12)/ALK(2p23)* associated with anaplastic large cell lymphoma; *SQSTM1(5q35)/ALK(2p23)* associated with *ALK*-positive large B-cell lymphoma; *KIF5B(10p11)/ALK*(2p23) associated with NSCLC; *STRN(2p22)/ALK(2p23)* associated

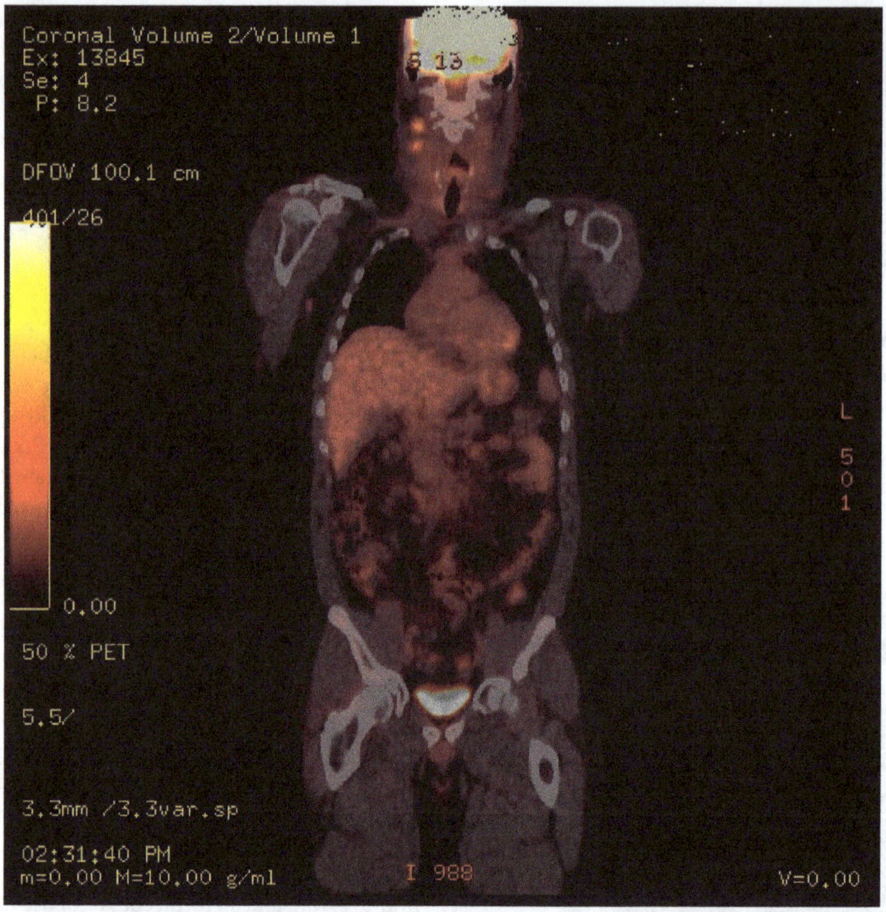

Figure 5: FDG-PET scan showing increase in uptake in two upper cervical lymph nodes.

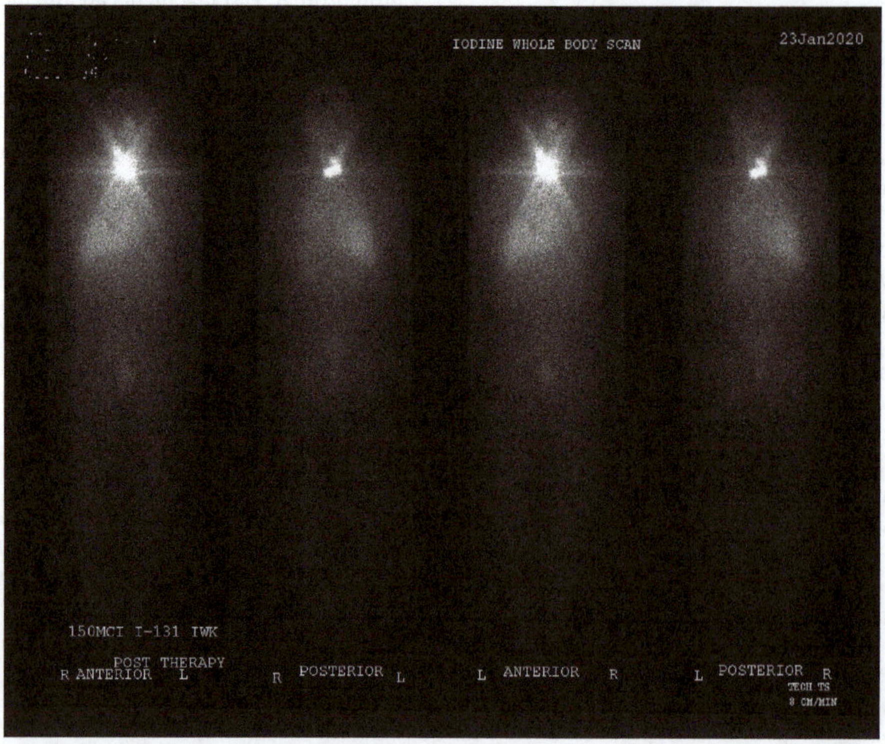

Figure 6: Whole body scan, one week posttreatment with 150 mCi I-131. It shows localized uptake in the neck area with no evidence of distant metastasis.

TABLE 1: Prevalence of *EML4/ALK* fusion.

Author (reference)	Year	Country	Study population	Sample size	Number of persons with kinase gene rearrangement (%)	Patients with *EML4/ALK* (number)	Findings	Follow-up (months)
Chu et al. [6]	2020	USA	PTC, PDTC, ANC	395	62 (16%)	1	Association seen between kinase gene fusion and clinical aggressiveness	6–480
Hamatani et al. [14]	2012	Japan	Atomic bomb survivors with PTC	105	10 (10%)	6	ALK fusion associated with radiation	NA
Agrawal et al. [15]	2014	USA	Patients with PTC	496	74 (15%)	4	>96% of PTCs have driver oncogenic mutation	NA
Kelly et al. [16]	2014	USA	PTC	256	4 (2%)	1	Compared to EML4-ALK, STRN-ALK is more common in PDTC	NA
Panebianco et al. [17]	2019	USA	PTC and PDTC	44	44 (100%)	17	Compared to EML4-ALK, STRN-ALK is more common in PDTC	2–108 months

PTC = papillary thyroid cancer; ATC = anaplastic thyroid cancer; PDTC = poorly differentiated thyroid cancer.

with DTC and breast cancer; *CLTC*(17q23)/*ALK(2p23)* and *TPM4(19p13)/ALK(2p23)* associated with anaplastic large cell lymphoma and inflammatory myofibroblastic tumors [13] (https://https://www.genecards.org/Search/Keyword?queryString=ALK%20EML); and Atlas of Genetics and Cytogenetics in Oncology and Haematology (atlasgeneticsoncology.org).

Our case's presentation was atypical for a well-differentiated FV-PTC in many aspects, including the rapid progression of clinical symptoms and signs, the extension beyond the thyroid and lymph nodes, and the persistence of high-volume local disease after thyroidectomy. Mutation analysis of the tumor tissue showed the presence of *EML4e13-ALKe20* fusion.

EML4-ALK fusion in thyroid cancer was first described in relation to exposure to ionizing radiation [14]. Hamatani et al. explored *EML4/ALK* and other *ALK* rearrangements in Atomic Bomb Survivors (ABS) of Hiroshima and Nagasaki who were diagnosed with PTC between 1956 and 1993. In the 25 ABS survivors with PTC with no detectable gene alteration in *BRAF, RAS, RET*, or *NTRK1*, *ALK* rearrangement was found in 10 out of 19 radiation-exposed PTCs (see Table 1). Five PTC cases with rearranged *ALK* were a fusion of *EML4* (exon 13) and *ALK* (exon 20), one case was a fusion of *EML4* (exon 20) and *ALK* (exon 20), and *ALK* partner genes in four cases have not been determined by the time of the publication and none in 6 patients with PTC without radiation exposure. Besides, solid/trabecular-like architecture in PTC was closely associated with *ALK* rearrangement in this cohort, being observed in 6 of 10 PTC cases with *ALK* rearrangements versus 2 of 15 cases with no *ALK* rearrangements [14].

Agrawal et al. in The Cancer Genome Atlas (TCGA) project performed a comprehensive multiplatform analysis of 496 PTCs. Fusions involving *ALK* presented in 4/484 (0.8%) tumors, including *EML4/ALK* [15].

Kelly et al. screened a total of 256 well-differentiated PTCs using whole-transcriptome RNA-sequencing analysis. The overall frequency of *ALK* fusion was four (1.6%) in 256 samples. *EML4-ALK* fusion was found in one tumor, and *ALK* fusions involving the striatin gene (*STRN-ALK*) were found in 3 tumors. In comparison, *STRN-ALK* was detected in three of 35 PDTCs (9%) and one of 24 ATCs (4%). All detected *ALK* fusions were *STRN-ALK*, and no additional cases of *EML4-ALK* were found [16].

Panebianco et al. showed in a series of 44 *ALK*-translocated thyroid neoplasms that *ALK* fusion-positive thyroid carcinomas are typically infiltrative PTCs with a common follicular growth pattern and may show tumor dedifferentiation, which is associated with increased mortality. The most common *ALK* fusion partners were *STRN* ($n = 22$) and *EML4* ($n = 17$). In 5 cases, novel *ALK* fusion partners were discovered. All 5 PDTCs carried the *STRN-ALK* fusion. Compared to *EML4-ALK, STRN-ALK* may be more common in PDTC, and ~10% of *ALK* fusions involve rare gene partners [17]. In the same study, Panebianco et al. showed that all 19 resected thyroid nodules with *ALK* fusions identified preoperatively by fine-needle aspiration were malignant [17].

Chu et al. investigated the correlation between genotype and tumor behavior in 62 kinase fusion-positive thyroid carcinomas, including 57 papillary thyroid carcinomas (PTCs), two poorly differentiated thyroid carcinomas (PDTCs), two undifferentiated thyroid carcinomas (ATCs), and one primary secretory carcinoma (SC). *ALK* rearrangements were found in one PDTC and two PTCs. The two PTCs, despite having different fusion partners (*STRN* and *EML4*), were morphologically similar (with multinodular growth and predominantly follicular architecture) [6].

Point mutation of *ALK* gene has been reported by Murugan and Xing, who identified two novel point mutations in exon 23 of the *ALK* gene, *C3592T* and *G3602A*, in patients with anaplastic thyroid cancer with a prevalence of 11.11% but found no mutations in the matched normal tissues or in well-differentiated thyroid cancer [18].

4. Conclusion

In summary, we presented a patient with aggressive DTC with a less common gene fusion involving the *ALK* gene (*EML4e13-ALKe20* fusion). Identification of *ALK* rearrangement in thyroid tumor is of particular interest due to crizotinib's effectiveness and other specific ALK inhibitors that have been shown to induce a remarkable response in one case of aggressive PTC and ATC [18, 19]. Kelly et al. demonstrated that crizotinib effectively inhibits thyroid cell proliferation driven by *STRN-ALK*, raising the possibility that *ALK* may serve as a therapeutic target for thyroid cancer [16]. Godbert et al. demonstrated a remarkable response to crizotinib in women with anaplastic lymphoma kinase-rearranged anaplastic thyroid carcinoma [20].

Precision medicine is an emerging approach for disease management that considers individual variability in presentation, progression, and response to treatment. Genetic mutation analysis and molecular markers are the cornerstones of precision medicine in cancer treatment, as many of these mutations are considered therapeutic targets for modern cancer medications.

The selective use of molecular diagnostics can help with DTC management, especially in patients with atypical presentations or more aggressive clinical courses.

References

[1] B. Hallberg and R. H. Palmer, "The role of the ALK receptor in cancer biology," *Annals of Oncology*, vol. 27, no. 3, pp. iii4–iii15, 2016.

[2] B. R. Haugen, E. K. Alexander, K. C. Bible et al., "2015 American thyroid association management guidelines for adult patients with thyroid nodules and differentiated thyroid cancer: the American thyroid association guidelines task force on thyroid nodules and differentiated thyroid cancer," *Thyroid*, vol. 26, no. 1, pp. 1–133, 2016.

[3] D. Chakravarty, E. Santos, M. Ryder et al., "Small-molecule MAPK inhibitors restore radioiodine incorporation in mouse thyroid cancers with conditional BRAF activation," *Journal of Clinical Investigation*, vol. 121, no. 12, pp. 4700–4711, 2011.

[4] J. A. Knauf, X. Ma, E. P. Smith et al., "Targeted expression of BRAFV600E in thyroid cells of transgenic mice results in papillary thyroid cancers that undergo dedifferentiation," *Cancer Research*, vol. 65, no. 10, pp. 4238–4245, 2005.

[5] K. A. Miller, N. Yeager, K. Baker, X.-H. Liao, S. Refetoff, and A. Di Cristofano, "Oncogenic Kras requires simultaneous PI3K signaling to induce ERK activation and transform thyroid epithelial cells in vivo," *Cancer Research*, vol. 69, no. 8, pp. 3689–3694, 2009.

[6] Y.-H. Chu, L. J. Wirth, A. A. Farahani et al., "Clinicopathologic features of kinase fusion-related thyroid carcinomas: an integrative analysis with molecular characterization," *Modern Pathology*, vol. 33, no. 12, pp. 2458–2472, 2020.

[7] I. Bongarzone, P. Vigneri, L. Mariani, P. Collini, S. Pilotti, and M. A. Pierotti, "RET/NTRK1 rearrangements in thyroid gland tumors of the papillary carcinoma family: correlation with clinicopathological features," *Clinical Cancer Research*, vol. 4, no. 1, p. 223, 1998.

[8] S. Morris, M. Kirstein, M. Valentine et al., "Fusion of a kinase gene, ALK, to a nucleolar protein gene, NPM, in non-Hodgkin's lymphoma," *Science*, vol. 263, no. 5151, pp. 1281–1284, 1994.

[9] M. Soda, Y. L. Choi, M. Enomoto et al., "Identification of the transforming EML4-ALK fusion gene in non-small-cell lung cancer," *Nature*, vol. 448, no. 7153, pp. 561–566, 2007.

[10] T. Takahashi, M. Sonobe, M. Kobayashi et al., "Clinicopathologic features of non-small-cell lung cancer with EML4-ALK fusion gene," *Annals of Surgical Oncology*, vol. 17, no. 3, pp. 889–897, 2010.

[11] A. T. Shaw and B. Solomon, "Targeting anaplastic lymphoma kinase in lung cancer: figure 1," *Clinical Cancer Research*, vol. 17, no. 8, pp. 2081–2086, 2011.

[12] L. A. Pikor, V. R. Ramnarine, S. Lam, and W. L. Lam, "Genetic alterations defining NSCLC subtypes and their therapeutic implications," *Lung Cancer*, vol. 82, no. 2, pp. 179–189, 2013.

[13] Z. Cao, Q. Gao, M. Fu, N. Ni, Y. Pei, and W.-B. Ou, "Anaplastic lymphoma kinase fusions: roles in cancer and therapeutic perspectives," *Oncology Letters*, vol. 17, no. 2, pp. 2020–2030, 2019.

[14] K. Hamatani, M. Mukai, K. Takahashi, Y. Hayashi, K. Nakachi, and Y. Kusunoki, "Rearranged anaplastic lymphoma kinase (ALK) gene in adult-onset papillary thyroid cancer amongst atomic bomb survivors," *Thyroid*, vol. 22, no. 11, pp. 1153–1159, 2012.

[15] Cancer Genome Atlas Research Network, "Integrated genomic characterization of papillary thyroid carcinoma- genome Atlas research network," *Cell*, vol. 159, no. 3, pp. 676–690, 2014.

[16] L. M. Kelly, G. Barila, P. Liu et al., "Identification of the transforming STRN-ALK fusion as a potential therapeutic target in the aggressive forms of thyroid cancer," *Proceedings of the National Academy of Sciences*, vol. 111, no. 11, pp. 4233–4238, 2014.

[17] F. Panebianco, A. V. Nikitski, M. N. Nikiforova et al., "Characterization of thyroid cancer driven by known and novel ALK fusions," *Endocrine-Related Cancer*, vol. 26, no. 11, pp. 803–814, 2019.

[18] A. K. Murugan and M. Xing, "Anaplastic thyroid cancers harbor novel oncogenic mutations of the ALK gene," *Cancer Research*, vol. 71, no. 13, pp. 4403–4411, 2011.

[19] M. J. Demeure, M. Aziz, R. Rosenberg, S. D. Gurley, K. J. Bussey, and J. D. Carpten, "Whole-genome sequencing of an aggressive BRAF wild-type papillary thyroid cancer identified EML4-ALK translocation as a therapeutic target," *World Journal of Surgery*, vol. 38, no. 6, pp. 1296–1305, 2014.

[20] Y. Godbert, B. Henriques de Figueiredo, F. Bonichon et al., "Remarkable response to crizotinib in woman with anaplastic lymphoma kinase-rearranged anaplastic thyroid carcinoma," *Journal of Clinical Oncology*, vol. 33, no. 20, pp. e84–e87, 2015.

37

Multiple Endocrine Neoplasia Type 1 with Concomitant Existence of Malignant Insulinoma: A Rare Finding

Randhir Sagar Yadav,[1] **Ashik Pokharel**,[2] **Deepshikha Gaire**,[3] **Shumneva Shrestha**,[1] **Ashbita Pokharel**,[1] **Sumita Pradhan**,[2] **and Prasan Bir Singh Kansakar**[2]

[1]*Maharajgunj Medical Campus, Institute of Medicine, Tribhuvan University, Kathmandu, Nepal*
[2]*Department of Gastrointestinal and General Surgery, Tribhuvan University Teaching Hospital, Kathmandu, Nepal*
[3]*Department of Pathology, Tribhuvan University Teaching Hospital, Kathmandu, Nepal*

Correspondence should be addressed to Randhir Sagar Yadav; sagar.randhir@gmail.com

Academic Editor: Keiji Iida

Multiple endocrine neoplasia type 1 (MEN1) is a rare syndrome of autosomal dominant inheritance defined by co-occurrence of two or more tumors originating from the parathyroid gland, pancreatic islet cells, and/or anterior pituitary. Insulinoma which has an incidence of 0.4% is a rare pancreatic neuroendocrine tumor. Malignant insulinoma is extremely rare, while primary hyperparathyroidism is a common occurrence in MEN1. We present a case of MEN1 syndrome with 2.6 cm insulinoma in the pancreatic head and parathyroid adenoma in a 56-year-old female who presented with symptoms suggestive of hypoglycemia like multiple episodes of loss of consciousness for four years. Classical pancreaticoduodenectomy was carried out, and the post-operative period was uneventful. Later, subtotal parathyroidectomy was performed, which showed parathyroid adenoma. Patients presenting with features of hypoglycemia should be vigilantly assessed for the presence of a sinister pathology.

1. Background

Multiple endocrine neoplasia type 1 (MEN1) is an autosomal dominant disorder characterized primarily by two or three principal MEN1-related endocrine tumors originating from parathyroid glands, endocrine gastroenteropancreatic (GEP) tract, and anterior pituitary [1]. Primary hyperparathyroidism is found in 90% of patients with MEN1 syndrome [1], whereas only 5–10% insulinomas present as a constituent of MEN1 [2]. Most of the insulinomas are benign; very rarely, they are malignant [3]. Whipple's triad along with supervised fasting serum insulin, C-peptide, and proinsulin thresholds/cutoffs along with imaging studies are vital in diagnosis and localization of mass [4]. Surgical resection is the mainstay of treatment of insulinoma [4] and parathyroid adenoma [1].

2. Case Presentation

A 56-year-old lady presented to us with a history of multiple episodes of loss of consciousness mostly on empty stomach for 4 years with 15–20 fainting attacks per year. She was hospitalized multiple times at local health facilities for hypoglycemia, and she was managed symptomatically. Except for some other neuroglycopenic and adrenergic symptoms of hypoglycemia, there were no other systemic complaints, findings, and significant medical or surgical history. Her family history revealed that her two brothers and two sons died of unknown diseases at a young age (20–37 years). Due to financial constraints, they were not able to undergo any medical investigation or treatment. The systemic examination was normal.

In the emergency room, Whipple's triad was seen (frequent episodes of hypoglycemia with a blood sugar of 34 mg/dl (normal 70–110 mg/dl) along with neuroglycopenic symptoms relieved on intravenous dextrose). The basal insulin and C-peptide were 39.3 IU/ml (normal 2.5–25.0 uIU/ml) and 4.85 ng/ml (normal 1.5–5.0 ng/m), respectively. The 72-hour supervised fasting was abandoned at 6 hours due to the development of sweating and dizziness (blood sugar 42 mg/dl). The fasting insulin (63.8 IU/ml) and C-peptide (6.82 ng/ml) were not suppressed suggesting insulinoma. She also had hypercalcemia (serum calcium 11.6 mg/dl; normal 8.3–10.3 mg/dl) with an increased parathyroid hormone (PTH) (344 pg/ml; normal < 53.5 pg/ml). Serum prolactin, thyroid stimulating hormone (TSH) and other hormonal and routine biochemical investigations were within the normal range. With suspicion of insulinoma and parathyroid adenoma, further imaging studies were performed to localize the lesion. Ultrasound of the abdomen showed a hypoechoic lesion in the pancreatic head (2.6 cm × 2.8 cm) while the left kidney was not visualized. Contrast-enhanced computed tomography (CECT) abdomen showed a hyperattenuating lesion in the pancreatic head (2.4 cm × 2.3 cm × 2.1 cm) communicating with the main pancreatic duct and bilateral adrenal hyperplasia (Figure 1). The lesion being situated in the pancreatic head did not reveal any abnormality on the upper GI endoscopy, while taking a biopsy was not possible. Esophagogastroduodenal scope-guided biopsy would have helped, but it was not available. Ultrasound of the neck showed a nodular lesion in the right lobe of the thyroid gland. Likewise, technetium-99m labeled hexakis-methoxyisobutyl isonitrile (^{99m}Tc MIBI) scan showed right inferior parathyroid adenoma (Figure 2). Brain magnetic resonance imaging (MRI) was normal.

Based on the clinical and investigation analyses, a diagnosis of MEN1 syndrome with insulinoma of the head of the pancreas and parathyroid adenoma was made. Classical pancreaticoduodenectomy (Whipple's procedure) was performed which showed 3 cm × 2 cm fleshy mass present in the pancreatic head (Figure 3) with no ascites, the pancreas was soft, and common bile duct measured about 12 mm. The pancreatic duct traversed through the tumor, so pancreatic resection was unavoidable. Her postoperative period was uneventful. Postoperative blood sugar, insulin, and C-peptide were 127 mg/dl, 8.9 IU/ml, and 2.28 ng/ml, respectively. Histopathological examination (HPE) revealed a well-differentiated neuroendocrine tumor (Figure 4) with a maximum tumor dimension of about 2.6 cm with lymph node metastasis. However, lymphovascular and perineural invasions were not identified. One out of seven lymph nodes resected was positive for tumor with TNM stage pT2N1. Due to the paucity of resources, immunohistochemical studies and positron emission tomography (PET) scan could not be performed. A year later, she underwent right hemithyroidectomy with excision of the right superior and inferior parathyroid glands at another center. The HPE showed infrathyroid parathyroid adenoma with nodular goiter with a hyperplastic nodule. Her biochemical parameters including blood glucose and PTH were within the normal range on regular follow-up visits, and she has been doing well clinically, and she was satisfied with the treatment and its response.

3. Discussion

The majority of insulinomas are sporadic, and only 5–10% insulinomas present as a constituent of MEN1 [2]. Most insulinomas unlike other pancreatic islet cell tumors (gastrinoma and VIPoma) are benign [3, 5] solitary [5]. The majority of insulinomas are less than 2 cm. Malignant insulinomas are rare. Thus, among reported cases of insulinoma, only 5–12% of cases were found malignant [3, 6–8].

The clinical presentations of insulinoma vary. Hypoglycemia is the most common presentation. Hypoglycemia manifests as neuroglycopenic as well as adrenergic symptoms. Neuroglycopenic patients present with neurological as well as psychiatric manifestations such as confusion, blurring of vision, seizure, agitation, and behavioral changes [9, 10]. Our patient also had multiple episodes of loss of consciousness due to hypoglycemia along with some neuroglycopenic and adrenergic symptoms.

Diagnosis of MEN1-associated lesions includes biochemical and hormonal evaluation, endoscopic, nuclear medicine, or other imaging studies. Moreover, clinical diagnostic criteria for MEN1 syndrome include the presence of two out of three tumors that are parathyroid, pituitary, or GEP tract tumors [1]. Whipple's triad is the classic approach of diagnosing an insulinoma while a supervised 72-hour fasting test for measurement of plasma glucose, insulin, C-peptide, and proinsulin during the onset of hypoglycemic symptoms remains the gold standard for diagnosis of insulinoma. With the availability of proinsulin assay, proinsulin cutoffs have emerged as a diagnostic tool. There is some consensus on the thresholds/cutoffs for insulin, C-peptide, and proinsulin to diagnose insulinoma [4]. Moreover, Hirshberg et al. has recommended a 48-hour fast instead of 72-hour fast [6]. Upon establishing a diagnosis, noninvasive diagnostic investigations such as transabdominal ultrasonography, computed tomography (CT), and MRI help in localization of the insulinoma. CT and MRI are the accepted first-line and second-line investigations, respectively, while MRI can potentially supersede CT in the coming days due to its higher sensitivity. Endoscopic ultrasonography and arterial stimulation venous sampling are superior to CT and MRI in preoperative localization but are invasive [4]. Our patient was diagnosed based on the clinical evaluation, plasma glucose, insulin, C-peptide, calcium, and parathyroid hormone level as well as imaging studies such as an ultrasound of the abdomen and neck, CECT abdomen, and ^{99m}Tc MIBI scan.

There are two major challenges in managing patients with malignant insulinoma. First is the tumor itself, which is metastatic, and second is severe hypoglycemia [6]. Identification of patients at risk of aggressive disease is a challenge in treatment [8]. Patients have characteristic inappropriately elevated levels of insulin and proinsulin levels at diagnosis [6], but it does not differentiate between a benign and malignant or less and more aggressive form of the disease [7, 8]. An insulinoma is considered malignant when there is a local invasion to the surrounding tissue or lymph node or liver metastasis [11]. The lymph node or liver are the most common sites of metastasis in malignant insulinoma [4, 7]. Regional lymph node involvement is not always linked to poor prognosis [8]. Similarly, liver metastasis is commonly but not always associated with poor prognosis [7]. There are no predictive factors to determine the aggressive nature of

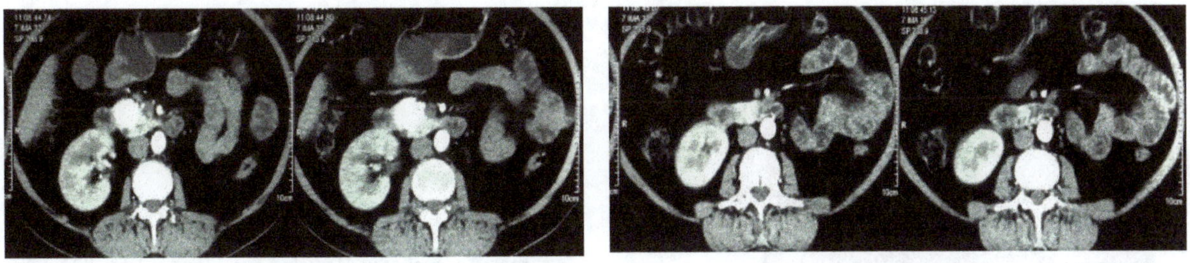

(a) (b)

FIGURE 1: Hyperattenuating lesion in the anterior plane of the head of the pancreas (2.4 cm × 2.3 cm × 2.1 cm), bilateral adrenal hyperplasia, and nonvisualization of the left kidney.

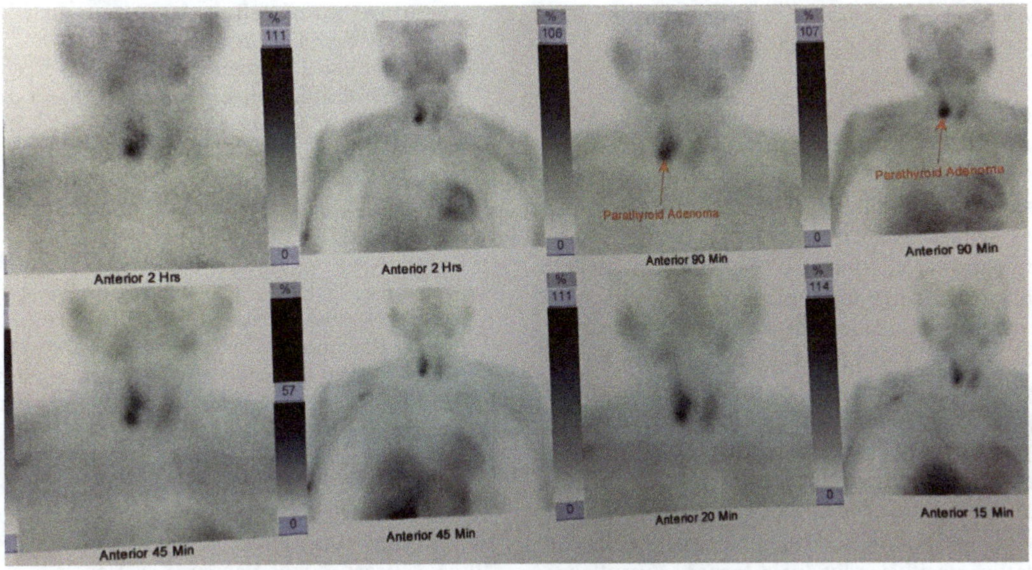

FIGURE 2: ^{99m}Tc MIBI scan showing right inferior parathyroid adenoma.

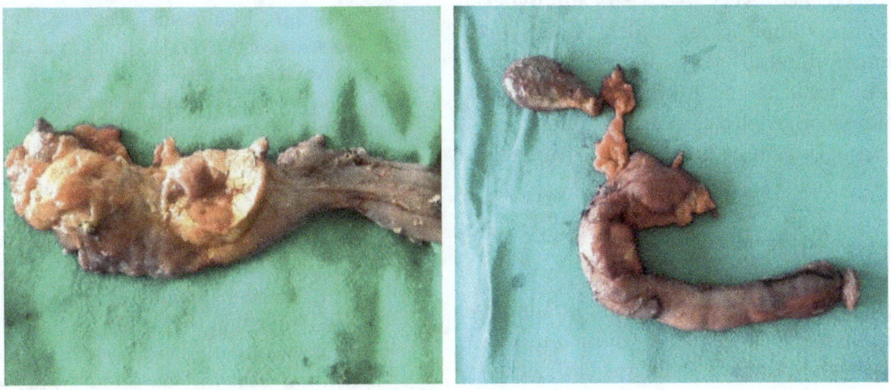

FIGURE 3: Postoperative specimen.

malignant insulinoma and its propensity to metastasis, while only about 2% of benign insulinoma metastasize later [8]. Surgical removal of the tumor remains the mainstay of treatment of insulinoma, which reverts the neurological sequelae of hypoglycemia [4, 7]. Aggressive surgical resection favors survival and quality of life [4]. Neuroendocrine tumors are the histologic findings from both primary and metastatic sites [7]. Our patient underwent classical pancreaticoduodenectomy without any further episodes of hypoglycemia then after. HPE of the resected pancreatic lesion showed a well-differentiated neuroendocrine tumor with a single lymph node involvement and thus confirmed malignant insulinoma in our patient.

Primary hyperparathyroidism is associated with 90% of MEN1 which presents with hypercalcemia in 100% patients [1]. A parathyroid lesion in MEN1 is almost always (99%)

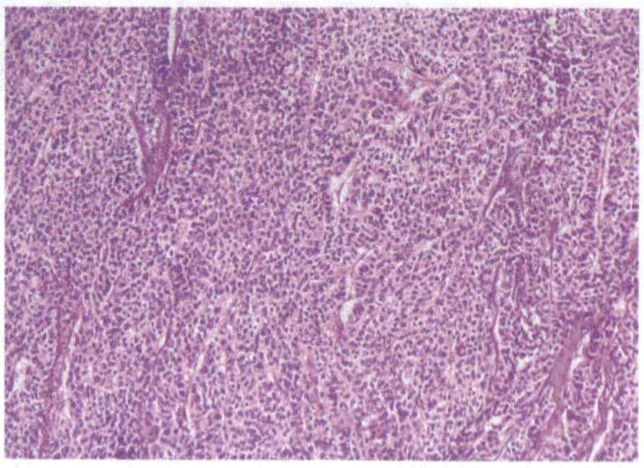

Figure 4: Well-differentiated neuroendocrine tumor; tumor cells arranged in trabeculae, cords, and lobules with vascular septa. These cells show mild nuclear atypia, fine stippled chromatin, inconspicuous nucleoli, and moderate amount of eosinophilic granular cytoplasm. Mitosis is infrequent (H&E X100).

benign adenoma or hyperplasia, while malignant parathyroid tumors are extremely rare [1]. Surgery is the preferred and most effective treatment. The timing of surgery depends on age, the severity of symptoms, PTH and calcium levels, and MEN1-associated endocrinopathies. [1] Our patient went for hemiparathyroidectomy a year later. In MEN1, besides tumors originating from parathyroid glands, endocrine gastroenteropancreatic tract, and anterior pituitary, nonfunctional adrenal and incidental thyroid lesions are found in 30–40% [12] and 25% [13], respectively. Hormonal and imaging studies revealed incidental nonfunctional adrenal and thyroid hyperplasias in our patient.

MEN1 presents with varied clinical features that warrant genetic testing for diagnosis in suspected cases and screen the family members for risk of development of the disease [14]. For mutation-positive individuals, focused surveillance for early identification of potentially malignant neuroendocrine tumors is recommended [1]. MEN1 carriers are recommended to be screened every 1-3 years for hyperparathyroidism, and other tumors as the clinical features are often mild for a longer duration [15]. A history of four undiagnosed deaths of her sons and brothers at early ages raises a strong suspicion of genetic association, but unfortunately, genetic testing was not done due to financial constraints.

4. Conclusions

Patients presenting with Whipple's triad should be further investigated with a high degree of suspicion for insulinoma. Eventhough MEN1 is a rare entity, a vigilant clinical approach to identify subtle clinical features of hypoglycemia along with localization and surgical removal of the resectable mass is imperative for treatment. Patients with an endocrine tumor should be investigated for the presence of other endocrine and/or neuroendocrine tumor(s) or syndrome.

Consent

Written informed consent was obtained from the patient.

Authors' Contributions

RSY and AP contributed equally to this work.

References

[1] A. Falchetti, F. Marini, E. Luzi et al., "Multiple endocrine neoplasia type 1 (MEN1): not only inherited endocrine tumors," *Genetics in Medicine*, vol. 11, no. 12, pp. 825–835, 2009.

[2] S. Pelengaris and M. Khan, "Oncogenic co-operation in beta-cell tumorigenesis," *Endocrine-related Cancer*, vol. 8, no. 4, pp. 307–314, 2001.

[3] F. J. Service, M. M. McMahon, P. C. O'Brien, and D. J. Ballard, "Functioning insulinoma-incidence, recurrence, and long-term survival of patients: a 60-year study," *Mayo Clinic Proceedings*, vol. 66, no. 7, pp. 711–719, 1991.

[4] T. Okabayashi, Y. Shima, S. Ito et al., "Diagnosis and management of insulinoma," *World Journal of Gastroenterology*, vol. 19, no. 6, pp. 829–837, 2013.

[5] D. H. Schussheim, M. C. Skarulis, S. K. Agarwal et al., "Multiple endocrine neoplasia type 1: new clinical and basic findings," *Trends in Endocrinology and Metabolism*, vol. 12, no. 4, pp. 173–178, 2001.

[6] B. Hirshberg, A. Livi, D. L. Bartlett et al., "Forty-eight-hour fast: the diagnostic test for insulinoma," *The Journal of Clinical Endocrinology and Metabolism*, vol. 85, no. 9, pp. 3222–3226, 2000.

[7] D. N. Danforth, P. Gorden, and M. F. Brennan, "Metastatic insulin-secreting carcinoma of the pancreas: clinical course and the role of surgery," *Surgery*, vol. 96, no. 6, pp. 1027–1037, 1984.

[8] B. Hirshberg, C. Cochran, M. C. Skarulis et al., "Malignant insulinoma," *Cancer*, vol. 104, no. 2, pp. 264–272, 2005.

[9] S. K. Agarwal, S. C. Guru, C. Heppner et al., "Menin interacts with the AP1 transcription factor JunD and represses JunD-activated transcription," *Cell*, vol. 96, no. 1, pp. 143–152, 1999.

[10] A. C. Jager, L Friis-Hansen, T. V Hansen et al., "Characteristics of the Danish families with multiple endocrine neoplasia type 1," *Molecular and Cellular Endocrinology*, vol. 249, no. 1-2, pp. 123–132, 2006.

[11] C. S. Grant, "Insulinoma," *Best Practice and Research Clinical Gastroenterology*, vol. 19, no. 5, pp. 783–798, 2005.

[12] M. Yoshida, M. Hiroi, T. Imai et al., "A case of ACTH-independent macronodular adrenal hyperplasia associated with multiple endocrine neoplasia type 1," *Endocrine Journal*, vol. 58, no. 4, pp. 269–277, 2011.

[13] R. V. Thakker, P. J. Newey, G. V. Walls et al., "Clinical practice guidelines for multiple endocrine neoplasia type 1 (MEN1)," *The Journal of Clinical Endocrinology and Metabolism*, vol. 97, no. 9, pp. 2990–3011, 2012.

[14] J. W. Cardinal, L. Bregman, N. Hayward et al., "A report of a national mutation testing service for the MEN1 gene: clinical presentations and implications for mutation testing," *Journal of Medical Genetics*, vol. 42, no. 1, pp. 69–74, 2005.

[15] J. Chudek, G. Piecha, T. Nieszporek, F. Marini, M. L. Brandi, and A. Więcek, "Novel 1113delC menin gene mutation in a Polish family with multiple endocrine neoplasia type 1 syndrome," *European Journal of Internal Medicine*, vol. 17, no. 6, pp. 447–449, 2006.

Euglycemic Ketoacidosis in a Patient with Metastatic Non-Small-Cell Lung Adenocarcinoma and Concomitant Pulmonary Embolism

Robert Sean O'Neill,[1] Lauren Tyack,[2] Mary Freeman,[2] and Hussein Soudy Hussein[1,3]

[1]*The Department of Medical Oncology, The Sutherland Hospital, Caringbah, NSW, Australia*
[2]*The Department of Endocrinology, The Sutherland Hospital, Caringbah, NSW, Australia*
[3]*The Department of Medical Oncology, St George Hospital, Kogarah, NSW, Australia*

Correspondence should be addressed to Robert Sean O'Neill; robert.oneill@health.nsw.gov.au

Academic Editor: Osamu Isozaki

Euglycemic ketoacidosis is a recognised side effect secondary to sodium-glucose cotransporter 2 inhibitor use in the treatment of type 2 diabetes mellitus; however, there is scarce evidence to suggest whether preexisting comorbid conditions contribute to the development of this potentially life-threatening complication. We describe a case of euglycemic ketoacidosis in a patient with type 2 diabetes mellitus in the context of empagliflozin use after a recent diagnosis of metastatic lung adenocarcinoma. The diagnosis was complicated by a pulmonary embolism and hospital-acquired pneumonia, and was subsequently established after an anion-gap metabolic acidosis was identified on arterial blood gas and serum ketone measurement. The patient required admission to the intensive care unit for fluid resuscitation and regular intravenous insulin to ensure resolution of acidosis and maintenance of normoglycaemia. The patient was discharged to home for outpatient single-agent pembrolizumab for treatment of his lung adenocarcinoma. This article highlights the importance or awareness of oral hypoglycaemic medications and their side effects, along with providing further evidence for the potential contribution of malignancy to the development of euglycemic ketoacidosis in a patient with type 2 diabetes mellitus.

1. Introduction

Sodium-glucose cotransporter 2 inhibitors (SGLT2i) are a new class of oral diabetic medications that have gained favour in recent times due to the reported favourable renal and cardiovascular outcomes; however, the full extent of their side-effect profile is not completely understood. The triad of euglycemia, ketosis, and anion-gap metabolic acidosis defines euglycemic ketoacidosis, a rare, yet lethal complication of SGLT2i therapy with rates ranging depending on the dose administered [1]. Diabetic ketoacidosis is known to occur in the context of depleted circulating insulin, a situation which can be precipitated by both a starvation state and an acute medical illness, which subsequently results in a state of catabolism highlighted by lipolysis, hyperglucagonemia, fatty acid oxidation, and finally ketosis. In the case of SGLT2i use, glycosuria is stimulated resulting in decreased serum glucose levels, producing euglycemia [2].

Here, we present the case of a male with type 2 diabetes mellitus (T2DM) and non-small-cell lung cancer (NSCLC) who developed euglycemic ketoacidosis in the context of empagliflozin use, after presenting with symptomatic hypercalcaemia, and was subsequently diagnosed with a pulmonary embolism.

2. Case Presentation

A 71-year-old male was referred to a metropolitan hospital for management of symptomatic hypercalcaemia. This was in the context of a recent diagnosis of metastatic stage IV lung adenocarcinoma and PDL-1 expression 50%, with baseline positron emission tomography (PET) scan demonstrating a left lingular lesion, and mediastinal and upper abdominal glucose avid nodes. In addition to this, avid disease was noted in the right hilum and bilateral supraclavicular regions. He had a background of invasive urinary bladder carcinoma previously treated with methotrexate, vinblastine sulfate, adriamycin, and cisplatin (MVAC) chemotherapy, formation of a ureteric ileostomy, and T2DM. With regard to the patient's diagnosis of T2DM, this was previously managed with diet and he had been diagnosed as an outpatient with a HbA1c of 9.0%. This had been escalated to oral metformin 500 mg twice daily, and in addition to this, empagliflozin 10 mg once daily had also been initiated three months prior to presentation due to labile blood sugar levels.

On preliminary assessment, he reported constipation and issues with short-term memory but was otherwise clinically well. Clinical examination demonstrated decreased air entry over his left lower lobe on thoracic auscultation. He was of short stature, weighing 75.3 kg with a body mass index (BMI) of 28.4 kg/m^2, and he reported nil changes in his ileostomy output preceding admission.

His calcium level was 3.0 mmol/L on admission which was managed with a single dose of zoledronic acid and intravenous fluids with resolution on day 2 of admission. On day 2 of admission, the patient developed a fever to 38.3 degrees Celsius and was commenced on intravenous antibiotics due to suspicion of hospital acquired pneumonia (HAP). On day 4 of admission, the patient developed tachypnoea and was hypoxic to 88% on room air. Computed tomography pulmonary angiogram (CTPA) (Figure 1) demonstrated bilateral pulmonary emboli, a significant left-sided pleural effusion, and straightening of the ventricular septum indicating right heart strain which was confirmed on transthoracic echocardiogram with an estimated mean pulmonary artery pressure of 42 mmHg and a dilated right ventricle with impaired systolic function reported. The patient was subsequently commenced on therapeutic anticoagulation and was escalated to high flow nasal prongs for ventilatory support. Due to ongoing tachypnoea despite high flow oxygen supplementation, an arterial blood gas was taken which demonstrated an anion-gap metabolic acidosis (pH 7.343, pCO_2 25.7 mmHg, base excess −11.0 mmol/L, HCO_3^- 13.6 mmol/L, and albumin-corrected anion gap 19.9 mmol/L) with bedside capillary glucose and ketones reported as 5.1 mmol/L and 7.4 mmol/L, respectively. Further investigation revealed that the patient's regular empagliflozin, a SGLT2i had been continued on admission.

The patient was commenced on an insulin and dextrose infusion and transferred to the intensive care unit (ICU) for further management. Repeat arterial blood gases were taken regularly throughout admission to the ICU, where he was maintained on a dextrose and insulin infusion until his metabolic acidosis resolved and normoglycemia, along with low-level serum ketonaemia maintained (Table 1). The patient's renal function remained normal throughout admission.

The patient underwent pleurocentesis on day 6 of admission for symptomatic relief with mild improvement in his oxygen requirement. Pleural fluid cytology was consistent with non-small-cell lung primary metastatic adenocarcinoma.

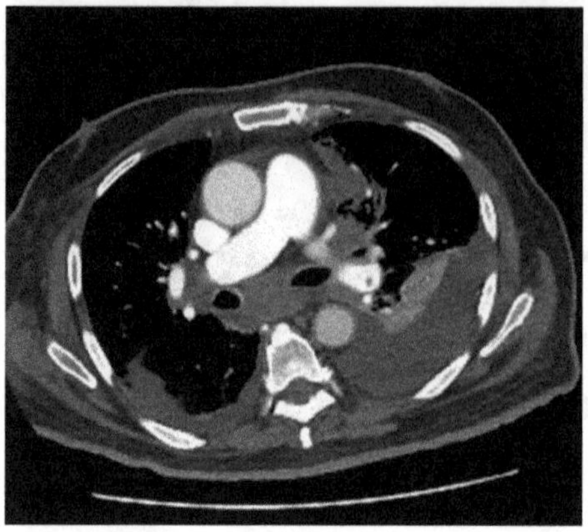

Figure 1: Transverse view of CTPA demonstrating bilateral pleural effusions with collapse consolidation and left pulmonary artery embolus.

The patient was subsequently discharged from the ICU on day 7 of admission, upon which his serum ketones had normalised and his BSLs were controlled on a supplemental subcutaneous insulin regime. He had an ongoing oxygen requirement; however. his tachypnoea had resolved. He was transitioned from a heparin infusion to therapeutic clexane for management of his bilateral pulmonary emboli, and his chest X-ray on discharge from the ICU demonstrated a stable appearance in his bilateral pleural effusions after pleurocentesis.

The remainder of the patient's admission was unremarkable. He was discharged on day 15 of admission with palliative oxygen therapy for symptomatic relief and was referred for outpatient treatment with single-agent pembrolizumab. Empagliflozin was withheld on discharge, and due to adequate BSL control as an inpatient, insulin was ceased with a view to recommence outpatient low-dose metformin.

3. Discussion

The concept of euglycemic ketoacidosis was first proposed in 1973, with causes such as gestational diabetes, reduced calorie intake, excessive alcohol consumption, acute pancreatitis, and chronic hepatitis being reported in the literature [1, 3]. In addition to this, the introduction of SGLT2i in the management of T2DM has resulted in emerging cases of euglycemic ketoacidosis [4]. This is postulated to occur through decreasing fasting and postprandial glucose levels resulting in decreased insulin production and subsequently has been shown to promote hyperglucagonemia, along with the propagation of a negative fluid and sodium balance [4, 5]. In addition to this, subsequent glycosuria as a result of the action of SGLT2i results in normoglycaemia, presenting the biochemical phenotype that is euglycemic ketoacidosis. The mechanism of action of SGLT2i is independent of insulin and can be used at any stage of illness in T2DM, and in addition to promoting normoglycaemia, they have favourable effects in reducing body weight, blood pressure,

Table 1: Blood gas from the point of assessment on day 2 of admission demonstrating resolving metabolic acidosis.

	0	5 hours	12 hours	15 hours	20 hours*
pH	7.343	7.348	7.391	7.365	7.384
pO_2 (mmHg)	75.3	110.0	70.9	85.7	34.3
pCO_2 (mmHg)	25.7	28.7	34.5	37.9	38.0
HCO_3^- (mmol/L)	13.6	15.4	20.5	21.1	22.2
Base excess (mmol/L)	−11.0	−9.1	−3.6	−3.4	−2.1
BGL (mmol/L)	4.7	9.7	6.8	7.1	7.0
Blood ketone level (mmol/L)	7.4	4.7	0.1	1.1	0.3

*Venous blood gas.

reducing atherosclerotic cardiovascular events in patients with established cardiovascular disease, reducing heart failure hospitalisation rates and progression of renal disease [6, 7].

Euglycemic acidosis occurring in the context of SGLT2i use in patients with malignancy is scarce, with previous reports documenting its incidence in the case of colorectal cancer [8], pancreatic cancer [9], and lung cancer [10]. Although previous data have demonstrated that SGLT2i-associated euglycemic ketoacidosis is not associated with any particular demographic or comorbid population, perhaps further prospective studies are required to determine whether malignancy can further predispose to the development of euglycemic ketoacidosis and, additionally, whether certain malignancies are associated with an increased risk.

The presented case presents a fortunate and timely diagnosis of euglycemic ketoacidosis in a patient with complex health comorbidities. It is the authors' opinion that, although this was not the reason for his presentation, the development of a HAP, subsequent pulmonary embolism, and his existing thoracic malignancy predisposed for the development of euglycemic ketoacidosis.

In patients with complex comorbidities presenting with an acute illness, clinicians should address the need for continuing SGLT2i use during admission and should have a high index of suspicious for the development of euglycemic ketoacidosis with their use. Complications of their continued use in a stress state can result in severe consequences in the unwell patient.

Consent

Written consent was obtained from the patient for the publication of this case report.

Authors' Contributions

RO, LT, MF, and HSH were involved in the direct care of the patient, drafting of the presented manuscript, editing of the presented manuscript, and submission.

References

[1] L. Barski, T. Eshkoli, E. Brandstaetter, and A. Jotkowitz, "Euglycemic diabetic ketoacidosis," *European Journal of Internal Medicine*, vol. 63, pp. 9–14, 2019.

[2] D. A. Milder, T. Y. Milder, and P. C. A. Kam, "Sodium-glucose co-transporter type-2 inhibitors: pharmacology and peri-operative considerations," *Anaesthesia*, vol. 73, no. 8, pp. 1008–1018, 2018.

[3] J. F. Munro, I. W. Campbell, A. C. McCuish, and L. J. P. Duncan, "Euglycaemic diabetic ketoacidosis," *BMJ*, vol. 2, no. 5866, pp. 578–580, 1973.

[4] A. L. Peters, E. O. Buschur, J. B. Buse, P. Cohan, J. C. Diner, and I. B. Hirsch, "Euglycemic diabetic ketoacidosis: a potential complication of treatment with sodium-glucose cotransporter 2 inhibition," *Diabetes Care*, vol. 38, no. 9, pp. 1687–1693, 2015.

[5] J. Rosenstock and E. Ferrannini, "Euglycemic diabetic ketoacidosis: a predictable, detectable, and preventable safety concern with SGLT2 inhibitors," *Diabetes Care*, vol. 38, no. 9, pp. 1638–1642, 2015.

[6] M. J. Davies, D. A. D'Alessio, J. Fradkin et al., "Management of hyperglycemia in type 2 diabetes, 2018. A consensus report by the American diabetes association (ADA) and the European association for the study of diabetes (EASD)," *Diabetes Care*, vol. 41, no. 12, pp. 2669–2701, 2018.

[7] T. A. Zelniker, S. D. Wiviott, I. Raz et al., "SGLT2 inhibitors for primary and secondary prevention of cardiovascular and renal outcomes in type 2 diabetes: a systematic review and meta-analysis of cardiovascular outcome trials," *The Lancet*, vol. 393, no. 10166, pp. 31–39, 2019.

[8] E. Papadokostaki and E. Liberopoulos, "Euglycemic diabetic ketoacidosis secondary to dapagliflozin in a patient with colon malignancy," *Case Reports in Endocrinology*, vol. 2019, Article ID 3901741, 4 pages, 2019.

[9] H. Sezer, O. Deyneli, Ç. Meriçöz, A. Esin, and E. Alper, "Empagliflozin-induced ketoacidosis in a patient presenting with new-onset type 2 diabetes mellitus due to indolent pancreatic cancer," *Endokrynologia Polska*, vol. 71, no. 3, pp. 283-284, 2020.

[10] J. Sexe, C. Mayes, and P. Tofts, "Euglycemic diabetic ketoacidosis in a lung cancer patient using empagliflozin," *Case Reports in Critical Care*, vol. 2020, Article ID 7437892, 3 pages, 2020.

39

Symptomatic Pituitary Metastasis as Initial Manifestation of Renal Cell Carcinoma: Case Report and Review of Literature

Gunjan Y. Gandhi[1,2] **Russell Fung,**[1,2] **Patrick E. Natter,**[3] **Raafat Makary,**[4] **and K. C. Balaji**[5]

[1]*Division of Endocrinology, University of Florida College of Medicine-Jacksonville, Jacksonville, FL, USA*
[2]*Department of Medicine, University of Florida College of Medicine-Jacksonville, Jacksonville, FL, USA*
[3]*Department of Radiology, University of Florida College of Medicine-Jacksonville, Jacksonville, FL, USA*
[4]*Department of Pathology and Laboratory Medicine, University of Florida College of Medicine-Jacksonville, Jacksonville, FL, USA*
[5]*Department of Urology, University of Florida College of Medicine-Jacksonville, Jacksonville, FL, USA*

Correspondence should be addressed to Gunjan Y. Gandhi; gunjan.gandhi@jax.ufl.edu

Academic Editor: Carlo Capella

Metastasis to the pituitary gland is extremely rare (~2% of sellar masses). Clinical, biochemical, and radiologic characteristics of pituitary metastasis are poorly defined and can be difficult to diagnose before surgery. We present an unusual case with pituitary metastasis as the first manifestation of renal cell carcinoma (RCC). A 70-year-old male presented with acute onset of weakness, dizziness, diplopia, and progressively worsening headache. The initial CT head revealed a heterogeneous sellar mass measuring 2.8 × 1.9 × 1.7 cm. A follow-up MRI showed the sellar mass invading the right cavernous sinus. The presumptive diagnosis was a pituitary macroadenoma. Physical examination revealed bilateral 6th cranial nerve palsy and episodes of intermittent binocular horizontal diplopia. Hormonal testing noted possible secondary adrenal insufficiency (AM serum cortisol: 3.3 mcg/dL, ACTH: 8 pg/mL), secondary hypothyroidism (TSH: <0.01 mIU/L, FT4: 0.7 ng/dL), secondary hypogonadism (testosterone: 47 ng/dL, LH: 1.3 mIU/mL, and FSH: 2.3 mIU/mL), and elevated serum prolactin (prolactin: 56.8 ng/ml, normal: 4.0–15.2 ng/ml). IGF-1 level was normal at 110 ng/mL (47–192 ng/mL). The patient was discharged on levothyroxine and hydrocortisone therapy with plans for close surveillance. However, his condition worsened over the next three months, and he was subsequently readmitted with nausea, vomiting, and hypernatremia secondary to diabetes insipidus. Repeat MRI pituitary showed an interval increase in the size of the sellar mass with suprasellar extension and a new mass effect on the optic chiasm. The sellar mass was urgently resected via a trans-sphenoidal approach. The tumor was negative for neuroendocrine markers and pituitary hormone panel, ruling out the diagnosis of pituitary adenoma and triggered workup for metastatic renal cell carcinoma, clear cell type. The diagnosis of renal cell carcinoma was confirmed by the diffuse and strong staining for renal cell carcinoma markers (Pax-8, RCC-1, and CD10). A follow-up CT scan noted large right renal mass measuring 11 × 10 × 11 cm. The patient underwent a cytoreductive robotic right radical nephrectomy for WHO/ISUP histologic grade II clear cell RCC, stage pT2b pNX pM1. He subsequently received fractionated stereotactic radiotherapy to the pituitary gland. He is presently stable with no radiological evidence of progression or new intracranial disease on subsequent imaging. Pituitary metastasis most commonly occurs from breast, lung, or gastrointestinal tumors but also rarely from renal cell carcinoma. Biochemical findings such as panhypopituitarism, acute clinical signs such as headache, visual symptoms, and diabetes insipidus and interval increase in sellar mass in a short time interval should raise suspicion for sellar metastasis.

1. Introduction

The sellar region is an uncommon site of metastatic disease. In 1857, L. Benjamin first described a case of metastasis to the pituitary gland in an autopsy of a patient with melanoma [1]. Since then, clinicians have become more aware of considering the pituitary gland as a potential site for metastatic disease [2, 3]. However, pituitary metastases are uncommon, occurring in 1% to 4% of all cancer patients in large autopsy studies, the most frequent primary tumors being breast and lung cancer [2, 4–6]. Most often, they are part of a generalized metastatic spread, especially skeletal [1, 7–10]. They tend to affect patients in the sixth or seventh decade of life [11, 12], with no clear sex predominance. Infrequently pituitary metastasis has been noted to be the first manifestation of an occult primary tumor or the only site of metastasis [7, 9, 10] and occurs in younger adults [7, 13].

Metastasis to the pituitary is often asymptomatic. Diabetes insipidus has traditionally been thought to be the most common symptom of pituitary metastases [7, 14], particularly when the posterior pituitary gland is affected. Anterior pituitary insufficiency and cranial nerve deficits have been less frequently described at presentation [15–17]. This has been attributed to a predisposition of metastasis to the posterior lobe and the pituitary stalk. Mild elevation of prolactin at levels less than 200 ng/ml, consistent with stalk compression, is not uncommon in pituitary metastasis [18]. There are no *sine qua non* radiological and clinical manifestations of sellar metastasis [19–21]. They may often mimic a pituitary adenoma [1, 9, 15, 16] or a variety of sellar lesions such as granuloma, abscess, cyst, aneurysm, tumor, and apoplexy [9, 18, 22–26]. This is especially true if there is no existing evidence of malignancy in the patient. Best practices of pituitary metastases treatment are not available as there is a lack of standardized therapy guidelines [10, 27–30]. The primary malignancy determines long-term prognosis. Local therapy aiming at symptom relief may be beneficial, and ensuring optimizing quality of life in accordance with patient's values and preferences is critical.

Renal cell carcinoma is a rare cause of pituitary metastases, with only a few cases having been reported thus far [28]. Anterior pituitary dysfunction may be more prevalent, and diabetes insipidus less commonplace in patients with renal cell carcinoma metastatic to the pituitary compared to ones associated with other primary malignancies [19, 27, 28]. We describe a case of a patient presenting with symptomatic pituitary metastasis from renal cell carcinoma. It is particularly revealing that pituitary metastasis was the first manifestation of cancer, and the absence of a known history of malignancy confused the diagnosis. We further describe the incidence, pathogenesis, diagnosis, and management of patients with pituitary metastasis by following the methods of Zhao et al. [31], He et al. [2], Castle-Kirszbaum et al. [3], and Gopan et al. [32].

2. Case Presentation

A 70-year-old male presented with a 5-day history of double vision that was described as horizontal diplopia. It was most often provoked with a quick lateral gaze and resolved with rest. He noted frontal headache, which was dull aching and always present. He noted some relief of pain with NSAIDs but never to full resolution. He also noted decreased energy and a feeling of weakness in legs. Past medical history was notable for diabetes mellitus not requiring treatment with medications, gastroesophageal reflux disease, hyperlipidemia, and tachycardia. He previously had meniscus surgery on his knee. Physical exam revealed bilateral 6th cranial nerve palsy and episodes of intermittent binocular horizontal diplopia. Initial CT head revealed a sellar mass involving the right cavernous sinus measuring 2.8 × 1.9 × 1.7 cm, confirmed by MRI demonstrating a heterogeneous sellar mass invading the right cavernous sinus with a leftward deviation of the infundibulum. There was a small amount of suprasellar extension with mild mass effect on the optic chiasm (Figures 1(a)–1(c)). The presumptive diagnosis was a pituitary macroadenoma. Hormonal testing noted possible secondary adrenal insufficiency (AM serum cortisol: 3.3 mcg/dL, ACTH: 8 pg/mL), secondary hypothyroidism (TSH: <0.01 mIU/L, FT4: 0.7 ng/dL), secondary hypogonadism (testosterone: 47 ng/dL, LH: 1.3 mIU/mL, and FSH: 2.3 mIU/mL), and hyperprolactinemia with mildly elevated prolactin levels (prolactin: 56.8 ng/ml, normal: 4.0–15.2 ng/ml). IGF-1 level was normal at 110 ng/mL (47–192 ng/mL). No acute neurosurgical involvement was planned. Formal visual field testing did not show visual field defects consistent with pituitary mass. The patient was discharged on hormone replacement therapy with levothyroxine 100 mcg daily and hydrocortisone 20 mg in the morning and 10 mg in the afternoon with plans for consideration of testosterone replacement therapy as an outpatient. His vision improved to some degree during hospitalization.

Repeat MRI in 3 months noted interval increase in the bulk of the tumor extending along the infundibulum, now measuring 0.7 cm in transverse width compared to 0.4 cm previously, and there was resulting interval mild increased mass effect on the optic chiasm at its central and left aspect (Figures 2(a)–2(c)). Besides, there was an interval increase in the tumor in the sella. The mass continued to extend to the right lateral aspect concerning for right cavernous sinus invasion with erosion into the clivus inferiorly. As a result of the growth of the sellar mass, neurosurgery planned surgical intervention. A few days later, the patient presented to the emergency room with severe acute headache, nausea, vomiting, polyuria, and polydipsia. The examination noted nystagmus and decreased abduction of the right eye. Sodium was mildly high, confirming diabetes insipidus requiring short-term DDAVP treatment. A repeat MRI did not indicate a significant change of the pituitary mass compared to MRI done a few days earlier. He was started on stress dose steroids in the form of hydrocortisone 50 mg IV every 8 hours. He underwent emergent endoscopic endonasal transsphenoidal resection of the pituitary lesion. The tumor was firm and hemorrhagic. Preliminary intraoperative pathology (frozen section) was suggestive of pituitary adenoma and tumor debulking performed as much as safely possible. He continued to have transient polyuria following surgery, requiring DDAVP until his discharge from the hospital. DDAVP did not have to be maintained as an outpatient as diabetes insipidus was mild.

Surprisingly, pathology of the resected pituitary mass after proper fixation showed metastatic renal cell carcinoma (Figures 3 and 4). The tumor histology was characterized by a nested Zellballen pattern of cells (on hematoxylin&eosin

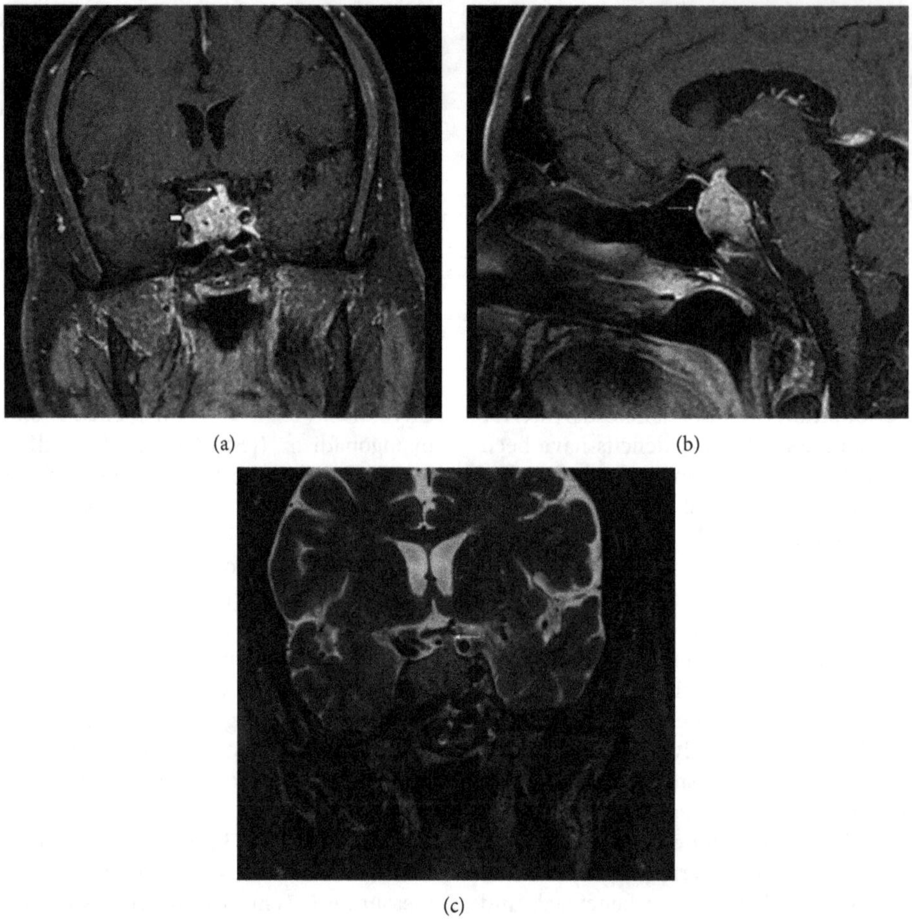

FIGURE 1: (a) Coronal postcontrast fat-saturated image demonstrates a heterogeneous sellar mass, which expands the sella (short thick arrow). There is also a slight suprasellar extension. The pituitary stalk is also involved and thickened (thin arrow). (b) Sagittal postcontrast fat-saturated image also demonstrates the heterogeneous sellar mass (thin arrow). (c) Coronal T2 image shows a mild mass effect on the optic chiasm from the thickened pituitary stalk (thin arrow).

and reticulin stains), separated by a delicate network of thin wall capillary vasculature. The tumor cells had relatively defined cell borders, clear and eosinophilic cytoplasm, round slightly pleomorphic nuclei with small prominent central nucleoli in several of the tumor cells. Mitoses were inconspicuous, and no tumor necrosis was seen. The tumor cell histomorphology was unusual for pituitary adenoma and triggered the immunohistochemical characterization of the tumor lineage (phenotype). Immunohistochemical stains were negative for neuroendocrine markers (chromogranin, synaptophysin, and neuron-specific enolase), pituitary hormones panel (TSH, ACTH, GH, prolactin, and nonspecific staining for FSH), and S100 and focally positive for CD56. The immunostain results were inconsistent with the diagnosis of pituitary adenoma. The clear cell morphology suggested metastatic renal cell carcinoma of clear cell type, which was confirmed by the diffuse and strong positive immunostains for renal cell carcinoma markers (Pax-8, RCC-1, and CD10). The Ki-67 proliferation marker labeled approximately 10% of the tumor cell nuclei.

Due to pathology findings, a CT scan of the abdomen was done that noted large heterogeneously enhancing solid mass, arising from the middle and lower thirds of the right kidney with prominent stellate central necrosis, measuring approximately $11 \times 10 \times 11$ cm. There was significant hyperemia in the perinephric fat with prominent vessels tracking along the lateral conal fascia. Haziness in the perinephric fat slightly concerned for early tumor spread. A 2 cm enhancing nodule in the left adrenal gland was also seen. PET/CT scan showed the renal mass to be not FDG avid. Minimal FDG uptake was seen of the left adrenal mass. As a result, a cytoreductive robotic right radical nephrectomy was performed, which confirmed WHO/ISUP histologic grade II clear cell renal cell carcinoma on pathology, stage pT2b pNX pM1 (Figure 5). The carcinoma did not involve margins and there was no lymphovascular invasion.

Repeat MRI of the sella noted subtotal resection of the pituitary mass. Repeat visual field testing indicated no defects. The patient subsequently received fractionated stereotactic radiotherapy to the pituitary metastasis at a dose of 30 Gy in 5 fractions. Repeat MRI 3 months after surgery and one year after surgery noted the sellar mass was stable with the thickened infundibulum causing mass effect upon the optic chiasm (Figures 6(a) and 6(b)). He has continued to require levothyroxine along with hydrocortisone and has been subsequently started on intramuscular testosterone

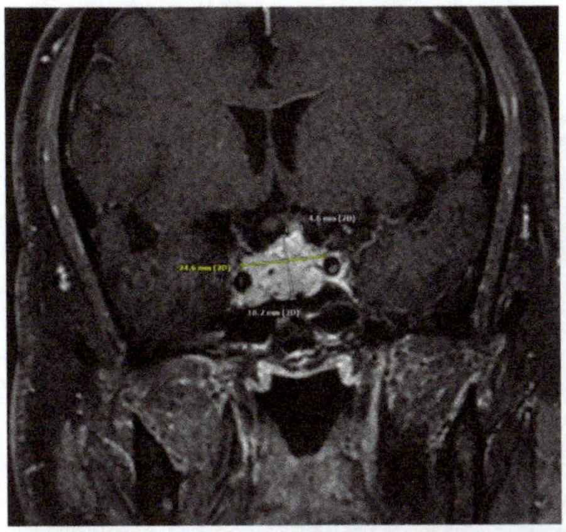

(a)

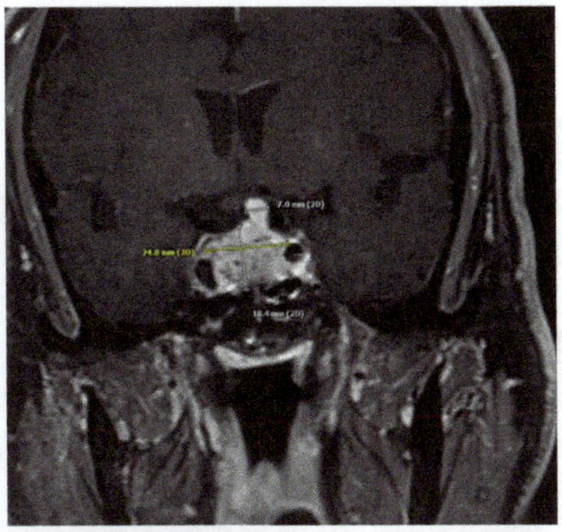

(b)

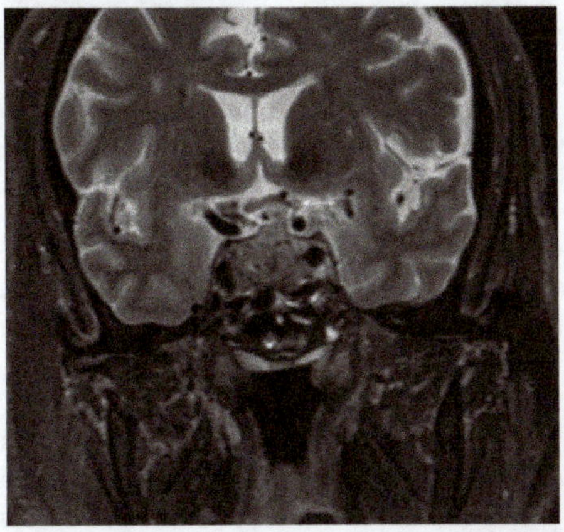

(c)

FIGURE 2: Coronal postcontrast image demonstrates the size of the mass upon initial imaging (a) also including the measurement of the mildly thickened pituitary stalk. At the time of follow-up imaging (b), the mass has slightly increased in size, which is most notable at the pituitary stalk, which now measures 7 mm in thickness, previously 4.6 mm. Also, note the mild increased mass effect on the optic chiasm (thin arrow) at the time of follow-up imaging on the coronal T2 image (c).

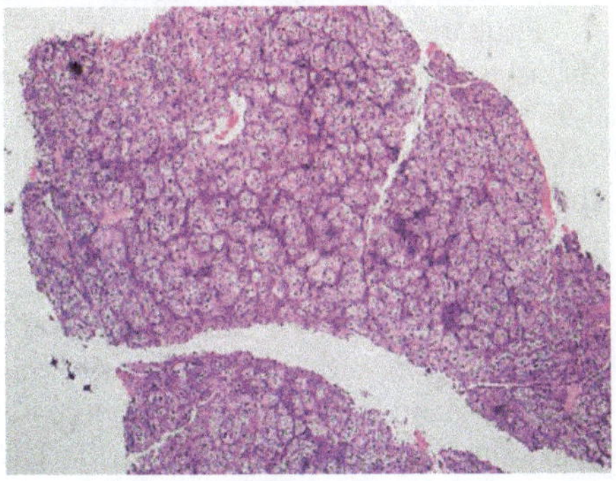

(a)

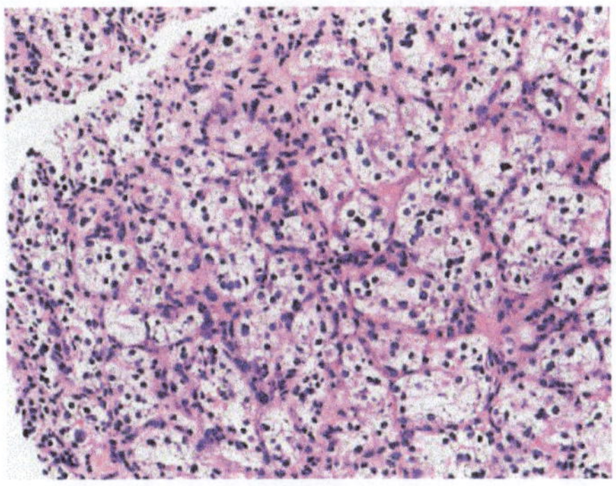

(b)

FIGURE 3: Pituitary tumor excision showing tumor nests of clear cells separated by fibrovascular septa (H&E stain: (a) ×2.5; (b) ×10).

injections. Subsequent imaging of the renal lesion has noted right retrocaval enhancing lesion concerning for metastatic lymph node from patient's previously identified right renal cell carcinoma along with slight interval enlargement of an enhancing left adrenal gland nodule with the possibility of a metastatic adrenal lesion. He has been offered options of tyrosine kinase inhibitor, immunotherapy with or without tyrosine kinase inhibitor, or surveillance. Stereotactic radiation to the adrenal area has also been discussed. The role of local treatment for the oligometastatic disease has been reviewed with the patient. The patient prefers to maintain his current quality of life and avoid additional treatment with

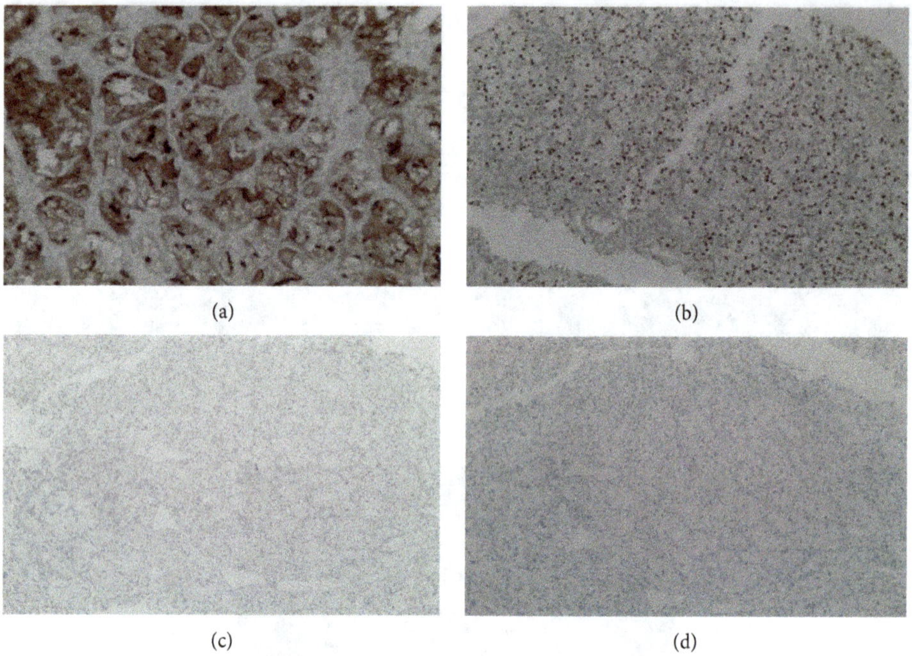

FIGURE 4: Immunohistochemical stains positive for renal cell carcinoma (a) and (b) and negative for neuroendocrine markers (c) and (d). (a) CD10 immunostain (×10). (b) PAX-8 immunostain (×5). (c) Synaptophysin (×2.5). (d) Chromgranin (×2.5).

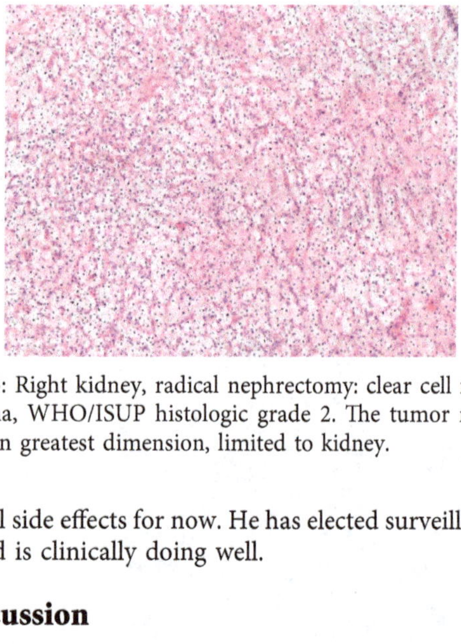

FIGURE 5: Right kidney, radical nephrectomy: clear cell renal cell carcinoma, WHO/ISUP histologic grade 2. The tumor measures 10.5 cm in greatest dimension, limited to kidney.

potential side effects for now. He has elected surveillance for now and is clinically doing well.

3. Discussion

Our case illustrates the importance of considering a broad differential diagnosis of a sellar mass. The differential diagnosis should include consideration of more commonly known conditions such as pituitary adenoma but also less frequent entities such as cysts, abscesses, granulomas, apoplexy, trauma, meningiomas, craniopharyngiomas, and aneurysm as well as pituitary metastasis amongst others. It is essential to consider that sellar symptoms may be the first manifestation of neoplastic diseases, such as in our patient in whom renal cell carcinoma was diagnosed after surgical pathology noted pituitary metastasis from renal cell carcinoma. It can closely mimic a benign pituitary adenoma symptomatically, as demonstrated in our case. Any clinical, biochemical, or imaging findings of pituitary pathology in a patient with known cancer, especially lung and breast, should raise suspicion for metastasis to the sella. Moreover, the development of diabetes insipidus or ophthalmoplegia from any pituitary lesion is suggestive of metastatic disease even in patients with no known primary malignancy. As in our case, an interval increase in sellar mass in a short time interval should also raise suspicion for sellar metastasis. Ultimately, pathology remains the gold standard for the diagnosis of pituitary metastasis.

Pituitary metastasis is rare. The incidence of pituitary metastasis among all intracranial metastases is 0.87%; it is 1.9% among all autopsied cancer cases in a large autopsy study [2]. In females, the most likely source of pituitary metastasis is the breast, while in men, metastases tend to be from the lung [33]. Two-thirds of metastasis to the sella originate from these primary sites, which could be as these are two of the more common malignancies. Although it is difficult to know the exact reason for affinity towards the pituitary for spread, the pituitary gland is rich in prolactin receptors that may attract cancerous breast cells [6]. Also, the gastrointestinal tract, prostate, kidney, thyroid, and pancreas primary tumors are possible sources of pituitary metastases [2, 3]. Renal cell carcinomas tend to very uncommonly spread to the pituitary gland [28, 32, 34, 35]. In a case series, Gopan et al. noted the average age of presentation for renal cell carcinoma metastatic to the pituitary gland to be 61 years, with most being male [32]. Of those with known renal cell carcinoma, the average interval between diagnosis and pituitary metastasis was approximately eight years [32]. Pituitary metastasis may be the initial presentation of an unknown primary tumor in up to 20–30% patients [36].

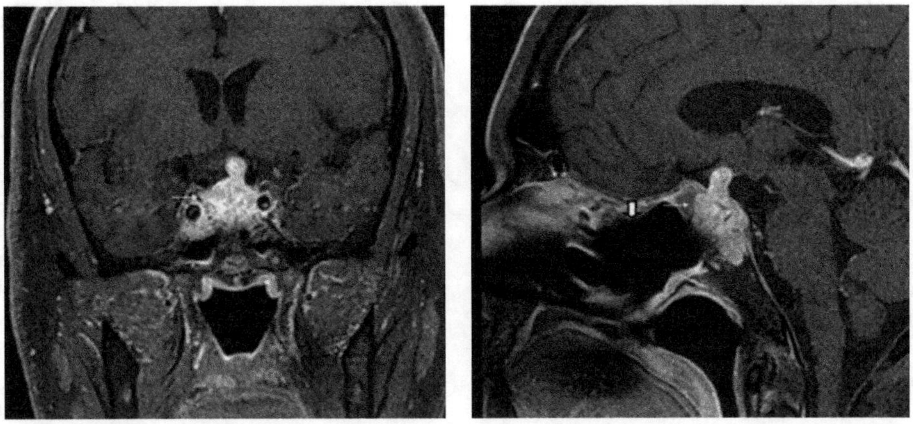

(a) (b)

FIGURE 6: Most recent postoperative scan demonstrates residual enhancing heterogeneous mass in the sella (thin arrow) on the coronal postcontrast image (a). The sagittal postcontrast image (b) also demonstrates the residual heterogeneous mass (thin arrow). Also, note the postsurgical changes in the adjacent sphenoid sinus and posterior ethmoid air cells from a trans-sphenoidal approach to the sella (short thick arrow).

The mechanism of metastasis to the pituitary gland is unclear. Still, it likely involves the following: (1) migration to the pituitary gland through a portal vessel system, (2) migration to the pituitary gland or sellar region via the internal carotid, (3) migration via the suprasellar cistern into the pituitary gland, and (4) migration from the skull base to the pituitary gland [5, 10, 29]. The most commonly involved site is the posterior lobe of the hypophysis (69–79%), followed by the anterior pituitary lobe, and then both the anterior and posterior hypophysis, and finally, the pituitary stalk [37].

Most patients with pituitary metastasis are asymptomatic [5, 8, 15, 38]. Some presenting symptoms include diabetes insipidus, hypopituitarism, visual field defects, ophthalmoplegia, and headache. Renal cell carcinoma has been noted to be strongly associated with visual field defects likely due to extension to the suprasellar cistern resulting in the compression of the optic chiasm and optic nerve [32]. Brisk worsening of vision may be a more useful gauge to separate sellar metastasis from pituitary macroadenomas as both conditions seem to have a high incidence of visual field defects [2, 39, 40]. Encroachment of cranial nerves in the cavernous sinus (three, six, four, and five) should raise suspicion for pituitary metastasis. Case series of patients with pituitary metastasis have noted cranial neuropathies to occur more commonly than in patients with pituitary macroadenomas [2, 3, 41]. Seizures associated with pituitary metastasis from small cell lung cancer have been described [42]. Headache is relatively common, seen in about one out of five patients with sellar metastasis [2]. No defining characteristics of headache have been noted in patients with pituitary metastasis. As renal cell carcinoma can have increased blood flow, there have been reports of pituitary apoplexy [43] and intraventricular hemorrhage causing hydrocephalus [44].

Diabetes insipidus is the most common symptom of pituitary metastases, particularly when the posterior lobe of the gland is affected. A large case series of pituitary metastases demonstrated that the posterior lobe was involved in more than 80% [8]. The main reason for this frequent involvement of the posterior pituitary lobe is related to its extensive contact with the adjacent dura mater and its direct arterial supply from the hypophyseal arteries, contrasting with the anterior lobe, which is supplied from the hypophyseal portal system [20]. Since diabetes insipidus is an infrequent symptom in pituitary adenoma, it can be particularly helpful in differentiating a metastatic tumor from a pituitary adenoma [9]. When compared to other pituitary metastasis, renal cell carcinoma tends to present more commonly with hypopituitarism and less often with DI [32, 45].

In a pooled study of patients with metastasis to the pituitary gland, hypopituitarism was seen in about a quarter of the patients [2]; this may be due to mass effect on the pituitary infundibulum and anterior pituitary lobe. An increase in prolactin is seen in a vast majority of patients with pituitary metastasis [46], but the degree of elevation is mild. It may be likely be related to the "stalk effect" rather than an actual prolactin-secreting tumor. Also, the prevalence of elevated prolactin level is relatively high in pituitary macroadenomas [46] and thus not helpful to differentiate between the two. When compared to nonfunctioning macroadenomas, deficiencies of anterior pituitary hormones, including ACTH, TSH, FSH, and LH, were significantly more common among patients with metastatic disease [46]. Isolated cases of neuroendocrine tumors (lung and pancreas) secreting GHRH and ACTH have been reported with functioning pituitary metastasis, causing acromegaly and Cushing's syndrome [47–49].

Pituitary metastasis appearance on imaging tends to overlap with other tumors, especially pituitary macroadenoma, and the imaging findings of metastasis are often nonspecific [50–53]. Invasion of adjacent structures such as the bony sella and cavernous sinuses is nonspecific and can be seen with pituitary metastasis or pituitary macroadenoma [50]. Multiple appearances have been reported previously. Metastasis can present with a "dumbbell" shaped mass with sellar and suprasellar components with an indentation at the level of the sellar diaphragm [17, 54]. It has been described that the indentation may be more prominent with metastasis at the sellar diaphragm due to rapid growth as compared to a pituitary macroadenoma, which could slowly expand the sellar diaphragm due to slower growth [17, 54]. Pituitary metastasis can also primarily involve the pituitary stalk with associated mass or thickening involving the stalk. One series demonstrated a pituitary stalk lesion in approximately 63.3% of patients. Metastatic disease in one radiological case review series was the most common adult infundibular tumor [55]. Another pattern of involvement that has been described is the pituitary infundibulum as a visible linear enhancement at the posterior inferior border of metastasis with a suprasellar component [17]. Diabetes insipidus, when associated with sellar metastasis, may be visible as a thickened pituitary stalk along with the absence of the usual high T1 signal intensity in the posterior pituitary lobe [54].

Treatment of metastasis to the pituitary requires a multidisciplinary approach. Treatment generally includes surgery, postoperative stereotactic radiosurgery, chemotherapy, and hormone replacement therapy. If a patient has an initial clinical presentation of deteriorated visual acuity and visual field impairment, which indicates compression of the optic nerve, surgery is often the first choice. The endoscopic endonasal trans-sphenoidal approach is the preferred surgical approach and can help improve headache, visual field defects, and cranial nerve deficits [29, 56]. The goal of surgery is to decrease the compression of optic chiasm caused by the often firm and vascular tumor and symptom relief as well as improving quality of life rather than improving survival [5, 10, 29, 57]. Surgery is often technically difficult due to possible invasion of tumor into cavernous sinuses. The gamma knife is a stereo-directional radiotherapy method that is used when lesions do not compress or only slightly compress optic nerves and optic chiasm. Piedra et al. [58] noted that the gamma knife approach could improve the symptoms of diabetes insipidus and minimize the deterioration of visual acuity and visual fields without causing hypopituitarism. Stereotactic radiosurgery thus represents an effective, safe, and noninvasive means of ameliorating the symptoms of pituitary metastasis in patients with limited survival. Hormone replacement therapy is critical under the guidance of an endocrinologist. Radiotherapy and chemotherapy are appropriate for patients with multiple metastatic lesions. Due to a better understanding of biology of renal cell carcinoma, clinicians now have a larger arsenal of targeted therapeutic options and immunotherapies available to them. One novel option is a tyrosine kinase inhibitor such as cabozantinib. Other options include a combination of nivolumab (antiprogrammed cell death 1 (PD-1)) and ipilimumab (anticytotoxic T-lymphocyte-associated antigen 4 (CTLA-4)). Combined use of atezolizumab (anti-PD-ligand 1 (PD-L1)) and bevacizumab (antivascular endothelial growth factor (VEGF)) has also been an effective therapy [59]. A recent network meta-analysis and systematic review by our group on first-line therapy for metastatic RCC demonstrated that a combination of pembrolizumab plus axitinib might be the preferred option based on efficacy and side effect profile compared with avelumab plus axitinib or atezolizumab plus bevacizumab [60]. Yang et al. [61] reported a case of pituitary metastasis from renal cell carcinoma; although the pituitary metastasis progressed, extracerebral metastasis showed a partial response to sorafenib treatment. Therefore, chemotherapy alone does not improve the treatment course of pituitary metastasis; surgery and postoperative radiotherapy are required. Some chemotherapeutic and immunotherapeutic regimens cross the blood-brain barrier and may provide a survival advantage, although evidence is limited to case reports [62, 63]. In addition to the role of cytoreductive nephrectomy in patients with metastatic renal cell carcinoma, there may be a role for treating primary renal carcinoma in presence of oligometastatic or progressive metastatic disease. There is a case report of improved outcome following partial nephrectomy in a patient with thyroid metastasis from renal cancer [64]. In addition to treating primary tumor in presence of metastatic renal cell cancer, the other strategy to improve outcome is metastasis-directed therapy especially in the setting of oligometastatic disease. Both surgical and radiotherapy approaches with or without adjuvant therapy such as immune check point inhibitors are described in the literature. However, currently there are no randomized phase III studies validating the metastases-directed local or regional therapy in patients with metastatic renal cell cancer [65–68]. While both minimally invasive and open approaches are effective in performing nephrectomy, the minimally invasive approach offers advantages of fewer complications and quicker postoperative recovery [69]. Moreover, available surgical expertise influences the choice of method and the surgeon at our institution was the first to perform and report on robotic nephrectomy [70].

The prognosis of pituitary metastasis, in general, is poor. Fassett et al. [52] retrospectively reviewed 36 cases of pituitary metastasis and found the average survival to be six months. Another study by Lin et al. noted a median survival of 4 months after diagnosis. Solitary or small metastasis, functional performance status, younger age, local therapy, including radiation therapy, and a longer interval from diagnosis of malignancy to pituitary metastasis have been linked to prolonged survival [57, 71]. With regards to specific primary malignancies metastatic to the pituitary, patients with renal cell carcinoma and melanoma survived longer when compared to patients with lung, colon, breast, prostate, liver, nasopharyngeal, and stomach malignancies [72].

In conclusion, sellar metastasis is uncommon and challenging to diagnose. Biochemical findings, such as panhypopituitarism, acute clinical signs such as headache, visual symptoms, and diabetes insipidus, and particularly rapid interval increase in pituitary mass in a short period, should raise suspicion for sellar metastasis. As in our case, pituitary symptoms may rarely be the first presentation of malignancy. Furthermore, in a patient with a known cancer history, there should be a heightened suspicion for metastasis to the pituitary gland. Treatment of pituitary metastases should be individualized and tailored to the patient's clinical condition, tumor histology, and presence of concomitant extrapituitary metastases. An important goal is symptom palliation and improving quality of life. A multidisciplinary approach to the disease (including involvement of an experienced radiologist, neurosurgeon, pathologist, endocrinologist, and urological oncologist) is necessary.

References

[1] M.-F. Chiang, M. Brock, and S. Patt, "Pituitary metastases," *Min-Minimally Invasive Neurosurgery*, vol. 33, no. 4, pp. 127–131, 1990.

[2] W. He, F. Chen, B. Dalm, P. A. Kirby, and J. D. W. Greenlee, "Metastatic involvement of the pituitary gland: a systematic review with pooled individual patient data analysis," *Pituitary*, vol. 18, no. 1, pp. 159–168, 2015.

[3] M. Castle-Kirszbaum, T. Goldschlager, B. Ho, Y. Y. Wang, and J. King, "Twelve cases of pituitary metastasis: a case series and review of the literature," *Pituitary*, vol. 21, no. 5, pp. 463–473, 2018.

[4] K. Kovacs, "Metastatic cancer of the pituitary gland," *Oncology*, vol. 27, no. 6, pp. 533–542, 1973.

[5] J. Komninos, V. Vlassopoulou, D. Protopapa et al., "Tumors metastatic to the pituitary gland: case report and literature review," *The Journal of Clinical Endocrinology & Metabolism*, vol. 89, no. 2, pp. 574–580, 2004.

[6] Y. H. Kim, B. j. Lee, K. J. Lee, and J. H. Cho, "A case of pituitary metastasis from breast cancer that presented as left visual disturbance," *Journal of Korean Neurosurgical Society*, vol. 51, no. 2, pp. 94–97, 2012.

[7] P. Sioutos, V. Yen, and E. Arbit, "Pituitary gland metastases," *Annals of Surgical Oncology*, vol. 3, no. 1, pp. 94–99, 1996.

[8] P. c. McCormick, K. d. Post, A. d. Kandji, and A. P. Hays, "Metastatic carcinoma to the pituitary gland," *British Journal of Neurosurgery*, vol. 3, no. 1, pp. 71–79, 1989.

[9] D. Ruelle, M. Palladino, and G. C. Andrioli, "Turbulenz: moden," *Zufall und Chaos*, vol. 36, no. 1, pp. 51–57, 1992.

[10] A. Morita, F. B. Meyer, and E. R. Laws, "Symptomatic pituitary metastases," *Journal of Neurosurgery*, vol. 89, no. 1, pp. 69–73, 1998.

[11] P. B. Nelson, A. G. Robinson, and J. A. Martinez, "Metastatic tumor of the pituitary gland," *Neurosurgery*, vol. 21, no. 6, pp. 941–944, 1987.

[12] P. U. Freda and K. D. Post, "Differential diagnosis of sellar masses," *Endocrinology and Metabolism Clinics of North America*, vol. 28, no. 1, pp. 81–117, 1999.

[13] I. Ito, T. Ishida, T. Hashimoto et al., "Hypopituitarism due to pituitary metastasis of lung cancer: case of a 21-year-old man," *Internal Medicine*, vol. 40, no. 5, pp. 414–417, 2001.

[14] W. A. Houck, K. B. Olson, and J. Horton, "Clinical features of tumor metastasis to the pituitary," *Cancer*, vol. 26, no. 3, pp. 656–659, 1970.

[15] C. L. Branch and E. R. Laws, "Metastatic tumors of the sella turcica masquerading as primary pituitary tumors," *The Journal of Clinical Endocrinology & Metabolism*, vol. 65, no. 3, pp. 469–474, 1987.

[16] J. Y. Delattre, C. Castelain, L. Davila, B. Schadeck, and M. Poisson, "Metastasis to the pituitary stalk in a case of breast cancer," *Revue Neurologique*, vol. 146, no. 6-7, pp. 455-456, 1990.

[17] O. Schubiger and D. Haller, "Metastases to the pituitary-hypothalamic axis," *Neuroradiology*, vol. 34, no. 2, pp. 131–134, 1992.

[18] M. P. Ntyonga-Pono, P. Thomopoulos, and J. P. Luton, "Pituitary metastases. 3 cases," *La Presse Médicale*, vol. 28, no. 29, pp. 1567–1571, 1999.

[19] J. M. Hwang, Y. H. Kim, T. M. Kim, and S. H. Park, "Differential diagnosis and management of a pituitary mass with renal cell carcinoma," *Journal of Korean Neurosurgical Society*, vol. 54, no. 2, pp. 132–135, 2013.

[20] R. Chaudhuri, C. Twelves, T. C. S. Cox, and J. B. Bingham, "MRI in diabetes insipidus due to metastatic breast carcinoma," *Clinical Radiology*, vol. 46, no. 3, pp. 184–188, 1992.

[21] S. H. Hyun, J. Y. Choi, K.-H. Lee, Y. S. Choe, and B.-T. Kim, "Incidental focal 18F-FDG uptake in the pituitary gland: clinical significance and differential diagnostic criteria," *Journal of Nuclear Medicine*, vol. 52, no. 4, pp. 547–550, 2011.

[22] E. L. Zager and T. E. Hedley-Whyte, "Metastasis within a pituitary adenoma presenting with bilateral abducens palsies: case report and review of the literature," *Neurosurgery*, vol. 21, no. 3, pp. 383–386, 1987.

[23] M. Neroni, M. Artico, F. S. Pastore, S. Esposito, and B. Fraioli, "Diaphragma sellae metastasis from colon carcinoma mimicking a meningioma. A case report," *Neurochirurgie*, vol. 45, no. 2, pp. 160–163, 1999.

[24] F. W. Hanna, O. M. Williams, J. S. Davies, T. Dawson, J. Neal, and M. F. Scanlon, "Pituitary apoplexy following metastasis of bronchogenic adenocarcinoma to a prolactinoma," *Clinical Endocrinology*, vol. 51, no. 3, pp. 377–381, 1999.

[25] S. Furuta, T. Hatakeyama, K. Zenke, and S. Fukumoto, "Pituitary metastasis from carcinoma of the urinary bladder mimicking pituitary apoplexy–case report," *Neurologia Medico-Chirurgica*, vol. 39, no. 2, pp. 165–168, 1999.

[26] A. W. McEvoy, N. Khan, and N. D. Kitchen, "Bitemporal hemianopia caused by metastatic carcinoma in a patient with Wegener's granulomatosis: an unexpected finding," *British Journal of Neurosurgery*, vol. 11, no. 6, pp. 579–581, 1997.

[27] R. Grossman, S. Maimon, R. Levite, and Z. Ram, "Multimodal treatment of hemorrhagic pituitary metastasis as first manifestation of renal cell carcinoma," *World Neurosurgery*, vol. 79, no. 5-6, pp. e1–e798, 2013.

[28] T. Yokoyama, A. Yoshino, Y. Katayama et al., "Metastatic pituitary tumor from renal cell carcinoma treated by fractionated stereotactic radiotherapy–case report," *Neurologia Medico-Chirurgica*, vol. 44, no. 1, pp. 47–52, 2004.

[29] M. Zoli, D. Mazzatenta, M. Faustini-Fustini, E. Pasquini, and G. Frank, "Pituitary metastases: role of surgery," *World Neurosurgery*, vol. 79, no. 2, pp. 327–330, 2013.

[30] V. Gilard, C. Alexandru, F. Proust, S. Derrey, P. Hannequin, and O. Langlois, "Pituitary metastasis: is there still a place for neurosurgical treatment?" *Journal of Neuro-Oncology*, vol. 126, no. 2, pp. 219–224, 2016.

[31] Y. Zhao, W. Lian, B. Xing et al., "Diagnosis, therapy, and therapeutic effects in cases of pituitary metastasis," *World Neurosurgery*, vol. 117, pp. 122–128, 2018.

[32] T. Gopan, S. A. Toms, R. A. Prayson, J. H. Suh, A. H. Hamrahian, and R. J. Weil, "Symptomatic pituitary metastases from renal cell carcinoma," *Pituitary*, vol. 10, no. 3, pp. 251–259, 2007.

[33] R. J. Weil, "Pituitary metastasis," *Archives of Neurology*, vol. 59, no. 12, pp. 1962-1963, 2002.

[34] C. K. Kramer, N. Ferreira, S. P. Silveiro, J. L. Gross, J. M. Dora, and M. J. d. Azevedo, "Pituitary gland metastasis from renal cell carcinoma presented as a non-functioning macroadenoma," *Arquivos Brasileiros de Endocrinologia & Metabologia*, vol. 54, no. 5, pp. 498–501, 2010.

[35] C. Wendel, M. Campitiello, F. Plastino et al., "Pituitary metastasis from renal cell carcinoma: description of a case report," *American Journal of Case Reports*, vol. 18, pp. 7–11, 2017.

[36] P. U. Freda, S. L. Wardlaw, and K. D. Post, "Unusual causes of sellar/parasellar masses in a large transsphenoidal surgical series," *The Journal of Clinical Endocrinology & Metabolism*, vol. 81, no. 10, pp. 3455–3459, 1996.

[37] R. J. Teears and E. M. Silverman, "Clinicopathologic review of 88 cases of carcinoma metastatic to the pituitary gland," *Cancer*, vol. 36, no. 1, pp. 216–220, 1975.

[38] M. B. Max, M. D. F. Deck, and D. A. Rottenberg, "Pituitary metastasis: incidence in cancer patients and clinical differentiation from pituitary adenorna," *Neurology*, vol. 31, no. 8, p. 998, 1981.

[39] I. H. Lee, N. R. Miller, E. Zan et al., "Visual defects in patients with pituitary adenomas: the myth of bitemporal hemianopsia," *American Journal of Roentgenology*, vol. 205, no. 5, pp. W512–W518, 2015.

[40] A. Hoellig, P. Niehusmann, S. Flacke, and R. A. Kristof, "Metastasis to pituitary adenoma: case report and review of the literature," *Central European Neurosurgery*, vol. 70, no. 03, pp. 149–153, 2009.

[41] R. Hollenhorst and B. R. Younge, "Ocular manifestations produced by adenomas of the pituitary gland-analysis of 1000 cases," in *Diagnosis and Treatment of Pituitary Tumors*, pp. 53–63, Excerpta Medica, Amsterdam, Netherlands, 1995.

[42] J. Fridley, G. Adams, V. Rao et al., "Small cell lung cancer metastasis in the pituitary gland presenting with seizures and headache," *Journal of Clinical Neuroscience*, vol. 18, no. 3, pp. 420–422, 2011.

[43] I. Quevedo, J. A. Rodríguez Portales, H. Rosenberg, and J. Mery, "Apoplexy in pituitary metastasis of renal cell carcinoma. Clinical case followed for 7 years," *Revista medica de Chile*, vol. 128, no. 9, pp. 1015–1018, 2000.

[44] J. Pallud, F. Nataf, T. Roujeau, and F.-X. Roux, "Intraventricular haemorrhage from a renal cell carcinoma pituitary metastasis," *Acta Neurochirurgica*, vol. 147, no. 9, pp. 1003-1004, 2005.

[45] H. Koshiyama, K. Ohgaki, S. Hida et al., "Metastatic renal cell carcinoma to the pituitary gland presenting with hypopituitarism," *Journal of Endocrinological Investigation*, vol. 15, no. 9, pp. 677–681, 1992.

[46] R. Al-Aridi, K. El Sibai, P. Fu, M. Khan, W. R. Selman, and B. M. Arafah, "Clinical and biochemical characteristic features of metastatic cancer to the sella turcica: an analytical review," *Pituitary*, vol. 17, no. 6, pp. 575–587, 2014.

[47] V. Chandra, L. W. McDonald, and R. J. Anderson, "Metastatic small cell carcinoma of the lung presenting as pituitary apoplexy and cushing's syndrome," *Journal of Neuro-Oncology*, vol. 2, no. 1, pp. 59–66, 1984.

[48] C. Nasr, A. Mason, M. Mayberg, S. M. Staugaitis, and S. L. Asa, "Acromegaly and somatotroph hyperplasia with adenomatous transformation due to pituitary metastasis of a growth hormone-releasing hormone-secreting pulmonary endocrine carcinoma," *The Journal of Clinical Endocrinology & Metabolism*, vol. 91, no. 12, pp. 4776–4780, 2006.

[49] N. Sanno, A. Teramoto, R. Y. Osamura et al., "A growth hormone-releasing hormone-producing pancreatic islet cell tumor metastasized to the pituitary is associated with pituitary somatotroph hyperplasia and acromegaly," *The Journal of Clinical Endocrinology & Metabolism*, vol. 82, no. 8, pp. 2731–2737, 1997.

[50] T. Altay, K. M. Krisht, and W. T. Couldwell, "Sellar and parasellar metastatic tumors," *International Journal of Surgical Oncology*, vol. 2012, Article ID 647256, 9 pages, 2012.

[51] D. Lin, B. Griffith, S. Patel, J. Rock, and H. Marin, "Pituitary metastasis from lung carcinoma presenting as a pituitary adenoma," *Applied Radiology*, vol. 47, no. 7, pp. 34–36, 2018.

[52] D. R. Fassett and W. T. Couldwell, "Metastases to the pituitary gland," *Neurosurgical Focus*, vol. 16, no. 4, pp. 1–4, 2004.

[53] R. Senetta, I. Castellano, D. Garbossa, A. Sapino, and P. Cassoni, "Pituitary metastasis of an unknown neuroendocrine breast carcinoma mimicking a pituitary adenoma," *Pathology*, vol. 45, no. 4, pp. 422–424, 2013.

[54] Y. Koshimoto, M. Maeda, H. Naiki, K. Nakakuki, and Y. Ishii, "MR of pituitary metastasis in a patient with diabetes insipidus," *AJNR. American Journal of Neuroradiology*, vol. 16, no. 4 Suppl, pp. 971–974, 1995.

[55] B. E. Hamilton, K. L. Salzman, and A. G. Osborn, "Anatomic and pathologic spectrum of pituitary infundibulum lesions," *American Journal of Roentgenology*, vol. 188, no. 3, pp. W223–W232, 2007.

[56] I. Feiz-Erfan, G. Rao, W. White, and I. McCutcheon, "Efficacy of trans-septal trans-sphenoidal surgery in correcting visual symptoms caused by hematogenous metastases to the sella and pituitary gland," *Skull Base*, vol. 18, no. 2, pp. 077–084, 2008.

[57] M. Habu, H. Tokimura, H. Hirano et al., "Pituitary metastases: current practice in Japan," *Journal of Neurosurgery*, vol. 123, no. 4, pp. 998–1007, 2015.

[58] M. P. Piedra, P. D. Brown, P. C. Carpenter, and M. J. Link, "Resolution of diabetes insipidus following gamma knife surgery for a solitary metastasis to the pituitary stalk," *Journal of Neurosurgery*, vol. 101, no. 6, pp. 1053–1056, 2004.

[59] M. B. Atkins and N. M. Tannir, "Current and emerging therapies for first-line treatment of metastatic clear cell renal cell carcinoma," *Cancer Treatment Reviews*, vol. 70, pp. 127–137, 2018.

[60] M. U. Alam, S. B. Jazayeri, S. Gautam et al., "Combination therapy for metastatic renal cell carcinoma: a systematic review and network meta-analysis," *American Journal of Clinical Oncology*, vol. 43, no. 7, pp. 477–483, 2020.

[61] L. Yang, S.-Y. Yu, and G.-Y. Hu, "Pituitary metastasis from a renal cell carcinoma progressed after sorafenib treatment," *Chinese Journal of Cancer*, vol. 32, no. 6, pp. 353–356, 2013.

[62] M. Payandeh, M. Sadeghi, and E. Sadeghi, "The complete response to targeted drugs without surgery or radiotherapy: a case of pituitary metastasis from renal cell carcinoma," *Acta Medica Iranica*, vol. 54, no. 9, pp. 617–619, 2016.

[63] Y. Park, H. Kim, E.-H. Kim, C.-O. Suh, and S. Lee, "Effective treatment of solitary pituitary metastasis with panhypopituitarism in HER2-positive breast cancer by lapatinib," *Cancer Research and Treatment*, vol. 48, no. 1, pp. 403–408, 2016.

[64] G. Cochetti, E. Puxeddu, F. D'Amico et al., "Laparoscopic partial nephrectomy of thyroid cancer metastasis: case report and review of the literature," *OncoTargets and Therapy*, vol. 2013, no. 6, pp. 355–360, 2013.

[65] M. Donini, S. Buti, F. Massari et al., "Management of oligometastatic and oligoprogressive renal cell carcinoma: state of the art and future directions," *Expert Review of Anticancer Therapy*, vol. 20, no. 6, pp. 491–501, 2020.

[66] A. Boni, G. Cochetti, S. Ascani et al., "Robotic treatment of oligometastatic kidney tumor with synchronous pancreatic metastasis: case report and review of the literature," *BMC Surgery*, vol. 18, no. 1, p. 40, 2018.

[67] G. Cochetti, E. Mearini, F. Barillaro, S. Fatigoni, and F. Roila, "Renal malignant solitary fibrous tumor with single lymph node involvement: report of unusual metastasis and review of the literature," *OncoTargets and Therapy*, vol. 2014, no. 7, pp. 679–685, 2014.

[68] G. Marulli, C. Breda, P. Fontana et al., "Pleurectomy-decortication in malignant pleural mesothelioma: are different surgical techniques associated with different outcomes? Results from a multicentre study," *European Journal of Cardio-Thoracic Surgery*, vol. 52, no. 1, pp. 63–69, 2017.

[69] T. Nazemi, A. Galich, S. Sterrett, D. Klingler, L. Smith, and K. C. Balaji, "Radical nephrectomy performed by open, laparoscopy with or without hand-assistance or robotic methods by the same surgeon produces comparable perioperative results," *International Brazilian Journal of Urology*, vol. 32, no. 1, pp. 15–22, 2006.

[70] D. K. Ornstein, "Feasibility of robotic radical nephrectomy-initial results of single-institution pilot study," *Yearbook of Urology*, vol. 2006, pp. 145-146, 2006.

[71] C. Y. Lin, W. K. Huang, F. T. Chung, and H. K. Chang, "Prognostic factors in cancer patients with symptomatic pituitary metastasis: a clinical case study," *Anticancer Research*, vol. 35, no. 2, pp. 983–987, 2015.

[72] H. M. Heshmati, B. W. Scheithauer, and W. F. Young, "Metastases to the pituitary gland," *The Endocrinologist*, vol. 12, no. 1, pp. 45–49, 2002.

40

A Rare Case of Uterine Leiomyosarcoma with Metastasis to the Thyroid Gland

Gabriel Irizarry-Villafañe,[1] Nadyeschka Rivera-Santana,[1] Michelle Mangual-García,[1] Alex González-Bóssolo,[1] Rafael Trinidad-Hernández,[2] Miosotis García-Maldonado,[3] and Víctor Carlo-Chévere[4]

[1]*Endocrinology Department, San Juan City Hospital, San Juan, Puerto Rico 00936, USA*
[2]*Building 1431 Ave Ponce de Leon, Suite 303, San Juan, Puerto Rico 00907, USA*
[3]*HRP Labs, 300 Manuel Domenech Street, San Juan, Puerto Rico 00918, USA*
[4]*Puerto Rico Pathology, 198 Calle Trinidad, San Juan, Puerto Rico 00917, USA*

Correspondence should be addressed to Gabriel Irizarry-Villafañe; gabriel_mdblue@yahoo.com

Academic Editor: Osamu Isozaki

Uterine leiomyosarcomas are aggressive tumors associated with a poor prognosis. These neoplasms have high metastatic potential, more frequently affecting the lungs, liver, and peritoneum. There are very few cases of metastasis to the thyroid described in the literature. We present the case of a 47-year-old female diagnosed with uterine leiomyosarcoma metastatic to the thyroid gland. In this case report, we want to emphasize the utility of ancillary studies to help differentiate a leiomyosarcoma from anaplastic thyroid carcinoma since cytologic evaluation alone can be challenging.

1. Introduction

The thyroid gland is one of the most vascular organs in the body, but metastases to this organ are rare [1, 2]. Epidemiologic studies state that of all the thyroid malignancies, approximately 2% to 3% are secondary to metastasis [3]. As reported by Pastorello and Saieg, adenocarcinomas predominantly from the kidney, breast, and lungs and squamous cells carcinomas mostly from the head and neck account for the most common metastatic cancers to the thyroid [2].

Leiomyosarcomas, as well as benign leiomyomas, can coexist in the same uterus [4]. Uterine leiomyosarcoma (LMS) which originates from the smooth muscle of the uterus is a rare aggressive tumor with the propensity for distant metastasis [5, 6]. Uterine LMS metastasic to the thyroid gland is a rare event, accounting for 1% of the reported metastatic cases [7]. As per our knowledge, there have been only six reported cases of this malignancy with metastasis to the thyroid gland [1, 8].

It is well documented that thyroid metastases may mimic primary thyroid malignancies. Primary and secondary thyroid leiomyosarcoma can resemble anaplastic thyroid carcinoma (ATC), as well as medullary thyroid cancer (MTC) and melanoma, since they all can present as spindle cell tumors on cytology [2, 8]. We present this case of a metastatic uterine leiomyosarcoma to the thyroid to review the differential diagnosis of spindle cell neoplasms. We want to discuss the best approach to accurately identify a metastatic leiomyosarcoma to the thyroid during the fine needle aspiration cytology (FNAC) evaluation utilizing the pertinent ancillary studies.

2. Case Presentation

A 47-year-old female presented to the endocrinologist for evaluation due to a thyroid mass found on neck ultrasound ordered by her primary care physician due to neck discomfort. The patient had a medical history of myomatous uterus and microcytic hypochromic anemia secondary to abnormal uterine bleeding (AUB), with a negative endometrial biopsy. The patient denied radiation exposure to the head or neck nor a smoking history. The family history was noncontributory. Upon further interview, the patient denied obstructive symptoms such as shortness of breath, hoarseness, dysphagia, or odynophagia. Physical examination found neither goiter nor lymphadenopathy, but it was remarkable for a palpable left thyroid nodule. Thyroid ultrasound showed a left upper lobe 2.4 cm solid hypoechoic nodule with irregular borders. Due to sonographic findings of a high suspicious nodule, the patient underwent ultrasound-guided fine-needle aspiration biopsy. The Diff-Quick stain showed marked cellularity of atypical spindle cells, dyscohesive, and in tissue aggregates with some binucleated cells (Figure 1). Immunohistochemical (IHC) studies performed were reported as positive for thyroglobulin and thyroid transcription factor-1 (TTF-1) and negative for calcitonin. On the pathology report, these findings were consistent with poorly differentiated thyroid carcinoma. The diagnosis of anaplastic thyroid carcinoma was suggested based mainly on cytologic parameters. Because of these findings, a total thyroidectomy was performed promptly due to the poor prognosis associated with this diagnosis. After total thyroidectomy was performed, hematoxylin-eosin staining showed a spindle cell tumor with frequent mitotic figures (Figure 2). IHC studies evidenced the presence of normal thyroid follicles, which stained positive for thyroglobulin and cytokeratin AE1/AE3, entrapped within fascicles of atypical spindle tumor cells. The tumor cells stained positive for smooth muscle actin (SMA) and desmin (Figure 3) and negative for cytokeratin and thyroglobulin. A diagnosis of metastatic high-grade leiomyosarcoma was made. Also, the patient was found to have multiple left lung nodules found on imaging which were evaluated by CT-guided core needle biopsy with findings compatible with metastatic leiomyosarcoma. This was based on the Diff-Quick stain showing increased cellularity of atypical spindle cells which, on IHC studies, also stained positive for SMA and desmin and negative for TTF-1 and S-100.

Due to the patient's history of AUB, a total abdominal hysterectomy with bilateral salpingo-oophorectomy was performed. Pathology confirmed the uterine corpus as the primary site as results revealed a uterine leiomyosarcoma of 11 cm with microvascular invasion strongly positive for SMA, desmin, epithelial membrane antigen (EMA), and caldesmon. Due to the diagnosis of uterine leiomyosarcoma stage IVB, the patient received surgical management and chemotherapy treatment. Despite aggressive treatment, in addition to radiation therapy, the patient's disease has progressively spread to other organs including the liver and stomach.

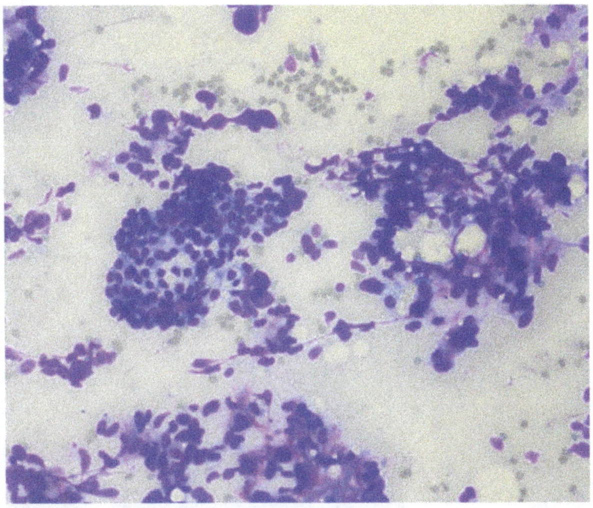

Figure 1: Thyroid nodule FNAB, Diff-Quick stain with marked cellularity of atypical spindle cells, dyscohesive, and in tissue aggregates with some binucleated cells.

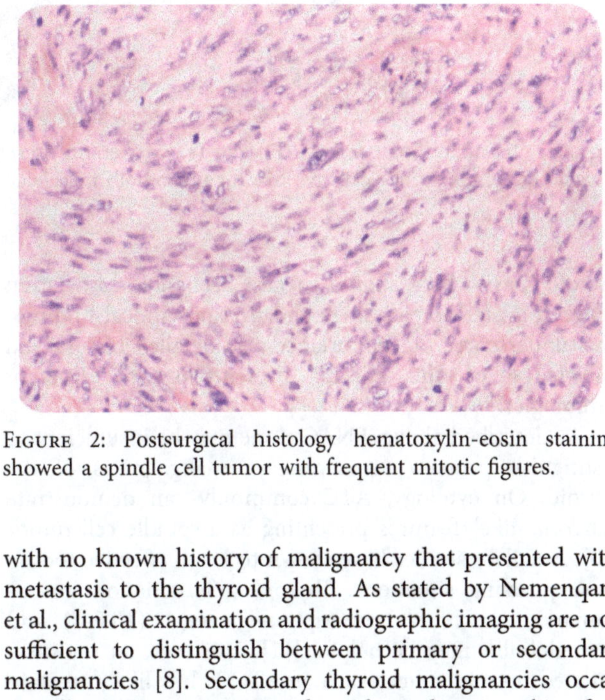

Figure 2: Postsurgical histology hematoxylin-eosin staining showed a spindle cell tumor with frequent mitotic figures.

3. Discussion

When evaluating a patient with a thyroid nodule, it is essential to consider metastasis among the differential diagnosis, whether symptomatic, asymptomatic, with a history of cancer, or the lack thereof. In our case, we portray a patient with no known history of malignancy that presented with metastasis to the thyroid gland. As stated by Nemenqani et al., clinical examination and radiographic imaging are not sufficient to distinguish between primary or secondary malignancies [8]. Secondary thyroid malignancies occasionally can imitate primary thyroid neoplasms, making fine needle aspiration cytologic diagnosis a challenging feat. The incorporation of ancillary studies to the FNAC is an important tool to achieve an accurate diagnosis.

Metastatic LMS and ATC are two entities that may have distinct clinical presentations although may be similar cytologically. ATC usually presents in older patients as an aggressive, rapidly enlarging thyroid mass with regional or distant spread. Uterine LMS, which is an aggressive neoplasm with a high tendency to metastasize, is most common in women over the age of forty and frequently presents with AUB [9]. As described in the literature, about 70% of patients with secondary thyroid malignancies presents with a palpable nodule [2]. Our patient was in her forties presenting with AUB of eight months of evolution and a palpable

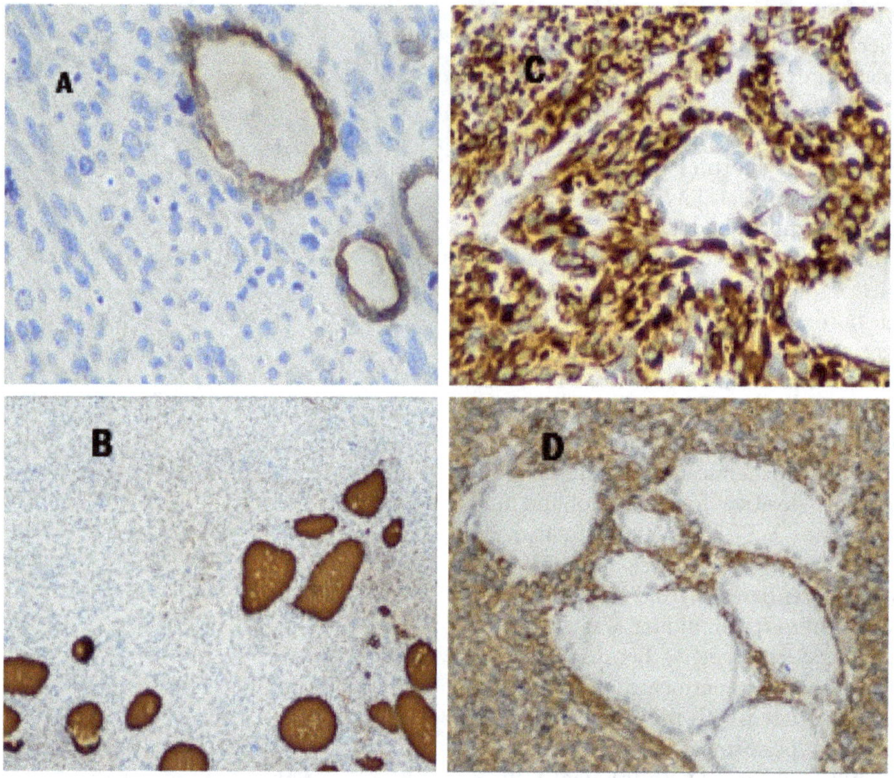

FIGURE 3: Immunohistochemical stains for (a) cytokeratin AE1/AE3 and (b) thyroglobulin showing entrapped thyroid follicles within fascicles of spindle tumor cells positive for (c) smooth muscle actin (SMA) and (d) desmin.

thyroid mass which should suggest a possible association between a uterine pathology and thyroid clinical findings. This underscores the importance of a detailed history and knowledge of the clinical presentation of different pathologies.

As described above, FNAC alone may be insufficient to distinguish primary vs. secondary malignancies of the thyroid. On cytology, ATC commonly can demonstrate "sarcoma-like" features presenting as a spindle cell tumor [10]. Ancillary studies have shown to be an effective tool in these puzzling situations. Thyroid differentiation immunomarkers such as transcription factor-1 (TTF-1) and thyroglobulin may be helpful [11]. However, an undifferentiated thyroid cancer such as ATC is less likely to stain positive for thyroglobulin or TTF-1, but most retain positivity for the transcription factor PAX-8 and the epithelial marker cytokeratin AE1/AE3 [12, 13]. The majority of leiomyosarcomas, as reported in the literature, stain positive for smooth muscle actin (SMA) and desmin [14]. It is pertinent to remember that medullary thyroid cancer can also present as a spindle cell tumor staining positive for TTF-1, keratins, and calcitonin [10].

In our case, the FNAC evaluation combined with a limited IHC study, which included thyroglobulin, TTF-1, and calcitonin, was not enough to differentiate between a LMS and a primary thyroid malignancy. As mentioned above, the FNAC was reported as positive in this high-grade tumor for these thyroid markers, except for calcitonin. These were falsely positive, due to staining of the normal thyroid follicular cells which were admixed with the neoplastic cells. Post-thyroidectomy histology marked positive for SMA and desmin but negative for TTF-1, CD34, cytokeratin AE1/AE3, and S-100 leading to the diagnosis of metastatic uterine LMS.

The FNAC is an excellent diagnostic tool for thyroid neoplasms. Nonetheless, in challenging cases such as this one, the IHC panel may be limited due to the scant cellularity that may be obtained in a cell block. Careful evaluation of the staining pattern and correlation with the morphologic findings of the staining cells is also of paramount importance to avoid false positives or false negatives, particularly in small biopsies such as FNA or core needle biopsies.

If the number of antibodies tested is felt to be insufficient for evaluation, a repeated FNA, or a core biopsy in selected cases, should be considered. A comprehensive approach, including both clinical and cytologic findings should be attempted, as each case will pose different challenges.

A detailed IHC panel should include SMA, desmin, cytokeratin pool AE1/AE3, and S-100 as a melanocyte marker combined with thyroid markers, in order to help distinguish a sarcoma from other spindle cell malignancies [2]. From the clinical point of view, some clues should be factored into the equation, for example, the presence or absence of the regional lymph node involvement. Since it is rare to find a high-grade primary thyroid malignancy without regional lymph node involvement, such a diagnosis without cervical adenopathy should alert to the possibility of a metastatic lesion. This knowledge may alert the pathology lab that additional markers are needed and may prompt the laboratory to request additional tissue.

Currently, there is no definite curative pharmacologic treatment for metastatic uterine leiomyosarcoma. Regarding the surgical treatment for distant metastatic leiomyosarcoma to the thyroid, there is a paucity of data. Nixon et al. describe that for patients with malignancies with localized small volume metastasis to the thyroid considered for surgical therapy, it may be managed with thyroid lobectomy with appropriate margins [15].

In conclusion, the diagnosis of metastasis to the thyroid gland can be difficult, and it is associated with poor prognosis [2]. Thyroid cancers most commonly are of a primary origin and of low-grade cytology [2, 6]. However, when confronting a high-grade thyroid lesion, this should prompt us to consider metastasis as the possible etiology of a thyroid nodule [2]. Spindle cell tumors on thyroid cytology can be due to anaplastic thyroid cancer, poorly differentiated thyroid cancers, MTC, and sarcomas, among other etiologies. We emphasize the importance of a detailed history and physical examination, knowledge of the differential diagnoses, and their presentations in addition to adequately accompanying FNAC with the pertinent ancillary studies in order to differentiate primary thyroid entities such ATC from metastatic spindle cell tumors such a leiomyosarcomas. There are scant data pertaining to the treatment of aggressive distant metastatic disease.

Consent

Written consent was obtained from the patient for publication of the case.

Authors' Contributions

Dr. Irizarry-Villafañe and Dr. Rivera-Santana were involved in the article review, manuscript writing, and revision. Dr. Mangual-García and Dr. González-Bóssolo are endocrinologists who were involved in manuscript revision. Dr. Trinidad-Hernández is an endocrinologist who was involved with patient care and manuscript revision. Dr. García-Maldonado and Dr. Carlo-Chévere are pathologists who were involved in manuscript revision.

References

[1] J. A. Eloy, M. Mortensen, S. Gupta, M. S. Lewis, E. M. Brett, and E. M. Genden, "Metastasis of uterine leiomyosarcoma to the thyroid gland: case report and review of the literature," *Thyroid*, vol. 17, no. 12, pp. 1295–1297, 2007.

[2] R. G. Pastorello and M. A. Saieg, "Metastases to the thyroid: potential cytologic mimics of primary thyroid neoplasms," *Archives of Pathology & Laboratory Medicine*, vol. 143, no. 3, pp. 394–399, 2019.

[3] L. Zhang, Y. Liu, X. Li, W. Gao, and C. Zheng, "Metastases to the thyroid gland," *Medicine*, vol. 96, no. 36, 2017.

[4] A. Sandberg, "Updates on the cytogenetics and molecular genetics of bone and soft tissue tumors: leiomyosarcoma," *Cancer Genetics and Cytogenetics*, vol. 161, no. 1, pp. 1–19, 2005.

[5] V. S. Vellanki, M. Rao, C. Babu Sunkavalli, R. N. Chinamotu, and S. Kaja, "A rare case of uterine leiomyosarcoma: a case report," *Journal of Medical Case Reports*, vol. 4, no. 1, 2010.

[6] C. Leath, W. K. Huh, J. M. Straughn, and M. G. Conner, "Uterine leiomyosarcoma metastatic to the thyroid," *Obstetrics & Gynecology*, vol. 100, no. 5, pp. 1122–1124, 2002.

[7] S. H. Tirumani, P. Deaver, A. B. Shinagare et al., "Metastatic pattern of uterine leiomyosarcoma: retrospective analysis of the predictors and outcome in 113 patients," *Journal of Gynecologic Oncology*, vol. 25, no. 4, p. 306, 2014.

[8] D. Nemenqani, N. Yaqoob, and H. Khoja, "Leiomyosarcoma metastatic to the thyroid diagnosed by fine needle aspiration cytology," *Journal of Pakistan Medical Association*, vol. 60, no. 4, pp. 307–309, 2010.

[9] P. Kaur, A. Kaur, A. Singla, and K. Kaur, "Uterine leiomyosarcoma: a case report," *Journal of Mid-life Health*, vol. 5, no. 4, p. 200, 2014.

[10] G. Conzo, G. Candela, E. Tartaglia et al., "Leiomyosarcoma of the thyroid gland: a case report and literature review," *Oncology Letters*, vol. 7, no. 4, pp. 1011–1014, 2014.

[11] H. Liu and F. Lin, "Application of immunohistochemistry in thyroid pathology," *Archives of Pathology & Laboratory Medicine*, vol. 139, no. 1, pp. 67–82, 2015.

[12] D. Nonaka, Y. Tang, L. Chiriboga, M. Rivera, and R. Ghossein, "Diagnostic utility of thyroid transcription factors pax8 and TTF-2 (foxE1) in thyroid epithelial neoplasms," *Modern Pathology*, vol. 21, no. 2, pp. 192–200, 2007.

[13] J. P. Solomon, F. Wen, and L. J. Jih, "Anaplastic transformation of papillary thyroid cancer in the retroperitoneum," *Case Reports in Pathology*, vol. 2015, Article ID 241308, 4 pages, 2015.

[14] J. C. Carvalho, D. G. Thomas, and D. R. Lucas, "Cluster analysis of immunohistochemical markers in leiomyosarcoma delineates specific anatomic and gender subgroups," *Cancer*, vol. 115, no. 18, pp. 4186–4195, 2009.

[15] I. J. Nixon, A. Coca-Pelaz, A. I. Kaleva et al., "Metastasis to the thyroid gland: a critical review," *Annals of Surgical Oncology*, vol. 24, no. 6, pp. 1533–1539, 2016.

41

Dramatic Response to First Line Single Agent Pembrolizumab in Anaplastic Thyroid Carcinoma

Valérie Spalart,[1] Barbara Legius,[2] Kurt Segers,[3] Johan Coolen,[4] Brigitte Maes,[5] and Lynn Decoster [2]

[1]*AZ Turnhout, Department of Internal Medicine, Turnhout, Belgium*
[2]*AZ Turnhout, Department of Pulmonology/Respiratory Oncology, Turnhout, Belgium*
[3]*AZ Turnhout, Department of Pathology, Turnhout, Belgium*
[4]*University Hospitals Leuven, Department of Radiology, Leuven, Belgium*
[5]*Jessa Hospital Hasselt, Laboratory for Molecular Diagnostics, Department of Clinical Biology, Hasselt, Belgium*

Correspondence should be addressed to Lynn Decoster; lynn.decoster@azturnhout.be

Academic Editor: Lucy Mastrandrea

Anaplastic thyroid carcinoma (ATC) is a deadly disease with very limited therapeutic options. There is an urgent need for new and efficacious drugs. Unfortunately accrual in clinical trials is problematic because of the rarity of the disease and often poor performance status at diagnosis. Recently some data have emerged suggesting a role for immunotherapy in the treatment of ATC. We describe the case of a 75-year-old patient with poor performance status and compromised airway and oesophagus at diagnosis, showing a rapid and dramatic response to first line single agent pembrolizumab. Disease progression in the brain occurred 16 months after initial diagnosis. At that time there was ongoing extracranial disease control.

1. Introduction

Anaplastic thyroid carcinoma (ATC) is a rare and aggressive disease representing 1-2% of all thyroid cancers but accounting for 50% of annual thyroid cancer related mortality. Approximately 50% of patients present with metastatic disease and treatment options are limited except for a subset of patients with BRAF-mutated tumors. Recent data suggest a potential role for immunotherapy in this disease desperate for new therapies. We describe a patient with poor performance status at presentation showing a rapid and dramatic response to first line single agent pembrolizumab.

2. Case Presentation

A 75-year-old female never smoker presented to the ear, nose and throat specialist with hoarseness, dry cough, difficulty swallowing and a 3 kg weight loss since 1 month.

5 years earlier she was treated with radioactive iodine for a toxic multinodular goiter. She also had a past medical history of a stage *Ic* well-differentiated serous papillary ovarian carcinoma treated with surgery and adjuvant chemotherapy.

On clinical examination, a multinodular and enlarged thyroid gland was palpated. A computed tomography (CT) scan of the neck and chest revealed a large mass (8 × 9 cm) in the anterior mediastinum involving the right thyroid lobe and causing deviation of both trachea and oesophagus. There were multiple pathologically enlarged cervical, supraclavicular and mediastinal lymph nodes as well as multiple bilateral lung metastases (Figure 1). Further staging revealed a bone metastasis in the right iliac crest. During bronchoscopy paralysis of the right vocal cord was noticed as well as invasion of the trachea with reduction of tracheal diameter estimated at 25%. No intracranial metastases were present on baseline brain CT imaging. A biopsy of a cervical lymph node was performed showing diffuse infiltration by an abnormal epithelial cell proliferation. The abnormal cells were large with large and hyperchromatic nuclei. Multiple mitotic figures were present as well as necrosis and several infiltrating lymphocytes. Immunohistochemical studies on the neoplastic cells were negative for thyroid transcription factor-1 (TTF-1), PAX-8,

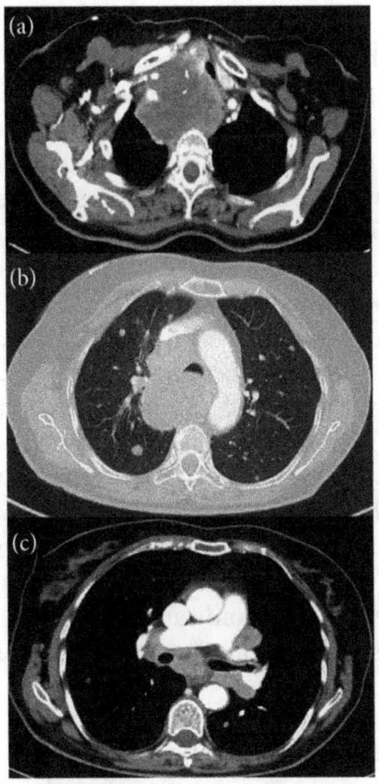

FIGURE 1: Baseline chest CT showing a large mass originating from the right thyroid lobe (a), with lung metastases (b), and hilar and mediastinal lymph nodes (c). (a), (c) images in mediastinal window. (b) image in lung window.

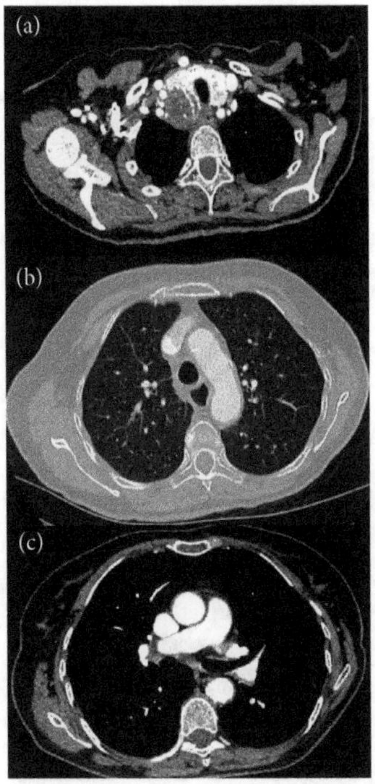

FIGURE 2: Chest CT after 3 cycles of pembrolizumab showing marked regression of primary tumor (a), lung metastases and (b), lymph nodes (c).

thyroglobulin, cytokeratin AE1/AE3, cytokeratin 7, CD 45, CD 34 and S-100. The pathological findings were compatible with an anaplastic large cell malignancy.

The case was discussed at the multidisciplinary tumor board and based on clinical presentation, imaging and pathology a diagnosis of primary anaplastic thyroid cancer was made. Next generation sequencing (NGS, TRUSEQ, MISEQ, ILLUMINA) was negative for molecular drivers. PDL1-staining was positive with a high expression (60% of tumor cells). At that point the clinical condition of the patient was rapidly deteriorating due to dysphagia with impaired food intake. The possibility of palliative stenting of the oesophagus was discussed with the gastroenterologist but was considered technically impossible. The patient was unfit for a clinical trial. Based on occasional case reports describing exceptional response to immunotherapy in patients with anaplastic thyroid cancer, the patient was offered the possibility of treatment with pembrolizumab. After only 2 cycles, the patient noticed a marked improvement of dysphagia and after 3 cycles, a near complete response was seen on CT (Figure 2). Thyroid function was thoroughly monitored during treatment and remained normal at all times.

After 8 cycles however, the patient developed a severe grade 4 colitis (bloody stools, severe dehydration with hypotension) requiring aggressive fluid resuscitation and treatment with systemic steroids. Due to further clinical deterioration infliximab was administered, after which gradual improvement occurred. 3 months after the last administration of pembrolizumab, there were no signs of tumor progression. As most guidelines recommend permanent discontinuation of immunotherapy after grade 4 gastro-intestinal toxicity, a watchful waiting approach was proposed with follow-up CT of the chest and neck every 3 months.

6 months later (16 months after diagnosis), the patient presented to the emergency department with gait difficulties, falling tendency to the left, left-sided facial palsy and hypoesthesia of the left upper arm. Magnetic resonance imaging (MRI) of the brain revealed a 19 × 18 × 19 mm lesion in the right thalamus. Stereotactic biopsy of this lesion was compatible with metastasis of known anaplastic large cell carcinoma. There were no signs of extra-cranial tumor progression (Figure 3). Stereotactic radiotherapy to the brain lesion was performed. However her neurological condition did not improve. Because of poor performance status, previous grade 4 gastro-intestinal toxicity and mainly intracranial treatment failure, a re-challenge with pembrolizumab was not considered nor was second line chemotherapy. The patient was referred for hospice care. She died 18 months after initial diagnosis.

3. Discussion

Anaplastic thyroid carcinoma (ATC) is a rare and aggressive disease with a median overall survival of less than 6 months and a 1-year survival of only 20%. In metastatic disease particularly, treatment options are limited [1]. The evidence for conventional chemotherapy is scarce as large randomized trials are lacking. Taxanes, doxorubicin and platin have shown some activity either as single agent or in combination, with response rates between 15% and 25% [2].

Lately promising results were reported with targeted therapies. In a single-arm, open-label study 17 ATC-patients

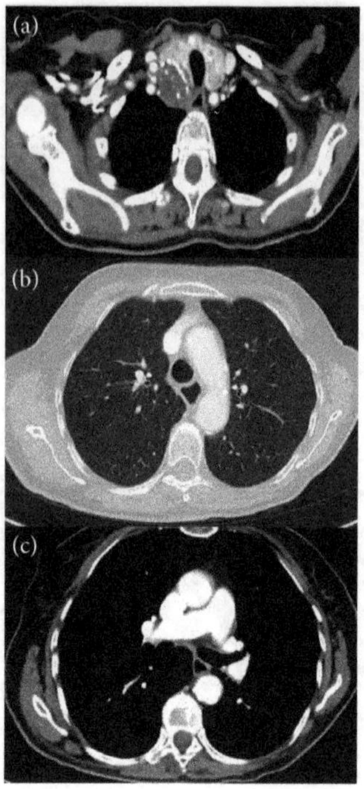

Figure 3: Chest CT 6 months after start of pembrolizumab showing ongoing response.

were treated with the multikinase-inhibitor lenvatinib. The objective response rate was 24%, the median progression-free survival (PFS) was 7.4 months and the median overall survival (OS) 10.6 months [3]. More importantly, in BRAF-mutated tumors, the combination of the selective kinase inhibitors (dabrafenib and trametinib) achieved a response rate of 69% and a 1-year survival of 80% [4]. Unfortunately resistance to these targeted therapies inevitably occurs.

The role of immunotherapy in ATC remains to be elucidated. Kolllipara et al. described an exceptional response with immunotherapy (nivolumab) in a patient with BRAF positive ATC who showed a mixed response to the BRAF-inhibitor vemurafenib [5]. In a small retrospective series of salvage pembrolizumab added to a kinase inhibitor at time of progression, partial response rate was 42% with a median OS from the start of pembrolizumab of 6.9 months [6]. Little is known about the role of single agent immunotherapy. In 30 ATC patients treated with the PD1-inhibitor spartalizumab, partial response was observed in less than 20% [7]. On the contrary, Khan et al. reported 2 out of 4 partial responses in ATC patients treated with pembrolizumab [8]. Currently 2 clinical trials are examining the role of immunotherapy-only in ATC patients (pembrolizumab in NCT02688608; nivolumab plus ipilimumab in NCT03246958).

In most ATC-trials however, accrual is hampered by the rarity of the disease and the often poor performance status at initial diagnosis. In a review article on diagnosis and management of ATC, Chintakuntlawar et al. state that it might therefore be reasonable to consider PD-1 inhibitors in these patients [1]. Occasional case reports might further build the evidence for the use of immunotherapy in a disease desperate for new treatment options.

We hereby describe a case of metastatic ATC treated with single agent pembrolizumab as first line therapy. Our case illustrates that a rapid and clinically meaningful response can be obtained even in a very sick patient with compromised airway and oesophagus. Clinical benefit occurred after only 2 cycles of pembrolizumab and near complete response was obtained after 3 cycles. Unfortunately, Pembrolizumab had to be discontinued because of grade 4 colitis and relapse occurred in the brain 14 months after initial diagnosis. At that moment there was ongoing extra-cranial disease control. As the initial impressive response to immunotherapy in our patient is intriguing we retrospectively assessed tumor infiltrating lymphocytes (TILs) on H&E slides from a metastatic lymph node. Stromal TILs (sTILs) could not be scored as no stroma was present in the biopsies. The percentage of intratumoral infiltrating lymphocytes (iTILS) was 30%. Whether PD-L1 or H&E based assessment of TILs (and at which cut-off) are predictive biomarkers in anaplastic thyroid cancer is a question that hopefully can be answered by ongoing or future clinical trials.

Author's Contributions

LD had the idea for the manuscript. VS and LD drafted the manuscript. LD and BL took part in the clinical management of the patient. JC was responsible for radiographic diagnosis. KS was responsible for pathological diagnosis. BM was responsible for molecular diagnosis. All authors contributed to and approved the final version of the manuscript.

References

[1] A. V. Chintakuntlawar, R. L. Foote, J. L. Kasperbauer, and K. C. Bible, "Diagnosis and management of anaplastic thyroid cancer," *Endocrinology and Metabolism Clinics of North America*, vol. 48, no. 1, pp. 269–284, 2019.

[2] M. E. Cabanillas, M. Zafereo, G. B. Gunn, and R. Ferrarotto, "Anaplastic thyroid carcinoma: treatment in the age of molecular targeted therapy," *Journal of Oncology Practice*, vol. 12, no. 6, pp. 511–518, 2016.

[3] M. Tahara, N. Kiyota, T. Yamazaki et al., "Lenvatinib for anaplastic thyroid cancer," *Frontiers in Oncology*, vol. 7, 2017.

[4] V. Subbiah, R. J. Kreitman, Z. A. Wainberg et al., "Dabrafenib and trametinib treatment in patients with locally advanced or metastatic BRAF V600-mutant anaplastic thyroid cancer," *Journal of Clinical Oncology*, vol. 36, no. 1, pp. 7–13, 2018.

[5] R. Kollipara, B. Schneider, M. Radovich, S. Babu, and P. J. Kiel, "Exceptional response with immunotherapy in a patient with anaplastic thyroid cancer," *The Oncologist*, vol. 22, no. 10, pp. 1149–1151, 2017.

[6] P. C. Iyer, R. Dadu, M. Gule-Monroe et al., "Salvage pembrolizulmab added to kinase inhibitor therapy for the treatment of anaplastic thyroid carcinoma," *Journal for Immunotherapy of Cancer*, vol. 6, no. 1, p. 68, 2018.

[7] L. J. Wirth, E. Eigendorff, J. Capdevila et al., "Phase I/II study of spartalizumab (PDR001), an anti-PD1 mAb, in patients with anaplastic thyroid cancer," *Journal of Clinical Oncology*, vol. 36, no. 15, pp. 6024–6024, 2018.

[8] S. A. Khan, P. Kurian, B. Mobley et al., "Relationship of anaplastic thyroid cancer high tumor mutation burden and MSI-H status with response to anti-PD1 monotherapy," *Journal of Clinical Oncology*, vol. 36, no. 15, pp. e18114–e18114, 2018.

42

Hyperandrogenism, Elevated 17-Hydroxyprogesterone and its Urinary Metabolites in a Young Woman with Ovarian Steroid Cell Tumour, not Otherwise Specified: Case Report and Review of the Literature

Felix C. K. Wong,[1] **Angela Z. Chan**,[2] **W. S. Wong**,[3] **Angel H. W. Kwan**,[4] **Tracy S. M. Law**,[4] **Jacqueline P. W. Chung**,[4] **Jeffrey S. S. Kwok**,[1] **and Angel O. K. Chan**[1]

[1]*Department of Chemical Pathology, Prince of Wales Hospital, The Chinese University of Hong Kong, Shatin, Hong Kong*
[2]*Department of Anatomical and Cellular Pathology, Prince of Wales Hospital, The Chinese University of Hong Kong, Shatin, Hong Kong*
[3]*Department of Medicine, North District Hospital, Sheung Shui, Hong Kong*
[4]*Department of Obstetrics and Gynaecology, Prince of Wales Hospital, The Chinese University of Hong Kong, Shatin, Hong Kong*

Correspondence should be addressed to Felix C. K. Wong; felix@cuhk.edu.hk

Academic Editor: Toshihiro Kita

We describe a case of a 24-year-old overweight woman who presented with hirsutism, secondary amenorrhea, clitoromegaly, and symptoms of diabetes mellitus (DM). While a diagnosis of polycystic ovary syndrome (PCOS) with its associated metabolic disturbances was initially considered, serum total testosterone, androstenedione and 17-hydroxyprogesterone (17-OHP) measured by liquid chromatography tandem mass spectrometry (LC-MS/MS) were significantly increased. As 17-OHP did not increase upon ACTH (Synacthen) stimulation and the urinary steroid profile (USP) was compatible with an ovarian source of 17-OHP excess rather than adrenal, non classical congenital adrenal hyperplasia (NCCAH) was unlikely and an androgen-secreting tumor was suspected. Transabdominal ultrasound revealed the presence of an enlarged right ovary with a polycystic ovary morphology and no discrete mass. Transvaginal ultrasound and [^{18}F]– fluorodeoxyglucose positron emission tomography–computed tomography (FDG PET–CT) enabled the localization of a right ovarian tumor. Laparoscopic right salpingo-oophorectomy was performed and a histological diagnosis of steroid cell tumor, not otherwise specified (SCT–NOS) was made. Hyperandrogenism and menstrual disturbances resolved postoperatively. A literature review revealed that 17-OHP-secreting SCT–NOS may uncommonly show positive responses to ACTH stimulation similar to 21-hydroxylase deficiency. Alternatively, USP might be useful in localizing the source of 17-OHP to the ovaries. Its diagnostic performance should be evaluated in further studies.

1. Introduction

Identifying the underlying cause and localizing the source of elevated androgens or their precursors in woman with hyperandrogenism can be challenging. In the setting of female hyperandrogenism, a significant elevation of 17-hydroxyprogesterone (17-OHP) is often suggestive of a diagnosis of congenital adrenal hyperplasia (CAH), most commonly 21-hydroxylase deficiency. Nevertheless, androgen-secreting tumors, which may be of adrenal or ovarian origin, may also be responsible for such finding. Investigations for an increased 17-OHP generally include serum androgen profile, ACTH stimulation test, urinary steroid profile (USP), and if biochemically compatible with 21-hydroxylase deficiency, confirmation by molecular testing of the CYP21A2 gene. Here we present the diagnostic challenges in a young woman with hirsutism and significantly elevated total testosterone, androstenedione and 17-OHP in whom the diagnosis of a hormone-secreting steroid cell tumour, not otherwise specified (SCT–NOS) was made.

TABLE 1: Pre- and postoperative laboratory results.

Tests (serum/plasma)	Concentration (before operation)	Concentration (2 weeks after operation)	Concentration (4 weeks after operation)	Reference interval
Luteinizing hormone (IU/L)	10.0	4.5	—	2.4–12.6 (follicular phase) 14.0–95.6 (ovulation phase) 1.0–11.4 (luteal phase)
Follicle-stimulating hormone (IU/L)	5.0	4.0	—	3.5–12.5 (follicular phase) 4.7–21.5 (ovulation phase) 1.7–7.7 (luteal phase)
Estradiol (pmol/L)	161	302	—	98–571 (follicular phase) 177–1153 (ovulation phase) 122–1094 (luteal phase)
Progesterone (nmol/L)	—	18.7	—	0.6–4.7 (follicular phase) 2.4–9.4 (ovulation phase) 5.3–86 (luteal phase)
Testosterone (nmol/L)	10.6	0.7	0.5	<1.7
Prolactin (mIU/L)	See footnote[a]	See footnote[a]	—	<496
Androstenedione (nmol/L)	28.2	4.2	3.0	1.1–6.5
DHEA-S[b] (μmol/L)	6.0	6.7	5.9	1.0–11.7
17-OHP (nmol/L)	52	4.3	0.7	0.6–4.0 (follicular phase) 1.0–6.0 (luteal phase)
Cortisol (1 mg overnight dexamethasone suppression test) (nmol/L)	21	—	—	<50
Fasting glucose (mmol/L)	7.2[c]	6.0	6.5	≥7.0: diabetes mellitus
HbA1c (%)	6.9[c]	—	—	≥6.5%: diabetes mellitus
CA125 (kU/L)	17	—	—	<35
Alpha-fetoprotein (μg/L)	8	—	—	<9
Human chorionic gonadotropin (IU/L)	<1	—	—	<1 (premenopausal non pregnant)

[a]Macroprolactin present, value within reference limits after PEG precipitation. [b]DHEAS: dehydroepiandrosterone-sulphate. [c]Results obtained at diagnosis, before initiation of anti-diabetic medication.

2. Case Presentation

A 24-year-old woman was referred to the gynecology clinic for a one-year history of secondary amenorrhea and symptoms of hyperandrogenism (acne and hirsutism) for two years. She had oligomenorrhea for one year prior to developing amenorrhea. She enjoyed good past health except for a referral for pediatric assessment for overweight [Body mass index (BMI) 24.9] at the age of 12 with no specific underlying cause identified. Menarche occurred at 12 years old. Examination revealed that she is overweight (BMI 26.0) with normal blood pressure. Acne was present but there was no obvious hirsutism (hair removal was done for cosmetic reasons). Other clinical features of Cushing's syndrome were absent. Pregnancy test was negative. Transabdominal ultrasound showed an enlarged (16.6 cm^3) right ovary with more than 12 small follicles (< 9 mm), which represents sonographic evidence of polycystic ovary based on the Rotterdam criteria [1]. The left ovary was normal in appearance and size (6.8 cm^3). Polycystic ovary syndrome (PCOS) was suspected and combined oral contraceptive pills were prescribed with a return of menstruation. Further laboratory testing however demonstrated a significant elevation of serum total testosterone (10.6 nmol/L), androstenedione (28.2 nmol/L), and 17-hydroxyprogesterone (17-OHP) (52 nmol/L) all measured by liquid chromatography tandem mass spectrometry (LC-MS/MS). 1 mg overnight dexamethasone suppression test was negative for Cushing's syndrome (Table 1). In view of the grossly elevated androgens and 17-OHP, PCOS was unlikely. In addition, the raised 17-OHP raised the possibility of non classical congenital adrenal hyperplasia (NCCAH). On further questioning and physical examination, the patient noticed deepening of her voice in the recent two years, and mild clitoromegaly was found. Furthermore, the patient complained of polyuria and polydipsia for 6 months and a diagnosis of diabetes mellitus was confirmed by laboratory tests (fasting glucose 7.2 mmol/L, HbA1c 6.9%). Metformin 250 mg twice daily was prescribed. 250 μg ACTH (Synacthen) stimulation test was performed to exclude NCCAH. While the baseline and stimulated 17-OHP concentrations were both compatible with NCCAH due to 21-hydroxylase deficiency (> 30 nmol/L based on the endocrine society clinical practice guideline [2]), a flat response was noted (Table 2), which was atypical of NCCAH. A 24-h urinary steroid profile (USP) by gas chromatography mass spectrometry (GC–MS) revealed moderate elevation of androgen metabolites (androsterone: 5855 μg/day, reference interval: 431–2037 μg/day; etiocholanolone: 2175 μg/day, reference interval: 198–1551 μg/day), and gross elevation of two of the

Table 2: ACTH (Synacthen) stimulation test.

	0 min	30 min	60 min	Reference interval
ACTH (pmol/L)	2.4	—	—	<10.2
Cortisol (nmol/L)	239	614	691	—
17-OHP (nmol/L)	46	35	37	—

three metabolites of 17-OHP (17-hydroxypregnanolone: 3358 μg/day, reference interval: 16–295 μg/day; pregnanetriol: 5338 μg/day, reference interval 132–1156 μg/day). 11-oxopregnanetriol, which is another metabolite of 17-OHP, was however normal (7 μg/day, reference interval: $< 44 \mu$g/day). Cortisol and corticosterone metabolites were not in excess. The USP findings suggested an ovarian source of 17-OHP rather than adrenal. Contrast computed tomography (CT) of the abdomen and pelvis showed a 2.6 × 2.3 × 2.5 cm ovoid enhancing soft tissue over the right adnexal region, commented to be likely the right ovary, with a small local surrounding fluid collection (Figure 1(a)). No adrenal mass was identified. Transabdominal pelvic ultrasound performed five months later showed an enlarged right ovary measuring 4.5 × 2.6 × 4.5 cm in size with a volume of 27.6 cm^3. There were more than 12 tiny follicles with sizes measuring up to 8 mm present at the periphery of the right ovary, representing sonographic evidence of polycystic ovary. The left ovary measured 2.6 × 2.2 × 2.0 cm in size with a volume of 5.8 cm^3. Similar to the CT scan obtained earlier, no obvious mass was found in either ovaries (Figure 1(b)). As NCCAH was less likely and severe hyperandrogenism was present, further imaging was arranged for the localization of an androgen-secreting tumor. Transvaginal ultrasound of the pelvis revealed a 2.6 × 2.4 × 2.2 cm hyperechoic solid tumor inside the right ovary with hypervascularity seen on Doppler and multiple follicles at the periphery of the right ovary (Figure 1(c)). The left ovary also appeared to be polycystic in appearance. Whole body [^{18}F]– fluorodeoxyglucose positron emission tomography–computed tomography (FDG PET–CT) scan with contrast showed a 2.6 × 2.3 × 2.5 cm mildly fluorodeoxyglucose–avid mass (SUV_{max} 2.9 g/ml) in the right ovary with homogeneous solid contrast enhancement and no calcification, fat or cystic component. There were no hypermetabolic lymph nodes seen in the abdomen and pelvis (Figure 1(d)). A diagnosis of an androgen-secreting tumor in the right ovary was made. Laparoscopic right salpingo-oophorectomy, diagnostic hysteroscopy and curettage of the uterus were performed. Peritoneal fluid was obtained for cytology. Intraoperatively, an enlarged right ovary measuring 4.5 × 4.5 cm was found. The left ovary had a polycystic ovary-like appearance with filmsy adhesions to the ovarian fossa and adhesiolysis was performed. The resected right ovary was cut open, revealing the presence of an orange-colored tumor inside.

Microscopic examination of the specimen revealed polygonal cells arranged in diffuse sheets with round nuclei, prominent nucleoli, and abundant granular eosinophilic to pale vacuolated cytoplasm. Mitotic figures were inconspicuous

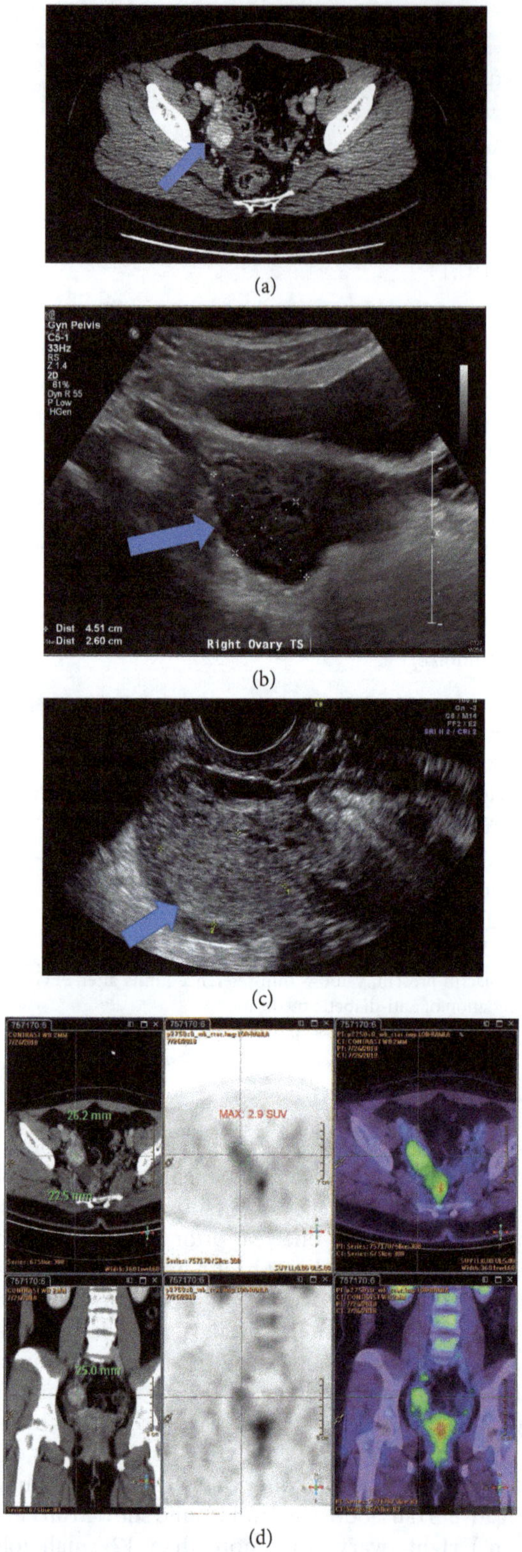

Figure 1: (a) Contrast CT scan of the abdomen and pelvis showed an enlarged 2.6 × 2.3 × 2.5 cm right ovary (blue arrow). (b) Transabdominal ultrasound showed an enlarged 4.5 × 2.6 × 4.5 cm right ovary five months after CT scan (blue arrow) (c) Transvaginal ultrasound showed a 2.6 × 2.4 × 2.2 cm hyperechoic solid tumor inside the right ovary (blue arrow) (d) FDG PET–CT scan with contrast showed a 2.6 × 2.3 × 2.5 cm mildly FDG-avid mass (SUV_{max} 2.9 g/ml) in the right ovary (tumor dimensions labelled).

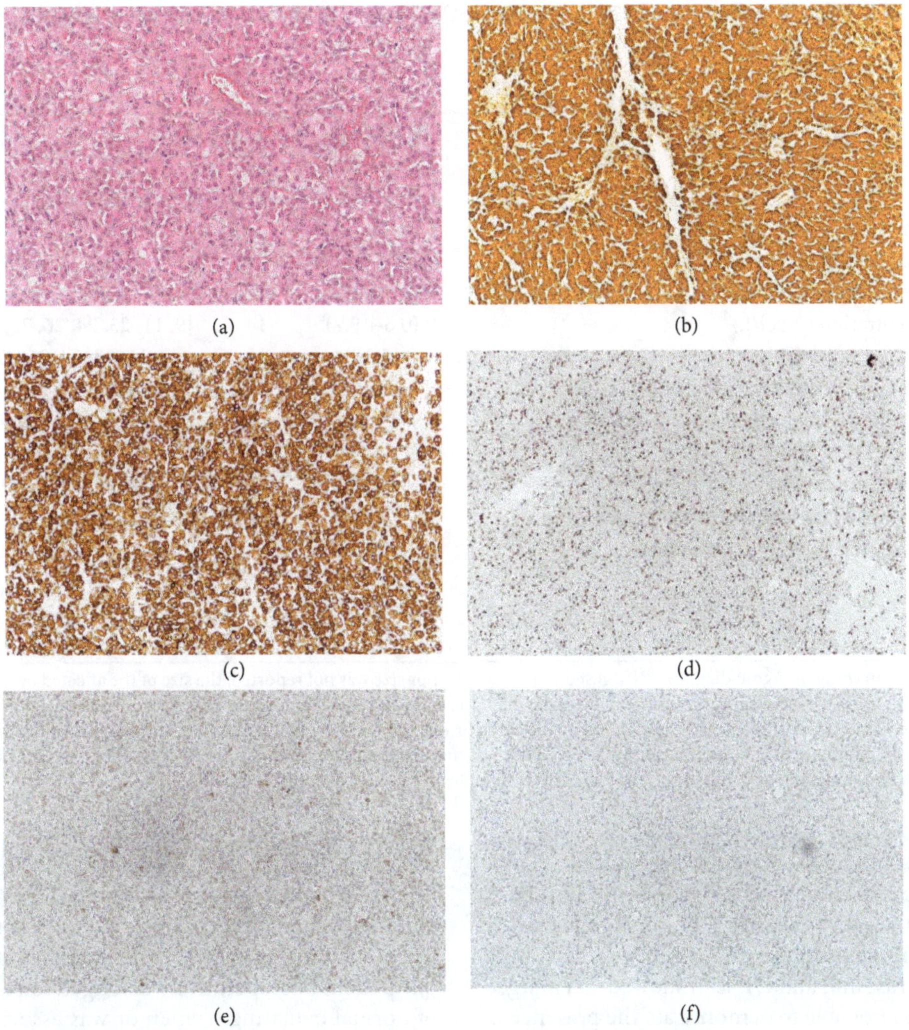

FIGURE 2: (a) Microscopic appearance of the tumor (20x magnification); (b) Calretinin immunostain (10x magnification): Positive; (c) Inhibin immunostain (10x magnification): Positive; (d) Androgen receptor immunostain (10x magnification): Positive; (e) Melan-A immunostain (10x magnification): Weakly positive; and (f) CD-99 (10x magnification) immunostain: Negative.

(<1 per 10 high power fields). No other negative prognostic features of steroid cell tumours (i.e., necrosis, haemorrhage, and nuclear atypia) were found. No Reinke crystals were identified. Immunostaining was positive for inhibin, calretinin, and androgen receptor, weakly positive for Melan-A, and negative for CD99 (Figure 2). The diagnosis was steroid cell tumor, not otherwise specified (SCT–NOS). Uterine curettage did not yield sufficient material for analysis. Cytology of the peritoneal fluid was negative for malignant cells.

The patient recovered uneventfully after the operation, with a normalization of testosterone, androstenedione and 17-OHP concentrations and attainment of a luteal phase progesterone concentration two weeks after the operation (Table 1). Postoperative HbA1c was 6.3–7.0% while she continued metformin at the same dosage (HbA1c at diagnosis was 6.9%, see Table 1). No obvious improvement in her glycemic control was seen after the operation. The patient regained spontaneous menstruation within one month after the operation with improvement in acne and subsequent menstrual cycles were regular and 28 days each. A transvaginal ultrasound performed five months postoperatively showed a persistent polycystic ovary (PCO) morphology of the left ovary with 20 antral follicles and an ovarian volume of 10 cm^3. She remained clinically well 9 months postoperatively.

3. Discussion

Androgen-secreting tumors are a rare cause of hyperandrogenism in women (0.2%) [3]. In contrast to PCOS in which the main presentation of hyperandrogenism is hirsutism, androgen-secreting tumors present with progressive and more severe hyperandrogenism leading to signs of virilization, e.g., clitoromegaly, deepening of voice, and male-pattern hair loss. Biochemically, these tumors are associated with total testosterone levels greater than 5.2 to 6.9 nmol/L [4–6]. Androgen-secreting tumors in female could be of adrenal or ovarian origin. While adrenal tumours are almost always detectable by CT scan [7, 8], ovarian androgen-secreting tumours may

Table 3: A summary of steroid cell tumors, not otherwise specified (SCT–NOS) with 17-OHP concentration reported (n = 21, including the current case). Please refer to Supplementary Table S1 for a detailed summary of all cases.

		n	Reference
Age (years)[b]	23 (3–68)[a]	21	[9, 11, 22–27, 29–35, 44–48]
Extraovarian (%)	14 (3/21)	21	
Tumor size (cm)[c]	4.9 (1–12)[a]	20	[9, 11, 22, 24–27, 29–35, 44–48]
Evidence of malignancy (%)	5 (1/21)	21	
Serum testosterone concentration (nmol/L)[d]	12 (1.2–37)[a]	21	[9, 11, 22–27, 29–35, 44–48]
Elevated testosterone concentration (%)	100 (21/21)	21	
Serum DHEA-S concentration (μmol/L)[d]	2.9 (0.6–19.7)[a]	14	[9, 11, 23, 24, 26, 27, 29–32, 44, 45, 48]
Elevated DHEA-S concentration (%)	28 (5/18)	18	[9, 11, 23, 24, 26, 27, 29–34, 44–48]
Serum androstenedione concentration (nmol/L)[d]	35 (6.3–78)[a]	15	[9, 23–27, 29, 31–35, 44, 45]
Elevated androstenedione concentration (%)	88 (14/16)	16	[9, 23–27, 29, 31–35, 44, 45, 47]
Serum 17-OHP concentration (nmol/L)[d]	48 (1.8–312)[a]	16	[9, 11, 23–27, 29–32, 35, 44, 45, 48]
Elevated 17-OHP concentration (%)	81 (17/21)	21	[9, 11, 22–27, 29–35, 44–48]
Positive 17-OHP response after 1-24 ACTH stimulation (%)[e]	20 (2/10)	10	[11, 25, 27, 29–31, 33–35]
Hormonal co-secretion (hormones other than androgens) (%)	33 (7/21)	21	[9, 11, 22–27, 29–35, 44–48]
Cortisol	10 (2/21)		
Estradiol	14 (3/21)		
Estradiol and cortisol	10 (2/21)		

[a] Results expressed as median (range). [b] Age at diagnosis. [c] Largest dimension. If tumor size was not reported, the size of the affected ovary was used. [d] For results reported as "larger than X units", the value of X was used. For cases in which the diagnosis was delayed, the values at the age of diagnosis was used. Cases with no values reported (stated as "normal"), suspected errors in reporting units or unknown conversion factor to SI units were excluded. [e] Defined as positive if commented to be increased from baseline by authors and peak 17-OHP >30 nmol/L. Otherwise, it was arbitrarily defined an increase in 17-OHP, at either 30 min or 60 min after ACTH stimulation, by equal to or more than 100% of the basal value, and a peak value >30 nmol/L.

be small and difficult to be localized, often requiring a combination of imaging techniques and a high index of suspicion, and venous sampling was sometimes performed to locate the source of androgen secretion [5, 6, 9, 10]. In our case, both transabdominal ultrasound and CT scan showed an enlarged right ovary but were not able to demonstrate the presence of a discrete tumor mass arising from the right ovary. Transvaginal ultrasound and FDG PET–CT scan were required to reveal its presence. Multiple imaging modalities should be utilized for tumor localization when androgen-secreting ovarian tumors are suspected on clinical and biochemical grounds to facilitate subsequent treatment.

The patient had a number of features which were compatible with PCOS with its associated metabolic disturbances, including the presence of PCO morphology on ultrasound, diabetes mellitus, overweight and slightly high LH : FSH ratio of 2 (LH: 10.0 IU/L, FSH: 5.0 IU/L). Nevertheless, the presence of clitoromegaly, deepening of voice and the significantly elevated serum 17-OHP and androgen levels prompted us to consider alternative diagnoses. The presence of polycystic ovaries has been reported in a patient with an androgen-secreting SCT–NOS [11] and an androgen-secreting Sertoli–Leydig cell tumor [12]. In both cases, there were enlargement of the involved ovaries leading to gross asymmetry of bilateral ovarian sizes, similar to our case. PCO morphology on ultrasound is a non-specific finding representing an arrest of follicle development in the antral follicle stage that could be secondary to hyperinsulinemia and/or hyperandrogenism [13, 14]. Apart from hyperandrogenism, our patient also had clinical evidence of insulin resistance (overweight and diabetes mellitus), and both factors might have contributed to the development of the PCO morphology. On the other hand, PCO morphology could be seen in ovulating normal women without evidence of PCOS and may be inconsequential [15, 16]. It is uncertain whether the persistence of the PCO morphology in the left ovary of our patient postoperatively belonged to part of the spectrum of normal ovulating women or was associated with ongoing insulin resistance. The possibility of co-existing PCOS in this patient was unlikely in view of the resolution of hyperandrogenism and return of normal menstruation after removal of the ovarian tumor.

Steroid cell tumors (SCTs), also known as lipoid cell tumors, are rare ovarian tumors presumably of stromal cell origin and account for 0.1% of ovarian neoplasms [17]. SCTs are classified as Leydig cell tumours when cytoplasmic crystals of Reinke are identified, or when they have a hilar location, nuclear clustering, fibrinoid necrosis of vessels and have associated hilus cell hyperplasia. They are classified as steroid cell tumour, not otherwise specified (SCT–NOS) when lacking the above features. About 80% of SCTs fall into the NOS category [18]. The average age of diagnosis of SCT–NOS was 43 years old. Steroid cell tumours are solid and can range from yellow, orange, red to brown or black. Histologically, these tumours are composed of medium to large polygonal cells with abundant granular eosinophilic (lipid-poor) to pale vacuolated (lipid-rich) cytoplasm, round nuclei, prominent central nucleolus, and variable amounts of intracytoplasmic lipochrome pigment. Nuclear atypia and mitotic activity are rare. The cells are most commonly arranged in diffuse sheets, but can also be seen in nests and cords. The stroma is usually scant and can be oedematous, myxoid or fibromatous if present. Occasional calcification, necrosis and haemorrhage can be seen. About one-third of SCT–NOS exhibit malignant behaviour. Predictive features of malignant behaviour include size >7 cm, >2 mitoses/ 10 high-power fields (HPFs), necrosis, haemorrhage, and significant nuclear atypia [19]. For immunohistochemistry, steroid cell tumours are positive for sex cord–stromal markers including inhibin, calretinin, steroidogenic factor-1, and CD99. They are also usually positive for Melan-A and negative for S100 and FOXL2 [20]. Around half of SCT–NOS are androgen-secreting [19]. Less commonly, co-secretion of androgens, estradiol and/or cortisol can occur [21–27].

We reviewed the literature for the association of high 17-OHP levels and SCT–NOS. A PubMed search for cases of SCT–NOS in English using the search string ("steroid cell tumor" or "steroid cell tumour" or "lipoid cell tumor" or "lipoid cell tumour") was performed. A review of full texts for SCT–NOS with pre-treatment 17-OHP results identified a total of 21 such cases. One case was excluded from data analysis as it was associated with underlying poorly controlled NCCAH due to 21-hydroxylase deficiency [28] (see Table 3 for a summary and Supplementary Table S1 for details). Including our case, all 21 included cases presented with high serum total testosterone concentrations, although the clinical presentation of one case was that of isosexual precocious puberty with mildly elevated serum total testosterone in a 3-year-old girl rather than virilization [24]. Most cases were clinically non malignant (95%). 17 of the 21 cases (81%) presented with elevated 17-OHP levels. Elevation of androstenedione was also common (88%), In contrast, elevation of DHEA-S was uncommon (28%). Furthermore, 7 cases (33%) were associated with hormone co-secretion: 2 cases were associated with cortisol co-secretion [22, 29], 3 cases was associated with estradiol co-secretion[24, 26, 27], and 2 cases were associated with estradiol and cortisol co-secretion [23, 25]. All 7 cases of hormone co-secretion were associated with elevated 17-OHP levels. Among the 17 cases with elevated 17-OHP levels, 5 were initially diagnosed as NCCAH resulting in a delay in diagnosis [23, 26, 30–32]. ACTH stimulation test was performed in 10 cases (including the current case) with elevated baseline 17-OHP levels. No response or insignificant changes were seen in eight cases (80%), including the current case [11, 25, 27, 29, 33–35], while positive 17-OHP responses to ACTH stimulation were observed in two cases (20%) (see legend of Table 3 for the definition of a positive response) [30, 31]. The expression of ACTH receptor may explain the positive 17-OHP response to ACTH stimulation in the minority of cases of SCT–NOS, as the expression of ACTH receptor mRNA was demonstrated in the tumoral tissue of one reported case of SCT–NOS with slightly elevated 17-OHP but not in the ovarian control tissue, although no ACTH stimulation test was performed [24]. Similarly, both 17-OHP responsiveness [36] and non-responsiveness [37] to ACTH stimulation have been reported in virilizing ovarian Sertoli–Leydig cell tumors. Alternatively, it is possible that the 17-OHP levels in these cases were spuriously increased in response to ACTH stimulation due to cross-reactivity of immunoassays with cortisol and/or other cortisol precursors. Therefore, while a significant increase in 17-OHP in response to ACTH stimulation is typical of CAH [38], this may also be seen in ovarian tumors with 17-OHP hypersecretion, predisposing one to make a wrong diagnosis of CAH in these patients [30, 31].

11-oxopregnanetriol, also known as pregnanetriolone, is a metabolite of 21-deoxycortisol, which is an adrenal-specific metabolite produced by the enzymatic action of 11β-hydroxylase on 17-OHP [39, 40]. In both classical and non-classical forms of 21-hydroxylase deficiency, all three metabolites of 17-OHP (11-oxopregnanetriol, 17-hydroxypregnanolone and pregnanetriol) would be elevated [39, 41, 42]. In contrast, an ovarian source of 17-OHP is associated with the elevation of 17-hydroxypregnanolone and pregnanetriol only [43] (hereinafter referred to as "ovarian pattern"), as exemplified in a report of a 35-year-old woman with an androgen- and 17-OHP-secreting SCT–NOS, in which the 17-OHP concentration was 100.5 nmol/L [44]. It appears that the "ovarian pattern" of 17-OHP metabolism in USP was maintained even at such a high 17-OHP concentration without an "overflowing" of 17-OHP metabolism to the production of 11-oxopregnanetriol. Therefore, obtaining a USP in the investigation of female hyperandrogenism with elevated 17-OHP could be helpful in determining the source of 17-OHP excess (ovarian versus adrenal) and excluding NCCAH. Although unproven, the diagnostic accuracy of USP might theoretically be affected by the ectopic expression of 11β-hydroxylase in SCT–NOS, as demonstrated by the presence of its mRNA in one reported case [24]. Therefore, further studies are required to evaluate the diagnostic accuracy of this test in differentiating the origin of 17-OHP hypersecretion.

4. Conclusion

In summary, we have described a hormonally active ovarian SCT–NOS in a 24-year-old woman resulting in significant androgen excess, hypersecretion of 17-OHP with a negative response to ACTH stimulation and an "ovarian pattern" of metabolites of 17-OHP detected in the urine. The case required careful consideration of the clinical, biochemical and radiological data to clinch the correct diagnosis. A literature review revealed that 17-OHP hypersecretion is commonly seen in SCT–NOS and some patients with SCT–NOS were misdiagnosed as having CAH. Both ACTH stimulation test and USP are helpful biochemical tests to determine the cause of 17-OHP hypersecretion in these patients.

References

[1] A. H. Balen, J. S. E. Laven, S.-L. Tan, and D. Dewailly, "Ultrasound assessment of the polycystic ovary: international consensus definitions," *Human Reproduction Update*, vol. 9, no. 6, pp. 505–514, 2003.

[2] P. W. Speiser, W. Arlt, R. J. Auchus et al., "Congenital adrenal hyperplasia due to steroid 21-hydroxylase deficiency: an endocrine society clinical practice guideline," *Journal of Clinical Endocrinology & Metabolism*, vol. 103, no. 11, pp. 4043–4088, 2018.

[3] R. Azziz, L. A. Sanchez, E. S. Knochenhauer et al., "Androgen excess in women: experience with over 1000 consecutive patients," *Journal of Clinical Endocrinology & Metabolism*, vol. 89, no. 2, pp. 453–462, 2004.

[4] L. Moltz, H. Pickartz, R. Sörensen, U. Schwartz, and J. Hammerstein, "Ovarian and adrenal vein steroids in seven patients with androgen-secreting ovarian neoplasms: selective catheterization findings," *Fertility and Sterility*, vol. 42, no. 4, pp. 585–593, 1984.

[5] C. I. Friedman, G. E. Schmidt, M. H. Kim, and J. Powell, "Serum testosterone concentrations in the evaluation of androgen-producing tumors," *American Journal of Obstetrics and Gynecology*, vol. 153, no. 1, pp. 44–49, 1985.

[6] D. R. Meldrum and G. E. Abraham, "Peripheral and ovarian venous concentrations of various steroid hormones in virilizing ovarian tumors," *Obstetrics and Gynecology*, vol. 53, no. 1, pp. 36–43, 1979.

[7] D. Cavlan, N. Bharwani, and A. Grossman, "Androgen- and estrogen-secreting adrenal cancers," *Seminars in Oncology*, vol. 37, no. 6, pp. 638–648, 2010.

[8] F. Cordera, C. Grant, J. van Heerden, G. Thompson, and W. Young, "Androgen-secreting adrenal tumors," *Surgery*, vol. 134, no. 6, pp. 874–880, 2003.

[9] E. Cserepes, N. Szücs, P. Patkós et al., "Ovarian steroid cell tumor and a contralateral ovarian thecoma in a postmenopausal woman with severe hyperandrogenism," *Gynecological Endocrinology*, vol. 16, no. 3, pp. 213–216, 2002.

[10] A. J. Weiland, J. J. Bookstein, R. E. Cleary, and H. L. Judd, "Preoperative localization of virilizing tumors by selective venous sampling," *American Journal of Obstetrics and Gynecology*, vol. 131, no. 7, pp. 797–802, 1978.

[11] K. Kale, A. R. Chauhan, and S. Kalappa, "Virilization secondary to androgen-secreting tumor of the ovary: a report of three cases and review of literature," *The Journal of Obstetrics and Gynecology of India*, vol. 69, no. S1, pp. 56–59, 2019.

[12] S. Puzigaća, G. Prelević, Z. Svetenović, S. Djuricić, D. Kokan, and U. Radivojević, "Sertoli-Leydig cell tumour (arrhenoblastoma) in a patient with polycystic ovary syndrome: clinical, ultrasonographic, hormonal and histopathological evaluation," *Serbian Archives of Medicine*, vol. 129, no. Suppl 1, pp. 51–55, 2001.

[13] S. Franks, J. Stark, and K. Hardy, "Follicle dynamics and anovulation in polycystic ovary syndrome," *Human Reproduction Update*, vol. 14, no. 4, pp. 367–378, 2008.

[14] R. L. Rosenfield and D. A. Ehrmann, "The pathogenesis of polycystic ovary syndrome (PCOS): the hypothesis of pcos as functional ovarian hyperandrogenism revisited," *Endocrine Reviews*, vol. 37, no. 5, pp. 467–520, 2016.

[15] M. K. Murphy, J. E. Hall, J. M. Adams, H. Lee, and C. K. Welt, "Polycystic ovarian morphology in normal women does not predict the development of polycystic ovary syndrome," *Journal of Clinical Endocrinology & Metabolism*, vol. 91, no. 10, pp. 3878–3884, 2006.

[16] D. Dewailly, M. E. Lujan, E. Carmina et al., "Definition and significance of polycystic ovarian morphology: a task force report from the androgen excess and polycystic ovary syndrome society," *Human Reproduction Update*, vol. 20, no. 3, pp. 334–352, 2014.

[17] L. Qian, Z. Shen, X. Zhang, D. Wu, and Y. Zhou, "Ovarian steroid cell tumor, not otherwise specified: a case report and literature review," *Molecular and Clinical Oncology*, vol. 5, no. 6, pp. 839–841, 2016.

[18] M. Paraskevas and R. E. Scully, "Hilus cell tumor of the ovary. A clinicopathological analysis of 12 Reinke crystal-positive and nine crystal-negative cases," *International Journal of Gynecological Pathology*, vol. 8, no. 4, pp. 299–310, 1989.

[19] M. C. Hayes and R. E. Scully, "Ovarian steroid cell tumors (not otherwise specified). A clinicopathological analysis of 63 cases," *American Journal of Surgical Pathology*, vol. 11, no. 11, pp. 835–845, 1987.

[20] M. W. Jones, R. Harri, D. J. Dabbs, and G. J. Carter, "Immunohistochemical profile of steroid cell tumor of the ovary: a study of 14 cases and a review of the literature," *International Journal of Gynecological Pathology*, vol. 29, no. 4, pp. 315–320, 2010.

[21] J. Wan, X. Chen, and X. Li, "Ovarian steroid cell tumor, not otherwise specified: a rare case of postmenopausal vaginal bleeding Oncology," *Letters*, vol. 8, no. 3, pp. 1187–1189, 2014.

[22] L. Zang, M. Ye, G. Yang et al., "Accessory ovarian steroid cell tumor producing testosterone and cortisol," *Medicine (Baltimore)*, vol. 96, no. 37, Article ID e37998, 2017.

[23] P. Gupta, S. Goyal, L. Gonzalez-Mendoza et al., "Corticotropin-independent Cushing syndrome in a child with an ovarian tumor misdiagnosed as nonclassic congenital adrenal hyperplasia," *Endocrine Practice*, vol. 14, no. 7, pp. 875–879, 2008.

[24] C. J. Lin, A. A. Jorge, A. C. Latronico et al., "Origin of an ovarian steroid cell tumor causing isosexual pseudoprecocious puberty demonstrated by the expression of adrenal steroidogenic enzymes and adrenocorticotropin receptor," *Journal of Clinical Endocrinology & Metabolism*, vol. 85, no. 3, pp. 1211–1214, 2000.

[25] J. Imperato-McGinley, R. E. Peterson, M. Y. Dawood et al., "Steroid hormone secretion from a virilizing lipoid cell tumor of the ovary," *Obstetrics and Gynecology*, vol. 57, no. 4, pp. 525–531, 1981.

[26] H. Azizlerli, R. Tanakol, T. Terzioğlu, F. Alagöl, and F. Dizdaroglu, "Steroid cell tumor of the ovary as a rare cause of virilization," *Mount Sinai Journal of Medicine*, vol. 64, pp. 130–135, 1997.

[27] Correro P. Benavent, Valls M. Sáenz, Cano A. García, Mendiguchia L. Jiménez, Moreno E. Moreno, and M. Luque-Ramírez, "An unusual circulating steroid profile in a virilized postmenopausal woman," *Diagnosis (Berl)*, vol. 5, no. 2, pp. 83–87, 2018.

[28] T. T. Thomas, K. R. Ruscher, S. Mandavilli, F. Balarezo, and C. M. Finck, "Ovarian steroid cell tumor, not otherwise specified, associated with congenital adrenal hyperplasia: rare tumors of an endocrine disease," *Journal of Pediatric Surgery*, vol. 48, no. 6, pp. e23–e27, 2013.

[29] R. J. Chetkowski, H. L. Judd, P. I. Jagger, R. K. Nieberg, and R. J. Chang, "Autonomous cortisol secretion by a lipoid cell tumor of the ovary," *JAMA*, vol. 254, no. 18, pp. 2628–2631, 1985.

[30] S. Yılmaz-Ağladıoğlu, Ş. Savaş-Erdeve, E. Boduroğlu et al., "A girl with steroid cell ovarian tumor misdiagnosed as non-classical congenital adrenal hyperplasia," *Turkish Journal of Pediatrics*, vol. 55, no. 4, pp. 443–446, 2013.

[31] M. Dumic, V. Simunic, J. Ilic-Forko et al., "Extraovarian steroid cell tumor "not otherwise specified" as a rare cause of virilization in twelve-year-old girl," *Hormone Research Pediatrics*, vol. 55, no. 5, pp. 254–257, 2001.

[32] A. C. Harris, P. E. Wakely, P. B. Kaplowitz, and R. D. Lovinger, "Steroid cell tumor of the ovary in a child," *Archives of Pathology & Laboratory Medicine*, vol. 115, no. 2, pp. 150–154, 1991.

[33] I. Lambrinoudaki, N. Dafnios, A. Kondi-Pafiti et al., "A case of postmenopausal androgen excess," *Gynecological Endocrinology*, vol. 31, no. 10, pp. 760–764, 2015.

[34] D. Smith, T. B. Crotty, J. F. Murphy, M. E. Crofton, S. Franks, and T. J. McKenna, "A steroid cell tumor outside the ovary is a rare cause of virilization," *Fertility and Sterility*, vol. 85, no. 1, pp. 227.e13–227.e16, 2006.

[35] E. Y. Adashi, Z. Rosenwaks, P. A. Lee, G. S. Jones, and C. J. Migeon, "Endocrine features of an adrenal-like tumor of the ovary," *Journal of Clinical Endocrinology & Metabolism*, vol. 48, no. 2, pp. 241–245, 1979.

[36] D. Mango, P. Scirpa, M. Liberati, E. Menini, A. Fabiano, and S. Mancuso, "Ovarian and peripheral steroid hormones in a case of Sertoli-Leydig cell tumor," *Journal of Endocrinological Investigation*, vol. 11, no. 7, pp. 521–525, 1988.

[37] G. Amato, G. Izzo, and A. Izzo, "A paradoxical inhibition of androgenic hyperproduction by a Sertoli-Leydig cell tumour ovary," *Human Reproduction*, vol. 10, no. 11, pp. 2967–2969, 1995.

[38] M. I. New, F. Lorenzen, A. J. Lerner et al., "Genotyping steroid 21-hydroxylase deficiency: hormonal reference data," *The Journal of Clinical Endocrinology & Metabolism*, vol. 57, no. 2, pp. 320–326, 1983.

[39] G. Rumsby and G. M. Woodward, *Disorders of Steroidogenesis: Guide to Steroid Profiling and Biochemical Diagnosis*, Springer, Berlin, Germany, 2018.

[40] J. Fiet, J.-M. Villette, H. Galons et al., "The application of a new highly-sensitive radioimmunoassay for plasma 21-deoxycortisol to the detection of steroid-21-hydroxylase deficiency," *Annals of Clinical Biochemistry*, vol. 31, no. 1, pp. 56–64, 1994.

[41] J. Honour, "Biochemical aspects of congenital adrenal hyperplasia," *Journal of Inherited Metabolic Disease*, vol. 9, no. Suppl 1, pp. 124–134, 1986.

[42] J. W. Honour and C. G. D. Brook, "Clinical indications for the use of urinary steroid profiles in neonates and children," *Annals of Clinical Biochemistry*, vol. 34, no. 1, pp. 45–54, 1997.

[43] J. W. Honour, "17-Hydroxyprogesterone in children, adolescents, and adults," *Annals of Clinical Biochemistry*, vol. 51, no. 4, pp. 424–440, 2014.

[44] J. W. Stephens, A. Fielding, R. Verdaguer, and O. Freites, "A steroid-cell tumor of the ovary resulting in massive androgen excess early in the gonadol steroidogenic pathway," *Gynecological Endocrinology*, vol. 24, no. 3, pp. 151–153, 2008.

[45] J. Lee, V. S. John, S. X. Liang, C. A. D'Agostino, and A. W. Menzin, "Metastatic malignant ovarian steroid cell tumor: a case report and review of the literature," *Case Reports in Obstetrics and Gynecology*, vol. 2016, Article ID 6184573, 5 pages, 2016.

[46] M. Varras, T. Vasilakaki, E. Skafida, and C. Akrivis, "Clinical, ultrasonographic, computed tomography and histopathological manifestations of ovarian steroid cell tumour, not otherwise specified: our experience of a rare case with female virilisation and review of the literature," *Gynecological Endocrinology*, vol. 27, no. 6, pp. 412–418, 2011.

[47] G. Boyraz, I. Selcuk, Z. Yusifli, A. Usubutun, and S. Gunalp, "Steroid cell tumor of the ovary in an adolescent: a rare case report," *Case Reports in Medicine*, vol. 2013, Article ID 527698, 3 pages, 2013.

[48] J. Swain, S. Sharma, V. Prakash, N. K. Agrawal, and S. K. Singh, "Steroid cell tumor: a rare cause of hirsutism in a female," *Endocrinology, Diabetes & Metabolism Case Reports*, vol. 2013, 2013.

43

Hyperparathyroidism Jaw Tumor Syndrome Presenting as Recurrent Femur Fractures in a Young Woman: A Rare Presentation of a Rare Disease

Piyumi S. A. Wijewickrama and Noel P. Somasundaram

Endocrinology Unit, National Hospital of Sri Lanka, Colombo, Sri Lanka

Correspondence should be addressed to Piyumi S. A. Wijewickrama; psw8624@gmail.com

Academic Editor: Carlo Capella

Background. Primary hyperparathyroidism usually occurs secondary to parathyroid adenoma, multiglandular hyperplasia, or parathyroid carcinoma. The patients usually present with incidentally discovered high calcium level and systemic or skeletal manifestations. In young patients with primary hyperparathyroidism, familial syndromes including multiple endocrine neoplasia types 1, 2, and 4 and hyperparathyroidism jaw tumor syndrome should be considered. *Case Description.* We present a case of a 22-year-old Sri Lankan woman who presented with femur fractures in a background of childhood nephroblastoma and maxillary fibro-osseous tumor. The patient had biochemical parameters suggestive of primary hyperparathyroidism with a parathyroid mass. The histology following excision of the mass revealed a parathyroid adenoma. Based on the associated clinical manifestations, hyperparathyroidism jaw tumor syndrome was suspected, and genetic studies reported a positive CDC73 mutation with a whole-gene deletion of exon 1–17. *Conclusion.* Hyperparathyroidism jaw tumor syndrome is an important diagnosis to consider in a young patient presenting with classic clinical features due to the risk of malignancy, familial involvement, and need to monitor for progressive systemic manifestations. As this is a rare disease, it can often be missed due to low degree of suspicion and the ability of the jaw tumor to mimic a metastatic deposit.

1. Background

The most common presentation of primary hyperparathyroidism (PHPT) is asymptomatic hypercalcemia, which is incidentally detected in 80% of the patients [1]. PHPT was first described about 90 years ago when the patients presented with classic symptoms depicted by "bones, stones, abdominal groans, and psychic moans," describing skeletal manifestations, nephrolithiasis, constipation and abdominal pain, and confusion [2]. While nephrolithiasis and skeletal manifestations are a direct result of excess parathyroid hormone (PTH) levels, anorexia, nausea, constipation, polydipsia, and polyuria are caused by hypercalcemia [3].

The skeletal manifestations are mainly due to reduced bone mineral density (BMD), which is more remarkable in the cortical bones such as forearm and hip than in the trabecular bones. The risk of hip fractures due to primary hyperparathyroidism has contrasting evidence. A large population-based cohort study carried out in Sweden with 19 years of follow-up revealed an increased risk of hip fractures in men but not in women [4]. Another population-based study showed a significantly increase in risks of vertebral, Colles', rib, and pelvic fractures in PHPT patients, but proximal femur fractures showed only a marginal rise in these patients, with female gender and increasing age identified as risk factors [5].

PHPT occurs mainly due to benign parathyroid adenoma in 80%, while multiglandular parathyroid hyperplasia contributing to 15–20% and parathyroid carcinoma to 0.5% [3]. The majority of PHPT patients present at the age of 55 to 60 years, and incidence among females is twice that of males [6]. In a young patient presenting with PHPT, familial syndromes including multiple endocrine neoplasia (MEN 1), MEN 2, MEN 4, and hyperparathyroidism jaw tumor syndrome (HPT-JT), familial isolated hyperparathyroidism should be looked for, which contribute to around 10% of PHPT cases [7].

HPT-JT is an autosomal dominant syndrome with incomplete penetrance. The patients present with parathyroid tumors, ossifying fibromas of jaw, and a variety of renal and uterine tumors [8, 9]. This is due to mutation of CDC73 tumor suppression gene, which encodes the protein named Parafibromin, which is responsible for the cell cycle arrest [8]. This is an exceedingly rare syndrome where a total of about 100 index cases of CDC73 mutation carriers have been identified to date, without a clear correlation between genotype and phenotype [7]. HPT-JT patients present with parathyroid carcinoma or adenoma at an earlier age of onset with a mean age of 33 years, and they are particularly at a higher risk of developing parathyroid carcinoma.

We report a case of a young female presented with recurrent low trauma femur fractures, with a significant past history of Wilms' tumor and maxillary tumor, who was ultimately diagnosed to have HPT-JT syndrome.

2. Case Description

A 22-year-old Sri Lankan woman was referred from the orthopedics unit to the endocrinology unit, National Hospital of Sri Lanka, for further evaluation of recurrent femur fractures. She first experienced a right sided subtrochanteric fracture following a low trauma injury at the age of 20 years (Figure 1), for which she underwent internal fixation. Thereafter, she experienced a left intertrochanteric femur fracture at the age of 22 years, 2 months prior to the current presentation.

She had an interesting past medical history. She was diagnosed to have a left side nephroblastoma at the age of 8 years, for which she underwent left side radical nephrectomy followed by chemotherapy. Thereafter, at the age of 14 years, she developed a right sided facial swelling and was found to have a maxillary tumor which was described during the surgery as a well-circumscribed mass lesion in the left maxilla, eroding the anterior wall of maxilla and lateral nasal wall. She underwent partial maxillectomy for this, and histology revealed features suggestive of fibrous dysplasia.

She did not have a history of chronic steroid use, hypogonadism, hyperthyroidism, rheumatoid arthritis, and exposure to cigarette smoking to suggest secondary causes for osteoporosis. She had neither any features of malabsorption nor inadequate exposure to sunlight to suggest a vitamin D deficiency causing these fractures. The histology of bone biopsies was negative for metastatic deposits.

She did not have a family history of hyperparathyroidism, renal, or uterine tumors. There was no past history or family history suggestive of MEN 1. Her general and systemic examinations were normal apart from the healing fracture sites.

Her investigation findings are summarized in Table 1.

Her investigations revealed high total calcium and urinary calcium excretion, with low serum phosphate level. She was found to have a vitamin D deficiency, which was corrected by vitamin D replacement. As high calcium and low phosphate were suggestive of a primary hyperparathyroidism, intact parathyroid hormone (PTH) was done after correcting vitamin D level, which was found to be very high at 1025 pg/ml (10–65 pg/ml), confirming the diagnosis of hyperparathyroidism.

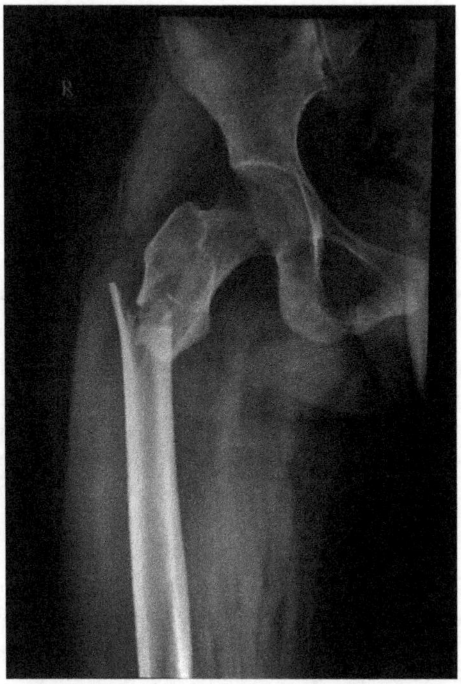

Figure 1: X-ray showing the right subtrochanteric fracture.

Table 1: Summary of investigations.

Investigations	Results	Normal range
Total calcium	3.57 mmol/l	(2.2–2.7)
Serum phosphate	0.55 mmol/l	(1.12–1.45)
Urine calcium excretion	10.8 mmol/l/24 h	(2.5–6.26)
Urine phosphate excretion	21.42 mmol/l/ 24 h	(12.9–4.2)
Serum alkaline phosphatase level	1633 μ/l	
Serum 25(OH) vitamin D level	7.51 μ/l	
Thyroid stimulating hormone	1.85 mIU/l	(0.4–4)
Free T4 level	0.99 ng/dl	(0.7–1.9)

Her left forearm dexa scan revealed osteoporosis with a Z score of −5.6, suggestive of active chronic hyperparathyroidism, leading to bone resorption and reduced bone mineral density with preferential involvement of cortical bone and increased risk of fracture [10].

Three-dimensional computed tomography (CT) of neck was carried out for localization, which revealed a 2.5 × 2.9 cm well-defined rounded mass with avid contrast enhancement posteroinferior to the left lobe of the thyroid gland, suggestive of a parathyroid mass (Figure 2). Nuclear imaging was not done as the facility was not available at our setting.

At this point, due to the constellation of nephroblastoma, maxillary tumor, and primary hyperparathyroidism with a

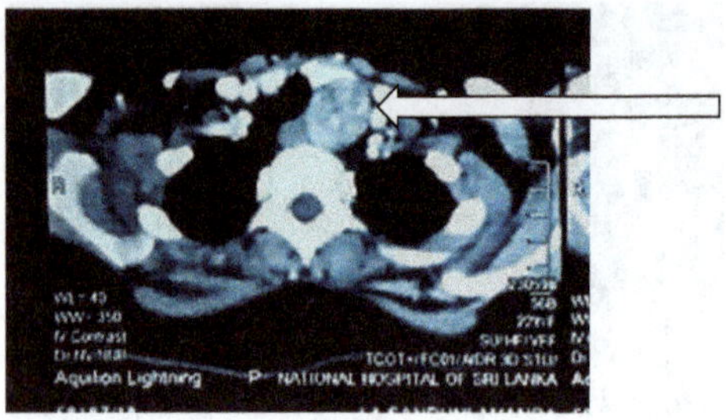

FIGURE 2: CT neck showing the left side parathyroid mass.

parathyroid mass, a possibility of hyperparathyroidism jaw tumor syndrome was suspected although a suggestive family history was not there. Therefore, the genetic studies were carried out via target region capture followed by next generation sequencing, using a specific indel detection tool, which revealed a positive CDC73 mutation with a large deletion of exon 1–17. This mutation was verified by reverse transcription polymerase chain reaction (RT-PCR), where exons 1, 10, and 17 were selected for verification. This confirmed the diagnosis of hyperparathyroidism jaw tumor syndrome (Table 2). MEN 1 and calcium sensitive receptor mutations were negative.

The patient underwent subtotal thyroidectomy with parathyroidectomy with removal of left lower parathyroid mass, which was a smooth, round, well-demarcated mass (Figure 3), and the remaining parathyroid glands were atrophied.

Immediate postoperative PTH level was reduced by more than 50%–76 pg/ml, suggesting successful removal of the parathyroid mass. The histology revealed encapsulated parathyroid adenoma composed of a proliferation of polygonal cells separated by fibrovascular septa, with round to ovoid nuclei with dispersed chromatin and inconspicuous nucleoli and moderate eosinophilic cytoplasm. Mitoses were rare, and there were also cystic areas. There was no evidence of vascular invasion, necrosis, or invasion into soft tissues of thyroid gland. These features were compatible with a parathyroid adenoma.

Currently, the patient is on calcium and calcitriol treatment and being followed up with serum calcium and phosphate levels with monitoring of urinary calcium excretion. Her imaging of the abdomen did not reveal a recurrence of nephroblastoma or uterine tumors. Biochemical screening of family members was negative, and genetic screening is underway.

3. Discussion

This case depicts a rare presentation of a rare disease. The typical initial presentation of individuals with HPT-JT is reported to be jaw and teeth deformities as a result of ossifying fibromas of mandible or maxilla [9]. In contrast, this patient's initial clinical manifestation was a nephroblastoma developed during childhood. Renal manifestations, including renal cysts, hamartoma, and nephroblastoma (Wilms' tumor), are well described but rare manifestations of HPT-JT syndrome. Wilms' tumors have been described in less than 3% of patients with the mutation, and despite a through literature survey, we did not come across cases where nephroblastoma has presented as the initial manifestation of HPT-JT syndrome as in this case [9, 11, 12].

TABLE 2: Characteristics of positive CDC73 mutation.

Gene	Nucleic acid alteration	Mutation location	Type
CDC73	EX 1–17 DEL	EX 1–17/CDS 1–17	Heterozygous

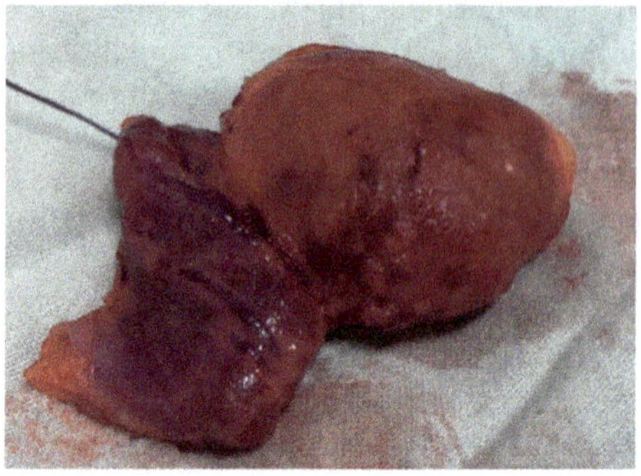

FIGURE 3: Macroscopic appearance of the excised parathyroid mass with hemithyroidectomy.

Ossifying fibromas of the jaw, which this patient developed as the second manifestation of the disease at the age of 14 years, is a well-described manifestation of HPT-JT syndrome, which is shown to occur in 50% of these patients, usually in the adolescent age [9, 11]. These are benign lesions which demonstrate locally invasive features. The distinction from brown tumors should be done histologically, and these lesions reveal features of fibrous dysplasia as seen in this patient. In this patient, as the maxillary tumor developed following the nephroblastoma, malignant metastatic deposit was suspected, which was excluded by histology. This sequence of clinical manifestations may have led to a delay in diagnosis as well.

The primary manifestation of hyperparathyroidism in this patient was bilateral low trauma femur fractures, which could have been contributed by the coexisting vitamin D deficiency. Vitamin D deficiency is known to be more prevalent among patients with primary hyperparathyroidism, due to multiple possible underlying mechanisms, such as increased conversion of 25-hydroxy vitamin D to 1,25-dihydroxy vitamin D and increased hepatic inactivation of 25-hydroxy vitamin D level [2, 13]. Therefore, patients with coexistent severe vitamin D deficiency usually have more biochemically and clinically severe PHPT as seen in our patient. Although parathyroid carcinomas have been reported relatively frequently in HPT-JT patients, our patient's histology was suggestive of a parathyroid adenoma. As HPT-JT syndrome patients are known to be susceptible for parathyroid carcinoma as well as high rate of recurrence of parathyroid disease, this patient warrants a close follow-up with frequent monitoring [14].

With regard to the types of CDC73 mutations reported in the literature, the majority of CDC73 mutations are frameshift, nonsense, and missense variants, as well as small deletions and insertions [7]. In contrast, our patient had a whole-gene deletion of exons 1–17 of CDC73 gene, which is reported infrequently in the literature [14–16]. In fact, gross deletions are reported only in 1% of the cases of CDC73 mutations, which makes this case more significant [15, 17].

Our patient's atypical sequence of clinical manifestations with initial development being a nephroblastoma prompted the clinicians to suspect metastatic deposits at each of subsequent developments of maxillary tumors and femur fractures, deviating them from considering this familial syndrome for several years, which contributed to a delay in diagnosis of the condition.

4. Conclusion

HPT-JT syndrome, although rare, is an important diagnosis to consider, especially in young patients presenting with classical constellation of clinical manifestations of parathyroid tumor, maxillary or mandibular tumors, and renal or uterine tumors, due to its risk of malignancy and importance of family screening. It needs close monitoring for new developments. The above case highlights an atypical presentation of this rare disease, which presented with nephroblastoma as the first clinical manifestations. Furthermore, this case is significant as the patient carries a rare type of mutation of a whole-gene deletion from exons 1–17 of CDC73 gene. To the best of our knowledge, this is the first genetically confirmed HPT-JT syndrome case reported from Sri Lanka.

References

[1] S. J. Silverberg and J. P. Bilezikian, "Evaluation and management of primary hyperparathyroidism," *The Journal of Clinical Endocrinology & Metabolism*, vol. 81, no. 6, pp. 2036–2040, 1996.

[2] M. D. Walker and S. J. Silverberg, "Primary hyperparathyroidism," *Nature Reviews Endocrinology*, vol. 14, no. 2, pp. 115–125, 2018.

[3] J. P. Bilezikian, M. L. Brandi, M. Rubin et al., "Primary hyperparathyroidism: new concepts in clinical, densitometric and biochemical features," *Journal of Internal Medicine*, vol. 257, no. 1, pp. 6–17, 2005.

[4] K. Larsson, S. Ljunghall, U. B. Krusemo, T. Naessén, E. Lindh, and I. Persson, "The risk of hip fractures in patients with primary hyperparathyroidism: a population-based cohort study with a follow-up of 19 years," *Journal of Internal Medicine*, vol. 234, no. 6, pp. 585–593, 1993.

[5] S. Khosla, L. J. Melton III, R. A. Wermers, C. S. Crowson, W. M. O'Fallon, and B. L. Riggs, "Primary hyperparathyroidism and the risk of fracture: a population-based study," *Journal of Bone and Mineral Research*, vol. 14, no. 10, pp. 1700–1707, 1999.

[6] M. L. Griebeler, A. E. Kearns, E. Ryu, M. A. Hathcock, L. J. Melton III, and R. A. Wermers, "Secular trends in the incidence of primary hyperparathyroidism over five decades (1965–2010)," *Bone*, vol. 7, pp. 1–7, 2015.

[7] K. Van Der Tuin, C. M. J. Tops, M. A. Adank et al., "CDC73-related disorders: clinical manifestations and case detection in primary hyperparathyroidism," *The Journal of Clinical Endocrinology & Metabolism*, vol. 102, no. 12, pp. 4534–4540, 2017.

[8] G. Masi, L. Barzon, M. Iacobone et al., "Clinical , genetic , and histopathologic investigation of CDC73-related familial hyperparathyroidism," *Endocrine Related Cancer*, vol. 15, no. 4, pp. 1115–1126, 2008.

[9] H. du Preez, A. Adams, P. Richards, and S. Whitley, "Hyperparathyroidism jaw tumour syndrome: a pictoral review," *Insights Into Imaging*, vol. 7, no. 6, pp. 793–800, 2016.

[10] K. Wood, S. Dhital, H. Chen, and R. S. Sippel, "What is the utility of distal forearm DXA in primary hyperparathyroidism?" *The Oncologist*, vol. 17, no. 3, pp. 322–325, 2012.

[11] M. R. Hobbs, A. R. Pole, G. N. Pidwirny et al., "Hyperparathyroidism-jaw tumor syndrome: the HRPT2 locus is within a 0.7-cM region on chromosome 1q," *The American Journal of Human Genetics*, vol. 64, no. 2, pp. 518–525, 1999.

[12] R. H. Scott, C. A. Stiller, L. Walker, and N. Rahman, "Syndromes and constitutional chromosomal abnormalities associated with Wilms tumour," *Journal of Medical Genetics*, vol. 43, no. 9, pp. 705–715, 2006.

[13] B. Moosgaard, P. Vestergaard, L. Heickendorff, F. Melsen, P. Christiansen, and L. Mosekilde, "Vitamin D status, seasonal variations, parathyroid adenoma weight and bone mineral density in primary hyperparathyroidism," *Clinical Endocrinology*, vol. 63, no. 5, pp. 506–513, 2005.

[14] A. Mehta, D. Patel, A. Rosenberg, M. Boufraqech, W. F. Simonds, and E. Kebebew, *NIH Public Access*, vol. 156, no. 6, pp. 1315–1325, 2015.

[15] J. C. Rubinstein, S. K. Majumdar, W. Laskin et al., "Hyperparathyroidism-jaw tumor syndrome associated with large-scale 1q31 deletion," *Journal of the Endocrine Society*, vol. 1, no. 7, pp. 926–930, 2017.

[16] R. Domingues, R. A. Tomaz, C. Martins, C. Nunes, and M. Joa, "Identification of the first germline HRPT2 whole-gene deletion in a patient with primary hyperparathyroidism," *Clinical Endocrinology*, vol. 76, no. 1, pp. 33–38, 2012.

[17] L. A. Muscarella, D. Turchetti, A. Fontana et al., "Large deletion at the CDC73 gene locus and search for predictive markers of the presence of a CDC73 genetic lesion," *Oncotarget*, vol. 9, no. 29, pp. 20721–20733, 2018.

44

Ketogenic Weight Loss Diet Rapidly Unmasks an Insulinoma

Erin Meier[1] **Lydia Winnicka**[2] **Michael Lau**[2] **Duc Vo**[3] **Alla Joutovsky,**[3] **and Mangalore Amith Shenoy**[2]

[1]*Department of Internal Medicine, NYU Winthrop, USA*
[2]*Department of Pulmonary and Critical Care Medicine, NYU Winthrop, USA*
[3]*Department of Pathology and Laboratory Medicine, NYU Winthrop, USA*

Correspondence should be addressed to Erin Meier; erin.meier@nyulangone.org

Academic Editor: J. Paul Frindik

The ketogenic diet, a diet high in fat and extremely low in carbohydrates, has recently gained momentum and is increasingly employed by patients in order to lose weight. We report a case of an otherwise healthy 47-year-old male who developed seizures and hypoglycemia shortly after initiating this diet. Biochemical testing confirmed hyperinsulinemic hypoglycemia and a subsequent abdomen MRI showed a pancreatic mass. The tumor was ultimately excised with pathology confirming an insulinoma. It was felt that his abrupt decrease in carbohydrate consumption led to the rapid unmasking of this tumor.

1. Introduction

The ketogenic diet is increasingly employed by the general public in order to lose weight. A standard ketogenic diet is typically very high in fat, with 65%–75% of calories coming from fat, and extremely low in carbohydrates, with 5%–10% of calories coming from carbohydrates. By significantly restricting carbohydrate intake, blood glucose and insulin levels drop, and the body's response is to use an alternate fuel source, namely fat, which can then lead to desired weight loss. Insulinomas are rare pancreatic tumors that pathologically secrete insulin and can cause significant hypoglycemia. We present a case of a 47-year-old male who began the ketogenic diet and within 1 week, developed severe hypoglycemia with eventual diagnosis of an insulinoma.

2. Case Report

A 47-year-old Hispanic male, with a BMI of 38 and no past medical history, presented to the Emergency Department (ED) with seizure activity. One-week prior, he had initiated a ketogenic diet in an attempt to lose weight. Prior to that, he did not follow any specific diet. He began predominantly consuming red meat, dairy, and eggs, and completely cut out grains, fruits, soda and juice. His goal was to consume as few carbohydrates as possible. During this time, he began to feel more weak and tired, but otherwise had no specific complaints. On the day of the presentation, he felt weaker and lay down to rest. His wife then observed him to become unresponsive and have rhythmic jerking movements, consistent with seizure activity. On arrival to the ED, he was lethargic but had normal vital signs and was saturating well on room air. He was found to have a glucose level of 42 mg/dL. His symptoms quickly improved with dextrose. Insulin level on presentation was 87.9 uIU/mL, with a c-peptide level of 8.9 ng/mL and a beta-hydroxybutyrate level of 0.06 mmol/L. Insulin antibody was negative. Given there was concern for an insulinoma, he underwent a prolonged fasting test, which confirmed the diagnosis of hyperinsulinemic hypoglycemia. Two hours into fasting, he felt lightheaded and was found to have a glucose level of 38 mg/dL, however, he had received intravenous dextrose two hours before. As it was difficult to maintain safe serum glucose levels whenever the dextrose infusion was stopped, he received multiple doses of diazoxide. Twenty-four hours after the dextrose infusion was stopped and the last dose of diazoxide was given, he began a second prolonged fasting test. Five hours after initiation, he became symptomatic with a glucose level of 56 mg/dL and a corresponding insulin level of 16.1 uIu/mL. Whipple's triad was documented at this time. Subsequently, a contrast-enhanced MRI of the abdomen and pelvis was done and revealed a 2.2×1.5 cm mass in the pancreatic neck/body, compatible with a neuroendocrine tumor (Figure 1).

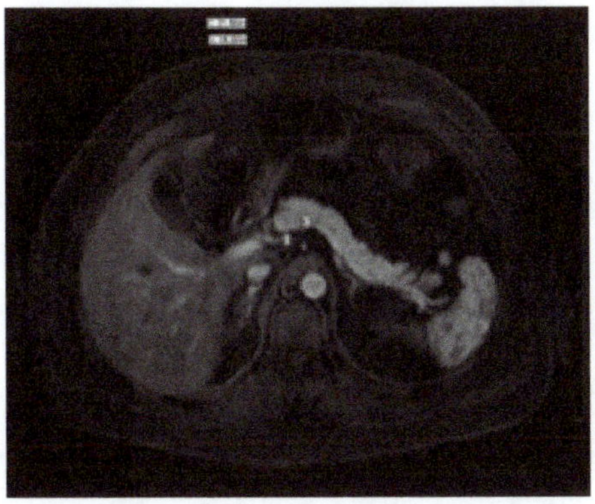

FIGURE 1: Magnetic resonance imaging T1 early arterial phase with arrow indicating mass.

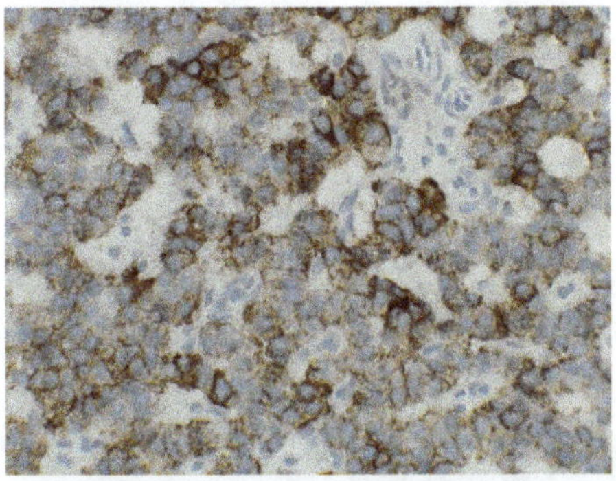

FIGURE 2: Neoplastic cells with positive cytoplasm stain for insulin, indicating an insulinoma.

Given prior biochemical testing, an insulinoma was felt very likely. Surgical enucleation of the mass was performed during hospital admission. Gross pathology revealed a 2 × 1.7 × 1.5 cm encapsulated mass with central hemorrhage. Light microscopy showed neoplastic cells with a trabecular architecture and a salt-and-pepper nuclear pattern, typical of neuroendocrine tumors. The neoplastic cells had a positive cytoplasmic stain for insulin (Figure 2).

In the post-operative period, he had no further episodes of hypoglycemia. Glucose levels remained between 70 and 120 mg/dL while in the hospital. No post-operative insulin level was obtained. At two months follow up, he again remained asymptomatic with no episodes of hypoglycemia.

3. Discussion

There has recently been increased public interest in a ketogenic diet as a means of weight loss. Originally proposed as a therapy for epilepsy, ketogenic diets have since been used in order to maintain or lose weight. Currently, the Obesity Medicine Association endorses a low or very-low carbohydrate diet as one option for weight loss [1]. The main tenant of this diet is that when carbohydrates are severely restricted, the body will enter a state of ketosis and will break down fat as a fuel source, which will lead to weight loss. In order to enter ketosis, blood glucose levels must decrease and glycogen stores must be depleted [2]. In the absence of glucose to trigger the release of insulin, insulin levels should then decrease. This combination will force the body into ketogenesis, which will convert fatty acids into ketones, namely acetate, acetoacetate, and beta-hydroxybutyrate, to use as an alternate fuel source. While on a strict ketogenic diet, insulin levels should be very low. Our patient had a pathological condition where his insulin levels were actually very elevated. As insulin halts the utilization of fat as fuel, he developed hypoglycemia abruptly upon eliminating carbohydrates from his diet. He was thus unable to utilize either glucose or fat as an energy source [3]. His beta-hydroxybutyrate level on admission was normal, indicating he had not been able to reach a state of ketosis, due to pathologically high insulin levels. Prior to initiating this diet, he did not have any apparent episodes of symptomatic hypoglycemia. He had presumably never restricted his carbohydrate intake before this point though.

Insulinomas are rare, insulin-secreting pancreatic tumors, with an incidence of approximately 1–4 per one million [4]. Though the biochemical diagnosis of an insulinoma is straightforward, there is a median duration of symptoms prior to diagnosis of 1.5 years, due to the often nonspecific presentation [5]. The symptoms of insulinomas, namely that of hypoglycemia, include confusion, diaphoresis, palpitations, and seizures. These symptoms may be attributed to other causes initially, and can lead to a delay in diagnosis. Once an insulinoma is considered, diagnostic criteria includes a prolonged fasting test, followed by imaging to localize the tumor [4]. The prolonged fasting test can detect up to 99% of insulinomas and must be performed in a controlled setting such as an intensive care unit [6]. Insulin levels, C-peptide levels, and glucose levels are measured once the patient experiences symptoms of hypoglycemia. Unfortunately, the first prolonged fasting test that our patient underwent was complicated by the fact that he had received intravenous dextrose within two hours of symptom onset. As reactive hyperinsulinemia resulting in hypoglycemia could not be ruled out, it was necessary to give diazoxide to our patient to inhibit insulin release, in order to allow discontinuation of any dextrose infusion. Diazoxide, which has both a hyperglycemic effect and lowers insulin levels, is commonly used as medical therapy in patients who are not surgical candidates or who refuse surgery. Other medical options include somatostatin analogs, which at high doses inhibit the secretion of insulin [7]. Our patient's second prolonged fasting test ended with a blood glucose of 56 mg/dL and insulin level of 16.1 uIU/mL. Although an insulin level of 16 uIU/mL can fall within the normal range, a glucose level of less than 50 mg/dL should result in a much lower insulin level, around 6 uIU/mL [7].

It is unclear how long our patient had an insulinoma, or when it would have been discovered, had he not started the ketogenic diet. Our patient did not retrospectively identify any symptoms of hypoglycemia, as most patients with insulinomas do. We believe his decision to begin the ketogenic diet directly led to the rapid diagnosis of his tumor. Understanding the physiology of the ketogenic diet led us to quickly suspect an insulinoma as the most likely diagnosis. Our case is the first to our knowledge of a ketogenic diet rapidly unmasking an insulinoma and illustrates the importance of taking a thorough history and understanding the physiologic implications of different popular diets.

4. Conclusion

The premise of the ketogenic diet is that with low carbohydrate intake, the body will convert fat into fatty acids and use ketone bodies as energy, which can lead to weight loss. However, if insulin levels are high, then fat cannot be converted into energy and the body will not be able to reach a state of ketosis. After beginning the ketogenic diet, due to the presence of an insulinoma, our patient was unable to utilize either glucose or fat as energy. He therefore quickly developed symptomatic hypoglycemia and presented to the ED with seizures. Though hypoglycemia can occur in all persons on carbohydrate-restricted diets, the ketogenic diet has a much greater carbohydrate restriction, and therefore more often leads to hypoglycemia. This, coupled with a previously undiagnosed insulinoma, lead to rapid symptom unmasking. Understanding the physiology of the ketogenic diet helped to make a prompt diagnosis of an insulinoma in our patient.

References

[1] H. E. Bays, W. McCarthy, S. Christensen et al., "Obesity Algorithm Slides, presented by the Obesity Medicine Association," 2019, https://obesitymedicine.org/obesity-algorithm/.

[2] A. Adam-Perrot, P. Clifton, and F. Brouns, "Low-carbohydrate diets: nutritional and physiological aspects," *Obesity Reviews*, vol. 7, no. 1, pp. 49–58, 2006.

[3] O. Owen, "Ketone bodies as a fuel for the brain during starvation," *Biochemistry and Molecular Biology Education*, vol. 33, no. 4, pp. 246–251, 2006.

[4] T. Okabayashi, Y. Shima, and T. Sumiyoshi, "Diagnosis and management of insulinoma," *World Journal of Gastroenterology*, vol. 19, no. 6, pp. 829–837, 2013.

[5] F. J. Service, M. M. McMahon, P. C. O'brien, and D. J. Ballard, "Functioning insulinoma—incidence, recurrence, and long-term survival of patients: a 60-year study," *Mayo Clinic Proceedings*, vol. 66, no. 7, pp. 711–719, 1991.

[6] J. Service and N. Natt, "The prolonged fast," *The Journal of Clinical Endocrinology & Metabolism*, vol. 85, no. 11, pp. 3973–3974, 2000.

[7] J. J. Shin, P. Gorden, and S. K. Libutti, "Insulinoma: pathophysiology, localization and management management," *Future Oncology*, vol. 6, no. 2, pp. 229–237, 2010.

45

Effect of Vandetanib Treatment on Cystic Changes in the Liver following Metastasis from Medullary Thyroid Carcinoma

Ai Matsui, Soji Toda, Daisuke Murayama, and Hiroyuki Iwasaki

Department of Breast and Endocrine Surgery, Kanagawa Cancer Center, Yokohama, Japan

Correspondence should be addressed to Ai Matsui; a-matsui@kcch.jp

Academic Editor: Osamu Isozaki

A number of causes are responsible for the development of cystic lesions in the liver. However, metastasis is a rare cause, and cystic metastasis from medullary thyroid carcinoma has not yet been reported. A 46-year-old Japanese man presented to our hospital with a mass in the left side of his neck. Neck and thyroid ultrasonography revealed a thyroid tumor with calcification and enlarged cervical lymph nodes. He had a family history of medullary thyroid cancer. Computed tomography revealed a tumor in the thyroid and multiple cysts in the liver. Total thyroidectomy with modified neck and upper mediastinum dissections were performed. After surgery, vandetanib treatment was initiated owing to tumor progression; following this, the liver cysts increased in size, abdominal distension appeared, and serum liver enzyme levels were found to be elevated. Percutaneous liver cyst puncture was performed to reduce abdominal distension; however, it was ineffective. The liver enzyme levels improved after replacing vandetanib with lenvatinib treatment. The liver cysts in this case were indicated to be associated with medullary thyroid carcinoma.

1. Introduction

Medullary thyroid carcinoma (MTC) accounts for 3%–5% of all thyroid malignancies [1, 2]. Approximately 75% of MTC cases are sporadic, while the remaining 25% are hereditary [2]. Metastases to the liver occur in 45% of patients with advanced MTC [1]; however, to the best of our knowledge, cystic metastasis from MTC has not been reported previously. Here, we report the case of MTC with liver cysts that increased in size during vandetanib treatment.

2. Case Presentation

A 46-year-old Japanese man presented to our hospital with a mass in his left neck. He had a palpable nodule in the thyroid and palpable left cervical lymph nodes. His anamnesis revealed irritable bowel syndrome. He had no previous history of thyroid disease or other endocrinopathy but had a family history of thyroid cancer; his mother and maternal uncle had thyroid cancer and pheochromocytoma, and a maternal cousin had MTC. Rearranged during Transfection (RET) mutation analysis was positive, and he was determined as having a RET mutation at codon 634 in exon 11.

Ultrasonography of the neck and thyroid revealed a thyroid tumor with calcification and enlarged cervical lymph nodes. Serum carcinoembryonic antigen (CEA) and calcitonin levels were 2,540 ng/ml and 35,100 pg/ml, respectively. Computed tomography scans revealed a 2.5 cm × 3.5 cm thyroid tumor and multiple cysts in the liver. Calcifications were also observed in the thyroid, lymph node, and liver. No adrenal tumor was observed (Figure 1).

Total thyroidectomy and modified neck and upper mediastinum dissections were performed. The pathologic diagnosis was medullary carcinoma (pT3N1bM1). Four months later, vandetanib treatment was initiated at a dose of 300 mg/day owing to progression of the liver metastasis. At 44 months after the initiation of vandetanib treatment, its dose was reduced to 200 mg/day owing to increased serum creatinine levels. After the dose reduction, the levels of CEA, calcitonin, and liver enzymes, such as aspartate aminotransferase (AST) and alanine aminotransferase (ALT), were found to be elevated. At 48 months after the initiation of

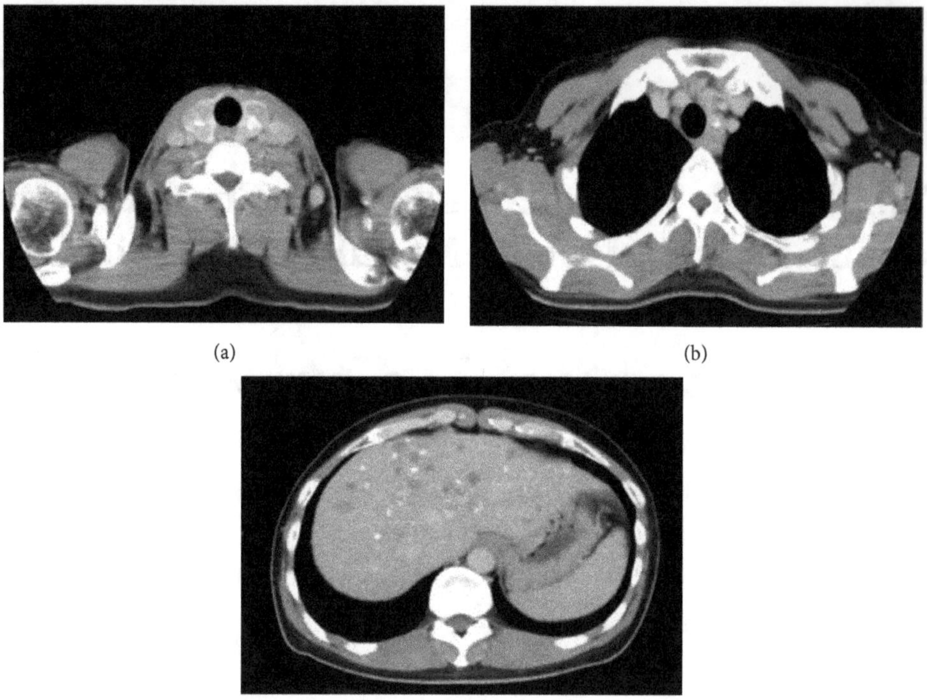

(a) (b) (c)

Figure 1: At the first visit to our hospital, computed tomography revealed a thyroid tumor (a), lymph node metastasis (b), and multiple cysts in the liver (c). The tumor was accompanied by calcification.

vandetanib treatment, abdominal distension appeared, and the liver cysts increased to a maximum diameter of 14 cm (Figure 2). Thus, the dose of vandetanib was increased to 300 mg/day. Percutaneous liver cyst puncture was performed to reduce abdominal distension, and aspiration biopsy cytology of the liver cyst indicated atypia of undetermined significance. Although serum AST and ALT levels were transiently worse, the patient was discharged a month after the drainage. After discharge, he experienced gastrointestinal perforation associated with an ulcer, and emergency surgery was performed. The postoperative course was good, and he was discharged two weeks after the surgery. However, the liver cysts had increased in size and the serum CEA and calcitonin levels were elevated; we considered these as signs of disease progression. Thus, vandetanib treatment was discontinued, and lenvatinib treatment was initiated at a dose of 12 mg/day owing to increased serum AST and ALT levels. At 8 weeks after the initiation of lenvatinib treatment, the serum CEA and calcitonin levels were decreased to 1589.5 ng/ml and 83,800 pg/ml, respectively, while the serum liver enzyme levels were within the normal range (Figure 3).

3. Discussion

MTC is a type of neuroendocrine tumor that arises from neural crest-derived parafollicular C-cells [1], which secrete calcitonin and CEA [2]. Calcitonin is a very specific tumor marker, whereas CEA is a non-specific tumor marker used for MTC surveillance [2]. The serum concentrations of these markers are directly related to C-cell mass [1].

Tyrosine kinase inhibitors (TKIs) are used for the treatment of MTC. Two TKIs, vandetanib and cabozantinib, prolonged progression-free survival compared with placebo in phase III clinical trials [3, 4]. Based on these phase III clinical trials, the U.S. Food and Drug Administration and the European Medicines Agency approved vandetanib and cabozantinib for the treatment of patients with advanced progressive MTC [1]. In Japan, the corresponding agency approved vandetanib, sorafenib, and lenvatinib for the treatment of advanced progressive MTC [5].

In this case, vandetanib treatment was initiated because liver metastasis had progressed, following which the liver cysts considerably increased in size. At the beginning of the treatment, we assumed that this change was attributable to the effect of vandetanib treatment. However, the disease course indicated that liver dysfunction might have been caused by vandetanib. As the liver cysts had considerably increased in size and the serum CEA and calcitonin levels were elevated, we assumed that vandetanib was ineffective for this patient. Therefore, vandetanib was discontinued and replaced with lenvatinib.

After shifting from vandetanib treatment to lenvatinib treatment, the liver enzyme and tumor marker levels did not increase, which indicated that the liver dysfunction was caused by disease progression and that vandetanib was ineffective for this patient. According to a randomized, double-blind phase III trial, liver dysfunction is not a common adverse event of vandetanib treatment [3].

This patient had multiple liver cysts at initial presentation to our hospital. The incidence of cystic liver lesions is reported to be as high as 5% of the population [6]. The most

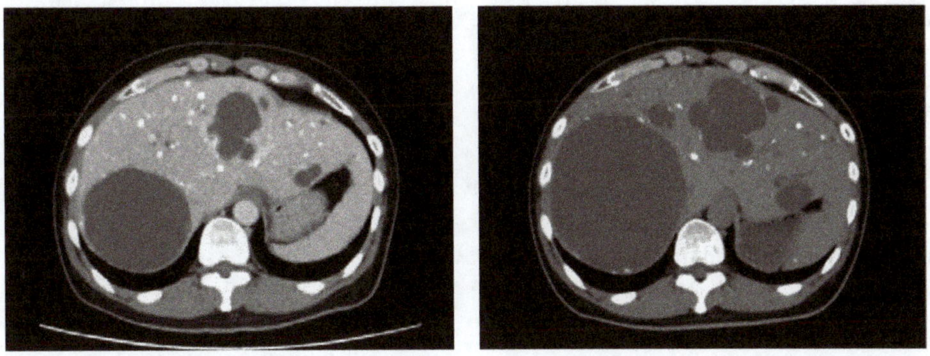

FIGURE 2: Computed tomography revealed that the liver cysts were increased in size after vandetanib treatment. (a) At 42 months after vandetanib treatment initiation. (b) At 48 months after vandetanib treatment initiation, abdominal distension developed.

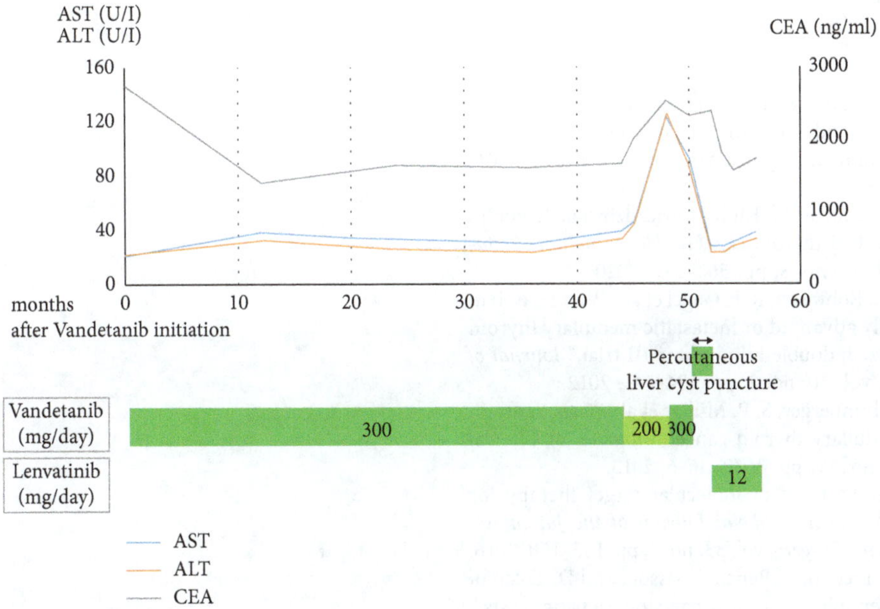

FIGURE 3: Clinical course and blood examination. AST: aspartate aminotransferase, ALT: alanine aminotransferase, and CEA: carcinoembryonic antigen.

common lesion type is benign simple cyst, and causes of cystic liver lesions include polycystic disease, parasite infection, abscess, or neoplasm. In cases of neoplasm, biliary cystadenoma and cystadenocarcinoma account for 5% of cystic lesions of the liver [7]. Cystic tumors, such as ovary and pancreatic cystadenocarcinomas, can metastasize to the liver. Although secondary neoplastic liver cysts are rare, cystic metastasis from gastrointestinal stromal tumors have been reported [8]. However, to the best of our knowledge, cystic metastasis from MTC has not been reported previously. In this case, despite initiating vandetanib treatment, the liver cysts increased in size and serum liver enzyme levels remained elevated. The cysts also caused abdominal distension; thus, we performed percutaneous liver cyst puncture. Aspiration biopsy cytology of liver cyst revealed atypia of undetermined significance as only few atypical cells were found. Moreover, we did not check the CEA and calcitonin level in the cystic fluid. Cyst puncture was ineffective, but after lenvatinib initiation, the liver cysts did not increase in size and serum liver enzyme levels improved owing to the antineoplastic effect of lenvatinib. Although the aspiration biopsy cytology of the liver cyst did not indicate metastasis, the cause of the liver cysts was believed to be the progression of the disease, as the cysts were found to be enlarged in the metastatic lesion and showed a tendency to improve with a change in the treatment.

This case indicated that cystic lesions of the liver may occur alongside MTC. It is also possible that increased liver cysts indicate disease progression, which may necessitate a change in treatment.

In conclusion, we reported the case of a patient with MTC and liver cysts that developed during vandetanib treatment. The liver cysts caused an increase in serum liver enzyme levels and abdominal distension. Percutaneous liver cyst puncture was ineffective, but treatment changes improved the serum liver enzyme, CEA, and calcitonin levels.

This case indicated that MTC may occur along with liver cysts, and an increase in the size of the liver cysts can cause elevation in serum liver enzyme levels. When the liver cysts increase in size and liver enzyme levels are elevated, the treatment may need to be changed.

Consent

Written informed consent was obtained from the patient for the publication of this case report and accompanying images.

Acknowledgments

The authors would like to thank Enago (https://www.enago.jp/) for the English language review. This study did not receive any funding.

References

[1] S. A. Wells Jr., S. L. Asa, H. Dralle et al., "Revised american thyroid association guidelines for the management of medullary thyroid carcinoma," *Thyroid*, vol. 25, no. 6, pp. 567–610, 2015.

[2] K. A. Araque, S. Gubbi, and J. Klubo-Gwiezdzinska, "Updates on the management of thyroid cancer," *Hormone and Metabolic Research*, vol. 52, no. 8, pp. 562–577, 2020.

[3] S. A. Wells Jr., B. G. Robinson, R. F. Gagel et al., "Vandetanib in patients with locally advanced or metastatic medullary thyroid cancer: a randomized, double-blind phase III trial," *Journal of Clinical Oncology*, vol. 30, no. 2, pp. 134–141, 2012.

[4] R. Elisei, M. J. Schlumberger, S. P. Müller et al., "Cabozantinib in progressive medullary thyroid cancer," *Journal of Clinical Oncology*, vol. 31, no. 29, pp. 3639–3646, 2013.

[5] S. Takahashi, "Development of molecular target therapy for medullary thyroid cancer," *Official Journal of the Japan Association of Endocrine Surgery*, vol. 33, no. 3, pp. 145–150, 2016.

[6] M. Caremani, A. Vincenti, A. Benci, S. Sassoli, and D. Tacconi, "Ecographic epidemiology of non-parasitic hepatic cysts," *Journal of Clinical Ultrasound*, vol. 21, no. 2, pp. 115–118, 1993.

[7] D. P. Vogt, J. M. Henderson, and E. Chmielewski, "Cystadenoma and cystadenocarcinoma of the liver: a single center experience," *Journal of the American College of Surgeons*, vol. 200, no. 5, pp. 727–733, 2005.

[8] R. E. Bechtold, M. Y. Chen, C. A. Stanton, P. D. Savage, and E. A. Levine, "Cystic changes in hepatic and peritoneal metastases from gastrointestinal stromal tumors treated with Gleevec," *Abdominal Imaging*, vol. 28, no. 6, pp. 808–814, 2003.

46

Outside the Thorax: Doege–Potter Syndrome Presenting as a Retroperitoneal Abdominal Mass

Daniel M. Berrebi[1] **Oksana Symczyk,**[2] **Taylor Cater,**[2] **Ayodele Adelanwa,**[3] **Patrick Bacaj,**[3] **Alan A. Thomay,**[4] **and Adnan Haider**[2]

[1]*School of Medicine, West Virginia University, Morgantown, WV, USA*
[2]*Department of Endocrinology, Department of Medicine, West Virginia University, Morgantown, WV, USA*
[3]*Department of Pathology, Anatomy and Laboratory Medicine, West Virginia University, Morgantown, WV, USA*
[4]*Department of Surgery, Division of Surgical Oncology, West Virginia University, Morgantown, WV, USA*

Correspondence should be addressed to Daniel M. Berrebi; dmberrebi@mix.wvu.edu

Academic Editor: Wei Wu

Objective. We present a case of refractory hypoglycemia, weight loss, and retroperitoneal solitary fibrous tumor. *Case report.* A 68-year-old female presented with symptomatic hypoglycemia, weight loss, and abdominal mass identified on CT scan of the abdomen. Blood work during symptomatic hypoglycemia was consistent with an IGF-2-producing tumor. The abdominal mass pathology was consistent with solitary fibrous tumor surrounding the adrenal gland, and resection resulted in complete resolution of hypoglycemia. *Discussion.* Understanding the biochemical mechanisms behind glucose regulation is necessary to diagnose and adequately treat Doege–Potter syndrome, a paraneoplastic syndrome observed in patients with solitary fibrous tumors. Solitary fibrous tumors can be characterized by specific histologic and immunohistochemical studies. *Conclusion.* This report describes the clinical workup of a patient presenting with hypoglycemia and a retroperitoneal tumor. This case is unique because of its presentation with severe, refractory hypoglycemia and the tumor's location in the retroperitoneum, given the majority of solitary fibrous tumors are found in the lungs originating from the pleura.

1. Case Report

A 68-year-old female patient presented to the emergency department with refractory neuroglycopenic symptoms. In the emergency room, her glucose level was noted to be <50 mg/dL on multiple occasions despite repeated administrations of IV dextrose and PO intake. She described a 3-week history of episodes characterized by confusion, diaphoresis, and severe weakness which were improved with ingestion of food. She also described a weight loss of 30 pounds over the last 4-5 months despite normal appetite. She had no history of type 1 or type 2 diabetes mellitus and did not use insulin or antidiabetic medications. Medical history included hypertension and gastroesophageal reflux, and she did not endorse a history of smoking, alcohol, or recreational drug use. No pertinent family history was identified. On physical examination, she was found to have a palpable, mildly tender right upper quadrant mass and palpable hepatomegaly. A CT scan demonstrated evidence of an 18.6 cm mass projecting inferior to the liver and superior to the right kidney, in the approximate location of the right adrenal gland (Figure 1). The mass was described as lobular and formed by 3 confluent mass lesions. No other suspicious lesions were described in the report. In addition, venogram showed severe extrinsic compression of the inferior vena cava secondary to the retroperitoneal mass.

Clinical workup of her hypoglycemia proceeded as follows (Figure 2). Hypoglycemia was initially prevented with a maintenance dextrose drip; however, this was discontinued to allow clinical observation of hypoglycemic episodes ideally proving or disproving Whipple's triad. Whipple's triad includes a venous glucose level less than

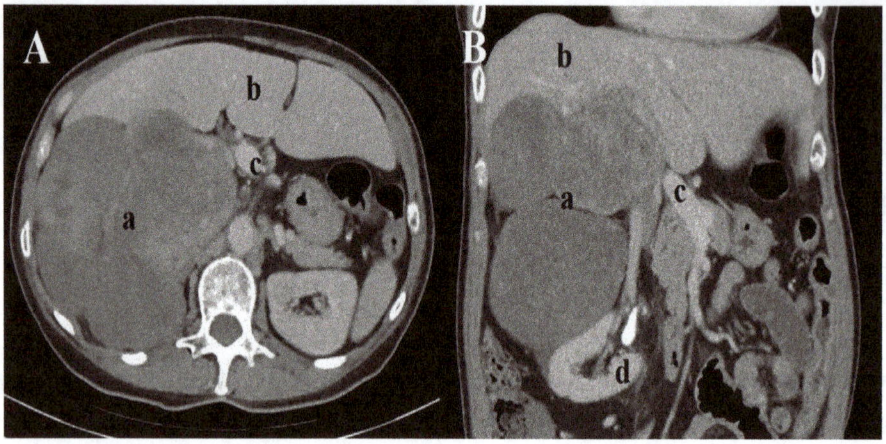

Figure 1: CT Scan of retroperitoneal mass. (a) Axial slice of contrast enhanced CT of the abdomen demonstrating a large right retroperitoneal tumor (A) with mass effect upon the right lobe of the liver (B) and displacement of the vena cava and porta hepatis (C) medially. (b) Coronal slice of contrast enhanced CT of the abdomen again showing the tumor, with displacement of the right kidney (D) inferiorly.

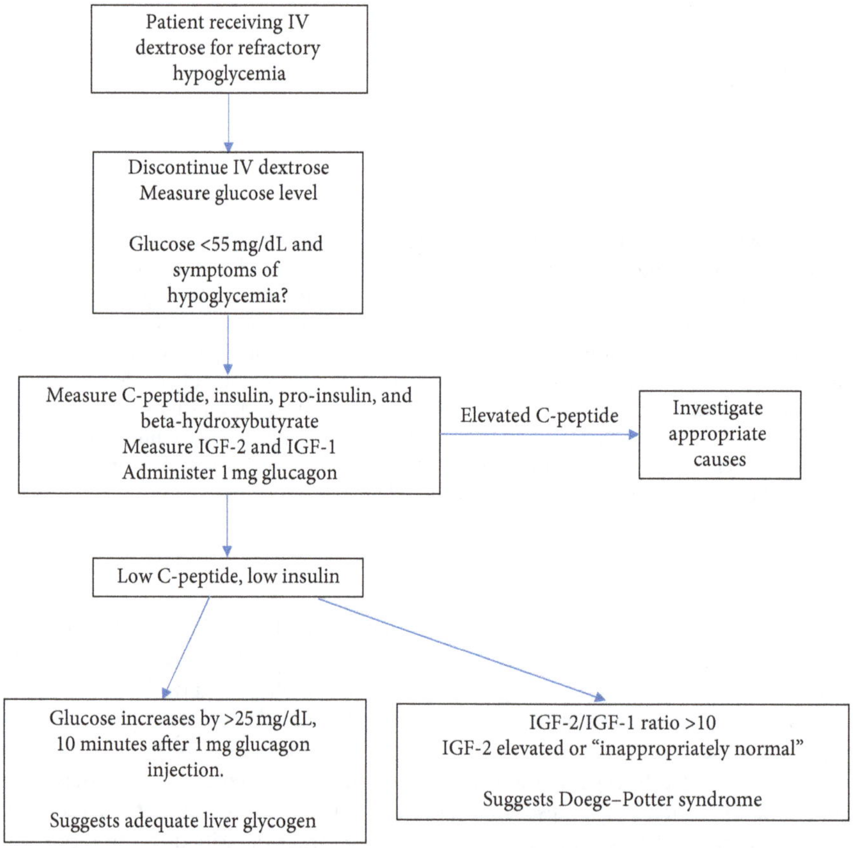

Figure 2: Clinical workup of Doege–Potter syndrome.

55 mg/dL, symptoms of hypoglycemia, and resolution of symptoms after glucose administration. Dextrose drip was discontinued, her glucose level decreased to 47 mg/dL, and she became symptomatic. At that time, C-peptide, insulin, pro-insulin, and beta-hydroxybutyrate levels were measured and all were found to be low, suggesting IGF-2 secretion. IGF-2 was measured during that hypoglycemic episode but resulted within the normal range. This is classified as inappropriately normal because IGF-2 levels are expected to be suppressed in the setting of hypoglycemia (Table 1). The patient was given a 1 mg dose of glucagon, and her glucose level increased to 82 mg/dL with resolution of symptoms. Increase in glucose value of greater then 25 mg/dl represent adequate glycogen stores in the liver, yet repeated and

Table 1: Relevant laboratory values and corresponding reference ranges.

Test	Result	Range
Plasma glucose after dextrose discontinuation	47 mg/dL	
C-peptide	0.1 ng/mL	0.9–7.1 ng/mL
Beta-hydroxybutyrate	0.10 mmol/L	<0.40 mmol/L
Pro-insulin	2.8 pmol/L	3.6–22 pmol/L
Insulin	<2.0 mIU/mL	2.5–24.0 mIU/mL
Insulin-like growth factor-2	382 ng/mL	333–967 ng/mL
Insulin antibodies	Negative	

persistent hypoglycemia infers that the patient's hepatocytes were not secreting glucose despite severe hypoglycemia. Dextrose drip was resumed to maintain safe glucose levels.

Screening for use of oral hypoglycemic agents to rule out factitious hypoglycemia was negative. Antibodies to insulin were also undetectable. Our surgical colleagues recommended ruling out adrenal hypersecretion, as elevated precursor hormones are often seen in rapidly dividing adrenocortical carcinoma. Serum renin, aldosterone, 11-deoxycorticosterone, and 17-hydroxyprogesterone were all within normal limits. 5-HIAA and urine metanephrine levels were normal as well, which lessened suspicion for pheochromocytoma or neuroendocrine tumor. Although these conditions are not classically associated with hypoglycemia, we felt it would be useful to exclude additional causes of a large retroperitoneal mass.

Given the in-depth negative workup other than the abdominal mass, the decision was made to pursue resection. The gross pathology specimen (Figure 3) showed a mass weighing 2270 gm. Following removal, the patient's hypoglycemia resolved and 2 days later, IGF-2 was re-measured and found to be significantly lower than that measured preoperatively. During recovery, she had episodes of hyperglycemia, which could be explained by the sudden decrease in IGF-2 levels triggering a new equilibrium for glucose homeostasis.

Unfortunately, IGF-1 level, which was drawn at the time of a hypoglycemic episode, could not be resulted because the sample was hemolyzed en route to the laboratory. By the time we were alerted, the patient was in pre-op for surgical resection. It would have been ideal to have this value, but this case highlights that clinical suspicion in the setting of appropriate imaging, low insulin, C-peptide, and beta-hydroxybutyrate, and an increase in glucose following glucagon injection point to an IGF-2-producing tumor. Finally, in the setting of an acutely ill patient, we anticipate a low/suppressed IGF-1 level.

A follow-up CT scan one month after surgery demonstrated interval resection of the previously noted large, lobulated right suprarenal mass. There were no findings to suggest residual or recurrent disease.

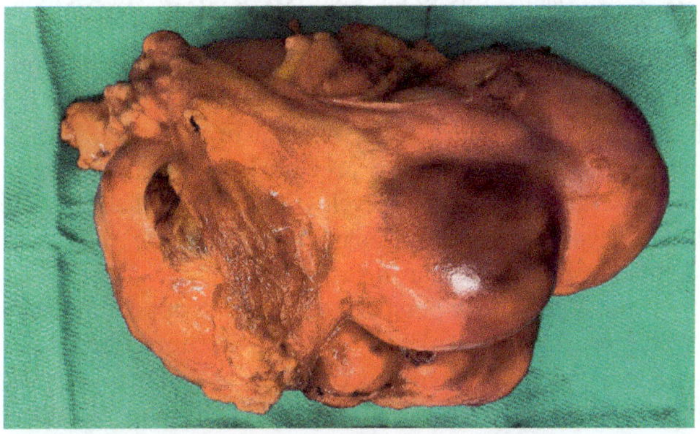

Figure 3: Gross image of solitary fibrous tumor. Specimen weighed 2270 grams with dimensions of 22.0 cm × 18.0 cm × 12.0 cm. Solitary fibrous tumors often appear as a well-circumscribed mass with tan-white homogeneous cut surfaces that can be cystic or hemorrhagic.

2. Discussion

Solitary fibrous tumors (SFTs) arise from mesenchymal cells and account for less than 2% of all soft tissue tumors [1]. SFTs usually manifest as slowly growing, asymptomatic masses and are benign in clinical course. Cases of aggressive SFTs with local invasion have been reported [2]. SFTs typically originate within the thorax but can arise anywhere, and to date, there have been fewer than 100 cases reported of retroperitoneal SFTs. Rarely, SFTs can present with paraneoplastic syndromes such as hypoglycemia, specifically referred to as the Doege–Potter syndrome, which was first reported in the 1930s [3, 4].

The effectiveness of the normal physiological reactions to falling blood glucose concentrations makes hypoglycemia an uncommon clinical event. The first response to falling serum glucose concentration is a decrease in the secretion of endogenous insulin. Once glucose concentrations fall below the normal physiological range, counter-regulatory hormones are released in response simulating glucagon, cortisol, catecholamine, and growth hormone secretion [5]. Together these effects stimulate hepatic glucose production and decrease glucose utilization in peripheral tissues. In the event of recurrent episodes of hypoglycemia, the glycemic threshold of physiological defenses shifts to a lower glucose concentration making diagnosis and treatment critical to prevent fatal consequences as a result of hypoglycemic unawareness [6].

Although hypoglycemia from non-islet cell tumors is very rare, when present it often results from overproduction of pro-insulin-like growth factor-2 (IGF-2) which is an incompletely processed high molecular weight protein. Due to its poor affinity to serum IGF-2 binding proteins, IGF-2 freely enters tissue eliciting its insulin-like effects and therefore leads to hypoglycemia [7, 8]. When glucose levels fall during a fasting state, compensatory mechanisms result in a rise in ketones such as β-hydroxybutyrate, as an alternative energy source for the brain [9, 10]. However, this rise in ketones is blunted by hypoglycemia stemming from IGF-2-producing tumors [11]. Just like insulin, IGF-2 stimulates uptake of glucose by skeletal muscles [12]. Continued stimulation of insulin receptors by IGF-2 leads to further suppression of free fatty acid release as well as inhibition of gluconeogenesis, glycogenolysis, and ketogenesis by the liver [11, 12]. Suppression of growth hormone and IGF-1 also results due to elevated IGF-2 levels. These effects in turn lead to an elevated IGF-2 to IGF-1 ratio. An IGF-2 to IGF-1 ratio of greater than 10 is typically revealing of non-islet cell tumor hypoglycemia (NICTH) [13]. Although the IGF-2 level was found to be normal in this case, IGF-2-producing NICTH has been previously reported with both normal and elevated IGF-2 levels [14]. We would classify the IGF-2 level as inappropriately normal in the setting of significant hypoglycemia in such cases.

From a pathology perspective, the gross appearance of a typical or conventional SFT is a well-circumscribed mass with tan-white homogeneous cut surfaces that can be cystic or hemorrhagic with sizes ranging from 1 cm to 20 cm (Figure 3). Histologically, SFTs are often described as having a "pattern-less pattern" (Figure 4) which refers to a storiform arrangement of neoplastic spindle cells in a stroma with variable amounts of collagen and large thin-walled branching "staghorn" appearing vessels and medium-sized vessels. A diagnosis of malignant SFT is rendered when the tumor displays high cellularity, high mitotic activity (more than 4 mitoses per 10HPF), cytological pleomorphism, and necrosis on histopathologic evaluation [15].

Immunohistochemically, CD34, Bcl-2, and CD99 SFT usually show a strong diffuse pattern of staining; however, in 5–10% of SFT, CD34 can be negative. These markers can also show positivity in other neoplasms of mesenchymal differentiation, limiting the utility of these markers, particularly CD34, in the workup of the differential diagnosis [16]. The most sensitive and specific marker for the diagnosis of both conventional and malignant SFTs is the detection of NAB2-STAT6 fusion by next-generation sequencing [17]. Immunohistochemical expression of the STAT6 protein in tumor cell nuclei is a sensitive and specific marker for SFT. Cytoplasmic expression of STAT6 can sometimes be seen in other neoplasms such as synovial sarcoma, well-differentiated and dedifferentiated liposarcomas, and desmoid fibromatosis. The distinguishing feature for SFTs lies in the pattern of expression. SFT exclusively shows a nuclear pattern of STAT6 expression, whereas these other neoplasms display a nuclear and cytoplasmic pattern of staining [18].

The only definitive treatment for NICTH is complete tumor resection. As in previously reported cases, our patient's symptoms completely resolved once the tumor was resected. Normalization of plasma glucose levels occurred shortly after tumor resection. Postoperatively, during the recovery phase, she experienced episodes of postprandial hyperglycemia. This was presumably secondary to residually suppressed insulin secretion from pancreatic β cells. This resolved with decreasing levels of IGF-2 and a re-equilibration in glucose homeostasis. A study by Le Jeune et al. [19] showed that the recurrence-free survival generally exceeds 90% [19].

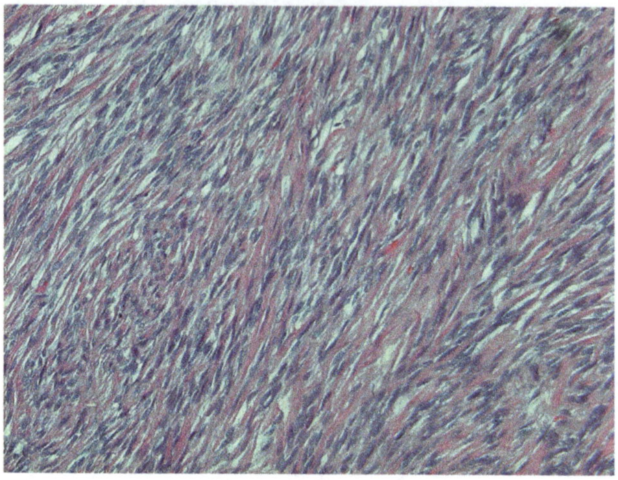

FIGURE 4: Histologic appearance of solitary fibrous tumor. Photomicrograph of solitary fibrous tumor at 100x magnification demonstrating the classic pattern-less pattern of uniform, spindled to ovoid fibroblastic cells.

In cases of incomplete resection or tumors that cannot be surgically removed, there are medical management options. Han et al. [20] describes the efficacy of various glucocorticoid regimens, which suppress production of IGF-2 and have been shown to improve hypoglycemia in a dose-dependent manner. In combination with steroids, some providers initiate growth hormone therapy, which may have a synergistic effect. In a patient with Doege–Potter syndrome and end-stage renal disease, Shekhar et al. [21] described use of dexamethasone and recombinant growth hormone to manage hypoglycemia; however, the patient became increasingly dependent on IV dextrose and eventually an attempt to de-bulk the tumor was made. Chemotherapy and radiation can be considered, but according to Han et al., IGF-2-producing solitary fibrous tumors often respond poorly to these interventions.

3. Conclusion

SFTs have been described in extrapleural sites such as the upper respiratory tract and the orbits but are most commonly found in the lungs originating from the pleura. If hypoglycemia is demonstrated in connection with a solitary fibrous tumor, it is referred to as the Doege–Potter syndrome. This case is unique because of its presentation with severe hypoglycemia and its location "outside the thoracic cavity."

Abbreviations

DPS: Doege–Potter syndrome
IGF-2: Insulin-like growth factor-2
SFT: Solitary fibrous tumor
NICTH: Non-islet cell tumor hypoglycemia.

Authors' Contributions

Daniel M. Berrebi and Oksana Symczyk contributed equally to this study and should be regarded as co-first authors.

References

[1] J. S. Gold, C. R. Antonescu, C. Hajdu et al., "Clinicopathologic correlates of solitary fibrous tumors," *Cancer*, vol. 94, no. 4, pp. 1057–1068, 2002.

[2] A. Vilaca, M. Monteiro, and T. Pimentel, "Solitary fibrous tumor: an uncommon cause of paraparesis and sciatic pain," *Journal of Medical Cases*, vol. 8, no. 6, pp. 196–199, 2017.

[3] K. W. Doege, "Fibro-sarcoma of the mediastinum," *Annals of Surgery*, vol. 92, no. 5, pp. 955–960, 1930.

[4] R. P. Potter, "Intrathoracic tumors," *Radiology*, vol. 14, no. 1, pp. 60-61, 1930.

[5] J. E. Sprague and A. M. Arbeláez, "Glucose counterregulatory responses to hypoglycemia," *Pediatric Endocrinology Reviews: PER*, vol. 9, no. 1, pp. 463–465, 2011.

[6] P. Iglesias and J. J. Diez, "Management of endocrine disease: a clinical update on tumor-induced hypoglycemia," *European Journal of Endocrinology*, vol. 170, no. 4, p. 147, 2014.

[7] A. Denley, E. R. Bonython, G. W. Booker et al., "Structural determinants for high-affinity binding of insulin-like growth factor II to insulin receptor (IR)-A, the exon 11 minus isoform of the IR," *Molecular Endocrinology*, vol. 18, no. 10, pp. 2502–2512, 2004.

[8] G. L. King, C. R. Kahn, M. M. Rechler, and S. P. Nissley, "Direct demonstration of separate receptors for growth and metabolic activities of insulin and multiplication-stimulating activity (an insulinlike growth factor) using antibodies to the insulin receptor," *Journal of Clinical Investigation*, vol. 66, no. 1, pp. 130–140, 1980.

[9] G. F. Cahill Jr., M. G. Herrera, A. P. Morgan et al., "Hormone-fuel interrelationships during fasting," *Journal of Clinical Investigation*, vol. 45, no. 11, pp. 1751–1769, 1966.

[10] C. A. Stanley and L. Baker, "Hyperinsulinism in infancy: diagnosis by demonstration of abnormal response to fasting hypoglycemia," *Pediatrics*, vol. 57, no. 5, pp. 702–711, 1976.

[11] F. Miraki-Moud, A. B. Grossman, M. Besser, J. P. Monson, and C. Camacho-Hübner, "A rapid method for analyzing serum pro-insulin-like growth factor-II in patients with non-islet cell tumor hypoglycemia," *The Journal of Clinical Endocrinology & Metabolism*, vol. 90, no. 7, pp. 3819–3823, 2005.

[12] Y. Dynkevich, K. I. Rother, I. Whitford et al., "Tumors, IGF-2, and hypoglycemia: insights from the clinic, the laboratory, and the historical archive," *Endocrine Reviews*, vol. 34, no. 6, pp. 798–826, 2013.

[13] T.-T. Tian, J.-T. Wu, X.-H. Hu et al., "Imaging findings of solitary fibrous tumor in the abdomen and pelvis," *Abdominal Imaging*, vol. 39, no. 6, pp. 1323–1329, 2014.

[14] C. Livingstone, "IGF2 and cancer," *Endocrine-Related Cancer*, vol. 20, no. 6, pp. 321–339, 2013.

[15] D. M. England, L. Hochholzer, and M. J. McCarthy, "Localized benign and malignant fibrous tumors of the pleura," *The American Journal of Surgical Pathology*, vol. 13, no. 8, pp. 640–658, 1989.

[16] M. Miettinen, "Immunohistochemistry of soft tissue tumours-review with emphasis on 10 markers," *Histopathology*, vol. 64, no. 1, pp. 101–118, 2014.

[17] L. A. Doyle, M. Vivero, C. D. Fletcher, F. Mertens, and J. L. Hornick, "Nuclear expression of STAT6 distinguishes solitary fibrous tumor from histologic mimics," *Modern Pathology*, vol. 27, no. 3, pp. 390–395, 2014.

[18] E. G. Demicco, K. Wani, P. S. Fox et al., "Histologic variability in solitary fibrous tumors reflects angiogenic and growth factor signaling pathway alterations," *Human Pathology*, vol. 46, no. 7, pp. 1015–1026, 2015.

[19] S. Le. Jeune, G. Des Guetz, H. Bihan, R. Cohen, J.-M. Coindre, and J.-J. Mourad, "Refractory hypoglycemia controlled by sorafenib in solitary fibrous tumor," *Journal of Clinical Oncology*, vol. 31, no. 9, pp. e118–e121, 2013.

[20] G. Han, Z. Zhang, X. Shen et al., "Doege–Potter syndrome: a review of the literature including a new case report," *Medicine (Baltimore)*, vol. 96, no. 27, 2017.

[21] S. Shekhar, J. Chen, and K. Desai, "Doege-Potter syndrome presenting as "end-stage renal Disease-associated hypoglycaemia": a primary presentation of retroperitoneal sarcoma," *BMJ Case Reports*, vol. 13, no. 8, 2020.

Permissions

All chapters in this book were first published by Hindawi Publishing Corporation; hereby published with permission under the Creative Commons Attribution License or equivalent. Every chapter published in this book has been scrutinized by our experts. Their significance has been extensively debated. The topics covered herein carry significant findings which will fuel the growth of the discipline. They may even be implemented as practical applications or may be referred to as a beginning point for another development.

The contributors of this book come from diverse backgrounds, making this book a truly international effort. This book will bring forth new frontiers with its revolutionizing research information and detailed analysis of the nascent developments around the world.

We would like to thank all the contributing authors for lending their expertise to make the book truly unique. They have played a crucial role in the development of this book. Without their invaluable contributions this book wouldn't have been possible. They have made vital efforts to compile up to date information on the varied aspects of this subject to make this book a valuable addition to the collection of many professionals and students.

This book was conceptualized with the vision of imparting up-to-date information and advanced data in this field. To ensure the same, a matchless editorial board was set up. Every individual on the board went through rigorous rounds of assessment to prove their worth. After which they invested a large part of their time researching and compiling the most relevant data for our readers.

The editorial board has been involved in producing this book since its inception. They have spent rigorous hours researching and exploring the diverse topics which have resulted in the successful publishing of this book. They have passed on their knowledge of decades through this book. To expedite this challenging task, the publisher supported the team at every step. A small team of assistant editors was also appointed to further simplify the editing procedure and attain best results for the readers.

Apart from the editorial board, the designing team has also invested a significant amount of their time in understanding the subject and creating the most relevant covers. They scrutinized every image to scout for the most suitable representation of the subject and create an appropriate cover for the book.

The publishing team has been an ardent support to the editorial, designing and production team. Their endless efforts to recruit the best for this project, has resulted in the accomplishment of this book. They are a veteran in the field of academics and their pool of knowledge is as vast as their experience in printing. Their expertise and guidance has proved useful at every step. Their uncompromising quality standards have made this book an exceptional effort. Their encouragement from time to time has been an inspiration for everyone.

The publisher and the editorial board hope that this book will prove to be a valuable piece of knowledge for researchers, students, practitioners and scholars across the globe.

List of Contributors

Michelle Ponder
University of Maryland Medical Center, 22 S Green St., RM N3E09, Baltimore, MD 21201-1554, USA

Elizabeth Lamos and Kashif Munir
Division of Endocrinology, Diabetes, and Nutrition, University of Maryland School of Medicine, 827 Linden Avenue, 2nd Floor, Baltimore, MD 21201, USA

Benedetta Zampetti, Emanuela Carioni and Daniela Dallabonzana
ASST Grande Ospedale Metropolitano Niguarda, Endocrinology Department, Milan, Italy

Roberto Attanasio and Renato Cozzi
Scientific Committee Associazione Medici Endocrinologi, International Chapter of Clinical Endocrinology, Milan, Italy

Iuliana Pauna and Marco Boniardi
ASST Grande Ospedale Metropolitano Niguarda, General Oncologic and Mini-invasive Surgery Department, Milan, Italy

Ėrika Mayumi Ikeda Cavamura
Academic of the Faculdade Pequeno Pr´ıncipe, Curitiba, Brazil

Fabiane Karen Miyake, Jéssica Yachio Wiezel and Luis Felipe Inglês Takada
Academics of the Faculdade Evangélica Mackenzie Paraná, Curitiba, Brazil

Laura Schwartz Maranho, Renata Cassitas Mendonça and Tamila Sohn Fagundes
Medical Residents of the Endocrinology Service at Hospital Universitário Mackenzie Paraná, Curitiba, Brazil

A. Zainal, O. Akinsola and K. Rajamani
Rochester Regional Health/Unity Hospital, USA

M. D. S. A. Dilrukshi, N. P. Somasundaram and D. D. K. Abeyaratne
Diabetes and Endocrinology Unit of National Hospital of Sri Lanka, Colombo 10, Sri Lanka

A. W. Wickramarachchi
National Hospital of Sri Lanka, Colombo, Sri Lanka

Brian Shine
Clinical Biochemistry, John Radcliffe Hospital, Oxford OX3 9DU, UK

Bahram Jafar-Mohammadi
Oxford Centre for Diabetes, Endocrinology and Metabolism, Churchill Hospital, Oxford University Hospitals NHS Foundation Trust, Oxford, UK

César Ernesto Lam-Chung
Department of Endocrinology and Metabolism, Instituto Nacional de Ciencias Médicas y Nutricion Salvador Zubirán, Vasco de Quiroga 15, Secci´on XVI, Tlalpan, México City 14000, Mexico

Diana Lizbeth Rodríguez-Orihuela, Jazmín De Anda González and Armando Gamboa-Domínguez
Department of Pathology, Instituto Nacional de Ciencias Médiócas y Nutricion Salvador Zubirán, Vasco de Quiroga 15, Seccion XVI, Tlalpan, México City 14000, Mexico

Nishant Sharma, Divya Ravi, Mehvish Khan, Metlapalli Venkata Sravanthi and Mark M. Aloysius
The Wright Center for Graduate Medical Education, 111 N Washington Ave, Scranton, PA 18503, USA

Antía Fernández-Pombo and David Araújo-Vilar
Division of Endocrinology, University Clinical Hospital of Santiago de Compostela, Spain
UETeM-Molecular Pathology Group, Department of Medicine, IDIS-CIMUS, University of Santiago de Compostela, Spain

José M. Cameselle-Teijeiro
Division of Pathology, University Clinical Hospital of Santiago de Compostela, Spain

Jose A. Puñal-Rodríguez
Division of Surgery, University Clinical Hospital of Santiago de Compostela, Spain

Lourdes Loidi
Fundación Galega de Medicina Xenómica, Santiago de Compostela, Spain

Roberto Peinó-García
Division of Endocrinology, University Clinical Hospital of Santiago de Compostela, Spain

Paloma Cabanas-Rodríguez
Division of Pediatrics, University Clinical Hospital of Santiago de Compostela, Spain

Miguel Garrido-Pumar
Division of Nuclear Medicine, University Clinical Hospital of Santiago de Compostela, Spain

Sandra Baleato-González and Enrique Flores-Ríos
Division of Radiology, University Clinical Hospital of Santiago de Compostela, Spain

X. Vandemergel
Department of Endocrinology, EpiCURA, Boussu, Belgium

Priyanka Lakshmanan
Department of Medicine Mount Sinai Morningside, Mount Sinai West Icahn School of Medicine, New York, NY, USA

Heena Asnani
Pravara Institute of Medical Sciences, Ahmednagar, India

David Knorr
Memorial Sloan Kettering Cancer Center, New York, NY, USA

Mio Yasukawa
Department of Breast and Endocrine Surgery, Kanagawa Cancer Center, 2-3-2 Nakao Asahi-ku, Yokohama, Kanagawa 241-8515, Japan

Yoichiro Okubo
Department of Pathology, Kanagawa Cancer Center, 2-3-2 Nakao Asahi-ku, Yokohama, Kanagawa 241-8515, Japan

Hiroyuki Hayashi
Department of Pathology, Yokohama Municipal Citizen's Hospital, 1-1 Mitsuzawanishicho Kanagawa-ku, Yokohama, Kanagawa 221-0855, Japan

Sofia Castro Oliveira, João Sérgio Neves, Pedro Souteiro, Paula Freitas and Davide Carvalho
Department of Endocrinology, Diabetes and Metabolism, Centro Hospitalar Universitário de São João (CHSJ), Porto, Portugal
Faculty of Medicine of Universidade do Porto (FMUP), Porto, Portugal
Instituto de Investigação e Inovação em Saúde, Universidade do Porto (i3S), Porto, Portugal

Sandra Belo and Ana Isabel Oliveira
Department of Endocrinology, Diabetes and Metabolism, Centro Hospitalar Universitário de São João (CHSJ), Porto, Portugal

Helena Moreira and Paulo Mergulhão Gomes
Unidade Polivalente de Cuidados Intermédios Geral (UPCIG), Centro Hospitalar Universitário de São João (CHSJ), Porto, Portugal

Lígia Coelho
Department of Maxillofacial Surgery, Centro Hospitalar Universitário de São João (CHSJ), Porto, Portugal

Cristina Sarmento
Department of Medical Oncology, Centro Hospitalar Universitário de São João (CHSJ), Porto, Portugal

Elsa Fonseca
Faculty of Medicine of Universidade do Porto (FMUP), Porto, Portugal
Department of Pathology, Centro Hospitalar Universitário de São João (CHSJ), Porto, Portugal
Instituto de Patologia e Imunologia Molecular, Universidade do Porto (IPATIMUP), Porto, Portugal

Celestino Neves
Department of Endocrinology, Diabetes and Metabolism, Centro Hospitalar Universitário de São João (CHSJ), Porto, Portugal
Faculty of Medicine of Universidade do Porto (FMUP), Porto, Portugal

Khaled Ahmed Baagar and Buthina Ibrahim Alowainati
Endocrine Department, Hamad Medical Corporation, Doha, Qatar

Paula Jeffs and Alex González-Bóssolo
Endocrinology Department, San Juan City Hospital, San Juan, PR 00921, USA

Styliani Laskou, Konstantinos Sapalidis and Isaak Kesisoglou
3rd Surgical Department, Aristotle University of Thessaloniki, AHEPA Hospital, Thessaloniki, Greece

Christos Topalidis and Triantafyllia Koletsa
Department of Pathology, Faculty of Medicine, Aristotle University of Thessaloniki, Thessaloniki, Greece

Chatchon Kaewkrasaesin
Division of Medicine, Taksin Hospital, Medical Service Department, Bangkok Metropolitan Administration, Bangkok, Thailand
Department of Medicine, Faculty of Medicine, Chulalongkorn University, Bangkok, Thailand

Patinut Buranasupkajorn, Sarat Sunthornyothin and Thiti Snabboon
Department of Medicine, Faculty of Medicine, Chulalongkorn University, Bangkok, Thailand
Excellence Center in Diabetes, Hormone and Metabolism, King Chulalongkorn Memorial Hospital, Thai Red Cross Society, Bangkok, Thailand

Paisith Piriyawat
Department of Neurology, Texas Tech University Health Sciences Center El Paso, El Paso, USA

Ibtissem Ben Nacef, Sabrine Mekni, Chedi Mhedhebi, Imen Rojbi, Mchirgui Nadia and Karima Khiari
Department of Endocrinology, Charles Nicolle Hospital, Tunis, Tunisia

Ines Riahi
Department of Otorhinolaryngology-Head and Neck Surgery, Charles Nicolle Hospital, Tunis, Tunisia

Aleksandra I. Pivovarova
Alabama College of Osteopathic Medicine, 445 Health Sciences Blvd, Dothan, AL 36303, USA
University of Mississippi Medical Center, 2500 N State St., Jackson, MS 39216, USA

Stephanie Patrick
Alabama College of Osteopathic Medicine, 445 Health Sciences Blvd, Dothan, AL 36303, USA
University of Tennessee Health Science Center, 910 Madison Ave, Memphis, TN 38163, USA

Punuru J. Reddy
Decatur Morgan Hospital, Department of Internal Medicine, 1201 7th St. SE, Decatur, AL 35601, USA

Somaya Safi, Yousra Benabdelfedil, Sara Derrou and Faycal El Guendouz
Department of Endocrinology, Moulay Ismail Military Hospital, Meknes, Morocco
Department of Fundamental Sciences, Laboratory of Human Pathology Biomedicine and Environment, Faculty of Medicine and Pharmacy of Fez (FMPF), Sidi Mohammed Ben Abdellah University (USMBA), Fez, Morocco

Sara Lomelino Pinheiro, Inés Damásio and Ana Figueiredo
Serviço de Endocrinologia, Instituto Portugués de Oncologia de Lisboa Francisco Gentil, Rua Professor Lima Basto, 1099-023 Lisboa, Portugal

Tiago Nunes da Silva and Valeriano Leite
Unidade de Investigação em Patobiologia Molecular, Instituto Portugués de Oncologia de Lisboa Francisco Gentil, Rua Professor Lima Basto, 1099-023 Lisboa, Portugal

Firas Warda
Division of Endocrinology, University of Florida College of Medicine-Jacksonville, Jacksonville, FL, USA
Department of Medicine, University of Florida College of Medicine-Jacksonville, Jacksonville, FL, USA

Madeline Fasen
Department of Medicine, University of Florida College of Medicine-Jacksonville, Jacksonville, FL, USA

Patrick Natter
Department of Radiology, University of Florida College of Medicine-Jacksonville, Jacksonville, FL, USA

Stacey Nedrud and Rui Fernandes
Department of Oral and Maxillofacial Surgery, University of Florida College of Medicine-Jacksonville, Jacksonville, FL, USA

Ahmad Alkhasawne
Division of Endocrinology, University of Florida College of Medicine-Jacksonville, Jacksonville, FL, USA
Department of Pathology and Laboratory Medicine, University of Florida College of Medicine-Jacksonville, Jacksonville, FL, USA

Hiroyuki Iwasaki, Soji Toda and Daisuke Murayama
Department of Breast and Endocrine Surgery, Kanagawa Cancer Center, Yokohama, Japan
Department of Breast and Endocrine Surgery, Kanagawa Cancer Center, 2-3-2 Nakao Asahi-ku, Yokohama, Kanagawa 241-8515, Japan
Department of Breast and Endocrine Surgery, Kanagawa Cancer Center, Yokohama, Japan

Hiroyuki Takahashi
Department of Oncology, Kanagawa Cancer Center, Yokohama, Japan

Nafiseh Sereshti and Bijan Iraj
Isfahan Endocrine and Metabolism Research Center, Isfahan University of Medical Sciences, Isfahan, Iran

Jinal K. Patel, Varun Reddy, Gauthier Stepman, Debra Angelo and Johnathan Frunzi
Department of Internal Medicine, HCA Healthcare/ USF Morsani College of Medicine GME: Medical Center of Trinity, Trinity, FL, USA

Darius A. Schneider, M. Zare, F. Behnia and M. Matesan
University of Washington, Department of Medicine, Seattle, WA, USA

T. Tylee
University of Washington, Department of Medicine, Seattle, WA, USA
Department of Radiology, Harborview Medical Center, Seattle, WA, USA

Alejandro Terrones-Lozano and Lesly Portocarrero-Ortiz
Instituto Nacional de Neurología y Neurocirugía Manuel Velasco Suárez (INNN) Neuroendocrinology, Mexico City, Mexico

Alan Hernández-Hernández, Edgar Nathal Vera and Gerardo Yoshiaki Guinto-Nishimura
Neurosurgery (INNN), Mexico City, Mexico

Jorge Luis Balderrama-Bañares
Endovascular Therapy (INNN), Mexico City, Mexico

Claudia Ramírez-Rentería
Unidad de Investigación en Endocrinología Experimental, Siglo XXI Instituto Mexicano del Seguro Social, Mexico City, Mexico

Judith de la Serna-Soto
Neuroanesthesia (INNN), Mexico City, Mexico

Alfredo Adolfo Reza-Albarran
Instituto Nacional de Ciencias Medicas y Nutrición, Mexico City, Mexico

Eleonora Molinaro, David Viola, Nicola Viola, Pierpaolo Falcetta, Francesca Orsolini, Paolo Vitti and Rossella Elisei
Unit of Endocrinology, Department of Clinical and Experimental Medicine, University Hospital of Pisa, Pisa 56124, Italy

Liborio Torregrossa
Unit of Pathology, Department of Surgical, Medical, and Molecular Pathology and Critical Care Medicine, University Hospital of Pisa, Pisa 56124, Italy

Paola Vagli
Diagnostic and Interventional Radiology, University Hospital of Pisa, Pisa 56124, Italy

Alessandro Ribechini
Endoscopic Section of Pneumology, University Hospital of Pisa, Pisa 56124, Italy

Gabriele Materazzi
Unit of Surgery, Department of Surgical, Medical, and Molecular Pathology and Critical Care Medicine, University Hospital of Pisa, Pisa 56124, Italy

Raed Aldahash
Department of Medicine, Ministry of National Guard Health Affairs, King Abdullah International Medical Research Center (KAIMRC), King Saud Bin Abdulaziz for Health Science, Riyadh, Saudi Arabia

Cheuk-Lik Wong, Chun-Kit Fok, Vicki Ho-Kee Tam and Lai-Ming Fung
Department of Medicine and Geriatrics, Caritas Medical Centre, Shamshuipo, Kowloon, Hong Kong

Yuk-Kit Chan
Department of Medicine and Geriatrics, Pok Oi Hospital, Yuen Long, e New Territories, Hong Kong

Madeline Mori
Western University of Health Sciences, Pomona, CA 91766, USA

Amanda Frugoli and Udesh Shah
Department of Graduate Medical Education, Community Memorial Hospital, Ventura, CA 93003, USA
Department of Internal Medicine, Community Memorial Hospital, Ventura, CA 93003, USA

Brad Barrows
Department of Pathology, Community Memorial Hospital, Ventura, CA 93003, USA

Tricia Westhoff
Department of Graduate Medical Education, Community Memorial Hospital, Ventura, CA 93003, USA
Department of Endocrinology, Community Memorial Hospital, Ventura, CA 93003, USA

David Westra
Department of Graduate Medical Education, Community Memorial Hospital, Ventura, CA 93003, USA
Department of Neurosurgery, Community Memorial Hospital, Ventura, CA 93003, USA

Marina Delli Colli, Bader N. Alamri and Juan Rivera
Division of Endocrinology and Metabolism, Department of Medicine, McGill University, Montreal, Quebec, Canada

Laura Palma
Division of Medical Genetics, Department of Specialized Medicine, McGill University, Montreal, Quebec, Canada

Elias G. Tzelepis, Elena Barengolts, Joseph Shulan and Yuval Eisenberg
Division of Endocrinology, Diabetes & Metabolism, University of Illinois at Chicago, Chicago, IL, USA

Steven Garzon
Department of Pathology, University of Illinois at Chicago, Chicago, IL, USA

Kaushik Mandal, Damilola Ashorobi, Alice Lee, Huijuan Liao, Salini C. Kumar and David S. Rosenthal
Division of Endocrinology, Nassau University Medical Center, 2201 Hempstead Turnpike, East Meadow, NY 11554, USA

Maryam Heidarpour and Hassan Rezvanian
Isfahan Endocrine and Metabolism Research Center, Isfahan University of Medical Sciences, Isfahan, Iran

Mohammad Ali Haghighatpanah
Isfahan University of Medical Sciences, Isfahan, Iran

Motahare Yadegarfar
University Hospitals of Leicester NHS Foundation Trust, LE1 5WW Leicester, UK

Amir Mohammad Mozafari
Medical Library and Information Sciences Department, Health Information Technology Research Center, School of Management and Medical Information Sciences, Isfahan University of Medical Sciences, Isfahan, Iran

Mehrbod Vakhshoori and Davood Shafie
Heart Failure Research Center, Cardiovascular Research Institute, Isfahan University of Medical Sciences, Isfahan, Iran

Hau Xuan Nguyen and Huy Le Trinh
Department of Oncology, Hanoi Medical University, Hanoi, Vietnam
Department of Oncology and Palliative Care, Hanoi Medical University Hospital, Hanoi, Vietnam

Hien Xuan Nguyen and Hung Van Nguyen
Department of Oncology, Hanoi Medical University, Hanoi, Vietnam

Quang Van Le
Department of Oncology, Hanoi Medical University, Hanoi, Vietnam
Department of Oncology and Palliative Care, Hanoi Medical University Hospital, Hanoi, Vietnam
Department of Head and Neck Surgery, National Cancer Hospital, Hanoi, Vietnam

Rodhan Khthir, Zainab Shaheen and Saroj Sigdel
Marshall University, School of Medicine, Huntington, WV, USA

Prasanna Santhanam
Johns Hopkins University, School of Medicine, Baltimore, MD, USA

Randhir Sagar Yadav, Shumneva Shrestha and Ashbita Pokharel
Maharajgunj Medical Campus, Institute of Medicine, Tribhuvan University, Kathmandu, Nepal

Ashik Pokharel, Sumita Pradhan and Prasan Bir Singh Kansakar
Department of Gastrointestinal and General Surgery, Tribhuvan University Teaching Hospital, Kathmandu, Nepal

Deepshikha Gaire
Department of Pathology, Tribhuvan University Teaching Hospital, Kathmandu, Nepal

Robert Sean O'Neill
The Department of Medical Oncology, The Sutherland Hospital, Caringbah, NSW, Australia

Lauren Tyack and Mary Freeman
The Department of Endocrinology, The Sutherland Hospital, Caringbah, NSW, Australia

Hussein Soudy Hussein
The Department of Medical Oncology, St George Hospital, Kogarah, NSW, Australia

Gunjan Y. Gandhi and Russell Fung
Division of Endocrinology, University of Florida College of Medicine-Jacksonville, Jacksonville, FL, USA
Department of Medicine, University of Florida College of Medicine-Jacksonville, Jacksonville, FL, USA
Division of Endocrinology, University of Florida College of Medicine-Jacksonville, Jacksonville, FL, USA
Department of Medicine, University of Florida College of Medicine-Jacksonville, Jacksonville, FL, USA

Patrick E. Natter
Department of Radiology, University of Florida College of Medicine-Jacksonville, Jacksonville, FL, USA

Raafat Makary
Department of Pathology and Laboratory Medicine, University of Florida College of Medicine-Jacksonville, Jacksonville, FL, USA

K. C. Balaji
Department of Urology, University of Florida College of Medicine-Jacksonville, Jacksonville, FL, USA

Rafael Trinidad-Hernández
Building 1431 Ave Ponce de Leon, Suite 303, San Juan, Puerto Rico 00907, USA

Gabriel Irizarry-Villafañe, Nadyeschka Rivera-Santana, Michelle Mangual-García and Alex González-Bóssolo
Endocrinology Department, San Juan City Hospital, San Juan, Puerto Rico 00936, USA
Endocrinology Department, San Juan City Hospital, San Juan, PR 00921, USA
Endocrinology Department, San Juan City Hospital, San Juan, PR 00921, USA

Miosotis García-Maldonado
HRP Labs, 300 Manuel Domenech Street, San Juan, Puerto Rico 00918, USA

Víctor Carlo-Chévere
Puerto Rico Pathology, 198 Calle Trinidad, San Juan, Puerto Rico 00917, USA

Valérie Spalart
AZ Turnhout, Department of Internal Medicine, Turnhout, Belgium

Barbara Legius and Lynn Decoster
AZ Turnhout, Department of Pulmonology/Respiratory Oncology, Turnhout, Belgium

Kurt Segers
AZ Turnhout, Department of Pathology, Turnhout, Belgium

Johan Coolen
University Hospitals Leuven, Department of Radiology, Leuven, Belgium

Brigitte Maes
Jessa Hospital Hasselt, Laboratory for Molecular Diagnostics, Department of Clinical Biology, Hasselt, Belgium

Felix C. K. Wong, Jeffrey S. S. Kwok and Angel O. K. Chan
Department of Chemical Pathology, Prince of Wales Hospital, The Chinese University of Hong Kong, Shatin, Hong Kong

Angela Z. Chan
Department of Anatomical and Cellular Pathology, Prince of Wales Hospital, The Chinese University of Hong Kong, Shatin, Hong Kong

W. S. Wong
Department of Medicine, North District Hospital, Sheung Shui, Hong Kong

Angel H. W. Kwan, Tracy S. M. Law and Jacqueline P. W. Chung
Department of Obstetrics and Gynaecology, Prince of Wales Hospital, e Chinese University of Hong Kong, Shatin, Hong Kong

Piyumi S. A. Wijewickrama and Noel P. Somasundaram
Endocrinology Unit, National Hospital of Sri Lanka, Colombo, Sri Lanka

Erin Meier
Department of Internal Medicine, NYU Winthrop, USA

Lydia Winnicka and Michael Lau
Department of Pulmonary and Critical Care Medicine, NYU Winthrop, USA

Duc Vo, Alla Joutovsky and Mangalore Amith Shenoy
Department of Pathology and Laboratory Medicine, NYU Winthrop, USA

Ai Matsui
Department of Breast and Endocrine Surgery, Kanagawa Cancer Center, Yokohama, Japan
Department of Breast and Endocrine Surgery, Kanagawa Cancer Center, 2-3-2 Nakao Asahi-ku, Yokohama, Kanagawa 241-8515, Japan

Daniel M. Berrebi
School of Medicine, West Virginia University, Morgantown, WV, USA

Oksana Symczyk, Taylor Cater and Adnan Haider
Department of Endocrinology, Department of Medicine, West Virginia University, Morgantown, WV, USA

Ayodele Adelanwa and Patrick Bacaj
Department of Pathology, Anatomy and Laboratory Medicine, West Virginia University, Morgantown, WV, USA

Alan A. Thomay
Department of Surgery, Division of Surgical Oncology, West Virginia University, Morgantown, WV, USA

Index

www.ingramcontent.com/pod-product-compliance
Lightning Source LLC
LaVergne TN
LVHW082124200926
848484LV00008B/2004